SYNOPSIS OF HUMAN PRENATAL DEVELOPMENT

1st Week — fertilization; cleavage, formation of inner cell mass, trophoblast, and blastocyst; implantation begins

2nd Week — amniotic cavity and bilaminar embryonic disc form; implantation is completed; trophoblast produces human chorionic gonadotrophic hormone; primitive placental circulation is established

3rd Week — trilaminar embryonic disc and head fold form; notochord and neural folds develop; primitive heart develops and begins to beat

4th Week — neural tube closes, and brain consists of 3 vesicles; eyes and ears begin to develop; trachea and lung buds become prominent; upper limb buds appear; approximate size about 5 mm at end of 4th week

5th Week — brain consists of 5 vesicles; face begins to develop; lower limb buds form

6th Week — gonads are prominent but undifferentiated; auricle of ear appears; finger rays develop

7th Week — heart becomes partitioned; eyelids begin to form; cloaca separates into urogenital and anorectal portions; toe rays develop

8th Week — testis and ovary distinguishable from each other; digits well developed; embryonic period ends at end of 8th week; approximate size about 30 mm at end of 8th week

9–16 Weeks — fetal period begins at beginning of 9th week; external genitalia show sexual differences; eyelids fuse; fetal movements detected; body hair appears; approximate size about 140 mm at end of 16th week

17–24 Weeks — teeth develop enamel and dentine; nail plates form; myelination begins in central nervous system; body covered with fine downy hair (lanugo); skin translucent; approximate size about 230 mm at end of 24th week

25–32 Weeks — eyelids reopen; testes descend; subcutaneous fat appears; fingernails reach fingertips, approximate size about 300 mm at end of 32nd week

33–38 Weeks — fat accumulates subcutaneously; skin wrinkles begin to disappear; lungs show functional capability

Birth — umbilical vessels close; lungs expand and fill with air; ductus arteriosus and foramen ovale of heart become functionally closed

HUMAN ANATOMY

Human Anatomy

SECOND EDITION

DORIS BURDA WILSON, PH.D.

Division of Anatomy
Department of Surgery
School of Medicine
University of California, San Diego

WILFRED J. WILSON, PH.D.

Department of Zoology
San Diego State University

With Illustrations by Ruth Valleau

New York Oxford
OXFORD UNIVERSITY PRESS
1983

Library of Congress Cataloging in Publication Data

Wilson, Doris Burda.
Human anatomy.

Bibliography: p.
Includes index.
1. Anatomy, Human. I. Wilson, Wilfred J.
II. Title.
QM23.2.W54 1983 611 82-42849
ISBN 0-19-503108-3

Printing (last digit): 9 8 7 6 5 4 3 2 1

Printed in the United States of America

Preface to the Second Edition

This second edition of *Human Anatomy* has been prepared in response to the success of our first edition and to the many helpful suggestions and encouragement which we have received from students, faculty, and our colleagues in the health sciences. In addition to a thorough review of each chapter and illustration, the major changes in this revision include a brief expansion of the chapter on the lymphatic system in order to include current information on immunologic aspects of this system, and additional functional correlations in the chapters on the cell, tissues, the endocrine system, the urinary system, and the reproductive system, as well as a modest expansion of the section on the history of anatomy in chapter 1, The Science and History of Anatomy.

We have added 45 new drawings, most of which are in color, as well as new micrographs, X-rays, and photographs of surface anatomy. Many micrographs also have been combined with additional drawings for orientation and clarification. The adjunct material now includes a Synopsis of Human Prenatal Development, a table of Units of Measure with measurements of various organs, and an expanded list of prefixes, suffixes, and root words. In order to provide greater accessibility and usage, this material has been placed on the end papers in the front and back of the book. In spite of these modifications, the overall size of this book has not increased, since it has been our intent to provide a concise, yet comprehensive, introduction to the structure, function, and clinical anatomy of the human body.

As was the case with our first edition, this new edition could not have been possible without the dedication and talent of our illustrator, Ruth Valleau. We also greatly appreciate the generosity of the authors and publishers who permitted us to borrow illustrations from their own publications. In addition to those already cited in the preface to the first edition, we would like to thank Dr. D. H. Cormack, Dr. L. V. Crowley, Dr. D. J. Gray, Dr. A. W. Ham, Dr. R. H. Kardon, Dr. R. G. Kessel, Dr. K. L. Moore, Dr. R. O'Rahilly, Dr. J. A. G. Rhodin, Dr. W. C. Sloan, Dr. R. T. Woodburne, the New York Academy of Medicine, and Turtox, Inc. We would also like to extend our appreciation to Juanita Smith and Leslie Oliver for secretarial assistance, and especially to Michael Cook, Jeffrey House, and the staff of the Oxford University Press for their support and commitment to this endeavor.

La Jolla, Calif. D. B. W.
September 1982 W. J. W.

Preface to the First Edition

This book is designed primarily for undergraduate students in the health sciences. With the increasing demand for qualified personnel in the allied medical professions such as nursing, physical therapy, X-ray technology, medical technology, inhalation therapy, and dental hygiene, large numbers of undergraduate students are enrolling in health science programs or exploring this area by taking medically oriented courses in human biology. Moreover, we see increasing numbers of students who, after receiving their undergraduate degree in the arts and sciences, decide upon a career in one of these allied professions. Even the undergraduate student who has chosen to pursue a research career in molecular biology often finds the need for a course in human structure as a background for his or her studies. Finally, we believe that many students, regardless of their chosen careers or areas of interest, are anxious to learn more about themselves as human organisms. We hope that this book will help to meet the needs of all these students and to generate an interest in pursuing further studies in the field of human biology.

The study of anatomy necessarily involves learning a considerable amount of facts, details, and terminology. We have found that much material can be assimilated and retained if it is related to function and to clinical situations. For this reason, medical implications have been incorporated directly into the body of the text wherever possible without disrupting the meaningful flow of information. In addition, separate sections on developmental and clinical anatomy have been included in several chapters to highlight and summarize pertinent aspects of each organ system.

Part I *(Levels of Organization)* includes a brief introduction to anatomical terminology and directional relationships as well as current information on the fine structure and molecular biology of cells and their organization into tissues. The chapter on early embryology traces the initial developmental events which show how tissue interactions produce an organ and how organs become functionally organized into organ systems.

Part II *(Systemic Anatomy)* is concerned with the gross, microscopic, developmental, and clinical anatomy of each organ system. The material presented in these chapters assumes that the reader has grasped the fundamental aspects of human structure presented in Part I.

Although it is convenient to study the human body from an organ system point of view, a regional approach is also important for understanding the structural and functional interrelationships of various organs. For this reason, the organ systems described individually in Part II are summarized and integrated into Part III *(Regional Anatomy)* which briefly considers three general regions of the body: the head and neck, the thorax and abdomen (including pelvis), and the limbs (upper and lower). Emphasis is placed here on clinical implications of these relationships.

Anatomy is basically a visual science, and we feel that the success of any anatomy book depends in large part on the quality of its illustrations. For this we are most grateful to our illustrator Ruth Valleau whose skill and devotion are evident throughout this book. We would also like to thank all the authors and publishers who so generously permitted us to borrow illustrative material extensively from their publications. Our particular gratitude goes to Dr. J. V. Basmajian, Dr. M. B. Bunge, Dr. R. P. Bunge, Dr. M. B. Carpenter, Dr. W. M. Copenhaver, Dr. E. D. Gardner, Dr. D. J. Gray, Dr. J. Langman, and Dr. R. O'Rahilly. We are also grateful for material borrowed from Dr. W. J. Banks, Dr. L. V. Crowley, Dr. D. W. Fawcett, Dr. M. D. Gershon, Dr. W. J. Hamilton, Dr. S. G. I. Hamilton, Dr. H. Kirkman, Dr. C. R. Leeson, Dr. T. S. Leeson, Dr. M. N. Nesbitt, Dr. J. A. G. Rhodin, Dr. L. L. Robbins, Dr. J. Royce, Dr. E. K. Sauerland, Dr. G. Simon, Dr. W. A. Stultz, Mr. J. Teague, the Editors of *Stedman's Medical Dictionary*, and the American Heart Association.

We would like to thank our colleagues, students, and friends for their suggestions, and in particular Dr. Eleanor Christensen and Laurel Finta for reading much of the manuscript. Our gratitude also goes to Juanita Doyle, Marleen Pibbs, and Renee Smith for secretarial assistance. Finally we are grateful to Sara A. Finnegan and the staff of The Williams and Wilkins Company and to Robert Tilley and the staff of the Oxford University Press for their assistance and support.

La Jolla, Calif. D. B. W.
October 1977 W. J. W.

CONTENTS

I

LEVELS OF ORGANIZATION

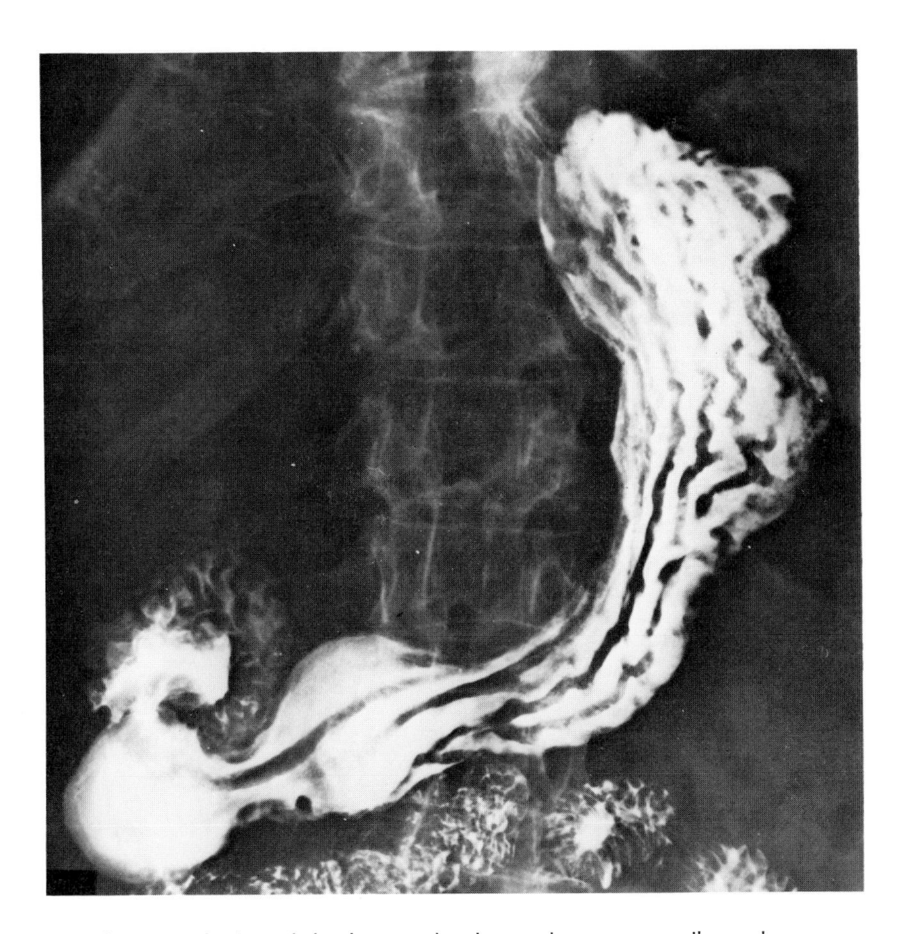

The complexity of the human body can be more easily understood if it is approached from the standpoint of different levels of organization. The following chapters present some fundamental aspects of human anatomy which should be mastered before proceeding to the anatomy of the organ systems presented in Part II.

1

The Science and History of Anatomy

Human anatomy has been studied for centuries dating back to the early Greeks and Egyptians. It is not surprising that there continues to be a prevailing and unmistakable interest in the human body, and we hope that your studies will leave you with a sense of appreciation and respect for its complexity and beauty. The science of anatomy also has considerable practical application: serving as a basis for understanding the form and function of the body in health and disease, as a means whereby artists have been able to convey substance and reality to the human figure, and as a vehicle for investigating our origins and relationships to other animals.

The word anatomy is derived from the Greek root words *ana* (up) and *tome* (cutting), and indeed our knowledge of human anatomy has depended in large part on "cutting up" (dissecting) the human body. The term anatomy commonly refers to studies on the human body, whereas comparative anatomy encompasses anatomical studies involving a broad spectrum of animals. As with most fields of study, anatomy can be subdivided into various categories and subspecialties, including gross anatomy, microscopic anatomy, and developmental anatomy.

GROSS ANATOMY

This approach to anatomy involves structures which can be seen with the naked eye. Various methods of study are used by gross anatomists, of which the most important has been (and still is) dissection of the human cadaver. However, a great deal of information can also be gleaned from studying surface contours of the body (surface or topographic anatomy) and from the study of X-rays (radiological anatomy), since these provide a means for observing living anatomy.

Radiological anatomy includes the use of plain X-rays (Fig. 1-1), as well as X-rays taken after the introduction of various opaque dyes into the blood stream **(angiography, angiocardiography)** (Fig. 1-2). Opaque substances such as barium can also be ingested, and their movement through organs can be followed by a series of X-ray films (Fig. 1-3) or by motion picture **(cineradiography)**. A relatively recent and exciting technique known as **computer tomography** scans the body with a series of X-rays taken from different angles and then combines them by means of a computer to provide a cross-sectional image similar to that which could only be obtained by an actual section through the body (Fig. 1-4).

Still another technique is **sonography,** based on the principles of radar, whereby ultrahigh frequency sound waves are directed into the body, and an image is obtained on the basis of echos produced by organs of varying densities. **Scintigraphy** involves the introduction of small amounts of radioisotopes into the body which is then scanned by a scintillation

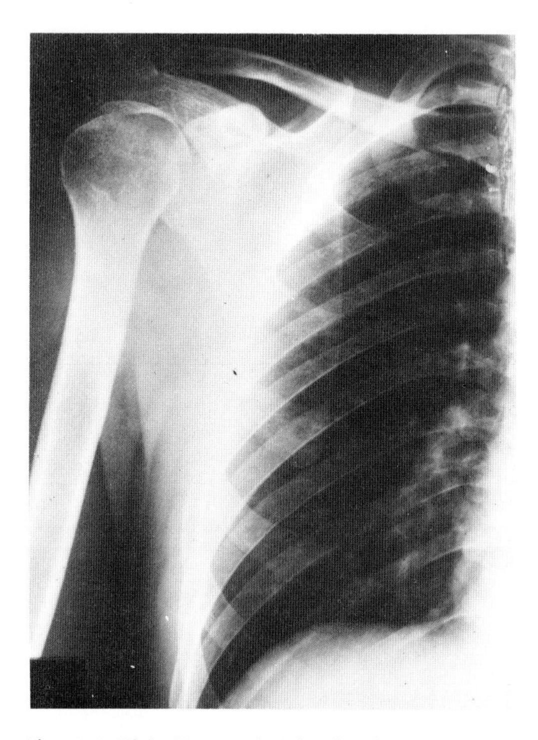

Fig. 1-1. Plain X-ray of right shoulder joint and right side of thorax. (From E. D. Gardner, D. J. Gray, and R. O'Rahilly, *Anatomy,* Ed. 4, W. B. Saunders, Co., Philadelphia, 1975.)

counter to detect the shape of organs where the isotope has become concentrated. Another technique for studying anatomy is **endoscopy** whereby the interior of some hollow organs such as the esophagus, intestines, and bronchial passageways can be viewed by passing a flexible, lighted tube within them and even removing bits of tissue for analysis. Obviously, all of the above methods are of use not only in studying normal living anatomy but more importantly as diagnostic tools in the detection of abnormal anatomy due to disease, injury, or congenital conditions.

MICROSCOPIC ANATOMY

This method depends on the use of a microscope to study structures which cannot be seen with the naked eye. There are basically two types of microscopy: light microscopy and electron microscopy, of which the latter is more powerful. Light microscopes adapted for low magnifications of surface structures are often called dissecting microscopes, while higher magnifications of surfaces can be obtained with a scanning electron microscope (Fig. 1-5). Deeper regions, however, can be seen only after a section has been made through the specimen so as to provide sufficient transparency for observation. Such sections are made with an instrument called a microtome after the specimen has been hardened either by freezing (frozen sections) or after infiltration with paraffin or a hard resin. The sections are usually stained so as to provide sufficient contrast to be viewed with the microscope. The study of structure by means of the light microscope is commonly referred to as **histology** whereas use of the electron microscope reveals **fine structure** (sometimes termed **ultrastructure**).

DEVELOPMENTAL ANATOMY

This is concerned with the prenatal development (embryology) and the postnatal development and maturation of an individual. Most studies of early development necessarily depend on microscopic observation, since the em-

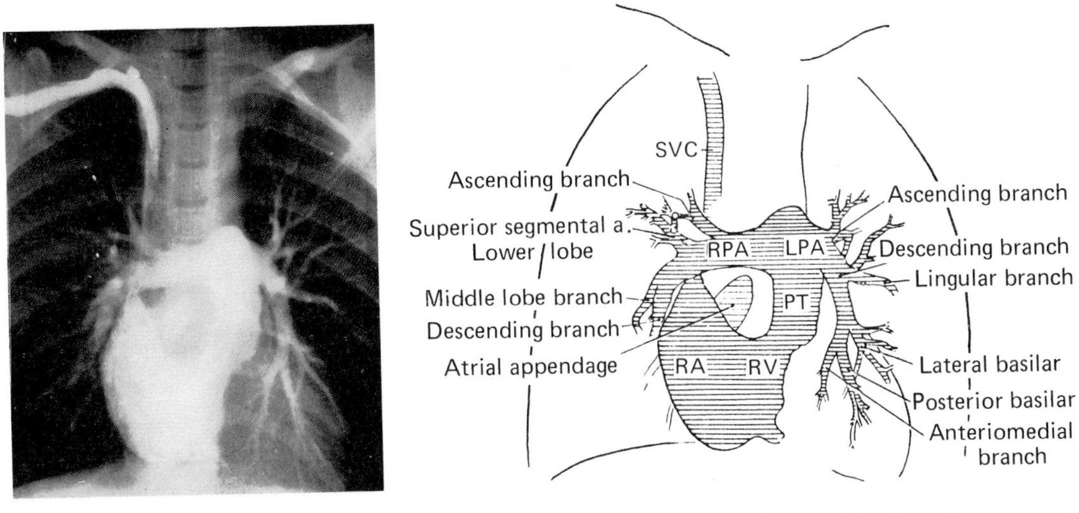

Fig. 1-2. *(left)* Angiocardiogram showing the heart and pulmonary vessels after injection of an opaque dye into the blood stream. *(right)* Diagram showing major structures outlined at left. (From L. R. Robbins (Ed.), *Golden's Diagnostic Radiology,* The Williams & Wilkins Co., Baltimore, 1968.)

bryo is so small. The study of the mechanisms of abnormal development leading to congenital malformations is known as **teratology.**

Various other categories of anatomy exist, such as **surgical anatomy** which approaches human structure from the viewpoint of surgical procedures, and **pathological anatomy** which utilizes gross and microscopic anatomy to study abnormal structure and function.

There are two basic approaches to the study of anatomy: by organ systems (systemic anatomy) and by regions (regional anatomy). **Systemic anatomy** views the body from the standpoint of groups of organs (organ systems) which work together in performing common functions. This is a particularly useful way to study the body since it emphasizes functional anatomy. Indeed, the study of one organ system in particular, the nervous system, has resulted in the establishment of the subspecialty known as neuroanatomy.

However, anatomy is also a study of spatial relationships among organs, and for this purpose **regional anatomy** is used to clarify the interrelationships of different organ systems in specific regions of the body such as the head, neck, thorax, abdomen, pelvis, and limbs. Re-

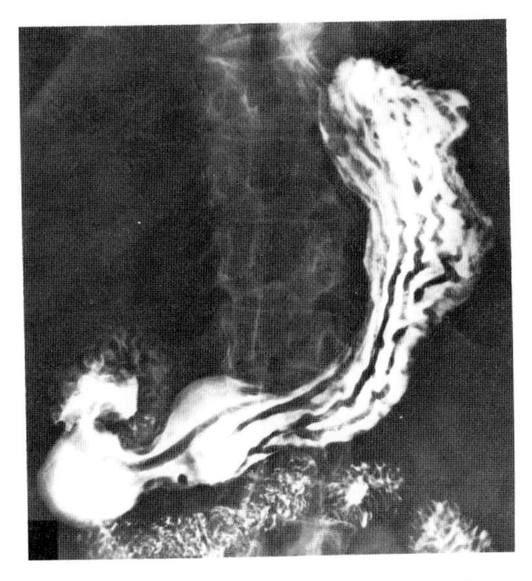

Fig. 1-3. An X-ray of the stomach after swallowing barium. (From E. D. Gardner, D. J. Gray, and R. O'Rahilly, *Anatomy,* Ed. 4, W. B. Saunders Co., Philadelphia, 1975.)

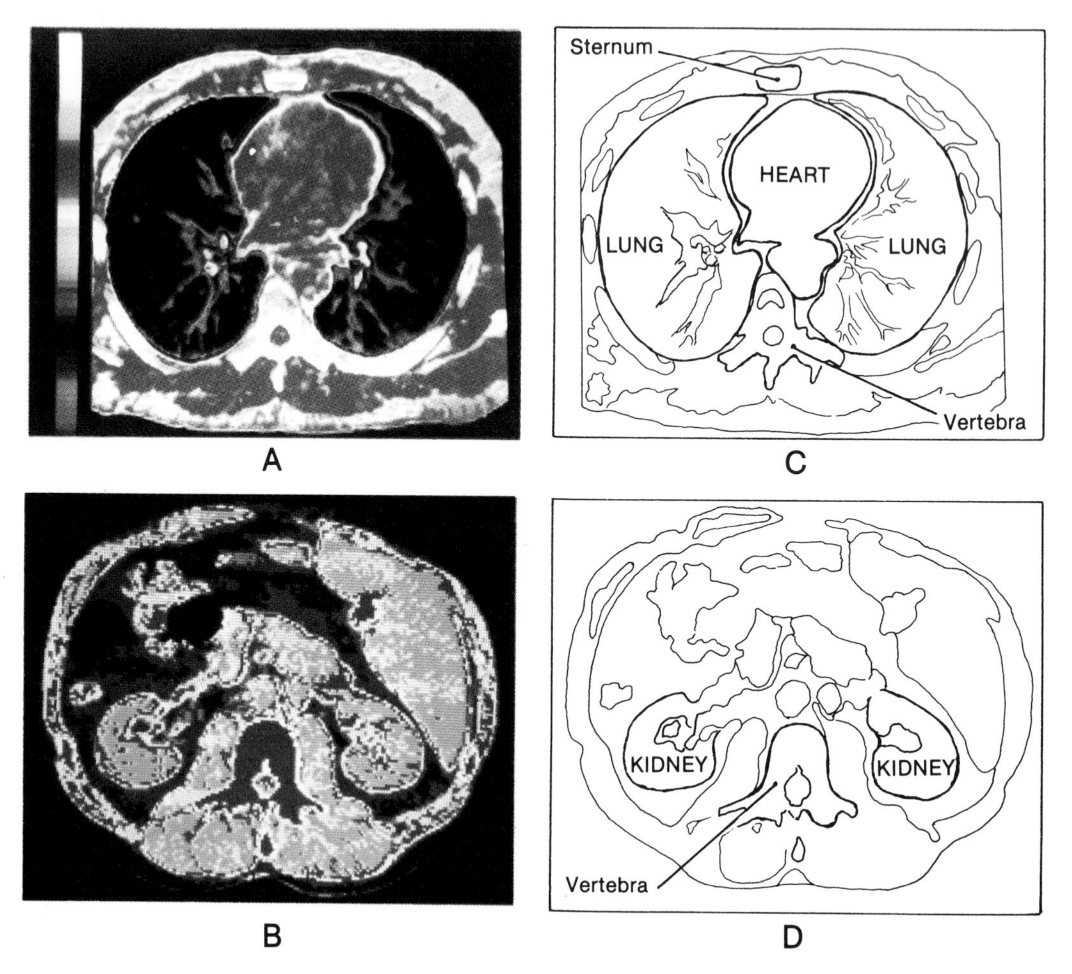

Fig. 1-4. Cross section of the thorax (A) and abdomen (B) as seen by computer tomography. (Produced with a Delta-Scan by Ohio-Nuclear, Inc., Solon, Ohio.) (C) Sketch of A; (D) Sketch of B.

gional anatomy is also best suited for dissection. (Although both approaches have their advantages and disadvantages, the format of the present book places greater emphasis on the systemic approach, but also includes three chapters on regional anatomy which hopefully will help to integrate the organ systems studied in earlier chapters.)

Whereas anatomy is fundamentally a visual science, *i.e.*, one learns from looking at structure, a great deal can also be learned from **palpation,** which involves feeling the contours of structures, and **auscultation,** which enables one to listen to sounds emanating from such organs as the heart, lungs, and intestines. **Percussion** consists of listening to vibrations produced by placing one finger against the body surface and striking the finger with a finger of the opposite hand. In this manner, solid or congested organs produce a dull sound, whereas hollow or air filled organs produce a resonance.

HISTORY OF ANATOMY

The early anatomists were basically gross anatomists, since adequate light microscopes were not perfected until the 17th century. Among the first anatomists were two Greeks, Hippocrates (about 400–377 B.C.) and Aristotle (384–322 B.C.), and an Egyptian, Herophilus (about 300 B.C.). Somewhat later Galen (A.D. 129–200), who served as a physician in Rome to Marcus Aurelius, produced two massive works: *On anatomical procedure,* consisting of sixteen books, and *On the uses of the parts of the body of man.* After Galen, Anatomy entered the Dark Ages during which little or no advancements were made other than translations of Galen's work. By the end of the 13th century, however, dissections were being performed at the University of Bologna, Italy.

During the 14th century human dissections were common in France and Italy, although they were done with great difficulty, since the use of alcohol as a tissue preservative was not recognized until the 17th century. In 1316 Mondino de' Luzzi (1270–1326), a faculty member at the University of Bologna, wrote the *Anothomia* which was the prototype of a dissection manual, and the field of Anatomy continued to be dominated by the Bologna School from the 13th to the 16th centuries.

During the 15th century, Anatomy became a scholarly pursuit, and much of the preceding anatomical works were translated into Latin, providing the basis for our anatomical nomenclature, as we know it today. However, the most well known anatomists during this time were artists, including Leonardo da Vinci (1452–1519), Albrecht Durer (1471–1528), and Michelangelo (1475–1564). Moreover, Leonardo da Vinci used dissections not only to perfect his depiction of the human form, but also to extend our knowledge of the structure and function of the human body.

During the first part of the 15th century, the Paris School of Anatomists was represented by Sylvius (Jacques Dubois, 1478–1555), who taught at the University of Paris and who was responsible for advancing and reorganizing anatomical nomenclature. One of his students was Andreas Vesalius, who was to become the most dominant figure in Anatomy during the 16th century.

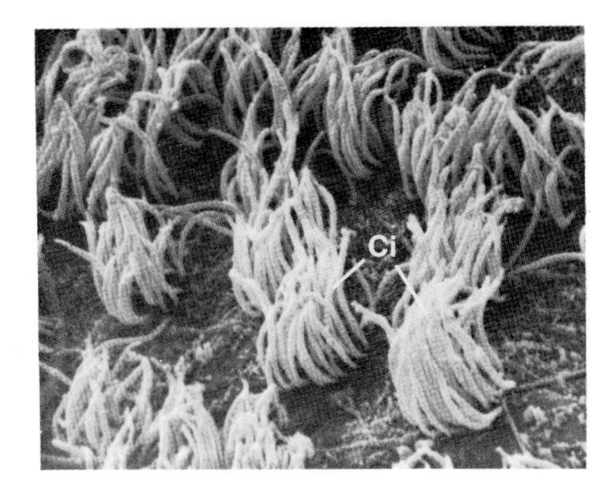

Fig. 1-5. A scanning electron micrograph of the inner surface of the brain, showing tufts of cilia (Ci). (From R. G. Kessel and R. H. Kardon, *Tissues and Organs: A Text-Atlas of Scanning Electron Microscopy,* W. H. Freeman and Company. Copyright © 1979.)

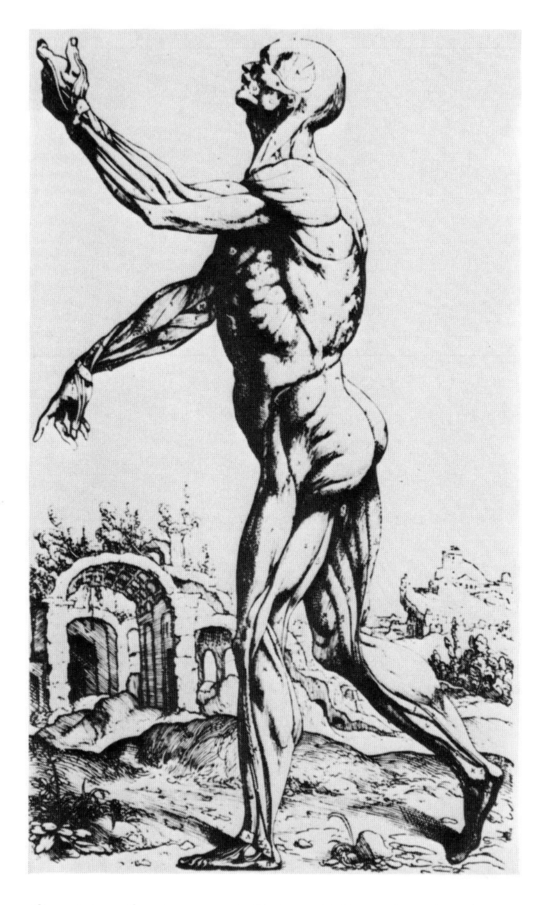

Fig. 1-6. The Second Plate of the Muscles from the Second Book of the *De Humani Corporis Fabrica* of Vesalius, published in 1543. (From *Icones Anatomicae of Andreas Vesalius,* The New York Academy of Medicine, 1934.)

Andreas Vesalius of Brussels (1514–1564) is often referred to as the Reformer of Anatomy. After studying in Paris, Vesalius became a Professor at the University at Padua, Italy, where he enthusiastically performed dissections before large audiences. His massive work *De Humani Corporis Fabrica (On the Workings of the Human Body)* was published in 1543. The illustrations in the *Fabrica*, consisting of seven books, show a remarkable combination of science and art (Fig. 1-6). With Vesalius, the University at Padua became dominant in the field of Anatomy, and a long line of Paduan anatomists emerged, including Fabricius ab Aquapendente (1537–1619), also noted as a comparative anatomist and embryologist, and Giulio Casserio (1561–1616).

Historically, the study of cells has paralleled the development of instruments and techniques used to observe their structure and test their functions. One of the earliest light microscopists was Robert Hooke (1635–1703), the English curator of experiments for the weekly meeting of the Royal Society of London. In 1665 he observed that a slice of cork was composed of a great many "little boxes" which he called cells. Observations on cells were refined by the Dutchman Anton van Leeuwenhoek (1632–1723), who perfected microscopes in the latter part of the 17th century. Many of van Leeuwenhoek's drawings based on observations made with the aid of single lens microscopes show cellular structures in both animal and plant tissues.

During the 17th century gross anatomy flourished not only in Italy, but also in France, Germany, Switzerland, and England. However, the study of anatomy was profoundly affected by the advent of a physiological approach as presented by the Englishman William Harvey (1578–1657) in his treatise *An anatomical dissertation on the movement of the heart and blood in animals.*

Although the field of modern embryology stems from the 18th century with Caspar Wolff (1733–1794), earlier anatomists, such as Fabricius and Marcello Malpighi (1628–1694) had already been intensely interested in embryology. During the 19th century the study of embryology was greatly advanced by Karl von Baer (1792–1876), Wilhelm His (1831–1904), and Wilhelm Roux (1850–1924).

The field of microscopic anatomy was furthered during the 19th century by two young German biologists, Matthias Schleiden (1804–1881) and Theodor Schwann (1810–1882), who formally stated the cell theory (actually a generalization rather than a theory) that all living things are composed of cells. Schleiden was first trained as a lawyer and later became a botanist. In 1838 he presented the theory that all higher plants are composed of individual units called cells. In 1839 Schwann, who was an animal physiologist and friend of Schleiden, extended the cell theory to animals. He also proposed that animals develop by forming new cells and that cells can be considered independent living units.

A further extension of the cell theory was made in 1858 by the German physician and pathological anatomist Rudolf Virchow (1821–1902), who stated that all cells come from preexisting cells. This formed the basis for the theory of biogenesis. Proof of this theory was furnished only a few years later in a series of classic experiments by the Frenchman Louis Pasteur (1822–1895). In proving biogenesis he was able to disprove the theory of spontaneous generation of living things from non-living substances, except perhaps when life first arose on this planet. Since the time of Pasteur, many scientists from many nations have contributed to our current understanding of the nature of cells, and the study of the structure and function of cells continues today as the field of cell biology.

It is not surprising that just as microscopic anatomy began to grow with the advent of the light microscope, so also did the field of cell biology eventually begin to flourish as the study of fine structure became possible with the advent of the electron microscope. However, although modern-day anatomists use increasingly sophisticated techniques for studying human structure, much of our basic understanding of anatomy, particularly gross anatomy, is still deeply rooted in work done hundreds of years ago.

2

Anatomical Terminology and Relationships

In order to understand structural and spatial relationships in the human body, it is necessary to use standardized anatomical terms. Although the seemingly endless number of these terms may at times be overwhelming and cumbersome, you can communicate with others and organize anatomical information much more easily if you understand the basis for this terminology.

Early anatomists often bestowed upon a structure the name of the individual who first identified it. These names are known as eponyms. Although eponyms are interesting from a historical point of view, they unfortunately give little clues as to what or where the structure is. (Moreover, the person whose name was assigned to a structure may not have been the first one who actually described it!) Some eponyms are still in use, but more descriptive terms are preferable. Thus the designation "rectouterine pouch" for the area between the rectum and uterus is more meaningful and easily remembered than the eponym "pouch of Douglas." However, some names such as "Eustachian tube" (named for a 16th century Italian anatomist) have become so firmly entrenched in our usage that it takes a certain amount of effort to use the less familiar but more descriptive term "pharyngotympanic tube."

Although anatomical terms have traditionally been designated in Latin, much of the terminology has been anglicized for convenience. For example, we use the word "muscle" instead of "musculus," and "artery" instead of "arteria." Yet, you will find that many specific names of structures are still in Latin, so that we refer to the "flexor digitorum profundus muscle" rather than the "deep muscle which flexes the digits." An understanding of the more common Latin and Greek root words, prefixes, and suffixes can thus help you to visualize and remember structures more easily .

Just like any language, anatomical terminology has gradually changed over the years. Indeed, anatomists have periodically gathered together to refine lists of terms, and in this manner a series of revisions has occurred. In 1955 a major revision took place in Paris and was known as the Nomina Anatomica (N.A.). It was recently re-evaluated in 1970.

ANATOMICAL RELATIONSHIPS

Anatomical Position of the Body

The anatomical position is arbitrarily designated with the body standing upright, the head, eyes, and toes pointing forward, and the upper limbs hanging downward with the palms facing forward (Fig. 2-1). In order to avoid confusion, all anatomical descriptions are based on this position, regardless of whether the body is lying down on its face (prone), on its back (supine), or on its side.

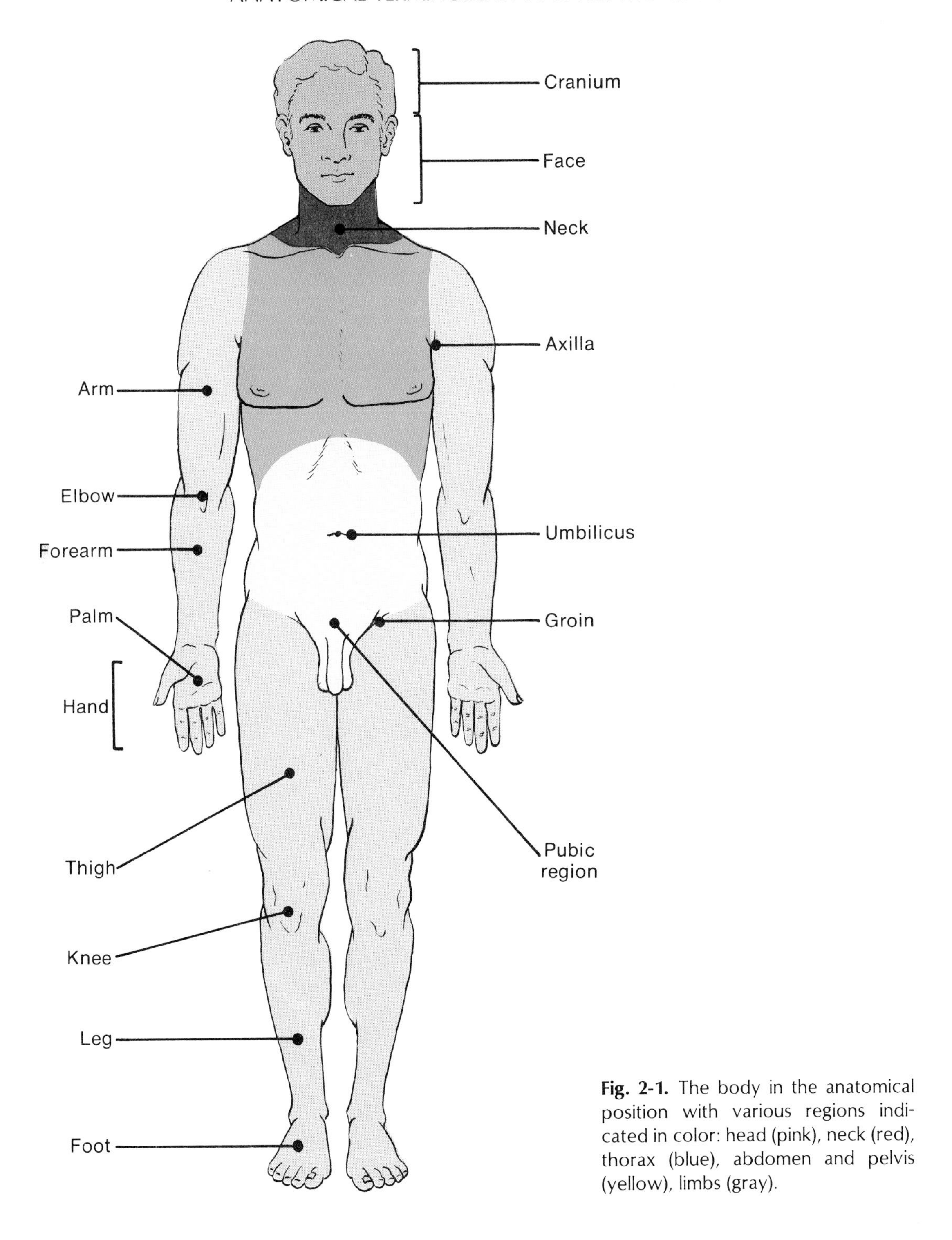

Fig. 2-1. The body in the anatomical position with various regions indicated in color: head (pink), neck (red), thorax (blue), abdomen and pelvis (yellow), limbs (gray).

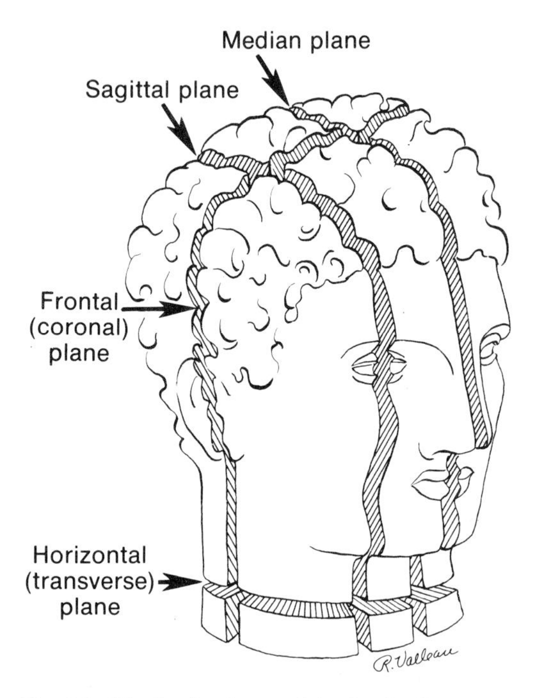

Fig. 2-2. The basic planes of the body, illustrated on the head and neck. (Modified after Gardner, Gray, and O'Rahilly.)

Regions of the Body

The body may be divided into four general regions: the head, neck, trunk, and limbs. The trunk may further be subdivided into the thorax and abdomen, including the pelvis. Within any particular region localized areas are given special names (Fig. 2-1). Further details on these regions are presented in Section III: Regional Anatomy (Chapters 17–19).

Body Planes

The **median plane** passes vertically through the body and divides it equally into right and left halves (Fig. 2-2). (On the surface of the body this is commonly referred to as the midline.) The median plane is sometimes redundantly designated as midsagittal. The term **sagittal** plane should be used only to denote a vertical plane parallel to the median plane. A vertical plane which is perpendicular (at a right angle) to the median plane is a **frontal** or **coronal** plane and thereby divides the body into front and back parts. The **horizontal** plane occurs at a right angle to both the median and frontal planes and divides the body into upper and lower parts. The term **transverse** means at a right angle to the long axis of any structure. The transverse plane thus often coincides with the horizontal plane, but can also coincide with other planes since some structures such as blood vessels pass in a variety of directions.

Directional Terms

The following terms of direction are important and should be learned carefully.

The front surface of the body is designated as **anterior** or **ventral,** while the back surface is **posterior** or **dorsal** (Fig. 2-3). (The terms anterior and posterior are used differently in animals which do not assume an upright position.)

The head region is at the **superior** or **cranial** end of the body, whereas the foot region is at the **inferior** or **caudal** end of the body.

Structures near the median plane are said to be **medial,** whereas those farther away are **lateral.**

The term **proximal** means close to the ori-

Fig. 2-3. Comparison of directional terms used for a four-footed animal whose body stands parallel to the ground *(left)* and those used for the human whose body stands in an upright position *(right).*

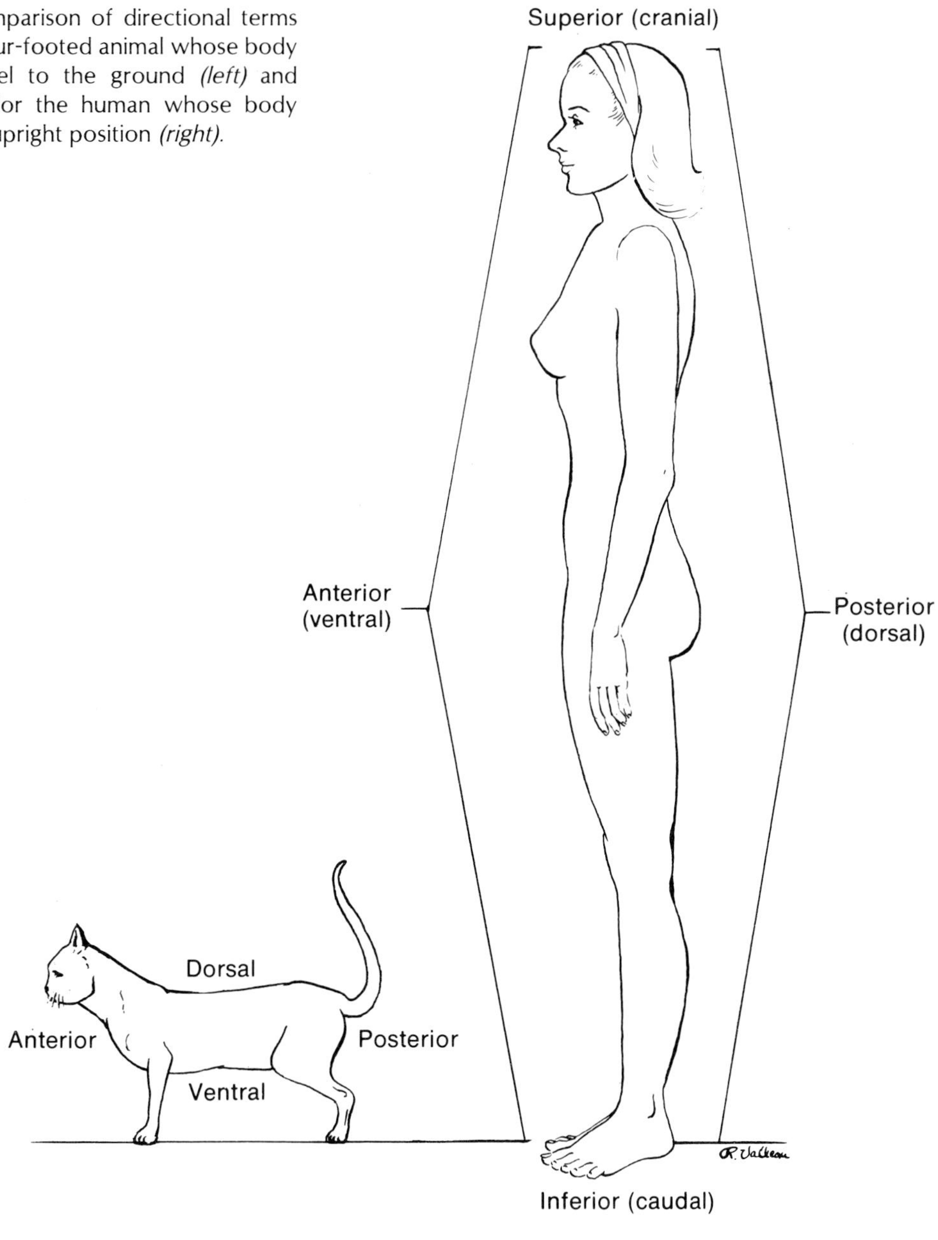

gin of a structure; **distal** means away from it. For example, the elbow is distal to the shoulder.

Internal means nearer to the center; **external** means farther from it.

Superficial refers to being near the surface, and **deep** is away from the surface. For example, the skin is superficial to the muscles.

In some regions of the body, special terms are used. Thus the anterior surface of the hand is **palmar (volar)**; the sole of the foot is **plantar.**

It is important to keep in mind that these positions are used in relation to one another. Thus a structure may be anterior to one organ but posterior to another.

Terms of Movement

The movement of body parts is given the following specific terms.

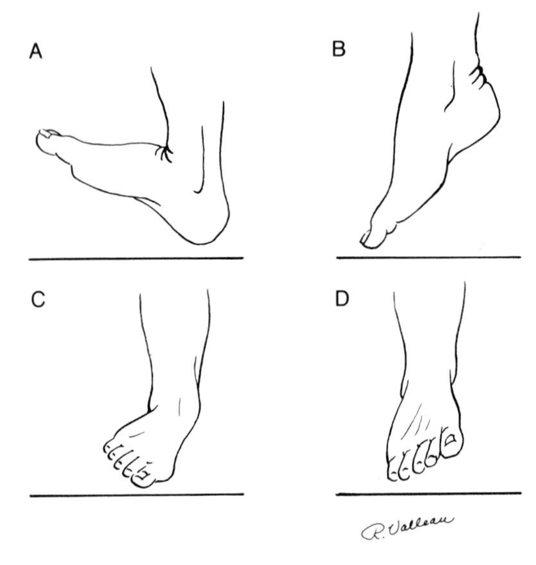

Fig. 2-4. Movements of the right foot. Solid line represents the horizontal plane, i.e., the ground. (A) Dorsiflexion (medial view), (B) plantar flexion (medial view), (C) eversion (anterior view), (D) inversion (anterior view).

Flexion consists of bending and thereby decreasing the angle between two body parts.

Extension involves straightening and increasing the angle between two body parts.

Abduction moves a body part away from the median plane.

Adduction moves a body part toward the median plane.

Rotation involves movement around a long axis.

Circumduction is a circular movement combining flexion, extension, abduction, and adduction.

In addition to the basic movements cited above, special movements involve the limbs:

Supination rotates the forearm and hand so that the palm faces forward (anteriorly). Thus, in the anatomical position the hands are supinated.

Pronation moves the forearm and hand so that the palm faces backward (posteriorly).

Dorsiflexion moves the foot upward (Fig. 2-4), as in walking uphill.

Plantar flexion moves the foot downward, as in walking downhill.

Inversion moves the sole of the foot inward.

Eversion moves the sole of the foot outward.

3

The Cell

The human body is composed of cells and materials produced by cells. All cells come from pre-existing cells; thus, the single-celled fertilized egg is the source for the trillions of cells that make up the adult human body. The cell is considered to be the basic functional level of organization even though each cell is composed of subunits called **organelles** which in turn consist of molecules. Cells exhibit all the basic characteristics of life. They interact with similar or different cell types to make up tissues, and cells are also the lowest level of organization that can be maintained outside of the body in a culture medium over a long period of time.

Cells of the human body are diverse in size, shape, composition, and function (Fig. 3-1). Some supportive cells (glial cells) in the central nervous system are only 2–3 micrometers (μm) in diameter, red blood cells (RBCs) are about 7 μm in diameter, and an ovum is about 100 μm. However, most human cells range between 5 and 50 μm in diameter. The length of cells also varies; some adult muscle cells may extend for several centimeters, and nerve cells may have processes (outgrowths) a meter or more long.

Some cells are round or oval (for example blood cells or ova); others are flattened, cubed, or columnar in shape such as those lining or covering surfaces, while others are stellate (star-shaped). The shape of a cell can be related to its stage of development or to its function and may change as development takes place or as functions change.

The internal composition of cells is also related to function. For example, cells which need large amounts of energy to perform special functions contain numerous energy generating structures (mitochondria). Other examples of differences in cell size, shape, composition, and function are presented in this and in subsequent chapters.

The cells of the body are quite diverse, and a typical or generalized cell is nonexistent; however, all cells do have certain features in common (Fig. 3-2). All cells contain **organelles** and **inclusions.** An **organelle** is a unit of living substance associated with a particular function. For example, a mitochondrion is an organelle associated with energy release and has a similar structure and function in all cells. **Inclusions** are temporary particles in cells which represent products of metabolism or ingested substances. They may consist of various materials such as proteins, carbohydrates, fats, or pigments.

It is useful to define some simple terms before we discuss specific cell structures and their functions. Those materials and activities occurring within cells are termed **intracellular,** those outside of the cell are **extracellular,** and those between cells **intercellular.** The term "**membrane**" (often used imprecisely by biologists) refers to a thin layer of material which

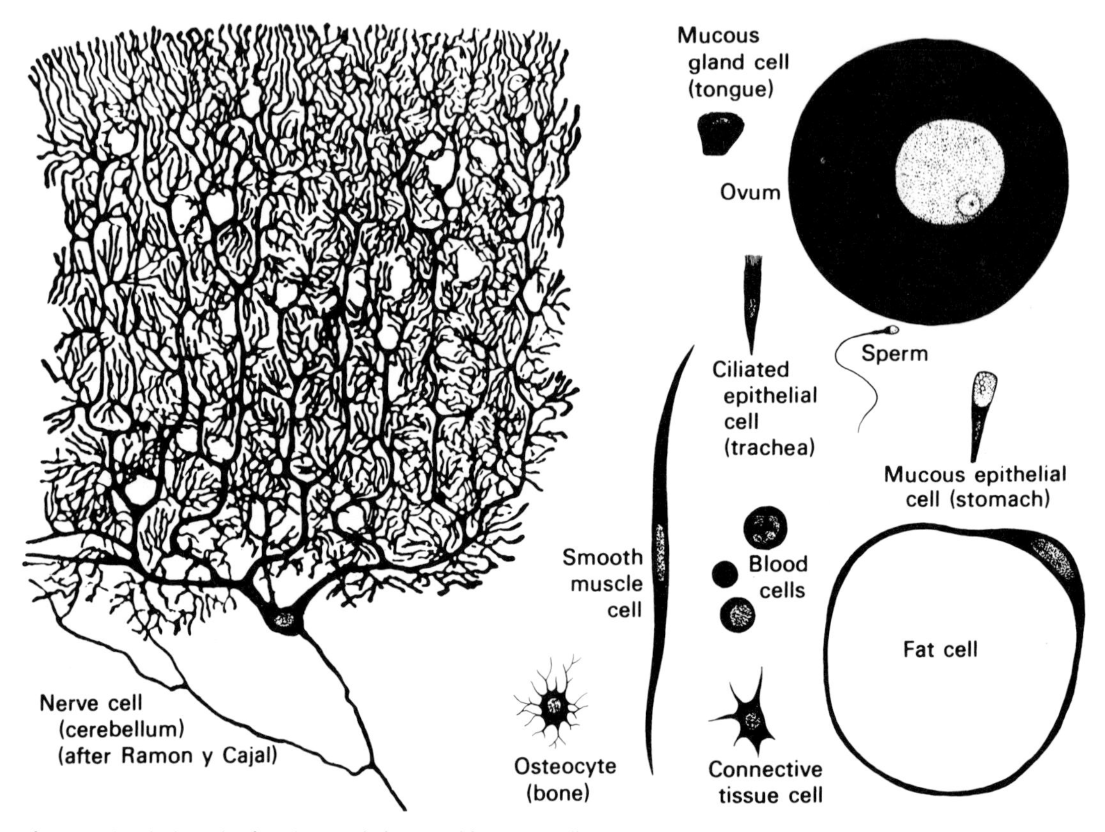

Fig. 3-1. Variations in the size and shape of human cells. (From W. M. Copenhaver, R. P. Bunge, and M. B. Bunge, *Bailey's Textbook of Histology,* Ed. 16, The Williams & Wilkins Co., Baltimore, 1971.)

covers a surface or divides a space or structure. At the cellular level a membrane varies between 60 and 120 Å in thickness. Above the cellular level anatomists broaden the definition of a membrane to include layers of other molecules, of cells, or of tissues.

Organelles and inclusions are located within two areas in the intracellular environment of a cell: (1) the **nucleus** and (2) the **cytoplasm,** including the outer limiting **plasma (cell) membrane.** The nucleus is concerned with control of relatively long-term biochemical activities and is the storage site for much of the genetic information in the cell. The cytoplasm is concerned with relatively short-term activities, receives messages from the nucleus, and communicates with the extracellular environment by means of the plasma membrane.

Nucleus

Usually there is one nucleus in each cell. However, cells may be binucleated as in some liver cells or multinucleated as in bone resorbing cells or in skeletal muscle cells. Some cells, such as circulating red blood cells, lack a nucleus. The nucleus may occupy a small fraction of a cell (example: nerve cells) or the bulk of a cell (example: sperm cell). The nucleus is usually round to oval but it may be lobed as in some white blood cells.

Nuclei of cells which are not undergoing division are delimited by a nuclear envelope which separates the nucleoplasm from the cytoplasm (Figs. 3-2 and 3-3). Suspended in the nucleoplasm of the nucleus is a dark staining material called **chromatin.** When cells prepare

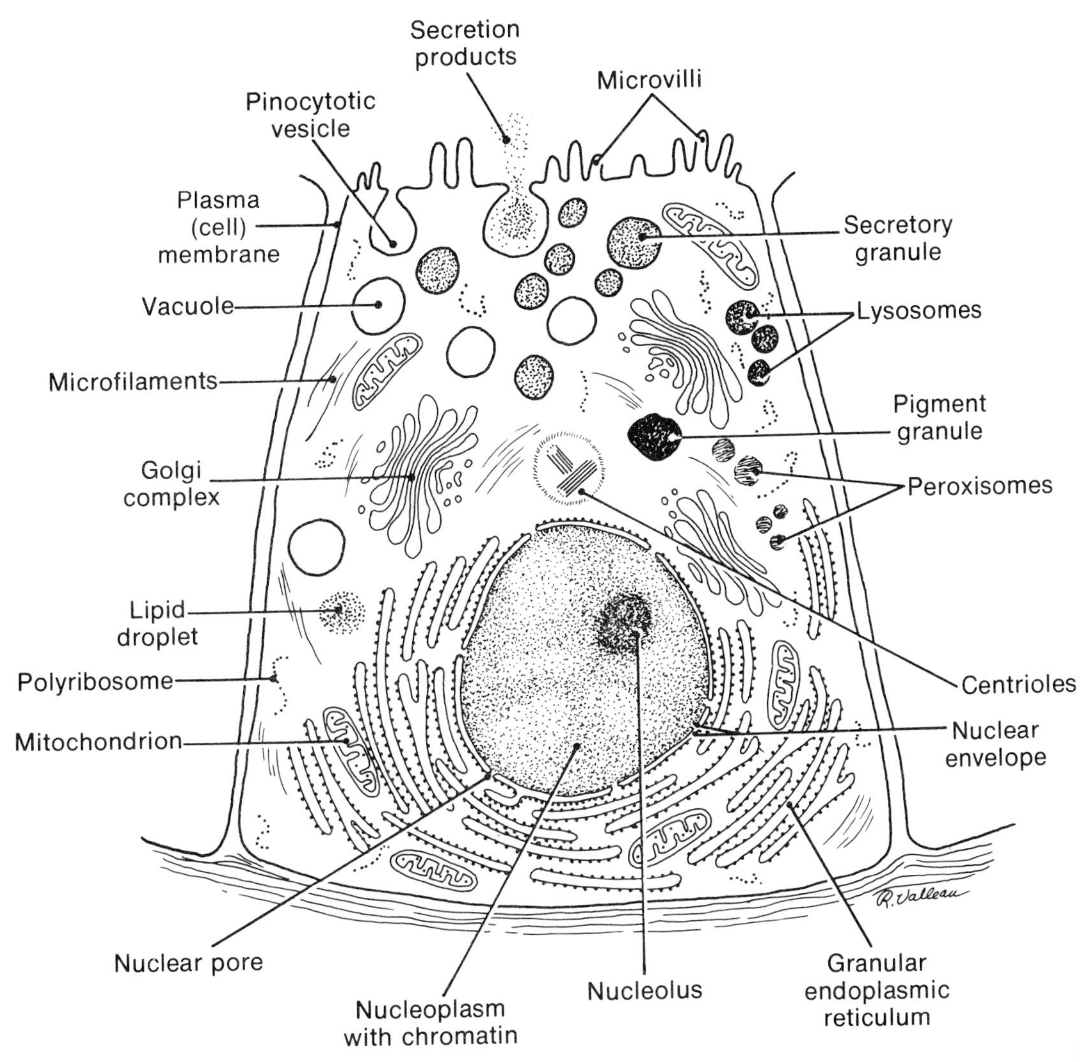

Fig. 3-2. Diagram of a cell as viewed highly magnified with the electron microscope. (Modified after *Bailey's Textbook of Histology*.)

for division the chromatin organizes into rodlike structures called **chromosomes.** The chromatin (and hence the chromosomes) contain the genetic material **deoxyribonucleic acid (DNA).**

The **nuclear envelope** consists of two membranes important in regulating nuclear-cytoplasmic interactions (Figs. 3-3 and 3-5). On the cytoplasmic side the outer membrane of the nucleus is studded with granules called ribosomes which contain **ribonucleic acid (RNA).** The outer membrane is also continuous with other intracellular membranes called the endoplasmic reticulum. On the nuclear side, the inner membrane of the nuclear envelope lacks ribosomes and is in direct contact with the nucleoplasm. **Nuclear pores** occur in the nuclear envelope at fairly regular intervals. They are more or less circular, are a few hundred angstroms in diameter, and probably allow substances, including large molecules, to pass to and from the nucleoplasm and cytoplasm.

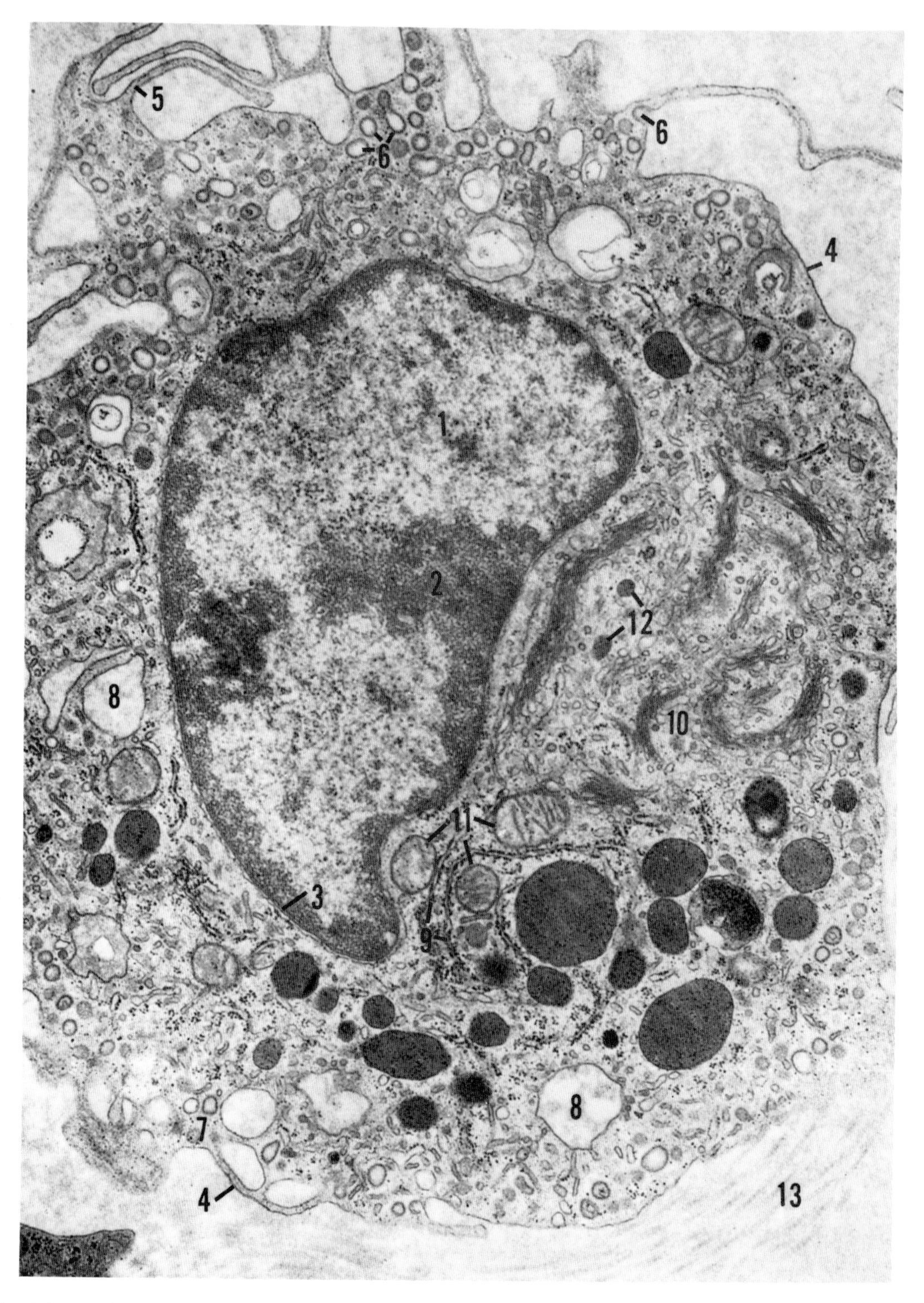

Fig. 3-3. An electron micrograph of a cell. *1, 2,* nuclear chromatin; *3,* nuclear envelope; *4,* plasma (cell) membrane; *5,* microvillus; *6,* pinocytic vesicles; *7,* phagocytic vacuoles; *8,* vacuoles; *9,* granular endoplasmic reticulum; *10,* Golgi complex; *11,* mitochondria; *12,* lysosomes; *13,* extracellular space. (Modified from *Histology: A Textbook and Atlas* by Johannes A. G. Rhodin. Copyright © 1976 by Johannes A. G. Rhodin. Reprinted by permission of the author and Oxford University Press, Inc.)

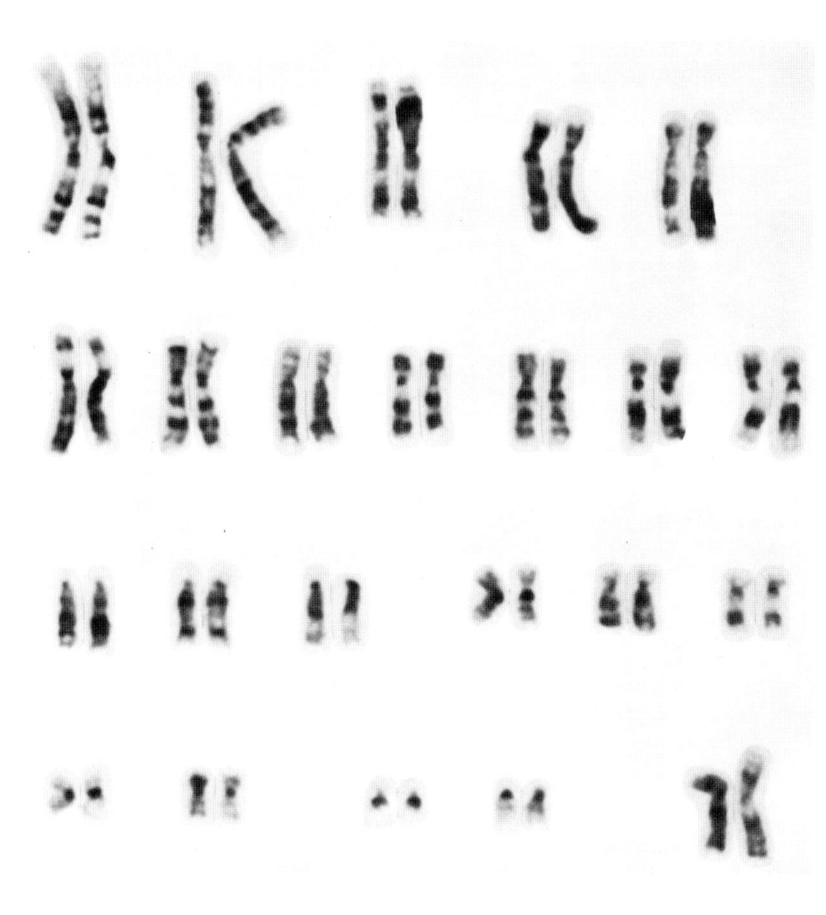

Fig. 3-4. The 23 pairs of human chromosomes, as seen in a karyotype. The dark bands on each chromosome represent areas of concentration of DNA material. (Chromosome preparation by Geoff Carson, courtesy of Dr. Muriel Nesbitt, University of California, San Diego.)

When cells are in the process of division the nuclear membranes fragment and then disappear, only to reappear again after the completion of the division process.

The **nucleoplasm** or nuclear sap is the background material of the nucleus which suspends the nuclear organelles. With the light microscope, nucleoplasm appears to be more or less fluid without distinct form; at the higher magnifications of the electron microscope, nucleoplasm is granular with distinct fibrils. The nucleoplasm is the site for many enzymatic reactions. For example, when DNA is synthesized or when messenger molecules are made, the nucleoplasm must supply the subunits, enzymes, and energy-releasing molecules for these reactions. The contents of the nucleoplasm and cytoplasm are in contact at the pore regions of the nuclear membranes and become confluent during cell division.

Chromatin and **chromosomes** contain DNA and structural protein. Chromatin appears granular with the light microscope and fibrillar with the electron microscope. These fibrils are really parts of chromosomes. In preparing for cell division, each of the 46 chromosomes becomes coiled into compact rodlike structures (Fig. 3-4). A chromosome which measures about 5 to 10 μm during cell division may contain an amount of DNA that would be several millimeters to several centimeters in length, if uncoiled and stretched out in one long molecule.

The **nucleolus** is a granular, densely staining structure within the nucleus (Figs. 3-2 and 3-5). It lacks membranes and has lightly staining zones of nucleoplasm extending into it. A nucleus usually contains only one nucleolus, although some cells may have more than one. It is composed of RNA and protein and is in-

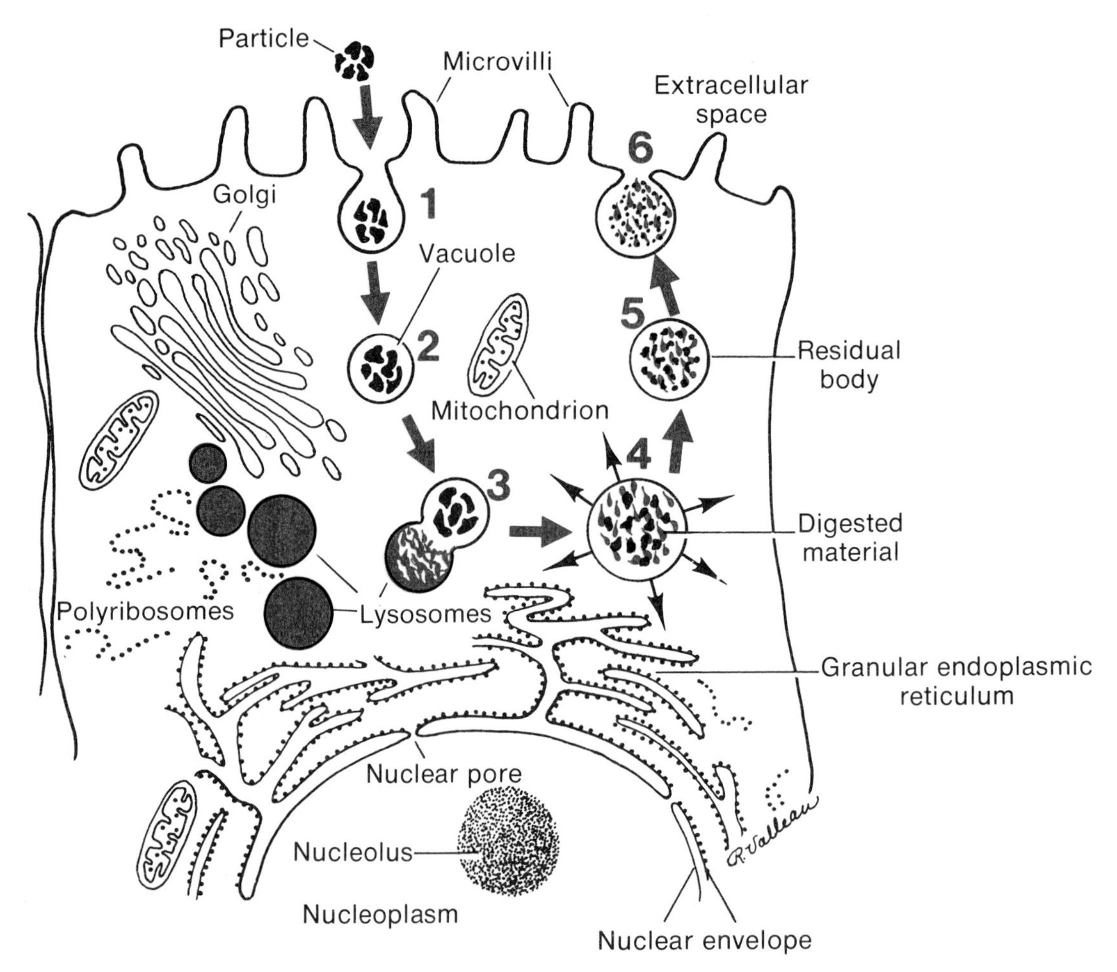

Fig. 3-5. Digestion of materials by an active cell. The black dots in the cytoplasm are ribosomes attached to the endoplasmic reticulum or in polyribosome chains which are sites for protein synthesis. *1,* A foreign body such as a bacterium or food particle is surrounded by the plasma membrane in the process of phagocytosis; *2,* formation of a vacuole containing the particle; *3,* the vacuole fuses with a lysosome containing digestive enzymes; *4,* digested materials move through the vacuole's membrane into the cytoplasm; *5,* undigested materials are left in a residual body; *6,* the residual body moves to the plasma membrane and dumps the undigested materials into the extracellular space.

volved in the assembly of ribosomes. During cell division the nucleoli of cells disappear only to reappear when cell division is completed.

Cytoplasm

The **cytoplasm** is that portion of a cell which is outside the nucleus and which contains background substance, as well as many organelles and inclusions, the nature and quantity of which determine a cell's function. The background substance of the cytoplasm consists of a filamentous latticework and is the site where many enzymatic reactions occur. It may range in consistency from quite fluid to quite gelatinous, depending on the type of cell and its state of activity. The structure and function of various organelles and inclusions will first be presented separately, and then their interactions with one another will be discussed in terms of the cell cycle and protein synthesis.

The **endoplasmic reticulum** (ER) as

viewed in electron micrographs is an extensive membrane system permeating the cytoplasm from the nuclear envelope to the outer cell membrane (Figs. 3-2, 3-3, and 3-5). It may be a **rough (granular) ER** studded with small granules termed **ribosomes** or a **smooth ER** which lacks ribosomes. The ER gives support to the cell, acts as a channel for transport, contains a variety of enzymes important in various metabolic activities, and is active in producing other membrane structures in the cell. Smooth ER connects with rough ER and seems to be active in cells which secrete steroids, such as in the hormone-secreting cells of the adrenal gland.

Ribosomes are small oval bodies about 150–250 Å in diameter. They contain RNA and protein and may be attached to the endoplasmic reticulum or distributed as free ribosomes in the cytoplasm. Ribosomes often become connected together in a **polyribosome** complex (Figs. 3-2 and 3-5). Cells which produce large amounts of proteins, such as digestive enzymes, for export out of the cell have large numbers of attached ribosomes; those which produce protein primarily for their own use tend to have more free ribosomes.

Mitochondria (singular: mitochondrion) are oval-shaped structures about 0.5–1.0 μm in diameter and up to 5–10 μm or more in length (Figs. 3-2, 3-3, and 3-5). They are more or less self-sufficient and contain their own DNA and ribosomes. Each mitochondrion is bounded by a double membrane, with the inner membrane folded inward as a series of projections termed **cristae.** Mitochondria are considered the powerhouses of cells since they are the sites where oxygen-dependent cellular respiration produces energy rich compounds such as adenosine triphosphate (ATP) necessary for cellular work. Very active cells such as those in kidney tubules, striated muscle tissue, and secreting glands, all contain large numbers of mitochondria.

The **Golgi complex (body)** as seen in electron micrographs consists of stacks of closely spaced membrane sacs situated near secretory surfaces (Figs. 3-2, 3-3, and 3-5). The membranes of these sacs lack ribosomes and are separated from each other by a usually constant distance of 200–300 Å. The Golgi complex is the site where polysaccharides are often assembled and added to proteins, where sulfates may also be added, and where these molecules are "packaged" into membrane bound vesicles. These vesicles then move to the cell surface for release from the cell or to other places within the cell so as to be utilized during intracellular digestion (Fig. 3-5).

Lysosomes are membrane-bound organelles in the cytoplasm which store digestive enzymes. Lysosomes are made by the Golgi complex and range in size from less than 1 μm to several μm, the average being about 0.5 μm in diameter. Lysosomes fuse with food vacuoles for intracellular digestion and also can discharge digestive enzymes directly into the extracellular environment. Although lysosomes function in most cells of the body, they are especially active in cells which fight infection and in those cells which are dying.

Peroxisomes (microbodies) are membrane-bound cytoplasmic organelles which are believed to be made by the endoplasmic reticulum. They range in size from 0.3 to 1.5 μm and average about 0.4 μm. They carry specialized digestive enzymes such as catalases which break down hydrogen peroxide. They usually have a crystal in their interior and are especially prominent in liver and kidney cells.

The terms **vacuole** and **vesicle** are imprecise. A vacuole is usually considered to be a rounded, membrane-bound structure, while a vesicle usually is a small vacuole. They can be defined either as organelles or as inclusions on the basis of their life span and function. Vacuoles may be formed by organelles such as the Golgi complex or endoplasmic reticulum. The plasma membrane is also active in vacuole formation (Fig. 3-5).

The **plasma membrane** (or **cell membrane**) is about 80 Å thick, separates the intracellular environment from the extracellular environment, and selectively allows materials to enter or leave the cell (Figs. 3-2 and 3-3). Because of its relative thinness and our inability to observe its structure directly, many models exist to explain membrane structure and func-

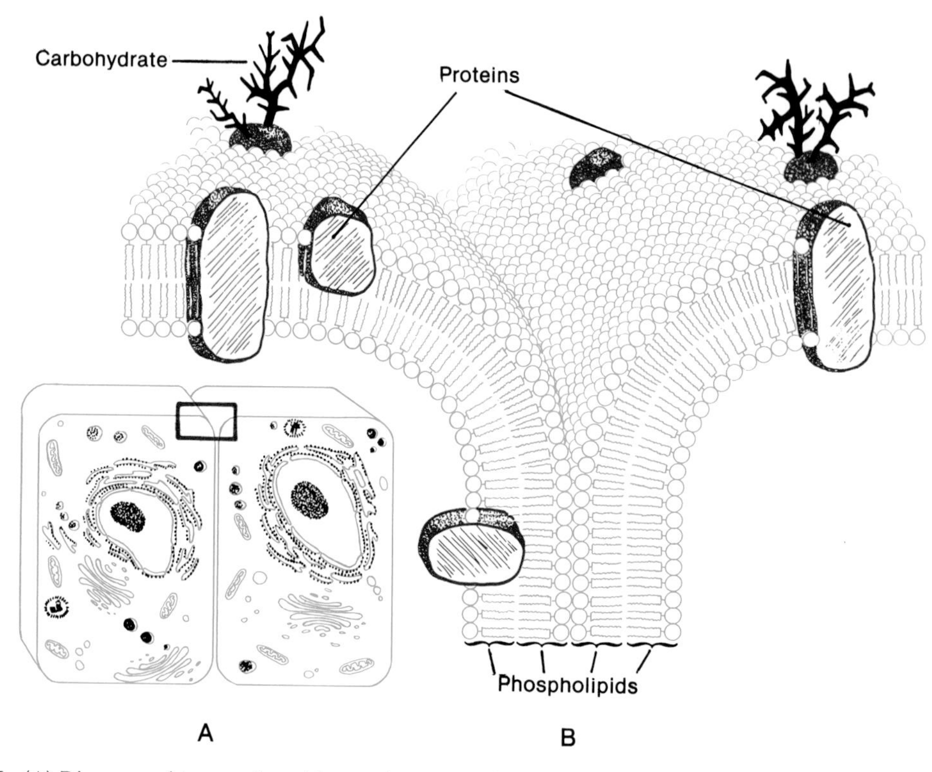

Fig. 3-6. (A) Diagram of two cells, with membranes outlined in blue. The area enclosed by the rectangle is shown at higher magnification in B, which depicts the fluid mosaic model of the two membranes shown in A.

tion. The plasma membrane and other membranes of the cell (such as those in mitochondria, the endoplasmic reticulum, and the Golgi complex) do have a more or less common thickness and are made of two layers of fatty molecules interspersed with larger protein molecules (Fig. 3-6). However, the variety of proteins, fats, and other molecules as well as differences in their orientation to each other can cause tremendous variations in the structure and function of membranes.

The plasma membranes of some cells of the body are specialized for transporting materials. Generally speaking, the amount of material which can be transported is proportional to the cell surface area. For example, intestinal lining cells which have to transport large volumes of molecules exhibit projections of the plasma membrane called **microvilli** (Figs. 3-2, 3-5, and 3-8). These fingerlike structures are not motile but have a core of protein filaments in their cytoplasm which are probably used for support.

The plasma membranes of many cells can absorb large molecules dissolved in fluids by forming pinocytotic vesicles which are then taken into the cell by a process called **pinocytosis,** or the plasma membrane may surround solid particles, such as groups of large organic molecules in the similar process of **phagocytosis** (Fig. 3-5). In either case the vesicles can then move into the cell's interior and become vacuoles. Small molecules in a vacuole can eventually pass through the vacuole membrane into the cytoplasm, or the vacuole may merge with cell organelles which carry digestive enzymes. Breakdown to smaller transportable molecules can then take place. The cytoplasm of a cell can also package into vacuoles various substances for secretion or waste products for removal from the cell. The vacuoles then can move to the plasma membrane, fuse with it, and dump their contents into the extracellular environment.

Microfilaments are composed of many different protein molecules, some of which are contractile. They may be found individually or in groups or incorporated into more complex structures such as **microtubules,** which are common in the cytoplasm of many cells. Microtubules are very thin protein cylinders approximately 200–300 Å in diameter and up to several micrometers in length. Each microtubule usually has 13 microfilaments arranged in a circular pattern. The functions of microtubules include: (1) control of cell shape (a "cytoskeletal" function), (2) cellular motion such as the movement of chromosomes within the cell or sending out motile projections from the surface of the cell, and (3) providing channels for transport of substances within the cell. Among the structures in which microtubules are found are **centrioles, basal bodies, cilia,** and **flagella.** Microtubules are also found in spindle fibers during cell division, nerve axons and dendrites (nerve cell processes), and pseudopods of ameboid cells.

Centrioles are cylindrical bodies about 0.2 μm in diameter and 0.5-2.0 μm in length. They occur in pairs oriented at right angles to each other in the cytoplasm adjacent to the nucleus (Fig. 3-2). With the light microscope they appear as two dots within a lightly staining homogeneous area called a **centrosome.** With the electron microscope, cross sections of centrioles are seen to be composed of 9 sets of microtubules arranged in a circular pattern. Each set is composed of 3 microtubules that extend the length of the centriole. Centrioles are involved in cell division and also can give rise to the **basal bodies** which are associated with cilia and flagella (see below).

Cilia and **flagella** are motile projections of cells. Cilia are 5–10 μm in length and about 0.2 μm in diameter. Several hundred may occur per cell (Fig. 3-7; see also Fig. 1-5). They are found projecting from the surfaces of cells lining the respiratory, reproductive, and central nervous systems. Flagella are much larger

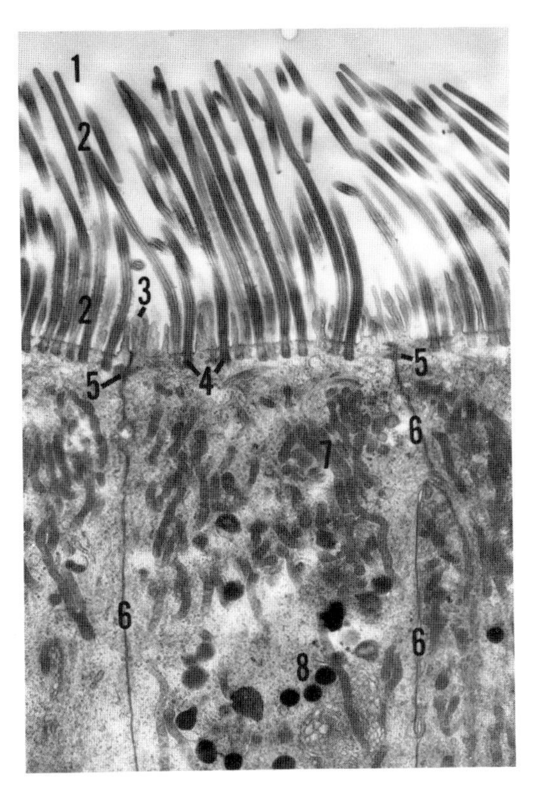

Fig. 3-7. Electron micrograph of cilia, as seen on the free surface of cells lining the lumen of the trachea. *1,* Lumen; *2,* cilia; *3,* microvilli; *4,* basal bodies; *5,* junctional complexes; *6,* cell borders; *7,* mitochondria; *8,* lysosomes. (From *Histology: A Text and Atlas* by Johannes A. G. Rhodin. Copyright © 1976 by Johannes A. G. Rhodin. Reprinted by permission of the author and Oxford University Press, Inc.)

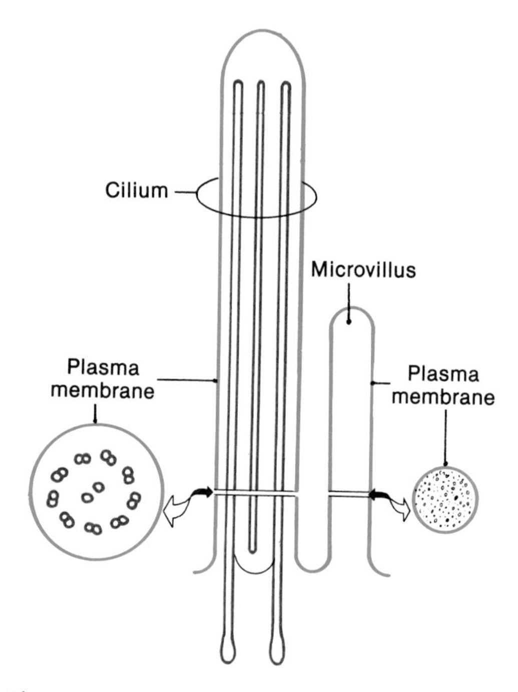

Fig. 3-8. Diagrammatic view showing differences between a cilium and a microvillus, as seen in vertical section and cross section.

(100–200 μm in length and about 0.2–0.5 μm in diameter) and are usually limited to one or two per cell. They are best seen in spermatozoa. In cross sectional views both cilia and flagella show a similar fine structure. Both are surrounded by an extension of the plasma membrane and consist of nine pairs of microtubules surrounding two central microtubules (Fig. 3-8). Cilia and flagella are produced by a specialized form of centrioles known as **basal bodies.** During cell differentiation centrioles reproduce and migrate to the plasma membrane of the cell. These centrioles are then basal bodies and produce the microtubular structures typical of cilia and flagella.

THE CELL CYCLE

The activities of organelles change as a cell proceeds from the time at which it is generated until the time when it will divide. In the last few years cell biologists have formulated a time table for these activities which are collectively called the "cell cycle." The total time involved in one cell cycle varies with the type of cell and its environment. Cells in culture or rapidly dividing embryonic cells may take just a few hours to complete one cell cycle. Moreover, some fully differentiated cells such as nerve cells may be held permanently in one phase of the cell cycle from before birth until the death of the individual.

The cell cycle can be conveniently divided into two phases: 1) interphase, which includes the period of time between one cell division and the next one, and 2) mitosis, when cell division actually occurs.

Interphase

In order to better relate cell activities to a time table, interphase of the cell cycle is subdivided into three discrete periods or phases: G_1 (first Gap), S (DNA synthesis), and G_2 (second Gap) (Fig. 3-9).

The **G_1 phase** of the cell cycle starts after new cells are formed by cell division. The G_1

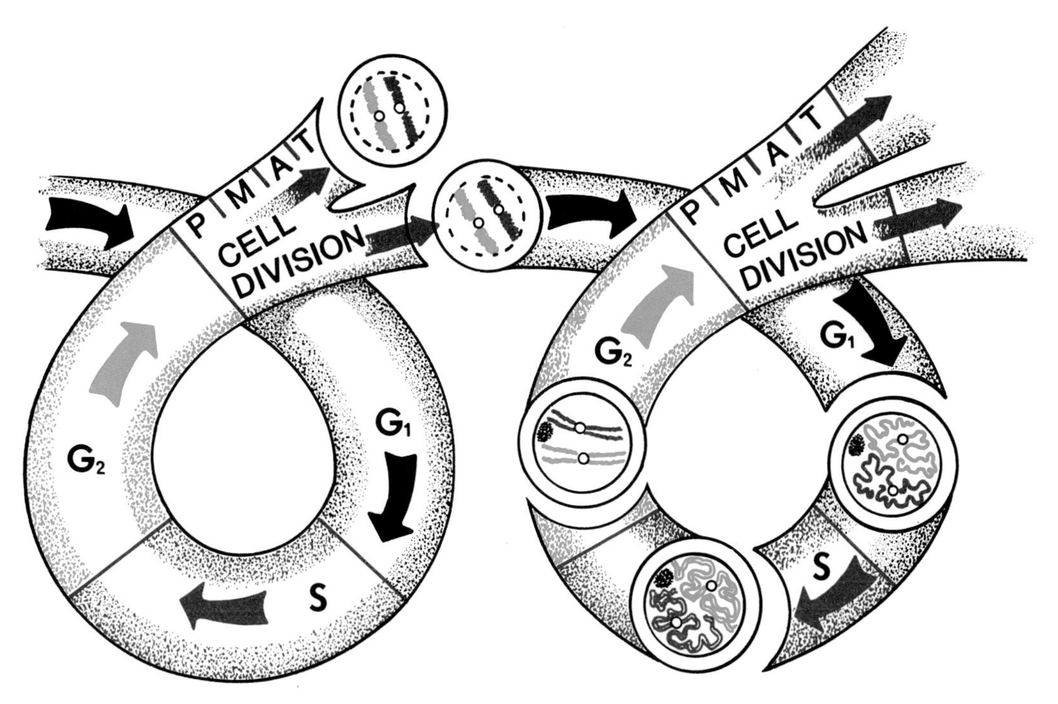

Fig. 3-9. Schematic diagram depicting two cell cycles. Chromosomes of the cells are shown at various phases of the cell cycle. (Human cells have 46 chromosomes in contrast to the 2 shown here.) During cell division chromosomes are fully contracted and a cell goes through prophase (P), metaphase (M), anaphase (A), and telophase (T). Chromosomes in the first gap phase (G_1) are single-stranded and fully dispersed. In the DNA-synthetic phase (S) the chromosomes become double-stranded, and in the second gap phase (G_2) the double-stranded chromosomes begin to contract as the cells prepare for cell division.

phase lasts 6–8 hours in the average cell, but can also be an extended holding phase for highly differentiated cells with long cell cycles. Much cellular growth occurs in this phase as evidenced by increased protein synthesis, the presence of well developed microvilli, and pinocytotic activity at the plasma membrane.

The **S phase** of the cell cycle follows the **G_1** stage. The S phase lasts about 6 hours in most cells, although in some very early embryonic cells it may last only a few minutes. This phase begins with the synthesis of DNA molecules representing the genetic material of the chromosomes; it ends with the completion of DNA synthesis. The plasma membrane has a very reduced number of microvilli and little pinocytotic activity indicating that intake of substances is restricted during this phase.

The **G_2 phase** of the cell cycle starts when DNA synthesis is completed. The G_2 phase in most cells lasts about 5 hours, is less metabolically active than is the G_1 phase, and prepares the cell for division. The plasma membrane has an increased number of microvilli, but not as many as in the G_1 phase. Little growth takes place unless the cell is preparing for those cell divisions which produce sperm or eggs.

Mitosis

The **M phase** or **mitosis** is that period of the cell cycle which begins when the chromosomes become distinctly visible. It ends after cell division is completed. Mitosis also includes **karyokinesis** (division of nuclear elements) and **cytokinesis** (division of the cytoplasm). The

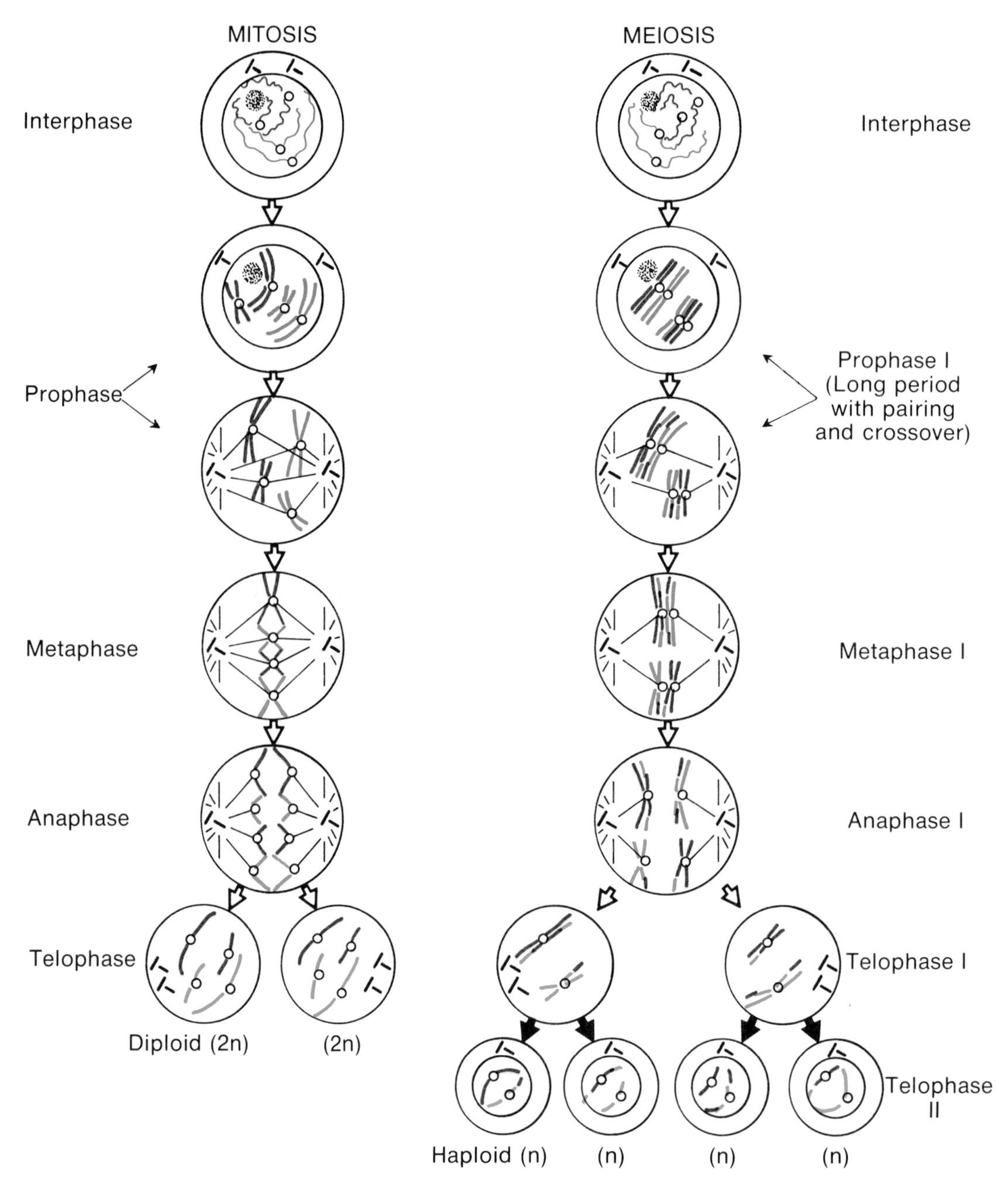

Fig. 3-10. Schematic diagram of mitosis *(left)* and meiosis *(right).* Each human diploid cell has 46 chromosomes in contrast to the 4 chromosomes shown. Each human haploid cell has 23 chromosomes in contrast to the 2 chromosomes shown. During prophase I of meiosis crossing over occurs. The *heavy black arrows* indicate that although prophase II, metaphase II, and anaphase II occur between telophase I and telophase II, these steps are not depicted in the diagram.

purpose of mitosis is to replace cells where needed. In the adult, mitosis is particularly prominent in cells lining the digestive tract, in the skin, and in cells which form blood cells. During mitosis the plasma membrane has extensive long microvilli which may possibly be a source for the additional membrane needed for cellular division.

The process of mitosis has been divided into 4 phases for descriptive purposes (Figs. 3-10 and 3-11). These phases are: **prophase, metaphase, anaphase,** and **telophase.** You should keep in mind that in living cells mitosis is a dynamic process and proceeds without sharp changes from one phase to the next.

Early in **prophase** the cell becomes rounder and the cytoplasm becomes more dense and viscous. The chromatin in the nucleus appears to condense into the elongated highly twisted structures called chromosomes. (In the human there are 46 chromosomes in the nucleus of each cell, except for the sex cells, which contain 23 chromosomes.) In prophase each chromosome consists of two highly coiled threads called **chromatids,** and the chromosome is thus described as being double-stranded. The chromatids are joined at a constricted point called the **centromere** or **kinetochore.** A chromatid, then, is a structure that *shares* a centromere with another chromatid.

The two chromatids that make up each chromosome progressively shorten and thicken. Meanwhile the nuclear envelope and the nucleolus become fragmented and disappear. In the cytoplasm there are two pairs of centrioles, and each pair moves to opposite poles of the cell. A system of microtubules, the astral rays, becomes radially arranged about each pair of centrioles. The astral rays and the centrioles together form the **aster** at each pole. A bundle of microtubules called the **spindle** forms between the asters.

In **metaphase** the 46 double-stranded chromosomes line up at the equator of the cell but do not pair with each other. Spindle microtubules attach to the centromeres, which then become duplicated, thereby allowing the 46

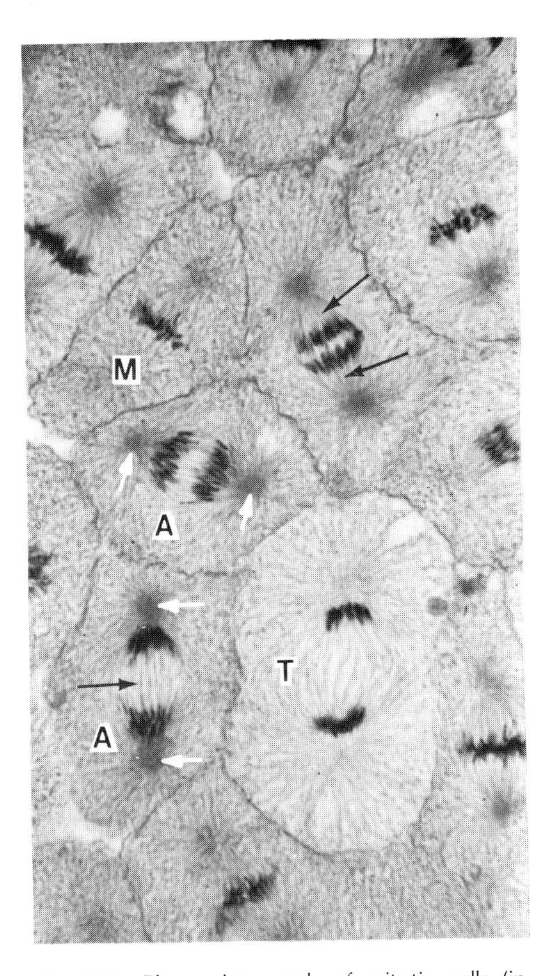

Fig. 3-11. Photomicrograph of mitotic cells (in whitefish blastula). A, anaphase, M, metaphase, T, telophase. Chromosomes (black) are attached to spindle fibers *(black arrows)* composed of microtubules which extend between asters *(white arrows).* (From Turtox, Inc., Chicago, Ill.)

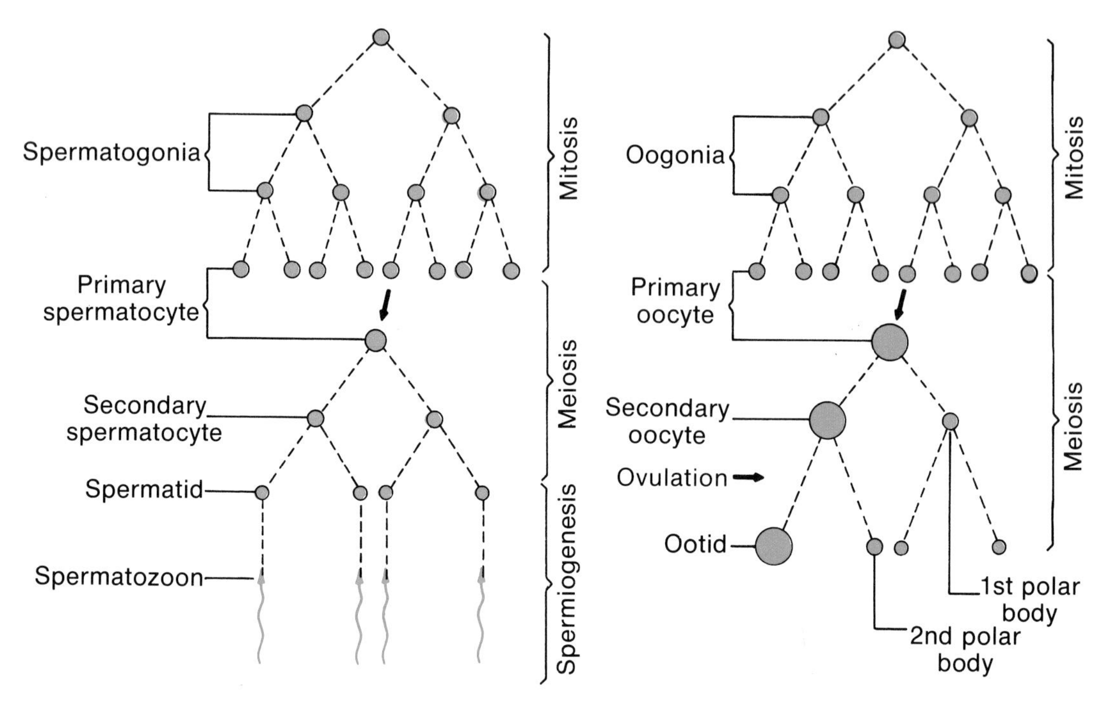

Fig. 3-12. Schematic diagram showing maturation of sperm *(left)* and oocytes *(right)*. The horizontal arrow indicates the point at which ovulation occurs.

double-stranded chromosomes to separate into 92 single-stranded chromosomes, each with its own centromere.

In **anaphase** the single-stranded chromosomes move apart and act as if they are repelled, or as if the microtubules of the spindle are pulling them. By the end of this phase each pole of the cell contains identical sets of 46 single-stranded chromosomes.

Telophase begins with indentation of the plasma membrane to constrict the cytoplasm at the equator of the cell. Division into two cells is usually completed in a minute or two. Centrioles then duplicate to produce two pairs of centrioles per cell. The events which occurred in prophase now take place in reverse. The nuclear envelope and nucleolus reappear, and the single-stranded chromosomes lengthen and revert back to chromatin.

Meiosis

Meiosis is a special process of cell division which occurs during the formation of sperm **(spermatogenesis)** and the formation of eggs **(oogenesis).** Meiosis consists of two cell divisions which reduce the chromosome number from 46 chromosomes **(diploid number)** to 23 chromosomes **(haploid number)** (Fig. 3-10). It also provides for a random sorting of the genetic material so that the new individual formed from the union of an egg and sperm will be different from either parent.

The specialized cells which are involved in meiosis are formed from **spermatogonia** in the testes and **oogonia** in the ovaries. These cells are initially produced by mitotic divisions. Some of these cells then undergo G_1 and S phases similar to those which occur prior to mitosis, but the G_2 phase is quite different in that it involves growth in size and extensive synthesis of RNA and protein. After this period of growth the cells are called **primary spermatocytes** or **primary oocytes.**

Prophase I (prophase of the first meiotic division) has 46 double-stranded chromosomes in the nucleus, although the double strands are not distinguishable with the light microscope.

Each double-stranded chromosome then finds and pairs with a like chromosome called a **homologue.** The 23 pairs of homologues shorten and thicken, and the double strands become apparent. Each pair of double-stranded chromosomes is called a **tetrad** since it consists of four strands (chromatids). At this time there may be an exchange of genetic material between chromatids of the paired chromosomes in a process called **crossing over.** Many of the events in prophase I of meiosis are similar to those in the prophase of mitosis. Thus the nuclear envelope and nucleolus disappear, the pairs of centrioles migrate to the poles of the cell to form asters, and a spindle is formed.

In **Metaphase I,** the 23 tetrads arrive at the equator of the cell. The two double-stranded chromosomes in each tetrad line up so as to have equal chances to migrate to either pole. Spindle fibers are attached to their centromeres, but the centromeres do not duplicate at this time.

In **Anaphase I,** the two double-stranded chromosomes from each tetrad separate and move toward the opposite poles of the spindle. At the end of this phase there is thus a complete set of 23 chromosomes clustered at each pole, and each chromosome consists of two strands (chromatids) joined by one centromere. However, if the phenomenon of crossing over occurs, these chromosomes are not quite the same as the chromosomes in early prophase I (Fig. 3-10).

Telophase I begins with the indentation of the plasma membrane to constrict the cytoplasm, thereby resulting in two cells. These cells are now called **secondary spermatocytes** in the male. In the female the division of cytoplasm is unequal so that a large **secondary oocyte** and a small **first polar body** are produced (Fig. 3-12). These cells duplicate their centrioles and proceed directly into the second meiotic cell division without an interphase period.

Prophase II involves the appearance of a new spindle with its two polar asters.

In **Metaphase II** the 23 double-stranded chromosomes become aligned at the equatorial plate (Fig. 3-10). The centromeres duplicate

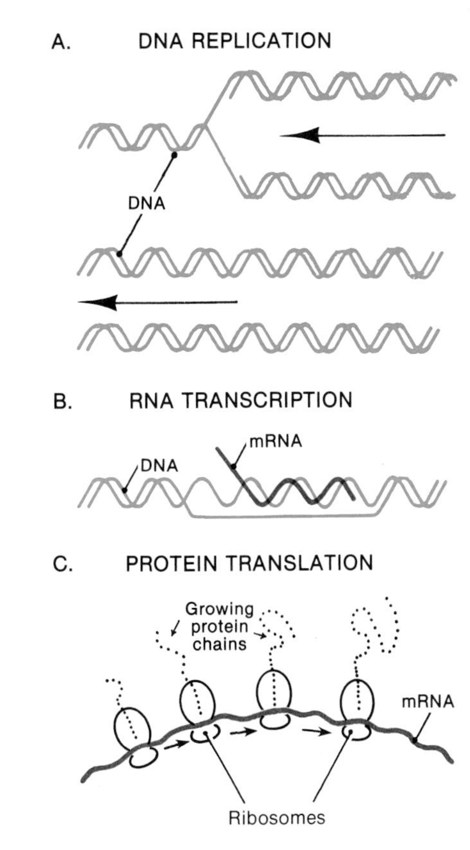

Fig. 3-13. A current understanding of interactions of genetic macromolecules within all cells. (A) Replication: DNA molecule is shown replicating into two molecules. This occurs in the chromosomes in the nucleus. (B) Transcription: an mRNA molecule (red) is synthesized and imprinted with a DNA code in the nucleus. (C) Translation: protein synthesis occurs whereby the information in mRNA is translated into specific protein molecules by the ribosomes located in the cytoplasm.

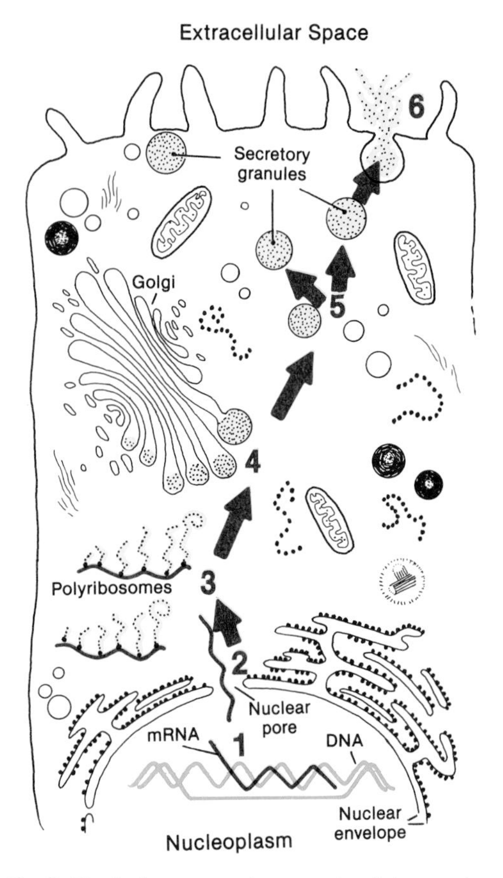

Fig. 3-14. A diagrammatic example of the synthesis and secretion of materials by a cell. 1, part of a DNA molecule in a chromosome unzips and imprints (transcribes) a code on a messenger RNA (mRNA) molecule for a specific kind of protein. 2, mRNA is transported from the nucleus through nuclear pores to the cytoplasm. 3, information in mRNA is translated by the ribosomes into specific protein molecules (yellow). 4, proteins are packaged along with other molecules into membrane-bound organelles by the Golgi complex. 5, membrane-bound organelles combine with vacuoles or are sent as secretion granules to the cell surface (6), where their contents are deposited into the extracellular environment.

and the 23 double-stranded chromosomes now separate into 46 single-stranded chromosomes.

In **Anaphase II** 23 single-stranded chromosomes move to each pole of the spindle.

Telophase II begins with indentation of the plasma membrane to constrict the cytoplasm into two new cells. In the male, these cells are now called **spermatids,** which undergo a metamorphosis to become **sperm (spermatozoa)** (Fig. 3-12). In the female, the division of cytoplasm is again unequal, so that a large **ootid** (ovum) and a small **second polar body** are produced. The second polar body, as well as remnants of the first polar body, have no known function and are eventually lost.

PROTEIN SYNTHESIS

Chromosomes are composed of subunits called **genes.** A gene is a region or segment of a DNA molecule. Genes control the production of specific protein molecules (Fig. 3-13). These proteins include enzymes necessary for specific metabolic reactions, components for structures such as membranes, and materials for export from the cell into the extracellular environment (Fig. 3-14).

In the S phase of the cell cycle the DNA molecule makes a copy of itself in a process called **replication.** Both copies of the DNA molecule are able to imprint a code on strips of special RNA molecules called messenger RNA (mRNA). This process is called **transcription.** In the G_1 and G_2 phases of the cell cycle, the mRNA strip is transported from the nucleus to the cytoplasm where a series of ribosomes (a polyribosome) "read" the coded message and translate it into a specific amino acid sequence to produce protein molecules. This process is called **translation.**

In addition to mRNA the DNA in the nucleus makes ribosomal RNA (rRNA) and transfer RNA (tRNA). Ribosomal RNA goes to the nucleolus where it is assembled into ribosomes which migrate to the cytoplasm. Transfer RNA molecules leave the nucleus and likewise pass to the cytoplasm where they help to bring amino acids to specific sites on the mRNA molecule to be assembled into proteins.

Most amino acids enter the cell by various means, including active transport and pinocytosis at the cell membrane. Before the amino acids can be reassembled into a new protein molecule, they must first be activated by ATP, an energy rich compound mostly produced in the mitochondria. Both rRNA and tRNA are made primarily during the G_1 phase of the cell cycle, are long lived, and can be used over and over again in the process of protein synthesis. In contrast, mRNA is usually short-lived.

4

Tissues

Tissues consist of many cells grouped together to perform similar functions. The individual cells are separated from one another by intercellular (extracellular) spaces of varying dimensions. This intercellular space may contain a variety of components including fluids (collectively termed tissue fluid), gels, and other organic and inorganic materials of varying densities.

Adult tissues are traditionally classified into four basic types: **epithelial, connective** (including blood and lymph), **muscle,** and **nervous.** Epithelial tissue contains very little intercellular space and serves to line cavities and cover surfaces. Connective tissue contains much intercellular space and plays a major role in supporting and binding together other tissues. Muscle and nervous tissues have little intercellular space and are highly adapted for contraction and communication, respectively. The four basic tissues interact with one another to form organs and organ systems.

EPITHELIAL TISSUE

Epithelial tissues are specialized for covering body surfaces or lining hollow structures. The individual cells of an epithelium are joined closely to one another by interdigitating cell membranes and specialized areas of contact called **junctional complexes** (Fig. 4-1). (These junctions have been called **terminal bars** by light microscopists.) One type of junctional complex is termed a **tight junction,** which acts as a seal and is particularly numerous near the central cavity (lumen) of a hollow organ. Since substances must therefore pass through the epithelial cells rather than between them in order to reach deeper tissues, epithelial cells act as barriers or mediators between two different environments. Another type of junctional complex is the **gap junction (nexus)** which allows ions or small molecules to pass rapidly from one cell to an adjacent cell and provides a means for cell to cell communication.

The structure of various epithelial cells reflects their specialized functions. In cells which absorb or transport large volumes of fluids, the cell surface is folded into numerous short fingerlike **microvilli.** Some cells show cellular specializations for engulfing materials (**pinocytotic** and **phagocytic vesicles**) or for releasing a variety of substances, while other cells have **cilia** which move particles along their surfaces (Fig. 4-2). Still other epithelial cell surfaces are modified so as to prevent dehydration or to protect deeper tissues. Epithelial cells may also be highly specialized to act as sensory receptors.

Epithelium is an avascular tissue, i.e., it is not penetrated by blood vessels but must depend on the diffusion of substances to and from blood vessels in the underlying connective tissues. At the interface between the epithelial

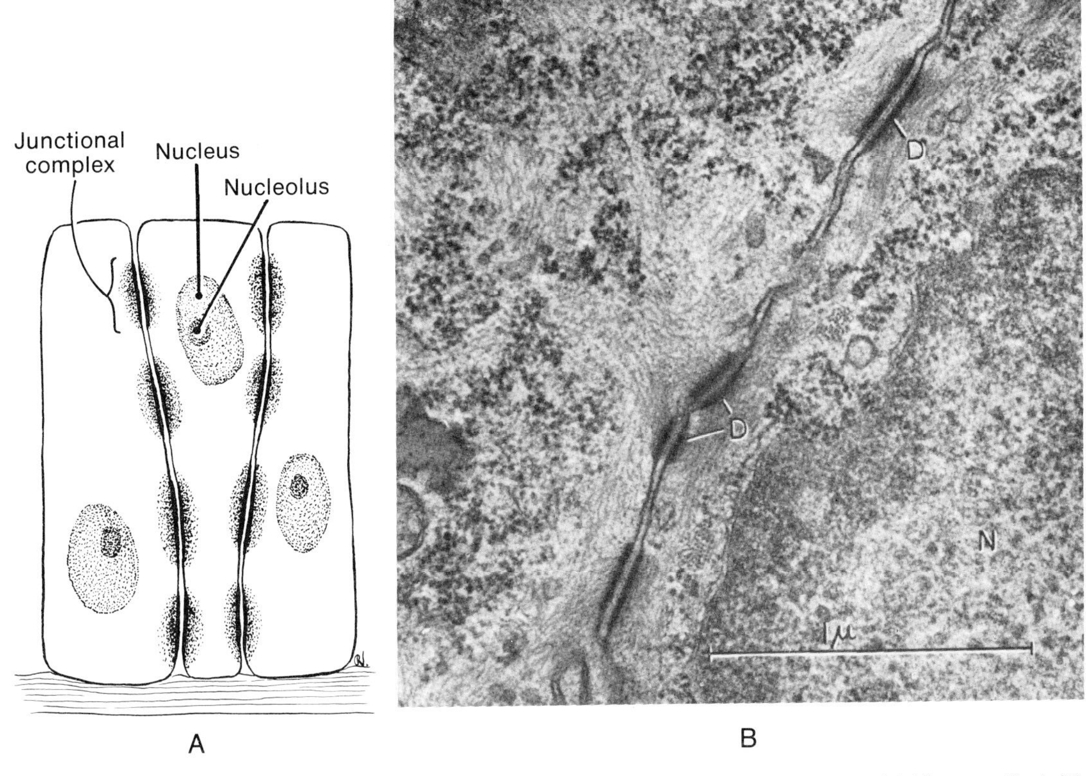

Fig. 4-1. (A) Sketch of three epithelial cells showing location of junctional complexes highly magnified. (B) Electron micrograph of junctional complexes, D, between epithelial cells; N, nucleus. (Courtesy of Dr. Keith Porter, from W. M. Copenhaver, R. P. Bunge, and M. B. Bunge, *Bailey's Textbook of Histology,* Ed. 16, The Williams & Wilkins Co., Baltimore, 1971.)

cells and connective tissue cells there is a concentration of noncellular material in the form of a **basement membrane (basal lamina)** (Fig. 4-2). Basement membranes can be of variable thickness and consist of a network of slender filaments in a complex matrix of polysaccharides and protein. The basement membrane maintains contact between the epithelium and connective tissue and also serves as a mediator for exchanging substances between the epithelial cells and underlying blood vessels. In regions such as the lining of the digestive and respiratory tracts, the combination of epithelium, basement membrane, and connective tissues is designated as a **mucous membrane.**

An epithelium can regenerate rapidly, especially in areas of constant wear and tear or when injured. The continuous repair of these tissues by cell division and growth is important in such areas as the epidermis of the skin and the lining of the digestive tract.

Glands

Some epithelial cells perform a secretory function, in which case they are termed **glands.** A **unicellular gland** consists of a single cell, of which a **goblet cell** is a good example (Fig. 4-2). A goblet cell produces **mucus** which accumulates and distends the apical region of the cell. The basal region remains narrow, thereby giving it a goblet or wine glass shape. Mucus serves an important function in moistening and lubricating cell surfaces, in trapping foreign particles, and in dissolving substances for absorption.

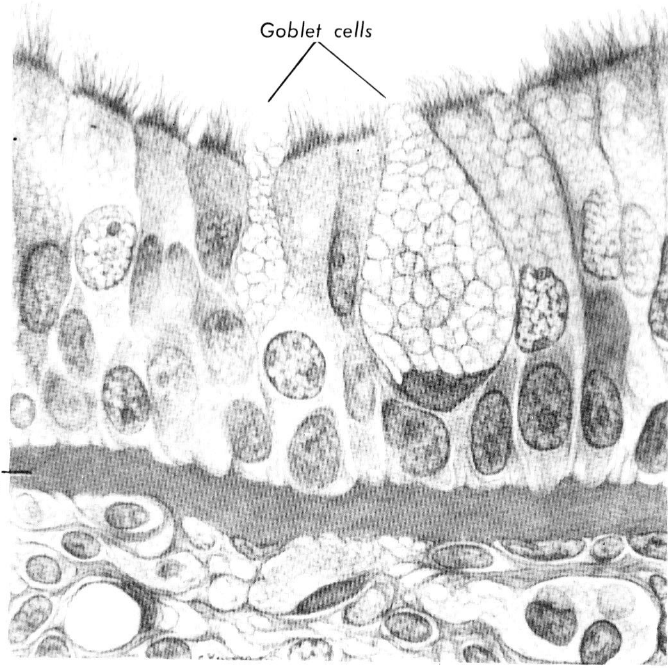

Fig. 4-2. Ciliated epithelial cells and goblet cells. Note the basement membrane lying deep to the epithelium. (From W. M. Copenhaver, R. P. Bunge, and M. B. Bunge, *Bailey's Textbook of Histology,* Ed. 16, The Williams & Wilkins Co., Baltimore, 1971.)

A **multicellular gland** is composed of several epithelial cells. During embryonic development most multicellular glands arise as invaginations or migrations of cells from the surface epithelium down into the connective tissue. These glands are composed of clusters of secretory epithelial cells which retain their communication with the surface via a system of ducts. Such glands are designated as **exocrine** glands, in contrast to ductless or **endocrine glands** which secrete their products (termed **hormones**) directly into the blood stream.

Multicellular glands may be classified as **simple** with a single secretory passageway or **compound** with a branched system of passageways (Fig. 4-3). In some cases the glands consist of slender tubes and are thus termed **tubular** glands; other glands may show sac-like bulges and are called **alveolar** (acinar) glands. Combinations of tubes and sacs are designated **tubuloalveolar** (tubuloacinar).

The epithelial cells of glands may secrete their products in a variety of ways. **Holocrine** glands contain cells which are discharged along with their secretions. Cells in **apocrine** glands lose only a portion of their cytoplasm at the time of secretion. **Merocrine** (eccrine) glands have cells with vesicles which discharge their contents onto the surface, but the cell itself remains intact.

Classification of Epithelia

Different types of epithelia can be identified on the basis of the structure and arrangement of their cells (Figs. 4-4 and 4-5). If the epithelium consists of one layer of cells it is a **simple** epithelium; if more than one layer is present it is **stratified.** Epithelia are further categorized according to the shape of their cells. Table 4-1 lists these features and the locations of the various types of epithelia.

Simple Epithelia

Simple squamous epithelium is composed of a single layer of flattened interlocking cells (Fig. 4-4). This epithelium is termed a **mesothelium** when it lines cavities such as the pericardial, pleural, and peritoneal cavities. It is

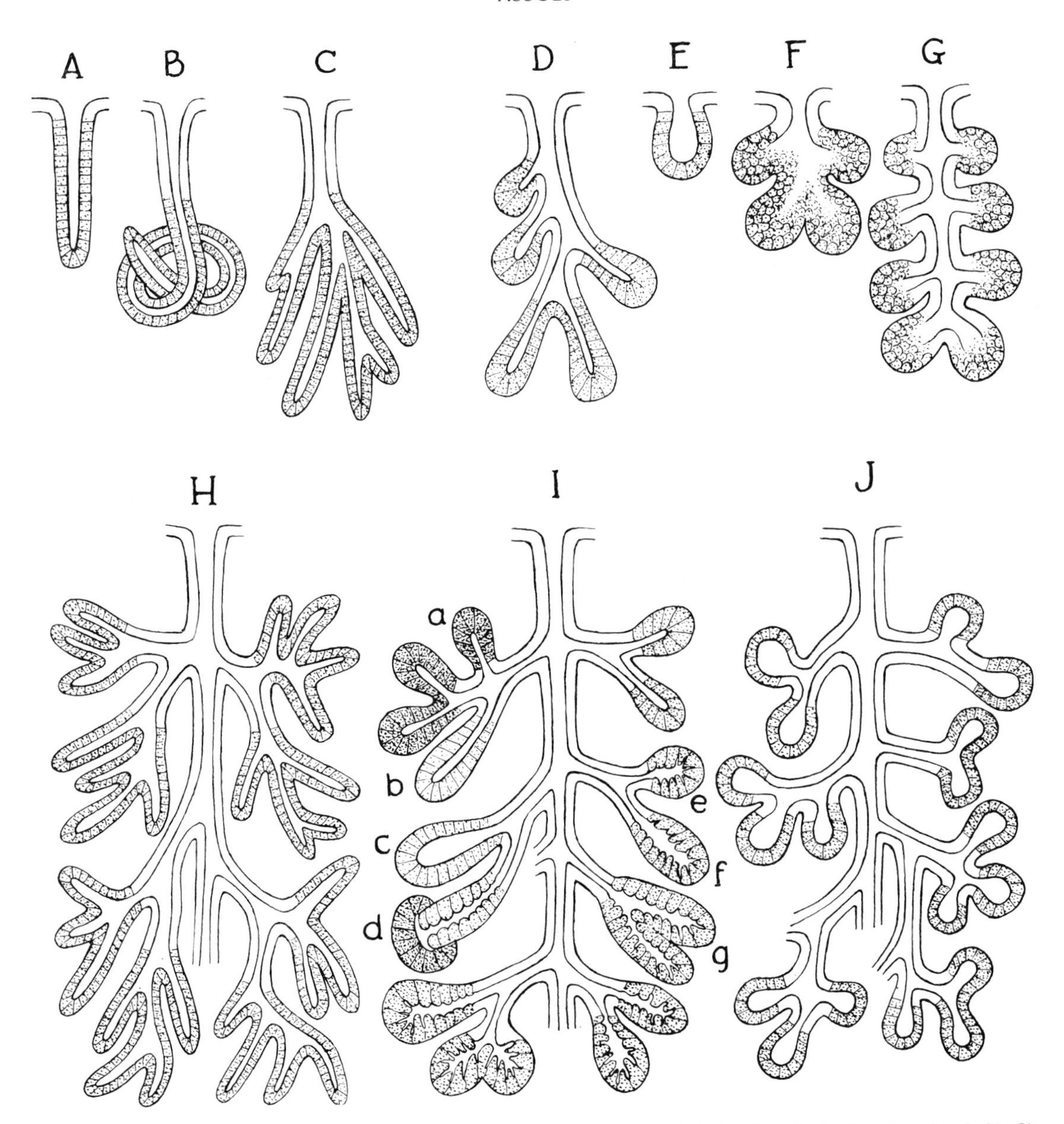

Fig. 4-3. Types of exocrine glands. (A–C) Simple tubular glands, (D) simple tubuloalveolar gland, (E–G) simple alveolar glands, (H) compound tubular gland, (I) compound tubuloalveolar gland showing variations in size and shape of terminations (a–g), (J) compound alveolar gland. (From W. M. Copenhaver, R. P. Bunge, and M. B. Bunge, *Bailey's Textbook of Histology,* Ed. 16, The Williams & Wilkins Co., Baltimore, 1971.)

termed an **endothelium** when it lines blood vessels and lymph vessels.

Simple cuboidal epithelium consists of a single layer of blockshaped cells. Their shape rarely approaches a perfect cube but may range between high simple squamous to low columnar. Simple cuboidal epithelium is found in many glands and in portions of many of their ducts.

Simple columnar epithelium is composed

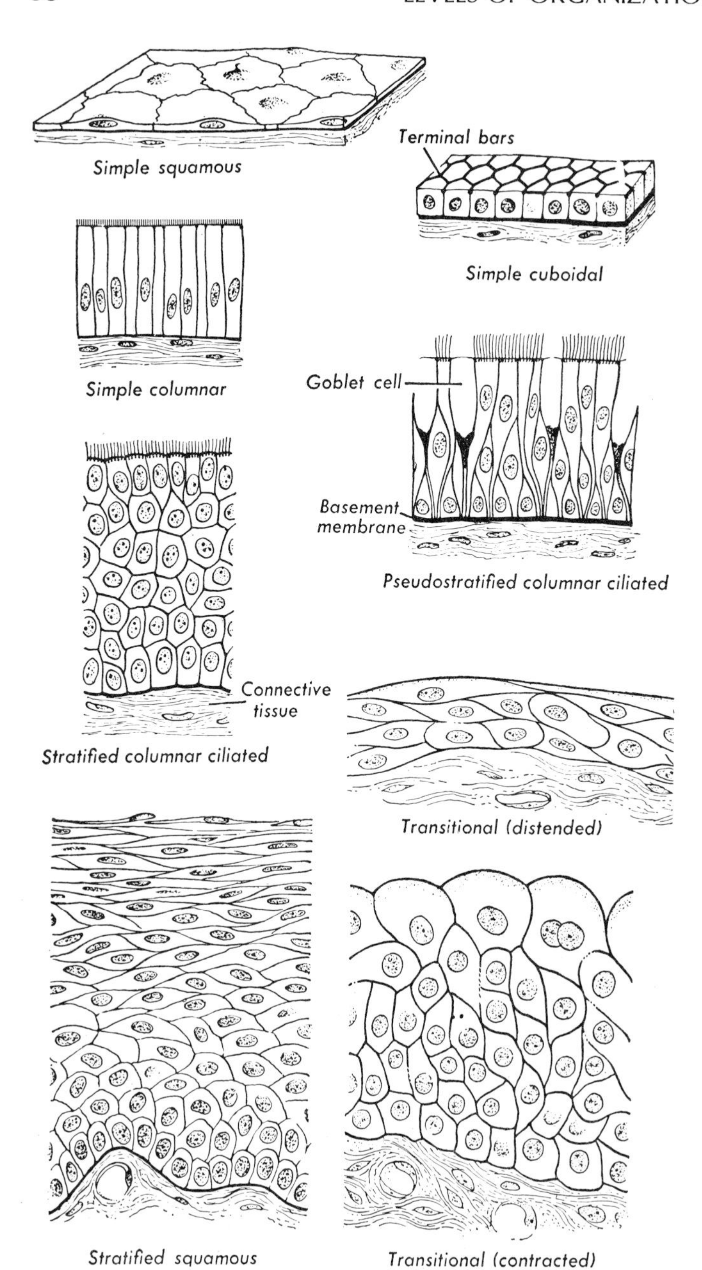

Fig. 4-4. Types of epithelium shown with underlying connective tissue. (From W. M. Copenhaver, R. P. Bunge, and M. B. Bunge, *Bailey's Textbook of Histology,* Ed. 16, The Williams & Wilkins Co., Baltimore, 1971.)

of a single layer of tall rectangular cells. The columnar cells in the small intestine have extensive microvilli for absorption of materials. Some columnar cells may be ciliated such as those which line parts of the uterine tubes.

Pseudostratified columnar epithelium contains several cell types. All cells rest on the basement membrane but their upper ends extend for varying distances. Nuclei of this tissue are usually at different levels, giving a falsely stratified appearance. Mucus-producing goblet cells are common in this epithelium. In some regions of the respiratory tract, the pseudostratified columnar epithelium is ciliated.

Stratified Epithelia

Stratified epithelia consist of several layers of cells and are classified according to the shape

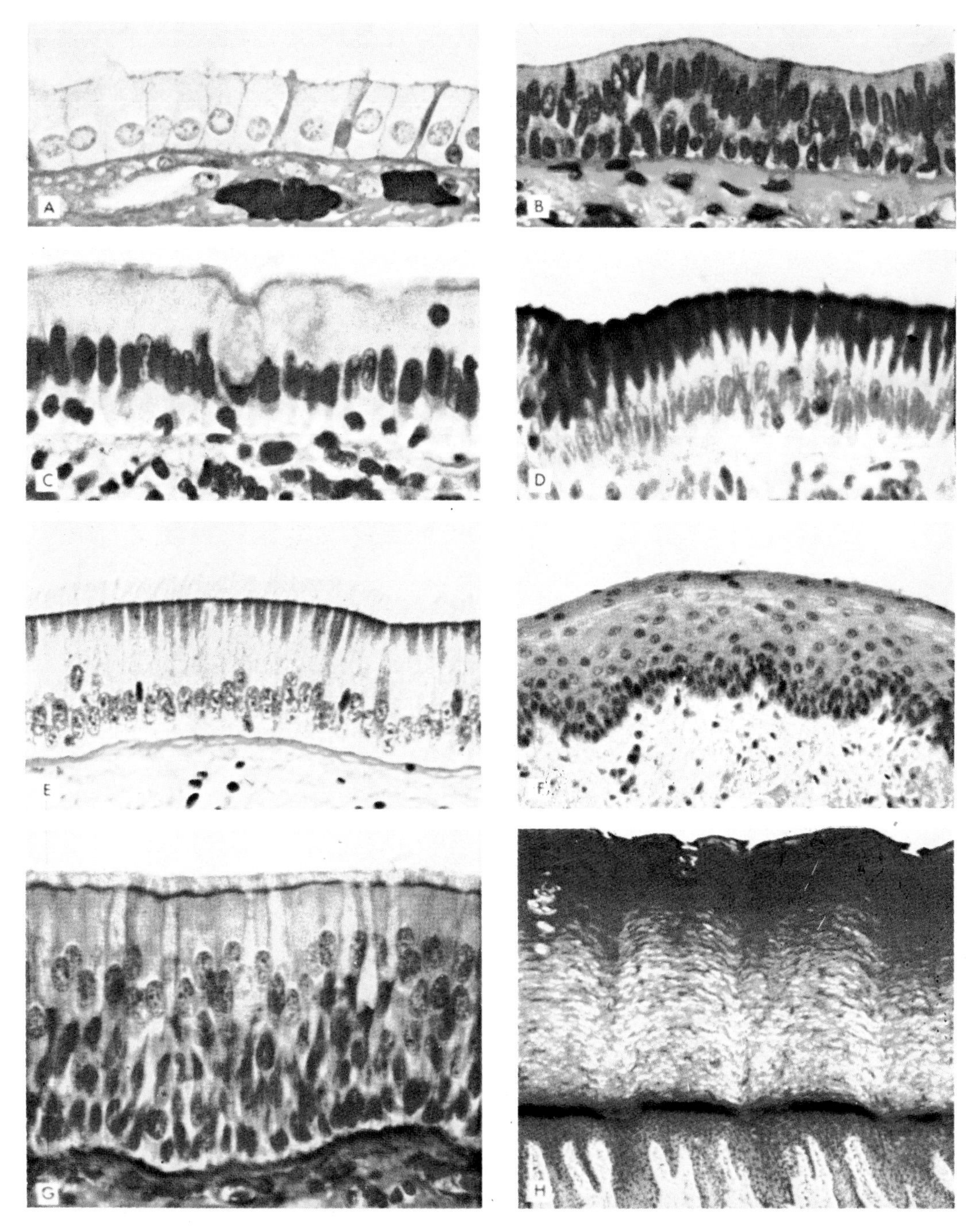

Fig. 4-5. Types of epithelia as seen with the light microscope and stained with different histological techniques. (A) Simple columnar, (B) stratified columnar, (C) simple columnar (with striated border), (D) simple columnar with mucous cells, (E) simple columnar with cilia, (F) stratified squamous, (G) pseudostratified ciliated columnar, (H) keratinized stratified squamous. (From W. Bloom and D. W. Fawcett, *A Textbook of Histology,* Ed. 10, W. B. Saunders Co., Philadelphia, 1975.)

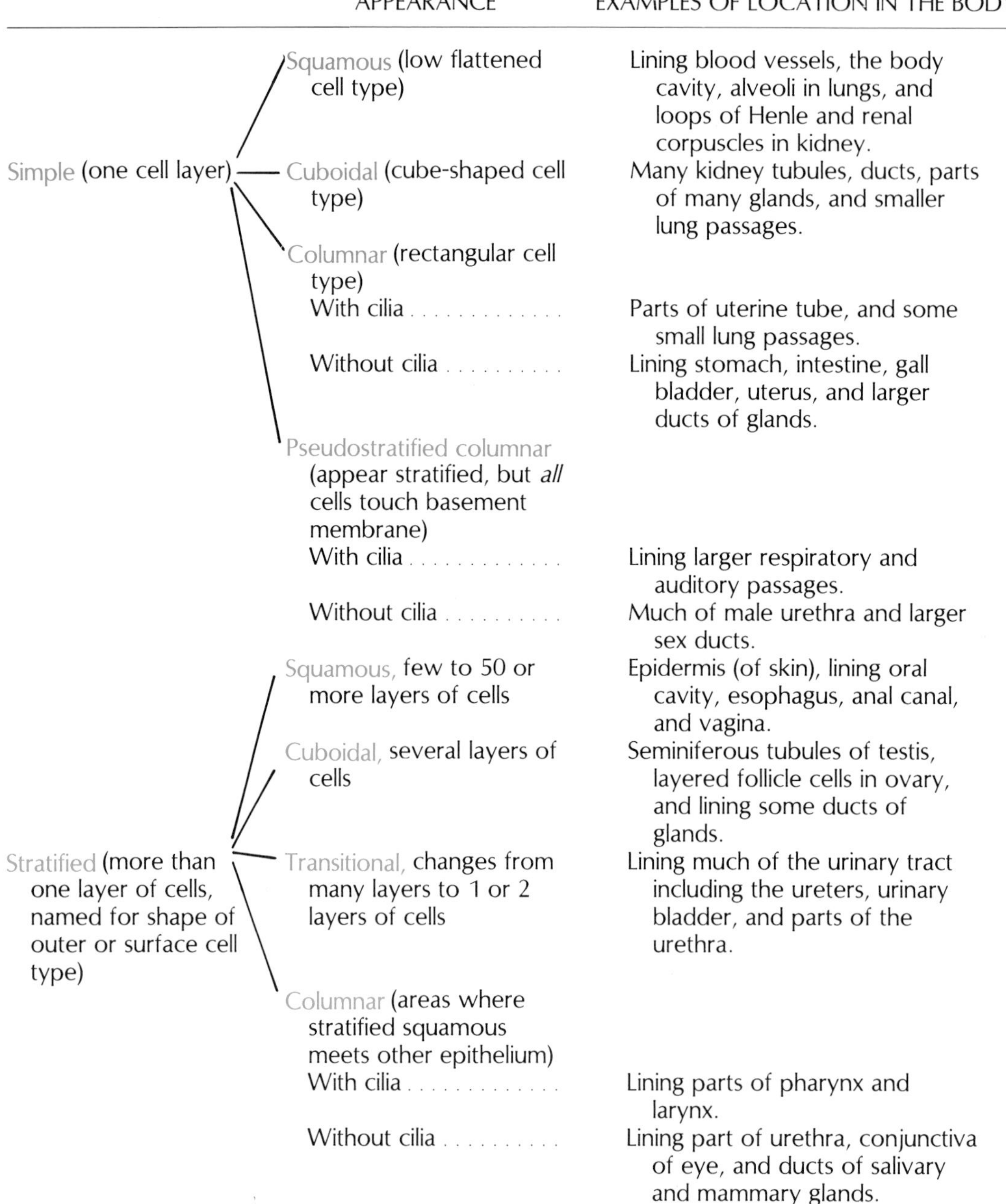

Table 4-1. Types of Epithelia

	APPEARANCE	EXAMPLES OF LOCATION IN THE BODY
Simple (one cell layer)	Squamous (low flattened cell type)	Lining blood vessels, the body cavity, alveoli in lungs, and loops of Henle and renal corpuscles in kidney.
	Cuboidal (cube-shaped cell type)	Many kidney tubules, ducts, parts of many glands, and smaller lung passages.
	Columnar (rectangular cell type)	
	With cilia	Parts of uterine tube, and some small lung passages.
	Without cilia	Lining stomach, intestine, gall bladder, uterus, and larger ducts of glands.
	Pseudostratified columnar (appear stratified, but *all* cells touch basement membrane)	
	With cilia	Lining larger respiratory and auditory passages.
	Without cilia	Much of male urethra and larger sex ducts.
Stratified (more than one layer of cells, named for shape of outer or surface cell type)	Squamous, few to 50 or more layers of cells	Epidermis (of skin), lining oral cavity, esophagus, anal canal, and vagina.
	Cuboidal, several layers of cells	Seminiferous tubules of testis, layered follicle cells in ovary, and lining some ducts of glands.
	Transitional, changes from many layers to 1 or 2 layers of cells	Lining much of the urinary tract including the ureters, urinary bladder, and parts of the urethra.
	Columnar (areas where stratified squamous meets other epithelium)	
	With cilia	Lining parts of pharynx and larynx.
	Without cilia	Lining part of urethra, conjunctiva of eye, and ducts of salivary and mammary glands.

of cells in the outermost layer (Figs. 4-4 and 4-5).

Stratified squamous epithelium is composed of numerous layers of cells, of which the deepest layer is high cuboidal to low columnar. As the cells multiply and move upward from the deep layer they become flattened. Cells in the upper layers no longer divide and may even lose their nuclei (such as those on the surface of the skin) or they may retain nuclei as in the stratified mucous membranes of the digestive and reproductive tracts.

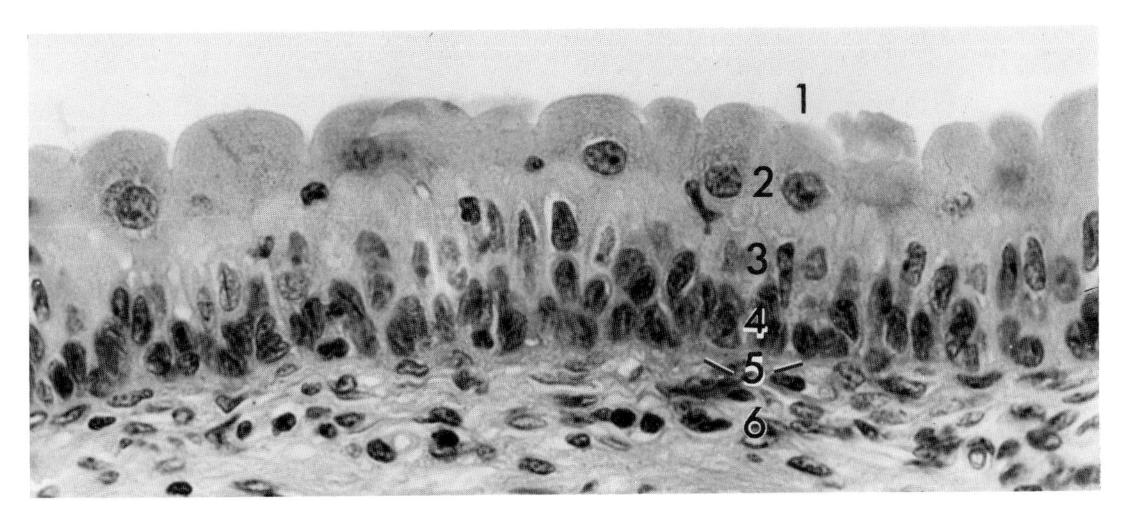

Fig. 4-6. Transitional epithelium from a urinary bladder, showing *1,* lumen of bladder; *2,* superficial epithelial cells; *3,* intermediate layers of epithelial cells; *4,* basal cells; *5,* basal lamina of epithelium; and *6,* underlying connective tissue. (From *Histology: A Text and Atlas* by Johannes A. G. Rhodin. Copyright © 1976 by Johannes A. G. Rhodin. Reprinted by permission of the author and Oxford University Press, Inc.)

Stratified cuboidal epithelium usually has a few layers of cells of fairly uniform size. It is found in diverse and highly specialized regions of the body such as follicles in the ovary, seminiferous tubules in the testis, and in ducts of sweat glands.

Transitional epithelium in the relaxed state may be classified as stratified cuboidal, since it has five to six layers of cube-shaped cells. However, when this tissue is stretched the number of cell layers is reduced to two or three, and the cells change their shape from cuboidal to a flattened cell type (Figs. 4-4, and 4-6). The relatively impermeable cells are held together by junctional complexes. Transitional epithelium is found lining much of the urinary tract.

Stratified columnar epithelium has few layers of cells. The outermost layer is columnar but other layers are somewhat cuboidal. This tissue is limited to regions of the body where stratified squamous epithelium becomes continuous with other epithelium.

CONNECTIVE TISSUE

Connective tissue provides support, protection, and a framework for the body. It is a widely distributed tissue which binds groups of cells and tissues together, provides packing material between and around organs, and serves as a pathway for vessels and nerves and as a source of undifferentiated cells which can develop into a variety of cell types. Some connective tissues also serve as storage depots for substances which are utilized by other tissues of the body.

An important feature of connective tissue is the large amount of intercellular space with varying composition and texture. The intercellular space is composed of a background material called **ground substance (matrix)** in which are embedded various non-cellular **fibers.** These fibers and ground substance are produced by the connective tissue cells. The nature, amount, and arrangement of the fibers, cells, and ground substance are often used as a means of classifying various types of connective tissue.

Embryonic connective tissue is often considered in a special category since it initially consists of irregularly shaped mesenchymal cells lying in a large amount of homogeneous ground substance. Fibers are eventually produced by the cells, and the ground substance becomes viscous and sticky. For this reason the embryonic tissue is often called **mucous connective tissue.** A good example of this tissue

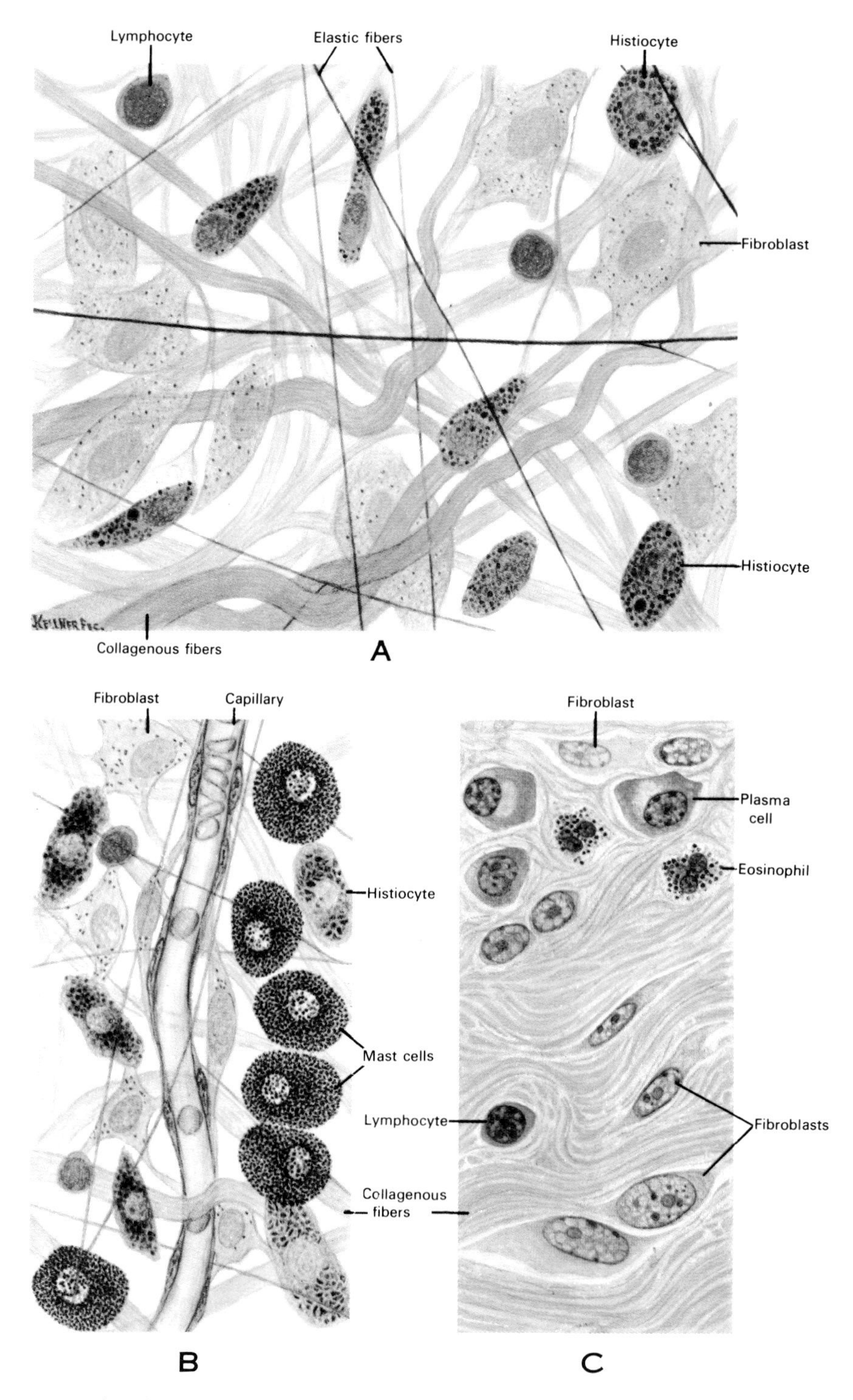

Fig. 4-7. Loose connective tissue stained variously to show different cell types and fibers. (From W. M. Copenhaver, R. P. Bunge, and M. B. Bunge, *Bailey's Textbook of Histology,* Ed. 16, The Williams & Wilkins Co., Baltimore, 1971.)

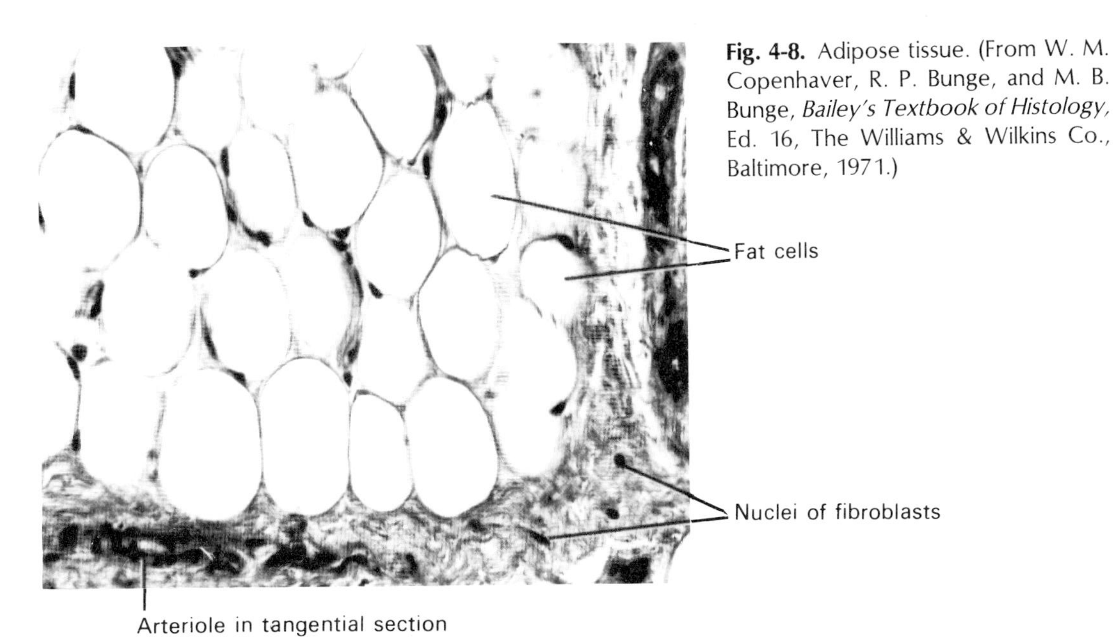

Fig. 4-8. Adipose tissue. (From W. M. Copenhaver, R. P. Bunge, and M. B. Bunge, *Bailey's Textbook of Histology,* Ed. 16, The Williams & Wilkins Co., Baltimore, 1971.)

type occurs in the umbilical cord where it is called **Wharton's jelly.**

Adult connective tissue can be classified into connective tissue proper, cartilage, bone, blood, and lymph. It is well to keep in mind that there is often a gradation between the various types of connective tissue, and occasionally one type may transform into another type.

Connective Tissue Proper

Loose Connective Tissue

This represents the basic plan for connective tissues in general, since it contains most of the cells and fibers which occur in other types of connective tissue (Fig. 4-7).

Cells. The common cell types in connective tissue are fibroblasts, macrophages, plasma cells, mast cells, and fat cells. The **fibroblasts** are spindle-shaped cells with branching processes and are among the most common cell types in loose connective tissue. As implied by their name, fibroblasts are responsible for forming fibers which are deposited in the ground substance. **Macrophages (histiocytes)** are large irregularly shaped cells commonly found in loose connective tissue and are important scavenger cells which engulf foreign material and cellular debris. They become particularly numerous in regions of inflammation. **Plasma cells** are less numerous than fibroblasts or macrophages but can be identified by their nucleus which has a "cart wheel" appearance and by their cytoplasm which stains deep blue with standard histological stains. Plasma cells produce antibodies. **Mast cells** occur near blood vessels and show large granules in their cytoplasm. They produce heparin (an anticoagulant) and histamine, which increases the size and permeability of small vessels. **Fat cells** contain a large droplet of fat which displaces the nucleus and most of the cytoplasm to a thin rim. Large accumulations of fat cells are referred to as **adipose tissue** (Fig. 4-8). In addition, various blood cells (eosinophils, neutrophils, and lymphocytes) often leave the blood vessels and pass out into the surrounding connective tissue, particularly at sites of infection and inflammation.

Fibers. Three types of fibers (collagenous, elastic, and reticular) are produced by the fibroblasts. **Collagenous fibers** are arranged in broad wavy bundles (Fig. 4-7). Each fiber consists of numerous smaller fibrils composed of

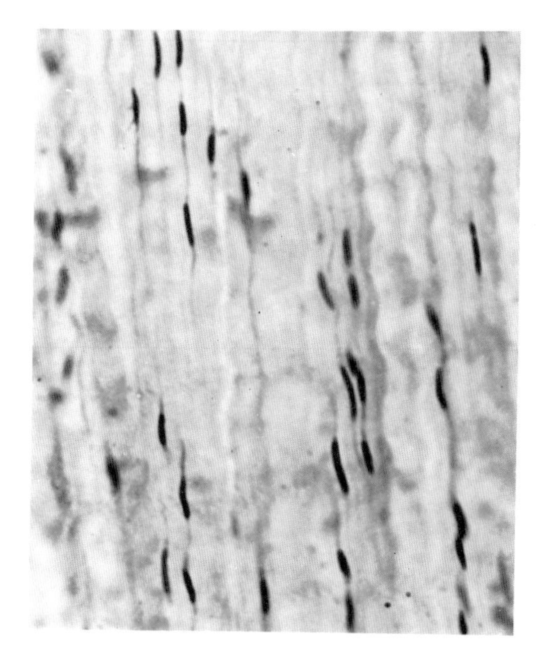

Fig. 4-9. Dense regular connective tissue. A longitudinal section of a tendon at low magnification. (From C. R. Leeson and T. S. Leeson, *Histology,* Ed. 3, W. B. Saunders Co., Philadelphia, 1976.)

collagen, a protein similar to albumin. If collagenous fibers are boiled, they yield gelatin and eventually glue. Collagenous fibers provide resilience and flexibility to connective tissue. Vitamin C is important in promoting collagen formation; thus a deficiency of this vitamin results in scurvy which is characterized by bleeding gums and easily damaged skin and mucous membranes. **Reticular fibers** are very thin, delicate strands similar in composition to collagenous fibers. Reticular fibers cannot be seen in ordinary histological preparations but become evident with the use of silver stains. Reticular fibers tend to be sparsely scattered in loose connective tissue. They form abundant networks in certain organs such as glands. **Elastic fibers** branch and interconnect with one another and are composed of **elastin,** a protein which enables them to be stretched. They can usually be seen only in material stained with a special dye (orcein).

Ground Substance. The ground substance is produced by some of the connective tissue cells and provides a medium for the diffusion

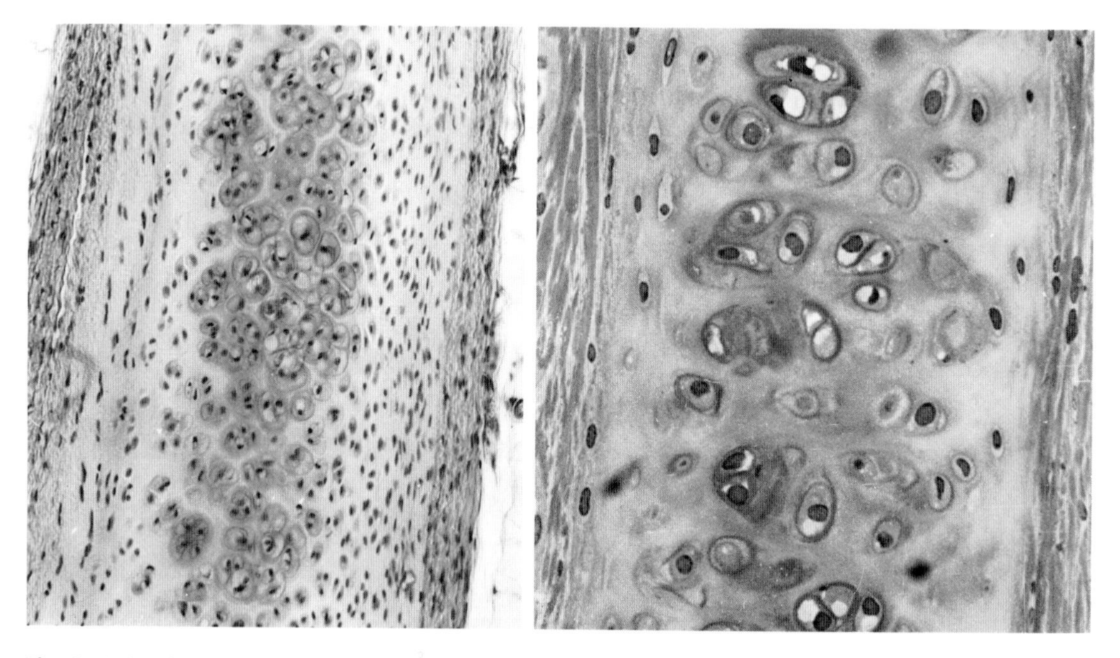

Fig. 4-10. Hyaline cartilage at low magnification *(left)* and high magnification *(right).* (From C. R. Leeson and T. S. Leeson, *Histology,* Ed. 3, W. B. Saunders Co., Philadelphia, 1976.)

of gases, nutrients, and wastes to and from the cells and blood vessels. This background material has a gel-like consistency and is composed of protein-carbohydrate complexes with varying amounts of water.

Dense Connective Tissue

This type of connective tissue is characterized by a large amount of densely packed collagenous fibers. If the fibroblasts are irregularly arranged and the collagenous fibers interlace and form an irregular network, this tissue type is termed **dense irregular** connective tissue. This is commonly found encapsulating many organs and making up the dermis of the skin. If the fibroblasts are arranged in parallel rows between which are bundles of longitudinally oriented collagenous fibers, then the tissue is termed **dense regular** connective tissue, examples being **tendons** and **ligaments** (Fig. 4-9). An **aponeurosis** is structurally similar to a ligament or a tendon except that it is a broad thin sheet of dense regular connective tissue. In some ligaments the dense regular connective tissue may consist predominantly of elastic fibers.

Reticular Connective Tissue

This type of connective tissue is characterized by a network of reticular fibers and a special cell type, the reticular cells. **Reticular cells** are phagocytic, but they are fixed in position, in contrast to macrophages which are mobile. This tissue is common in organs of the lymphatic (lymphoreticular) system.

Adipose Tissue

A large accumulation of fat cells in loose connective tissue is called adipose tissue (Fig. 4-8). The fat serves not only as a food reserve for the body but also as an insulator against cold. It also protects against abrasion in regions where organs lie against one another.

Pigmented Connective Tissue

In some regions of the body, the connective tissue may contain pigmented cells called **chromatophores.** These tend to occur in the dermis of the skin in the anal region, as well as in the choroid of the eye.

Cartilage

Cartilage provides support and protection, as well as flexibility. The mature cartilage cells are called **chondrocytes** and are usually arranged in clusters. Networks of collagenous fibers are embedded in a firm ground substance produced by the cartilage cells and composed of a protein-carbohydrate complex conjugated with sulfur. Cartilage tissue is surrounded by a dense irregular connective tissue called a **perichondrium** ("around the cartilage"). Blood vessels in the perichondrium do not normally penetrate the cartilage ground substance. Therefore, the chondrocytes receive nutrients and get rid of their waste products by means of diffusion through the ground substance and the walls of blood vessels in the perichondrium. The perichondrium is also important in providing new cells for repairing cartilage in the event that it is torn or damaged.

There are three types of cartilage, the most common of which is hyaline. **Hyaline cartilage** is translucent and contains fine collagenous fibers which form an interlacing network between the cartilage cells (Fig. 4-10). This type of cartilage constitutes much of the skeleton in the fetus, and is retained as a covering on the ends of long bones in the adult. Hyaline cartilage also is an important component of the major air passages of the respiratory system.

Fibrocartilage (fibrous cartilage) is characterized by a preponderance of collagenous fibers arranged in thick bundles which provide additional strength (Fig. 4-11). One location of fibrocartilage is in the intervertebral discs which act as shock absorbers between the vertebrae. Fibrocartilage also helps to connect the dense connective tissue of tendons and ligaments with the hyaline cartilage at the ends of bones and joints.

Elastic cartilage contains a dense network of elastic fibers providing considerable flexibility, as well as strength (Fig. 4-12). This can be demonstrated in the flaplike auricle of the ex-

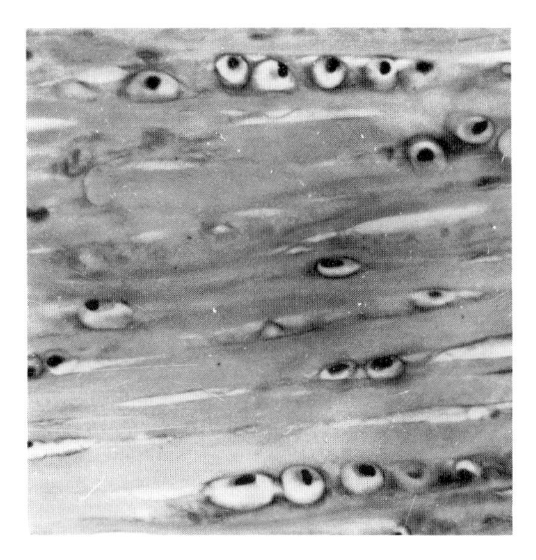

Fig. 4-11. Fibrocartilage showing chondrocytes and bundles of collagenous fibers. (From C. R. Leeson and T. S. Leeson, *Histology,* Ed. 3, W. B. Saunders Co., Philadelphia, 1976.)

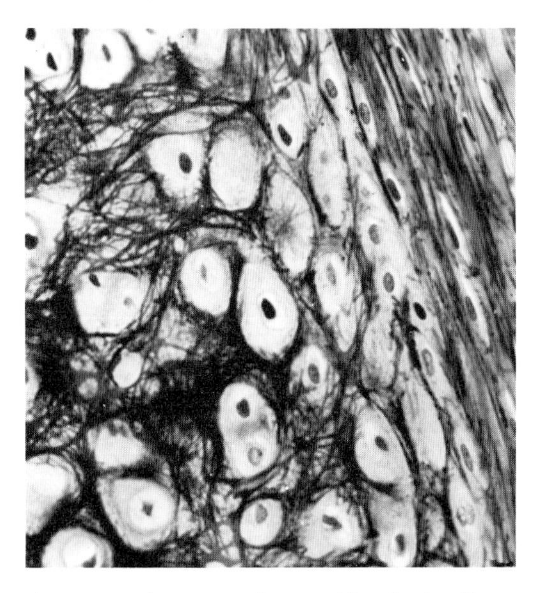

Fig. 4-12. Elastic cartilage with elastic fibers stained black. (From C. R. Leeson and T. S. Leeson, *Histology,* Ed. 3, W. B. Saunders Co., Philadelphia, 1976.)

ternal ear, which can be bent over but fortunately easily returns back to its original shape.

Bone

Bone (osseous) tissue is a dense rigid form of connective tissue characterized by the presence of inorganic salts in the intercellular ground substance produced by bone cells. Mature bone cells are called **osteocytes,** each of which is situated in a tiny cavity, the **lacuna** (Fig. 4-13). Radiating outward from the lacuna are tiny, fluid containing channels (**canaliculi**). The osteocytes send out slender cytoplasmic projections into the canaliculi and thereby manage to exchange substances with the canalicular fluid. This is necessary because of the extreme density of the ground substance preventing direct diffusion of substances to and from the cells.

The ground substance (**matrix**) of bone contains numerous collagenous fibers and is composed of a sulfated carbohydrate-protein complex in which inorganic salts (calcium phosphate and calcium carbonate) have been deposited in the form of hydroxyapatite crystals. If the organic component of osseous tissue diminishes (as may occur with age), the bone becomes brittle; if there is an insufficient amount of inorganic salts (as in such calcium deficiency diseases as rickets), the osseous tissue becomes pliable and cannot bear weight without bending. The ground substance is arranged in thin layers termed **lamellae,** and the osteocytes within the lacunae are usually situated between the lamellae (Fig. 4-13).

Adult bone is organized into two general types depending on the relative amounts of space and bone tissue. **Spongy bone** exhibits large irregular spaces between thin spicules and plates of bony tissue (Fig. 4-13). **Compact bone** is dense and contains an elaborate system of thin canals which interconnect with one another and which carry blood vessels and nerves. In compact bone the lamellae are arranged concentrically around a central channel known as a **Haversian canal** (Fig. 4-13). These canals lie parallel to one another and intercommunicate via transverse and oblique channels as well

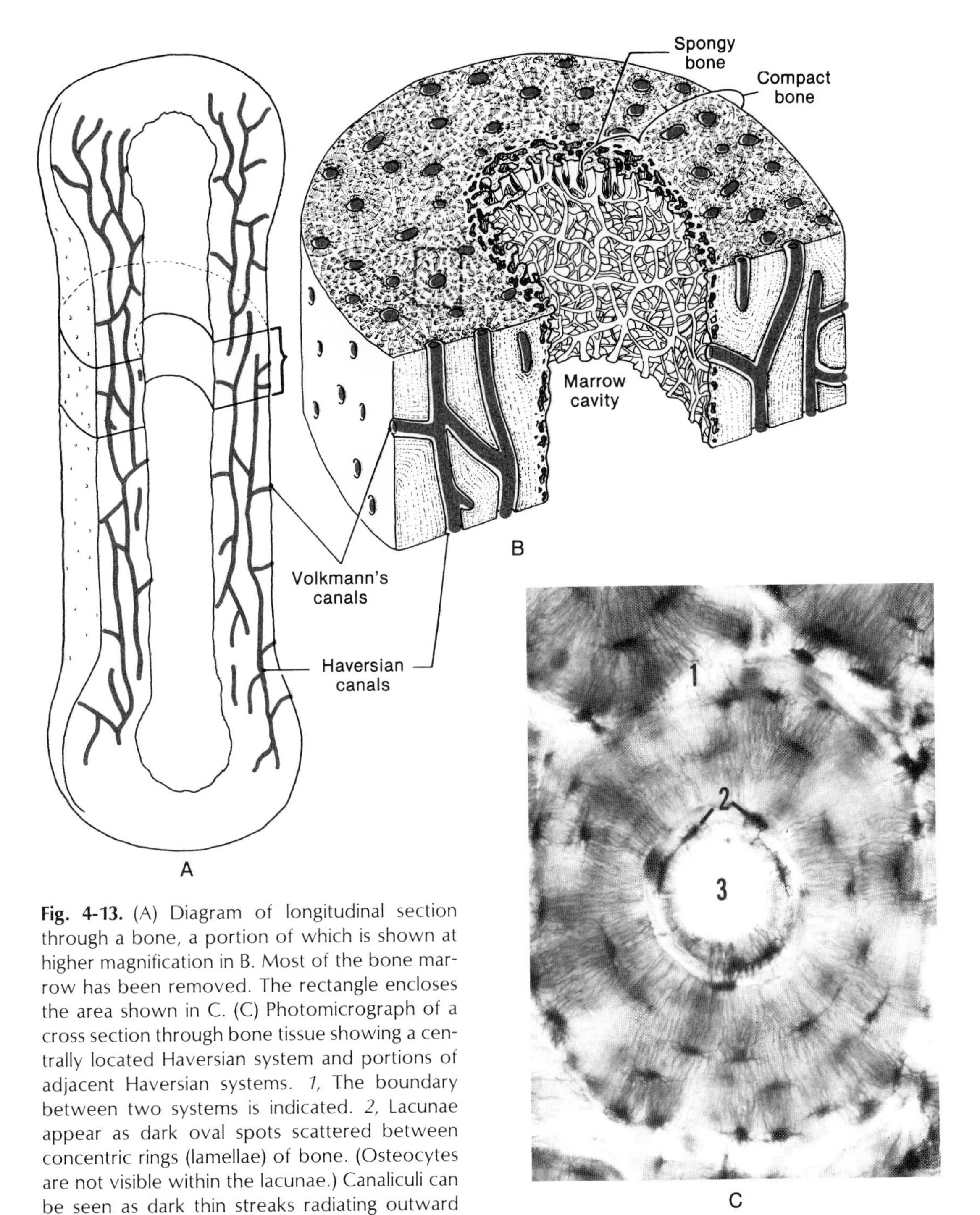

Fig. 4-13. (A) Diagram of longitudinal section through a bone, a portion of which is shown at higher magnification in B. Most of the bone marrow has been removed. The rectangle encloses the area shown in C. (C) Photomicrograph of a cross section through bone tissue showing a centrally located Haversian system and portions of adjacent Haversian systems. *1,* The boundary between two systems is indicated. *2,* Lacunae appear as dark oval spots scattered between concentric rings (lamellae) of bone. (Osteocytes are not visible within the lacunae.) Canaliculi can be seen as dark thin streaks radiating outward from each lacuna. *3,* The Haversian canal is centrally located. (From *Histology: A Text and Atlas* by Johannes A. G. Rhodin. Copyright © 1976 by Johannes A. G. Rhodin. Reprinted by permission of the author and Oxford University Press, Inc.)

as with the network of tiny canaliculi. Although the canaliculi are too small to permit the passage of blood vessels and nerves, substances can diffuse back and forth between the vessels and canalicular fluid, which in turn nourishes the osteocytes via their cytoplasmic projections. In cross-section a Haversian canal and its concentric lamellae are termed a **Haversian system** (**osteon**) (Fig. 4-13C). A further discussion of the structure, function, and development of bones is presented in Chapter 7: The Skeletal System.

Blood

Blood is a special type of connective tissue in which the formed elements (cells and fragments of cells) are suspended in a fluid intercellular material called **plasma**. The blood brings nutrients and oxygen to the body tissues and carries away metabolic wastes. It also transports special cell products such as hormones from one region of the body to another. Although the blood is confined within larger blood vessels, certain blood cells and constituents of the plasma can migrate out from the smaller blood vessels (capillaries) into the surrounding connective tissues. This serves a useful purpose in bringing defense elements to the sites of infection.

Formed Elements of the Blood

The blood cells are subdivided into two groups: red blood cells (erythrocytes) and white blood cells (leukocytes). In addition there are small fragments of cells, the blood platelets (Fig. 4-14).

Mature **red blood cells** are small in size (about 8 μm in diameter) and lack nuclei. They contain the protein hemoglobin which is important in carrying oxygen to the tissues. Red blood cells normally do not leave the blood vessels.

White blood cells are variable in size and contain nuclei. They are capable of migrating out through the walls of capillaries and are an important line of defense against infections.

The most numerous type of white cell is the **neutrophil,** whereas **eosinophils** and **basophils** are less common. These three types are often grouped together as **granulocytes** because of the tiny granules in their cytoplasm. In contrast, **agranulocytes** lack granules and consist of two cell types: monocytes and lymphocytes. **Monocytes** are large white blood cells capable of transforming into phagocytes. **Lymphocytes** are smaller and are related to plasma cells in that they are involved in immunological reactions. The total number of white blood cells as well as the percentage of each cell type are important indicators of whether an infection is present or not. A normal percentage of the total white cells, as determined by a differential count, would be:

Neutrophils	60–70%
Eosinophils	2–4%
Basophils	0.5–1%
Monocytes	3–8%
Lymphocytes	20–25%

Platelets are fragments of cells which are derived from giant cells (**megakaryocytes**) located in the bone marrow. They are important in causing blood to clot in the event a blood vessel is injured.

Blood Plasma

The blood plasma is composed of fluid in which a variety of substances is dissolved or suspended, including protein (globulin and albumins), salts, carbohydrates, fats, and urea. Blood plasma carries waste products and hormones. When it clots, certain of its proteins precipitate and form **fibrin.** The remaining fluid is then called **serum.**

Blood Formation and Destruction

Blood cells are produced by a process termed **hemopoiesis.** Red blood cells and granulocytes (neutrophils, eosinophils, and basophils) are formed in the bone marrow (myeloid tissue); agranulocytes (lymphocytes and monocytes) are produced mainly in lymphatic organs. Aged blood cells are destroyed by phagocytosis primarily in the spleen, although some white blood cells are also removed from the circulation at other sites such as the liver. A

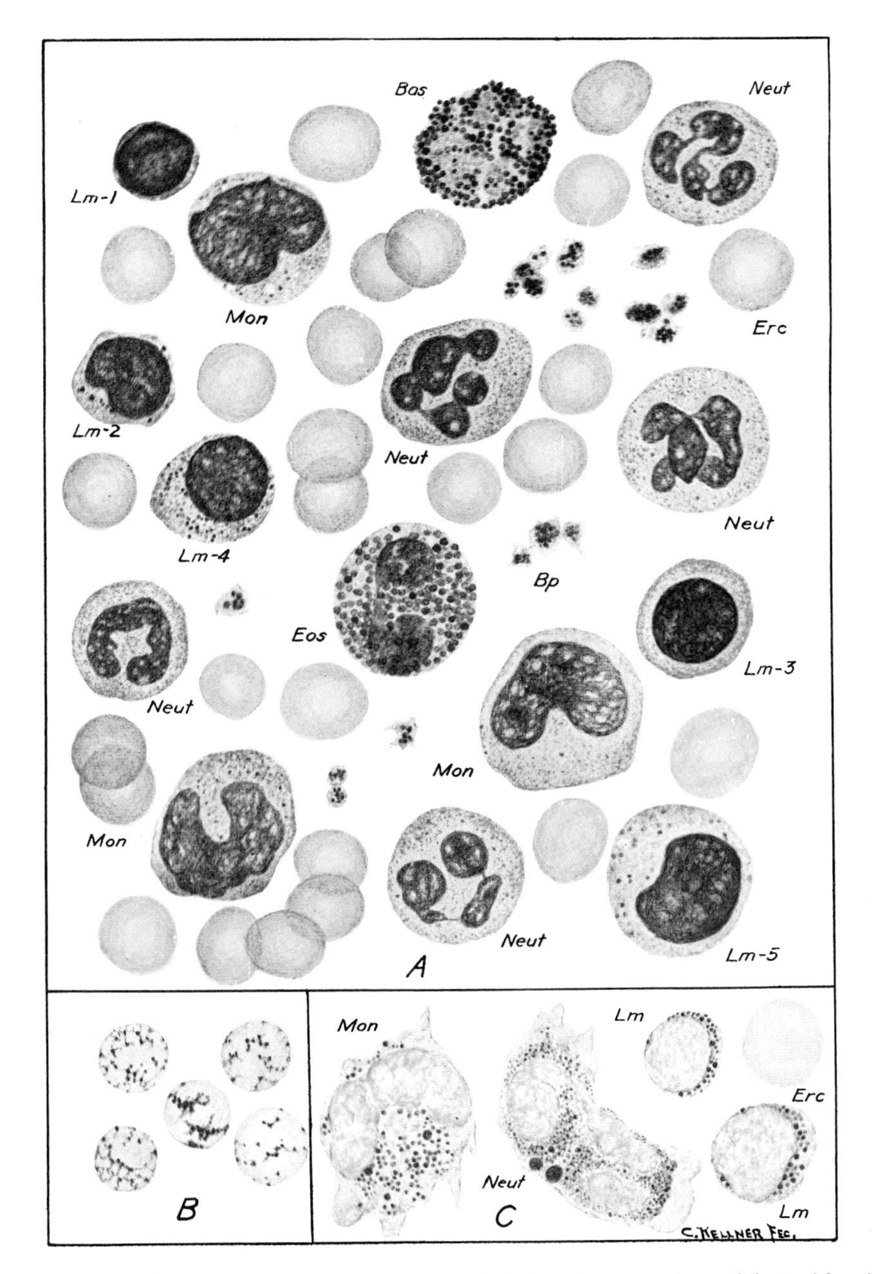

Fig. 4-14. (A) various cell types in normal human blood. Wright's stain. *Bas,* basophil; *Bp,* blood platelets, *Eos,* eosinophil; *Erc,* erythrocytes; *Lm*-1–5, lymphocytes; *Mon,* monocytes; *Neut,* neutrophils. (B,C) appearance of blood cells after use of special stains. In (B) the cells are immature red blood cells. (From W. M. Copenhaver, R. P. Bunge, and M. B. Bunge, *Bailey's Textbook of Histology,* Ed. 16, The Williams & Wilkins Co., Baltimore, 1971.)

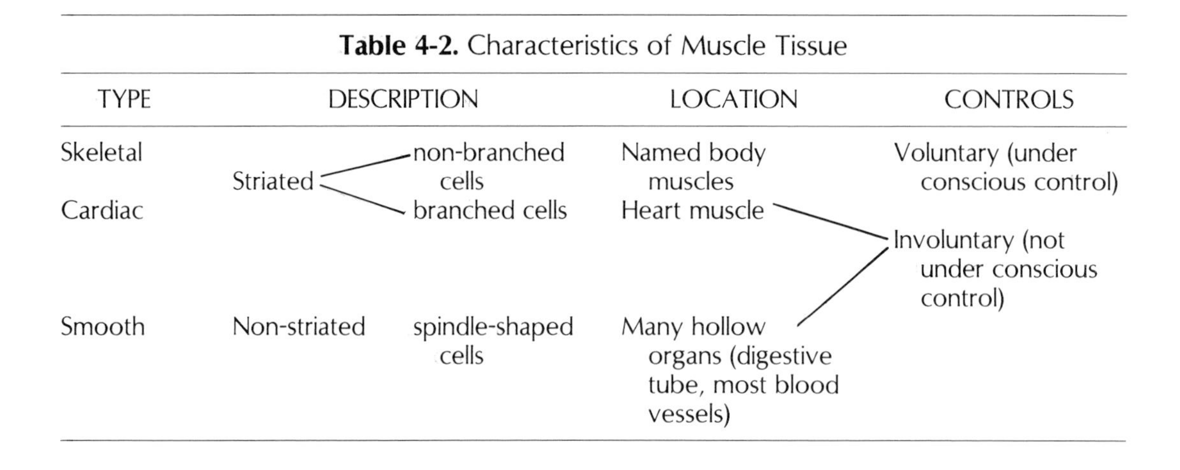

Table 4-2. Characteristics of Muscle Tissue

TYPE	DESCRIPTION		LOCATION	CONTROLS
Skeletal	Striated	non-branched cells	Named body muscles	Voluntary (under conscious control)
Cardiac		branched cells	Heart muscle	Involuntary (not under conscious control)
Smooth	Non-striated	spindle-shaped cells	Many hollow organs (digestive tube, most blood vessels)	

fine balance exists between blood formation and destruction. For example, anemia is characterized by a decrease in the number of red blood cells or in the amount of hemoglobin which they carry. This condition can result from a variety of factors including a deficiency in red blood cell production, hemorrhage, overly active red blood cell destruction, or a lack of sufficient iron to produce hemoglobin. An imbalance in blood cell formation can also be harmful, as in the case of leukemia, where there is an overproduction of white blood cells at the expense of red cells.

Lymph

Lymph may be classified as a connective tissue in which the majority of cells are lymphocytes suspended in the fluid **lymph plasma.** A small number of granulocytes are present in lymph, but red blood cells are lacking. Lymph is carried in lymph vessels which absorb tissue fluid from the extracellular spaces. The composition and function of lymph is further dealt with in Chapter 10: The Lymphatic System.

Reticuloendothelial "System"

Phagocytic cells are extensively distributed throughout the body and are often grouped together as the reticuloendothelial system. These cells include reticular cells in the lymphatic system and in the liver (where they are called Kupffer cells), macrophages in the bone marrow and in the loose connective tissue, and monocytes which migrate from the blood into the connective tissue.

MUSCLE TISSUE

Muscle tissue is highly specialized for contraction and also provides bulk to the frame of the body. It interacts with nervous, epithelial, and connective tissues to move materials within the body, to hold body parts in place, to move body parts in relation to each other, and to move the body from place to place. The biochemical reactions which take place when a muscle contracts produce heat as a by-product, thus helping to maintain body temperature. Three different types of muscle tissue are found in humans: skeletal, cardiac, and smooth. Table 4-2 outlines some of their major features.

The basic cellular unit of all three types of muscle is the **muscle fiber.** A muscle fiber is a cell containing many of the organelles found in other cells. However, the cytoplasm of a muscle cell is sometimes called **sarcoplasm,** and the plasma membrane may be called the **sarcolemma.**

Skeletal Muscle

A skeletal muscle is composed of elongated **fibers** (cells) (Fig. 4-15), some of which may extend the whole length of the muscle. A connective tissue covering on the outside of the entire muscle is called the **epimysium,** which sends connective tissue partitions, the **perimysium,** inward to surround bundles of muscle fibers called **fasciculi** (Fig. 4-16). The perimysium in turn sends delicate connective tissue strands inward to surround each muscle fiber as the **endomysium.** The epimysium, perimysium, and endomysium provide a pathway along which blood vessels and nerves are carried inward from the outside of the muscle.

Skeletal muscle fibers may be more than 30 cm long and 10–60 μm in diameter. Although the sarcolemma (plasma membrane) of each muscle fiber is covered externally by a basement membrane and connective tissue fibers, the light microscope cannot resolve these structures, but instead shows the whole area as a dark staining line. In the sarcoplasm just beneath the sarcolemma there are numerous oval nuclei (Fig. 4-15). Some muscle fibers may contain thousands of nuclei.

A dominant feature of a skeletal muscle fiber when viewed with the light microscope is the series of alternating light and dark bands which run perpendicular to the length of the fiber (Fig. 4-15). Skeletal muscle is thus designated as striated. It is also called voluntary muscle because it is under voluntary control.

When viewed with the electron microscope the sarcoplasm (cytoplasm) of a skeletal muscle fiber shows numerous densely packed **myofibrils,** each about 1 μm in diameter, running the length of the fiber (Fig. 4-16). Between the myofibrils are many mitochondria for energy production, ribosomes for synthesis of new proteins, granules containing carbohydrates and lipids, a Golgi complex, lysosomes, plus various other organelles and inclusions.

Each myofibril contains alternating **light** (**I**) and **dark** (**A**) bands, and it is the alignment of these bands with those of adjacent myofibrils which gives the characteristic striated appearance to the fiber when viewed with the light

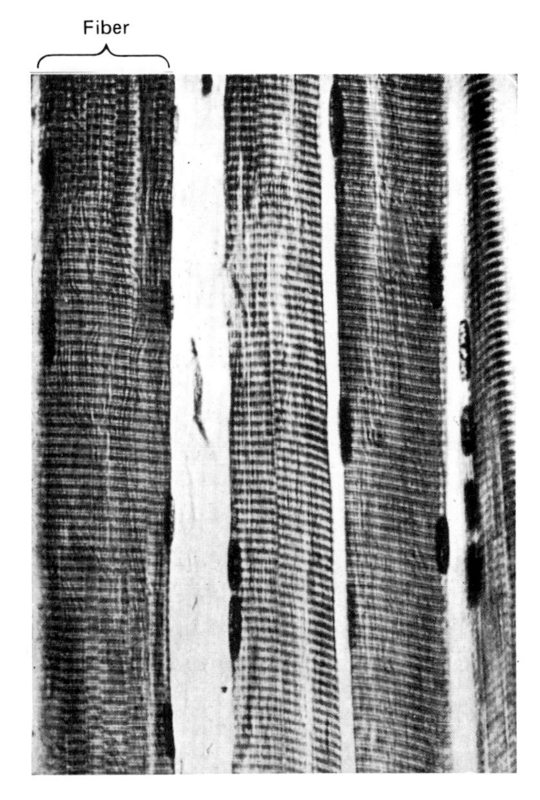

Fig. 4-15. Skeletal muscle as seen with the light microscope. (From W. M. Copenhaver, R. P. Bunge, and M. B. Bunge, *Bailey's Textbook of Histology,* Ed. 16, The Williams & Williams Co., Baltimore, 1971.)

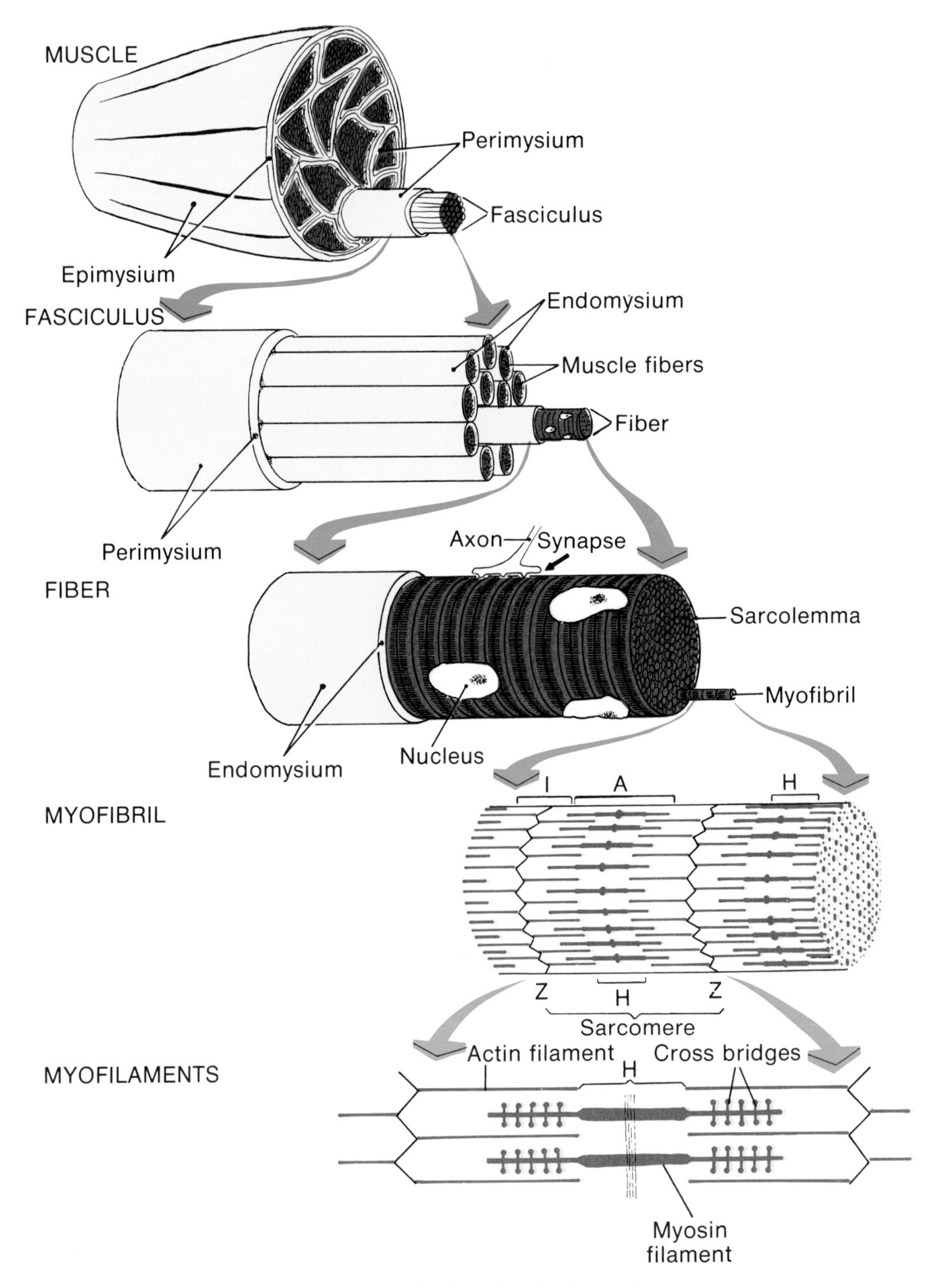

Fig. 4-16. Organization of skeletal muscle.

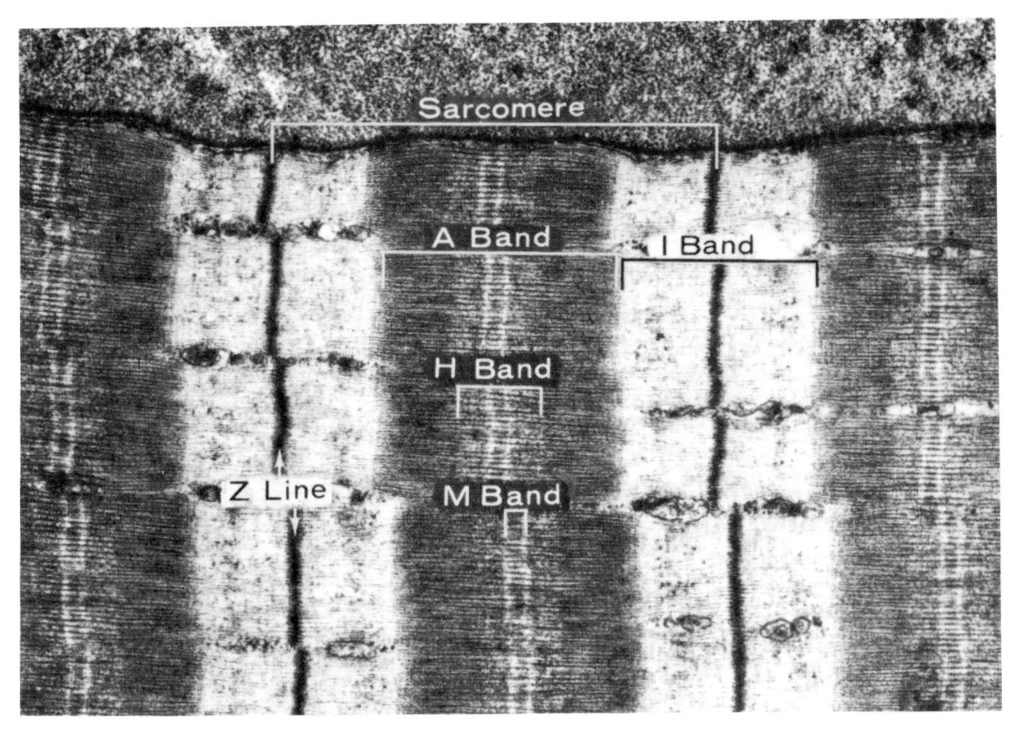

Fig.4-17. Electron micrograph of skeletal muscle showing five myofibrils cut longitudinally (From W. Bloom and D. W. Fawcett, *A Textbook of Histology,* Ed. 10, W. B. Saunders Co., Philadelphia, 1975.)

microscope. The electron microscope shows quite distinctly that each I band is transected by a dark area called the **Z band,** whereas each A band has a lighter staining area within it called an **H band** (Figs. 4-16 and 4-17). (Each H band in turn shows a dark streak termed an **M band.**)

The region of the fiber between two Z bands is called a **sarcomere** and is a functional unit of contraction. In the resting fiber the sarcomere is about 2.5-3 μm in length and includes the A band with one-half of an I band on each side of it. As the fiber contracts the sarcomere shortens to about 2 μm and the I and H bands shorten and then disappear, while the A band remains unchanged in length and abuts against the two Z bands.

Each myofibril contains hundreds of **myofilaments,** of which there are two sizes. The larger filaments are composed of molecules of the protein **myosin**. The smaller filaments are composed mostly of molecules of the protein **actin.** It is the arrangement of the myosin and actin filaments which produces the various bands described above. The A band consists of myosin and actin filaments, except for the region of the H band, where only myosin filaments are present. The region of the A band containing myosin and actin filaments is also called the **cross bridge** area since it is the site where the filaments interact and where many of the biochemical reactions necessary for muscle contraction occur. The I band is composed solely of actin filaments, which are attached to the Z band.

When a nerve impulse arrives at the end of a nerve fiber the impulse is chemically transmitted across a narrow space to the sarco-

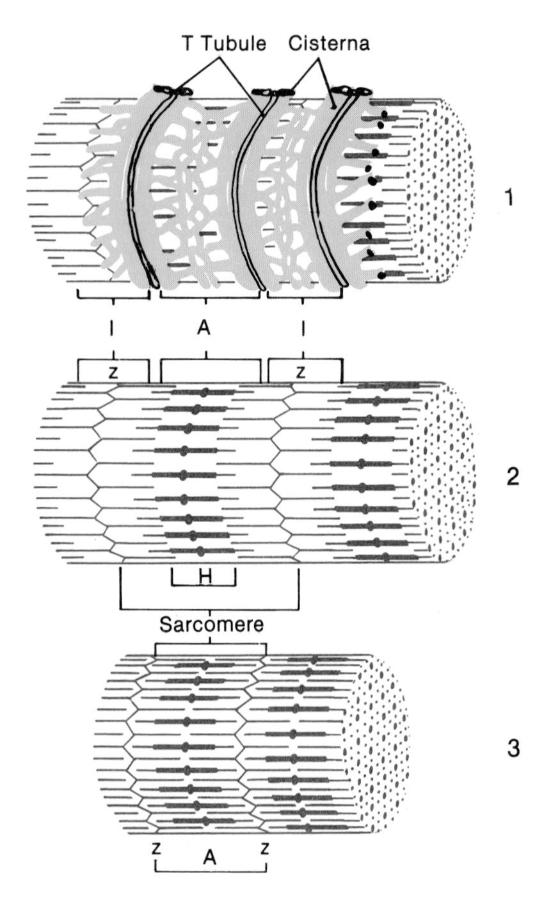

Fig. 4-18. *1,* A myofibril showing triads at the junction of the A-I bands. Each triad consists of a T tubule lying between two cisternae. *2,* The triads have been removed. Note the sarcomere. *3,* When contraction occurs, the sarcomere shortens as the microfilaments slide over each other.

lemma of a muscle fiber. The impulse travels along the sarcolemma and inward into the muscle fiber along invaginations of the sarcolemma called **T tubules** (Fig. 4-18). (The T tubules are located at the junctions between the A and I bands and are flanked by cisternae of the endoplasmic reticulum, thus forming a triad.) The impulse in the T tubules causes a release of calcium ions (Ca^{++}), and this is thought to activate the enzyme **ATPase** which in turn acts on **ATP** from the mitochondria in order to release the energy necessary for contraction. Contraction occurs when the actin filaments slide between the myosin filaments (Fig. 4-18).

When a muscle atrophies, there is initially a progressive loss of myofilaments (actin and myosin) followed by reduction and resorption of sarcoplasm, and finally a replacement of the muscle fibers by connective tissue. The severity of **muscle atrophy** depends on the degree to which the process occurs. There are many causes for muscular atrophy, such as old age, disuse, malnutrition, and disease.

Genetic diseases such as **muscular dystrophy** affect the very young as well as some adults by acting directly on skeletal muscle fibers and causing them to atrophy. Diseases such as poliomyelitis and many injuries which affect the nervous system act indirectly on the muscle fibers by preventing them from contracting and thus causing them to atrophy through disuse. However, a certain amount of this atrophy can be prevented with physical therapy by which the muscles are moved passively.

Development of Skeletal Muscle

Adult skeletal muscle fibers are derived from mesenchyme cells of the embryo. The mesenchyme cells become spindle shaped, begin to synthesize myofilaments around a central nucleus, and are thus transformed into **myoblasts.** The myofilaments aggregate into bundles called myofibrils with striations typical of the adult fiber. The myoblasts then fuse end to end, lose their adjoining cell membranes, and form the multinucleated adult muscle

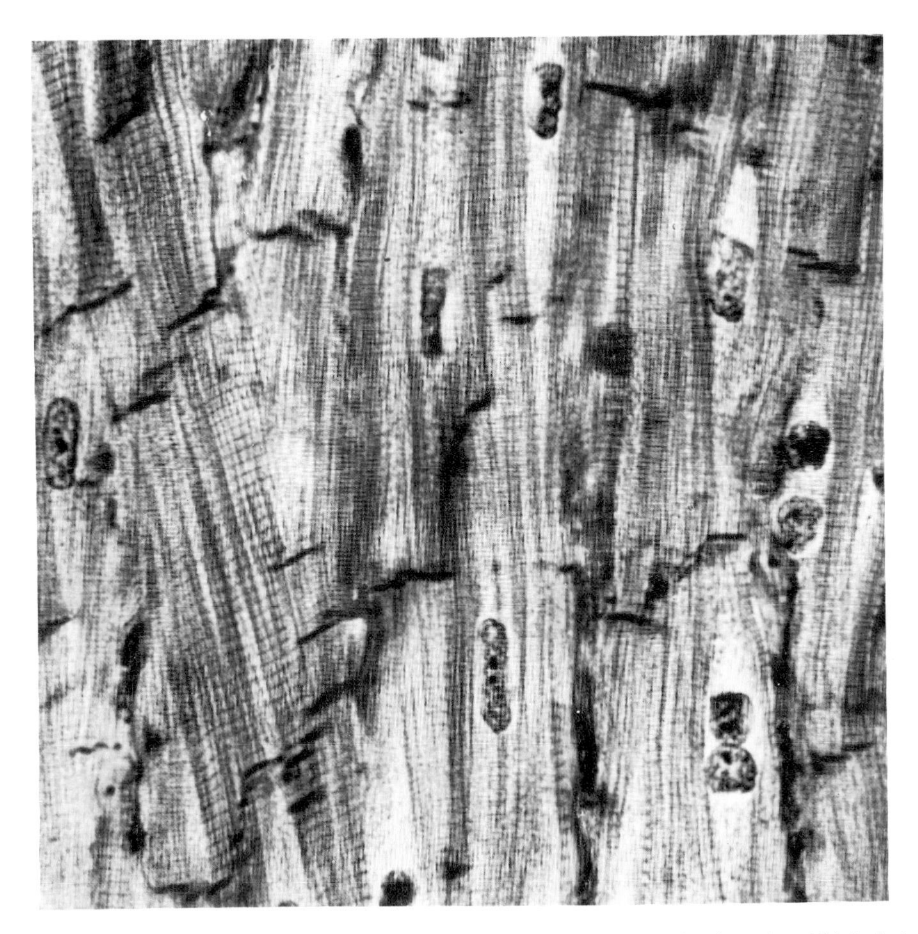

Fig. 4-19. Cardiac muscle fibers as seen with the light microscope, longitudinal section. Thick dark streaks across the fibers are intercalated discs. (From W. M. Copenhaver, R. P. Bunge, and M. B. Bunge, *Bailey's Textbook of Histology,* Ed. 16, The Williams & Wilkins Co., Baltimore, 1971.)

fiber. The final number of fibers is reached sometime before birth, although increase in fiber length and fiber diameter continues into adult life. Skeletal muscle is capable of limited regeneration, but if damage to the area is severe, connective tissue replaces the damaged muscle fibers.

Cardiac Muscle

Cardiac muscle is composed of striated fibers (cells) each of which has one centrally located nucleus. These fibers are about 75 μm in length and about 15 μm in diameter, and the light microscope shows them arranged as a network of branched fibers. At the ends of the cells the sarcolemmas from two adjacent fibers are thickened and appear together as a dark streak called an **intercalated disc** (Fig. 4-19). Connective tissue with blood vessels and nerves is found in the spaces between the cardiac cells.

The striations in cardiac muscle fibers are identical to those seen in skeletal muscle with A, I, H, and Z bands present. In cardiac muscle the pattern of actin and myosin myofilaments is also the same as in skeletal muscle; however, myofibrils are less distinct and may be branched. Mitochondria are numerous and indicative of the relatively high metabolic activity of cardiac muscle tissue. T tubules are pres-

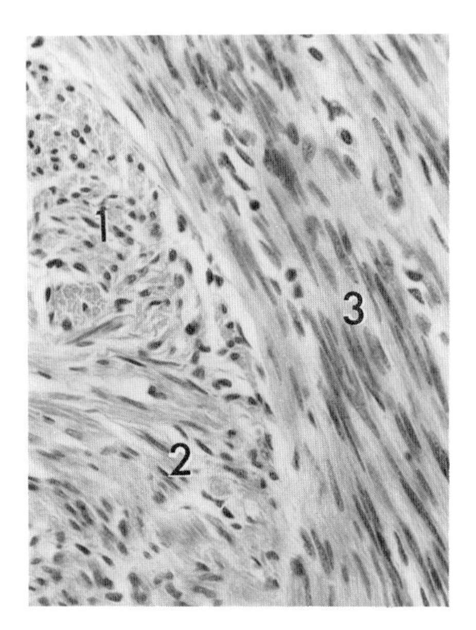

Fig. 4-20. Smooth muscle as seen with the light microscope and cut in three different planes: *1*, cross sectioned; *2*, obliquely sectioned; and *3*, longitudinally sectioned. (From *Histology: A Text and Atlas* by Johannes A. G. Rhodin. Copyright © 1976 by Johannes A. G. Rhodin. Reprinted by permission of the author and Oxford University Press, Inc.)

ent but occur at the Z band regions rather than at the A-I junctions typical of skeletal muscle. In the region of the intercalated disc the cell membranes adhere closely to one another and not only prevent the cells from pulling apart but also permit electrical impulses to flow easily from one cell to another. For this reason, the heart behaves physiologically as if it were composed of one highly specialized multinucleate cell without end cell membranes. Contraction of cardiac muscle fibers is involuntary, i.e., it is not under conscious control.

Some cardiac muscle cells are specialized for conducting contraction impulses. Those which are of large diameter and contain fewer myofibrils are termed **Purkinje fibers.**

Development of Cardiac Muscle

Cardiac muscle cells are derived from mesenchyme cells of the embryo. The cells are initially star-shaped and then begin to stick to each other at the sites of future intercalated discs. Cells continue to divide, clump together, and eventually develop myofilaments, at which time the cells are known as myoblasts. Cell division continues after birth, but gradually ceases shortly thereafter. Increase in cell size continues into adolescence and young adulthood, and is responsive to increases in the work load of the heart. If the blood vessels supplying oxygen and nutrients to cardiac muscle cells are blocked, the cells will die. Connective tissue then replaces these cells and forms scar tissue. Regeneration of heart muscle does not occur in the adult human.

Smooth Muscle

Smooth muscle tissue is composed of nonstriated, spindle-shaped cells, each of which contains a single nucleus (Fig. 4-20). The cells vary in size from about 15 μm (as in the smooth muscle of a small blood vessel) to over 500 μm (as in the uterus in a pregnant woman). Smooth muscle cells are often found in small tightly packed bundles (fasciculi), between which is some loose connective tissue carrying blood vessels and nerves. Within each fasciculus the muscle cells are separated from one another by basement membranes, fine connective tissue fibers, and varying numbers of nerve endings, although many cells have regions where their plasma membranes are in intimate contact. Here, electrical impulses probably pass freely from cell to cell, much as occurs at the intercalated discs of cardiac muscle.

In smooth muscle cells the single nuclei are elongate or ovoid and are centrally placed. Along with the nucleus, the organelles such as mitochondria, endoplasmic reticulum, and lysosomes are oriented parallel to the long axis of the cell. Smooth muscle cells lack myofibrils and their characteristic striations, but many small filaments composed of the protein actin are oriented in the long direction of the cell. The thicker filaments of myosin characteristic of striated muscle cells are not as readily apparent, although more or less equal amounts of actin and myosin can be demonstrated in the cytoplasm of smooth muscle cells using biochemical techniques.

Smooth muscle cells are found in many regions of the body, including the walls of the digestive tract, and in many blood vessels (where the smooth muscle may cause constriction and thus regulate blood pressure). Smooth muscle cells also occur in the ducts of glands, and in hollow organs in the urinary and reproductive systems. They are also found in the iris of the eye where they regulate the size of the pupil, and in the skin as the **arrector pili** muscles which pull at the hair follicles to produce the familiar "goose bumps."

Development of Smooth Muscle

Smooth muscle cells are formed from primitive mesenchyme cells in the embryo. As the protein molecules actin and myosin are synthesized, the mesenchyme cells become transformed into spindle-shaped myoblast cells and eventually into mature smooth muscle cells. Adult cells are able to undergo limited mitosis in order to repair torn or diseased smooth muscle tissue.

NERVOUS TISSUE

Nervous tissue is important in providing a rapid means of communication among different parts of the body and in enabling an individual to be in touch with and respond to the environment. There are basically two categories of nervous tissue: (1) **neurons,** which transmit nerve impulses and (2) **supporting cells,** which do not transmit impulses but which assist and provide sustenance for the neurons.

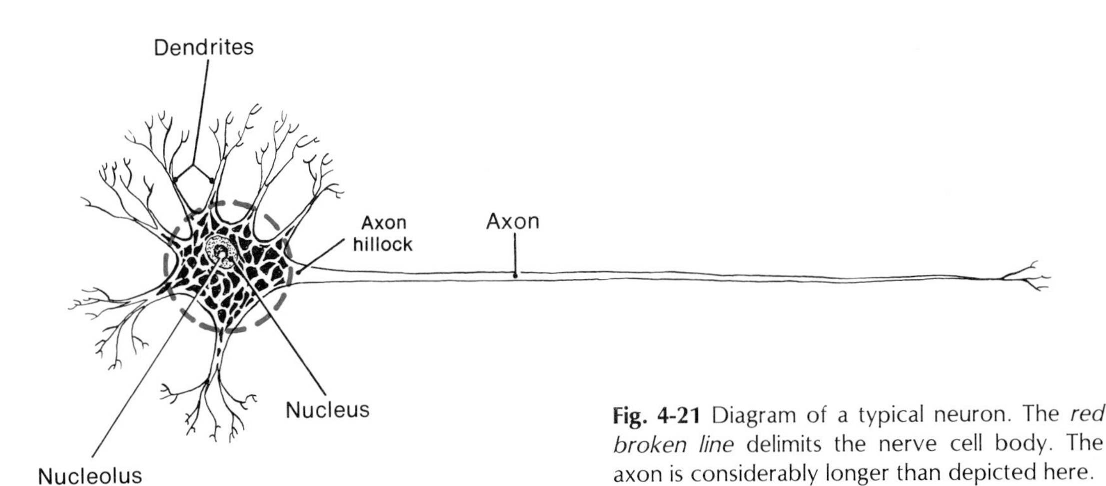

Fig. 4-21 Diagram of a typical neuron. The *red broken line* delimits the nerve cell body. The axon is considerably longer than depicted here.

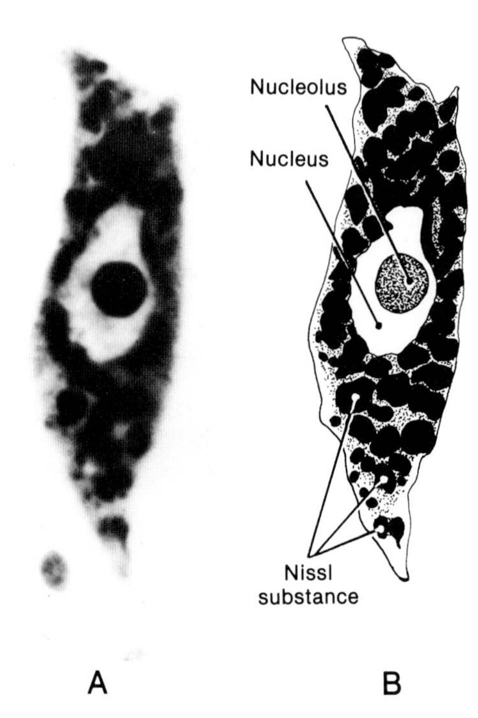

Fig. 4-22. (A) A neuron stained to show the Nissl substance. (From E. D. Gardner, *Fundamentals of Neurology,* Ed. 6, W. B. Saunders Co., Philadelphia, 1975.) (B) Sketch of neuron shown in A.

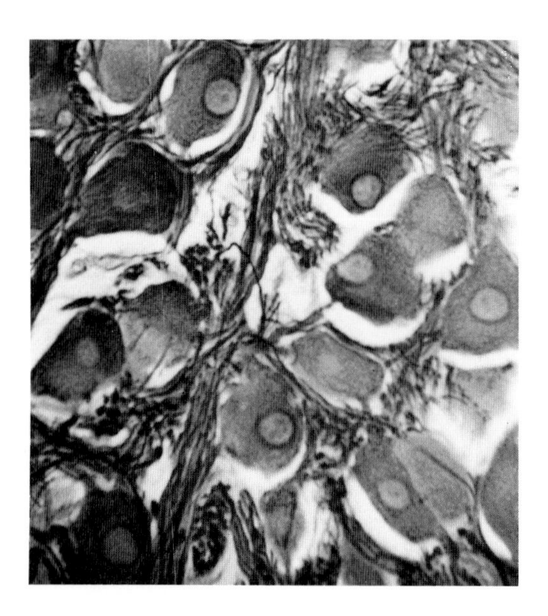

Fig. 4-23. Microscopic section of a ganglion showing groups of nerve cell bodies. (Courtesy of Dr. Hadley Kirkman, Stanford University.)

Neuron

A neuron consists of a nerve cell body and protoplasmic extensions called processes (Fig. 4-21). The lightly staining nucleus of the nerve cell body contains a dark prominent nucleolus. The cytoplasm exhibits a variety of organelles, including mitochondria, a Golgi complex, lysosomes, microtubules, microfilaments, and a highly developed endoplasmic reticulum with ribosomes (granular ER). The latter appears in the light microscope as clumps of darkly stained material called **Nissl substance** (Figs. 4-21 and 4-22).

The numerous short processes which extend out a short distance from the nerve cell body are termed **dendrites** and contain the same organelles as those found in the cytoplasm of the cell body. Most neurons also have a longer process, the **axon,** which extends for a considerable distance and which lacks Nissl substance. (The point at which the axon originates from the cell body is termed the **axon hillock.**)

The axon is maintained by materials produced in the nerve cell body. If an axon is severed, the distal portion will degenerate, whereas the proximal portion survives. Axons and their sheath-like coverings together are often called **fibers.**

Clusters of nerve cell bodies outside of the brain and spinal cord are termed **ganglia** (singular: ganglion) (Fig. 4-23), and bundles of fibers are called **nerves.** Within the brain and spinal cord clusters of nerve cell bodies are designated as **nuclei,** and the bundles of fibers as **tracts.**

Most neurons have numerous processes and are thus lableled **multipolar** neurons (Fig. 4-24). Those with two processes are the relatively rare **bipolar** neurons such as those in the retina of the eye. **Unipolar** neurons occur in the spinal ganglia and are characterized by having only one process which divides into two branches a short distance from the nerve cell body.

Supporting Cells

The non-neuronal supporting cells in the brain and spinal cord are termed **neuroglia** ("nerve glue"). These are classified as astrocytes, oligodendrocytes, microglia, and ependyma.

Astrocytes are star-shaped cells which are designated as **protoplasmic astrocytes** if they have numerous branched short processes, and **fibrous astrocytes** if they have a few long processes. Since these processes often end on the walls of blood vessels as perivascular "feet," it is possible that these cells mediate the exchange of substances between blood vessels and neurons (Fig. 4-25).

Oligodendrocytes are very small cells with a few processes which may also form perivascular "feet." Some of these cells are situated around nerve cell bodies of neurons, in which case they are called **satellite cells.** Others become elaborately wrapped around the long processes of neurons and serve as an insulator for them.

Microglia are small dense cells which often cluster near blood vessels. Microglia play a role as phagocytes in the brain and spinal cord and increase in number when nervous tissue is injured in order to get rid of cellular debris.

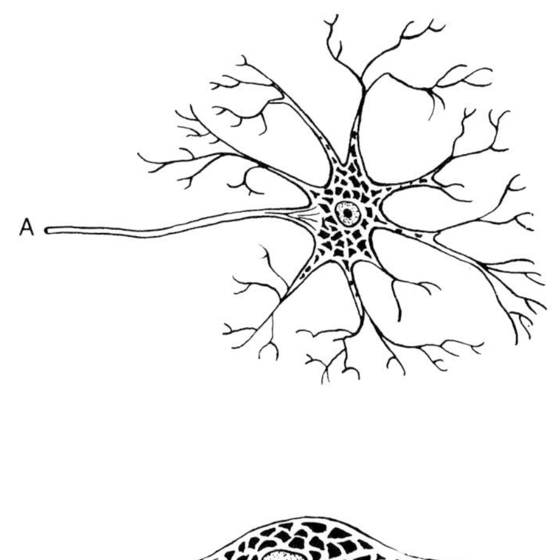

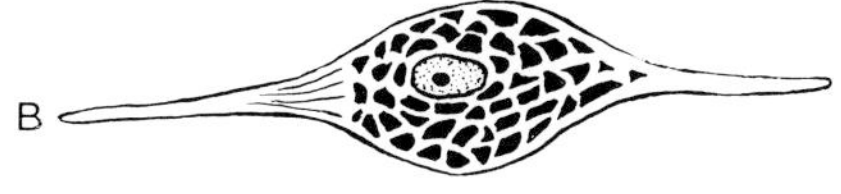

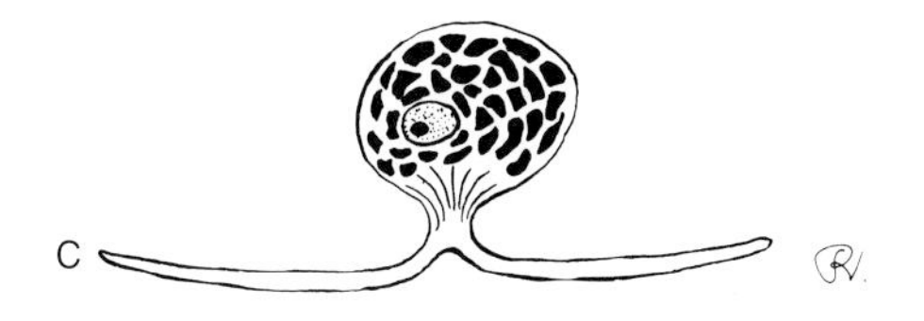

Fig. 4-24. Three types of neurons. (A) Multipolar (most common), (B) bipolar (relatively rare), (C) unipolar (in spinal ganglia).

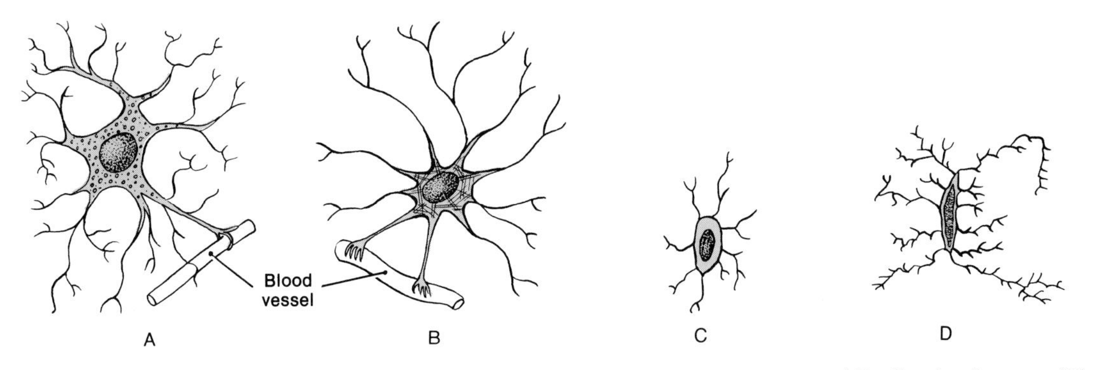

Fig. 4-25. Neuroglial cell types. (A) Protoplasmic astrocyte, (B) fibrous astrocyte, (C) oligodendrocyte, (D) microglial cell. (Modified after Penfield.)

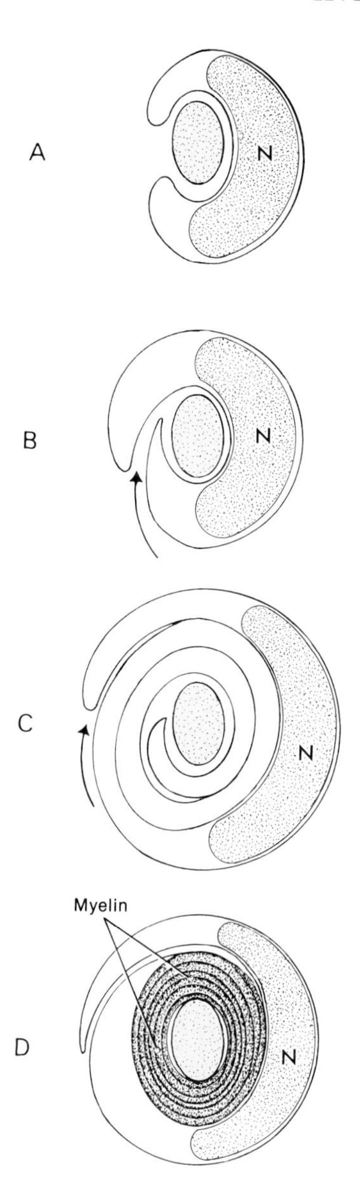

Fig. 4-26. A series of diagrams showing myelin sheath formation. An axon (yellow) is gradually surrounded by compressed plasma membranes of the Schwann cell. N, nucleus of Schwann cell.

The **ependyma** consists of epithelial-like ependymal cells which line cavities in the brain and spinal cord. The cells are low columnar in shape, and some may be ciliated and specialized for secretion.

Outside of the brain and spinal cord the supporting cells in the nervous tissue include satellite and Schwann cells. **Satellite cells** are small cells arranged around nerve cell bodies; **Schwann cells** provide nerve cell axons with a sheath-like covering, the **neurilemma.** Some Schwann cells rotate numerous times around the axons to form layers of plasma membrane (Fig. 4-26). The compressed layers of membranes represent **myelin,** and such fibers are said to be **myelinated** (Fig. 4-27). In contrast, those fibers surrounded by Schwann cells which do not rotate are said to be **unmyelinated.** In myelinated fibers the Schwann cells are situated in a row along the nerve fiber, and each Schwann cell represents a segment of myelin. Between each segment is a small gap called the **node of Ranvier** (Fig. 4-28).

When a nerve fiber (an axon or dendrite) is not transmitting an impulse it is said to be "resting." The inside of a resting fiber has a negative electrical potential relative to that of the outside of the fiber. This **resting potential** results from the fact that the plasma membrane of a resting fiber allows potassium ions to enter freely but actively pumps out sodium ions, thereby maintaining a slightly negative charge inside the fiber. When the fiber is stimulated (chemically, electrically, etc.), the permeability of the membrane briefly changes and allows sodium to pass inward. The inside of the fiber thus becomes positive relative to the outside. This change is known as **depolarization** and occurs as a wave (the **nerve impulse**) along the membrane. **Repolarization** occurs when sodium is once more pumped out and potassium flows in.

The speed of nerve impulses can range from a few meters per second to more than 100 meters per second. Impulses travel more quickly along fibers of large diameter and along those which are myelinated. It is thought

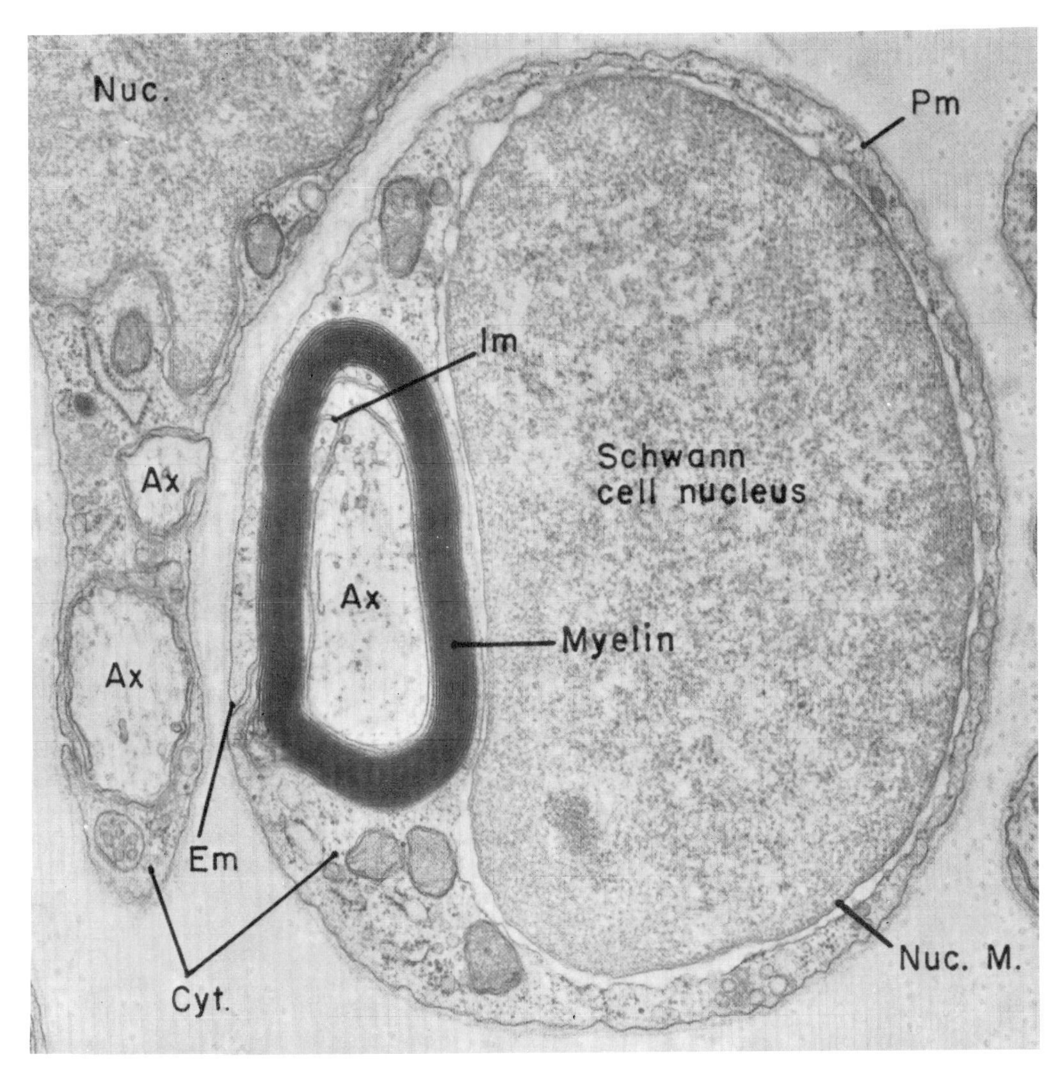

Fig. 4-27. Electron micrograph of a myelinated axon (Ax). Cyt., cytoplasm of Schwann cell; Pm, plasma membrane; Nuc. M., nuclear membrane; Em, external membrane of sheath; Im, internal membrane of sheath. At left are two unmyelinated axons and the nucleus of another Schwann cell *(upper left corner).* (Courtesy of M. B. Bunge and R. P. Bunge, from M. B. Carpenter, *Human Neuroanatomy,* Ed. 7, The Williams & Wilkins Co., Baltimore, 1976.)

that the myelin provides the means whereby the impulse can jump from node to node and thus achieve more speed than can occur along unmyelinated fibers. The vital role of myelin in nerve transmission is illustrated by the fact that demyelinating diseases, such as **multiple sclerosis,** produce severe neurological impairment due to the loss of myelin.

The Synapse

Neurons communicate with one another or with effector organs (muscle cells or gland cells) by means of specialized junctions known as synapses. A synapse may occur between an axon of one neuron and the dendrite or cell body of another. (Occasionally axon to axon

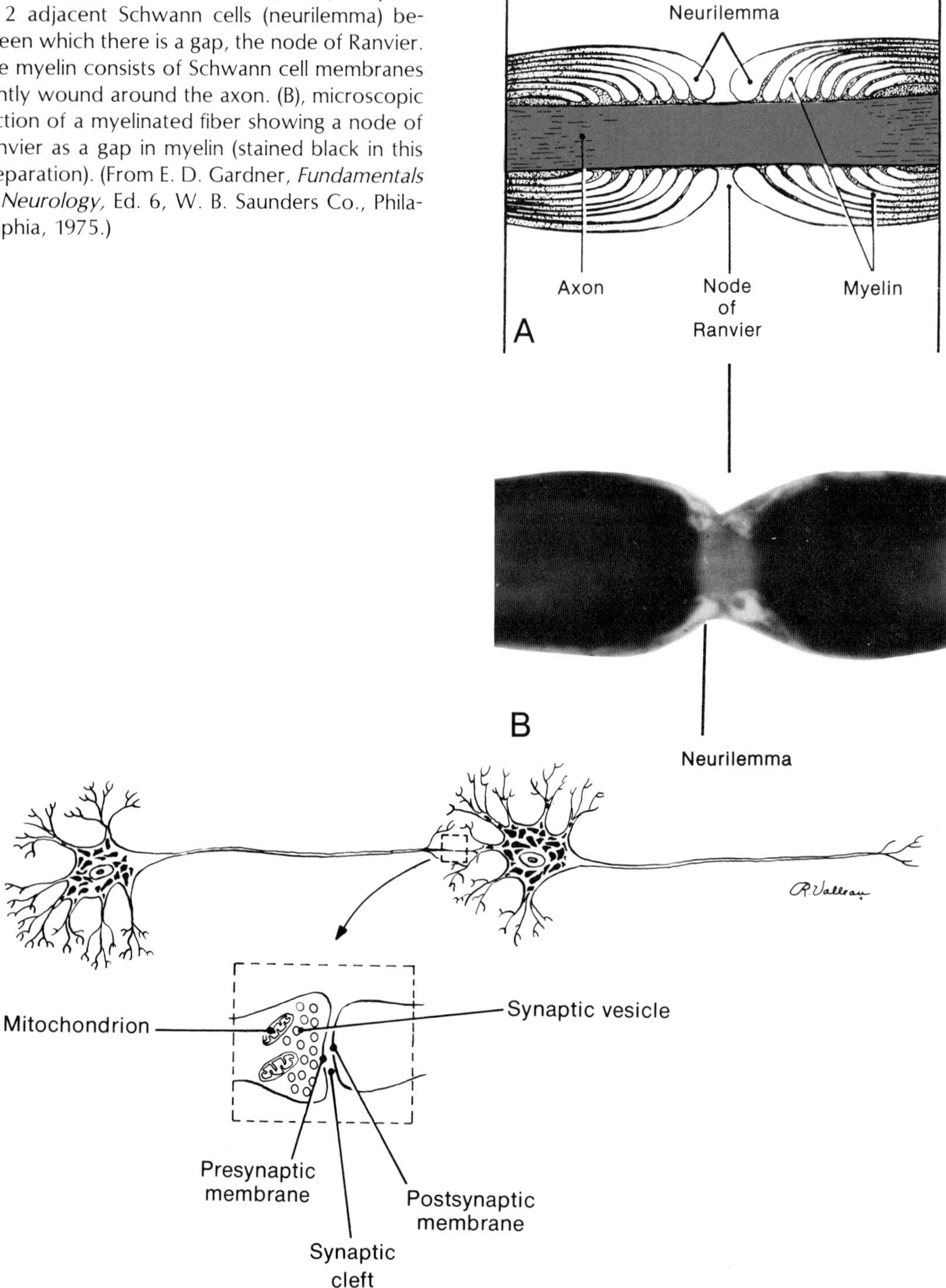

Fig. 4-28. (A), sketch of an axon (in red) and parts of 2 adjacent Schwann cells (neurilemma) between which there is a gap, the node of Ranvier. The myelin consists of Schwann cell membranes tightly wound around the axon. (B), microscopic section of a myelinated fiber showing a node of Ranvier as a gap in myelin (stained black in this preparation). (From E. D. Gardner, *Fundamentals of Neurology*, Ed. 6, W. B. Saunders Co., Philadelphia, 1975.)

Fig. 4-29. Two neurons, with the synaptic area enclosed in the rectangle. The *arrow* points to a higher magnification of the synaptic area.

synapses also occur, particularly at the proximal end of one axon; these synapses are usually inhibitory.) A **neuromuscular (myoneural) junction** occurs between an axon and a muscle cell membrane (sarcolemma), while a **neuroglandular junction** occurs between an axon and a gland cell membrane.

In the region of a synapse the axonal ending is enlarged and the plasma membrane is known as the **presynaptic membrane** (Fig. 4-29). A **synaptic cleft** of about 200–300 Å separates the presynaptic membrane from the **postsynaptic membrane** of the cell which receives the impulse. The end of the axon contains tiny **synaptic vesicles** filled with a chemical termed a **neurotransmitter,** such as acetylcholine, norepinephrine, and serotonin. As a nerve impulse reaches the end of the axon it causes these vesicles to discharge their neurotransmitter substance into the synaptic cleft; thus, synaptic transmission is chemical rather than electrical and is slower than electrical transmission. The neurotransmitter then causes the impulse to be reinitiated in the postsynaptic membrane of the cell receiving the impulse. Synapses are always unidirectional since the neurotransmitter is released only from the synaptic vesicles at the end of the axon, and the neurotransmitter affects only the postsynaptic membrane.

Additional information on the microscopic anatomy and organization of nervous tissue is included in Chapter 12: The Nervous System.

5

Early Embryology

One of the mysteries of life is how a complex multicellular organism such as the human develops from a single cell, the fertilized **egg.** Although much development occurs before birth, especially during the first 2 months of prenatal life, there is also substantial growth and maturation which continue to take place postnatally.

Prior to fertilization the egg develops in the ovary and is surrounded by a gelatinous covering termed the **zona pellucida,** as well as several layers of cells, the innermost of which are the **corona cells.** Just before the egg is released from the ovary a tiny cell (termed the **first polar body**) buds off from the egg and becomes situated between the surface of the egg and the zona pellucida (Fig. 5-1). At the time of ovulation the egg, polar body, zona pellucida, and corona cells are expelled as a unit from the ovary and collected into the nearby portion of the uterine tube (oviduct) where fertilization can take place, provided that sperm are present. The egg most likely is capable of being fertilized only during the first 24–30 hours after ovulation, after which time the unfertilized egg will degenerate and be absorbed. If the egg is fertilized, a second polar body is formed and the egg becomes a **zygote,** which is a diploid cell containing the haploid set of chromosomes from the egg and the haploid set from the sperm. The sperm also provides a pair of centrioles which become involved in the formation of the spindle for the first mitotic division of the zygote.

The zygote divides mitotically into 2 cells (**blastomeres**) about 30 hours after fertilization. The blastomeres divide repeatedly, reaching 8 cells at about 60 hours. Eventually, a ball of cells, the **morula,** is produced (Fig. 5-1). This process of mitotic division is known as **cleavage** and differs from ordinary cell division in that the large zygote becomes subdivided into progressively smaller and smaller cells without any intervening periods of cellular growth.

The morula soon becomes reorganized into an outer layer of **trophoblast cells** surrounding an inner cavity with an eccentrically located cluster of cells termed the **inner cell mass,** most of which will become the embryo proper. The entire structure is now known as a **blastocyst.**

The cleavage and morula stages occur as the developing embryo travels through the uterine tube and finally reaches the uterus approximately 3 days after fertilization. During this time the corona cells detach from the morula and degenerate. The blastocyst forms in the uterus and floats freely in the uterine cavity for a few days. Prior to implantation, the zona pellucida is lost. The blastocyst then adheres to the uterine wall, and the process of implantation begins (Fig. 5-2).

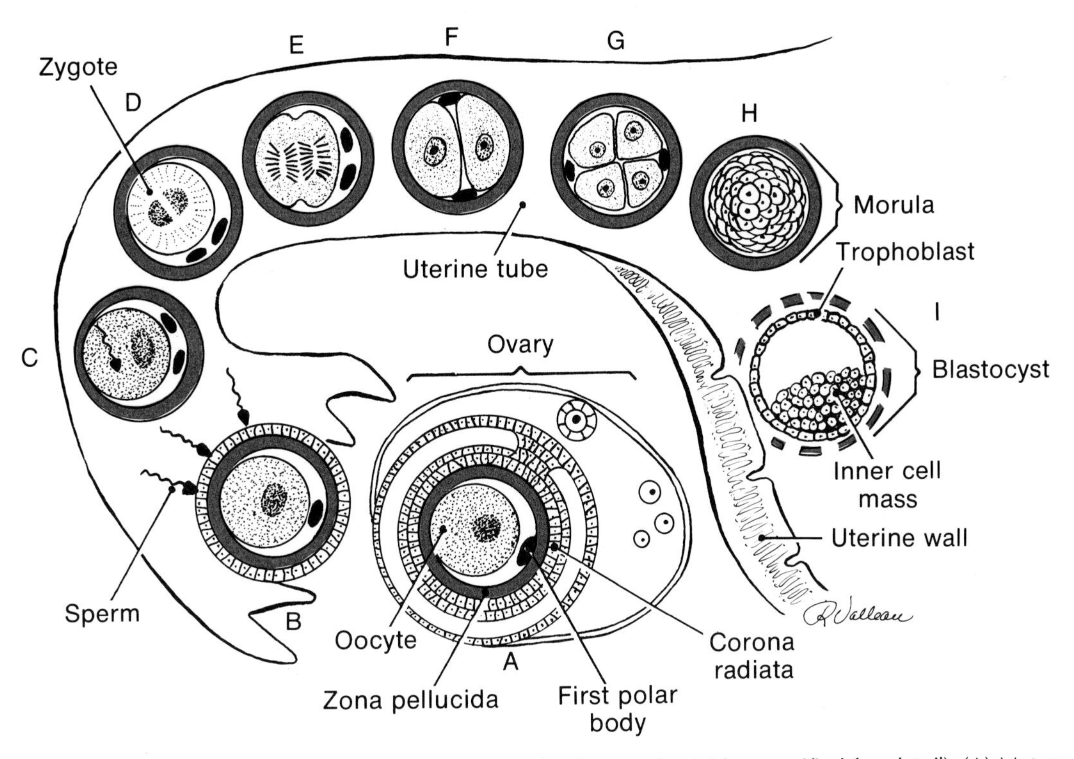

Fig. 5-1. Early development of the human embryo. (Each stage is highly magnified for detail). (A) Mature oocyte with first polar body in ovary, (B) ovulated egg collected into nearby uterine tube and surrounded by sperm, (C, D) fertilization and formation of the zygote, (E, F, G) cleavage, (H) formation of the morula, (I) the blastocyst in the uterus. (Modified after Langman.)

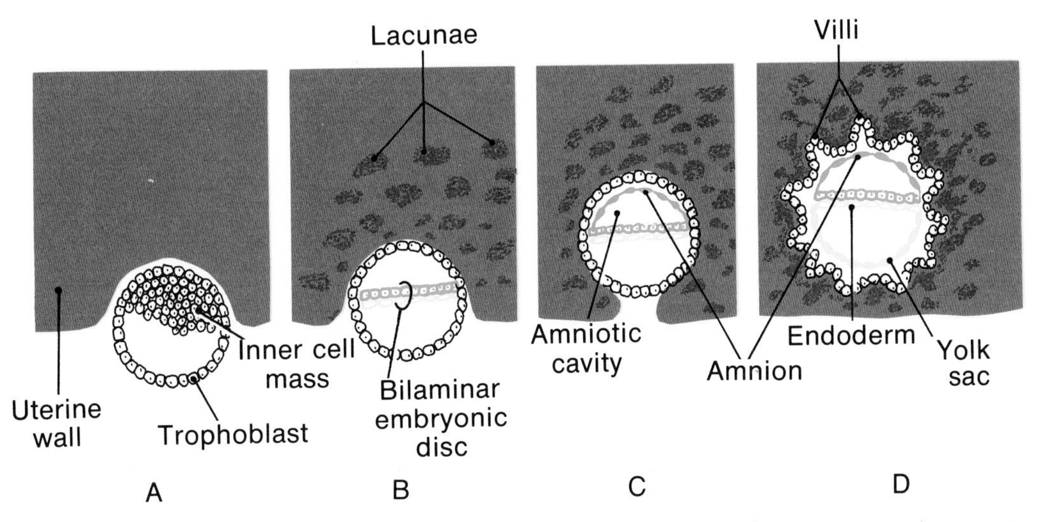

Fig. 5-2. Implantation of the embryo into the wall of the uterus. (A) The blastocyst comes in contact with the lining of the uterus, (B) the inner cell mass becomes organized into a bilaminar embryonic disc. Uterine arteries release blood into lacunae, (C) the amnion forms above the embryonic disc, (D) villi develop from the trophoblast and project into the lacunae, and yolk sac projects downward from the lower layer (endoderm) of the embryonic disc.

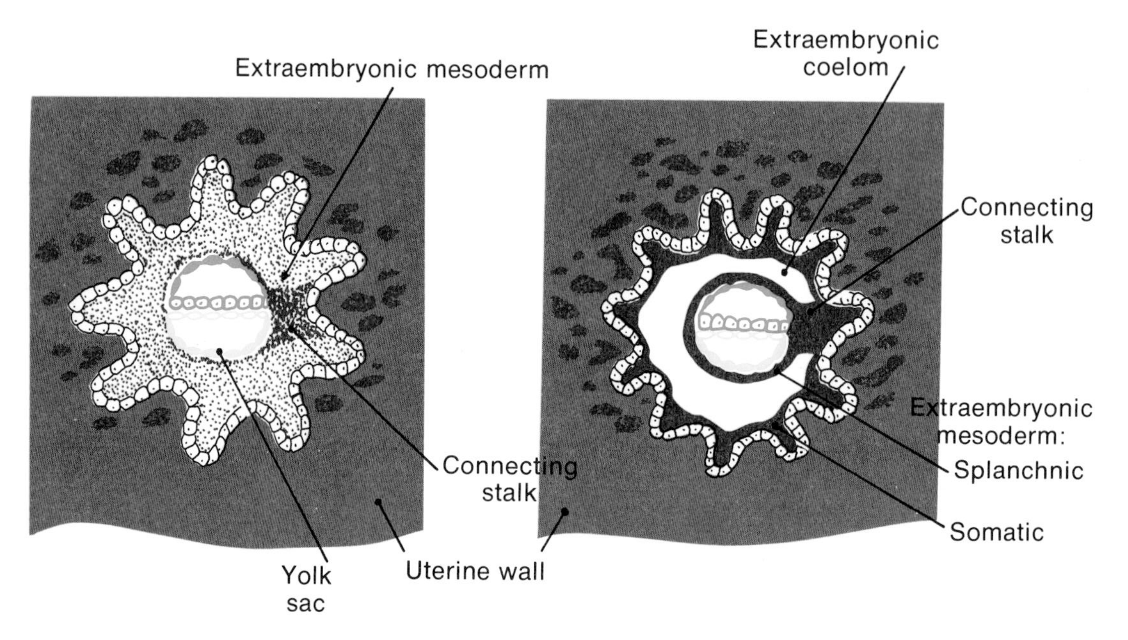

Fig. 5-3. Formation of extraembryonic mesoderm, coelom, and connecting stalk between the 9th and 13th day of gestation. (A) Extraembryonic mesoderm develops between the trophoblast and amnion and yolk sac; (B) extraembryonic mesoderm splits to form somatic and splanchnic layers and the extraembryonic coelom. The connecting stalk attaches the caudal end of the embryo to the trophoblast.

Implantation takes place from the 6th through the 11th day after fertilization and involves the gradual invasion of the blastocyst into the lining of the uterus. During this period the trophoblast cells digest their way into the uterine lining and eventually cause some blood vessels of the uterus to discharge blood into small spaces or **lacunae** between the uterine cells (Fig. 5-2). The trophoblast cells form fingerlike projections **(trophoblastic villi)** which project into these little pools of maternal blood and are thus able to absorb and transport nutrients and oxygen inward to supply deeper cells of the blastocyst.

The inner cell mass also undergoes changes and begins to pull away from the overlying trophoblast cells. The inner cell mass then differentiates into the **bilaminar embryonic disc,** consisting of an upper layer of columnar cells and a lower layer of flattened cells (Fig. 5-2*B*). Meanwhile, a new layer of cells forms a dome over the embryonic disc. This dome is the **amnion,** and fluid soon accumulates in the **amniotic cavity,** lying below the amnion and above the bilaminar embryonic disc. The disc will develop into the body of the embryo, whereas most of the remaining structures of the blastocyst will become extraembryonic membranes which serve to support and sustain the metabolic activities of the embryo.

The lower layer of the embryonic disc develops into the **endoderm** layer, and it becomes continuous with a sac-like structure projecting downward from the embryonic disc (Fig. 5-2*D*). This is the **yolk sac,** which in humans is a rudimentary structure, since the maternal tissues provide the source of nourishment for the human embryo. The upper layer of the embryonic disc gives rise to other tissues which will be described later.

The trophoblast again generates additional cells which push inward between the trophoblast and amnion and yolk sac (Fig. 5-3). These cells form the **extraembryonic mesoderm** which soon develops isolated spaces among its loosely scattered cells. The spaces eventually coalesce to form a single **extraembryonic coelom** around the amnion and yolk sac, except for one region where the extraembryonic mesoderm remains intact as a **connecting stalk** between the trophoblast and what will be the caudal end of the developing embryo. The formation of the extraembryonic coelom splits the extraembryonic mesoderm into two portions: one portion lines the trophoblast and covers the amnion and is termed the **extraembryonic somatic mesoderm,** while the other covers the yolk sac and is called the **extraembryonic splanchnic mesoderm.** By this time approximately 2 weeks have elapsed since fertilization, the blastocyst is completely implanted beneath the surface of the uterine lining (Fig. 5-4), and the mother may suspect that she is pregnant since her menstrual period fails to occur.

The bilaminar embryonic disc becomes converted into a **trilaminar embryonic disc** by the formation of a third layer of cells, the **intraembryonic mesoderm.** This begins in the caudal region of the embryonic disc where a slit known as the **primitive streak** develops in the dorsal midline of the disc (Fig. 5-5*A*). The primitive streak is an active area where some of the surface cells of the disc sink downward and migrate laterally and cranially to become the intraembryonic mesoderm sandwiched between the overlying cells and underlying endoderm layer (Fig. 5-5*B*). Those cells which remain on the surface become the **ectoderm** layer of the disc. This process of cellular migration and relocation is known as **gastrulation.**

As the mesoderm passes forward from the region of the primitive streak, a rod of mesodermal tissue becomes discernible in the midline. This is the **notochordal process** (or future **notochord**) which apparently provides some temporary support to the early embryonic body; however, most of the notochord eventually degenerates, except for a remnant (nucleus pulposus) which is retained in each intervertebral disc. On either side of the notochord the intraembryonic mesoderm forms a solid mass of tissue which becomes subdivided into three

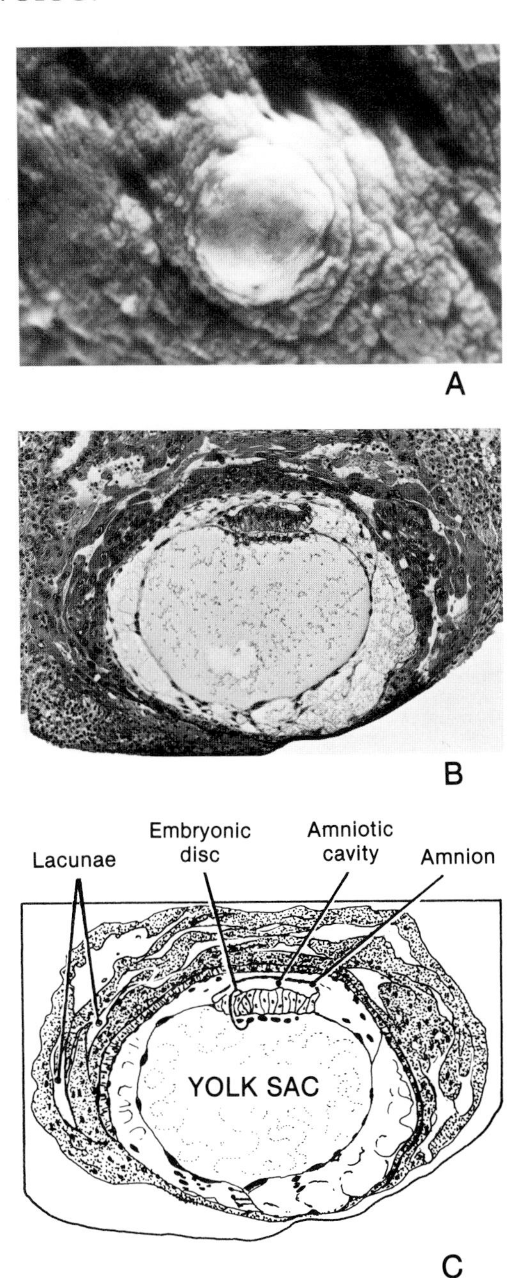

Fig. 5-4. An 11- to 12-day human embryo. (A) Surface view of the uterine lining showing the implantation site as a raised area (near the center of the photograph) just beneath the surface. (B) Microscopic section through the implantation site (courtesy of the Carnegie Institution of Washington, Department of Embryology, Davis Division). (C) Sketch of section shown in B.

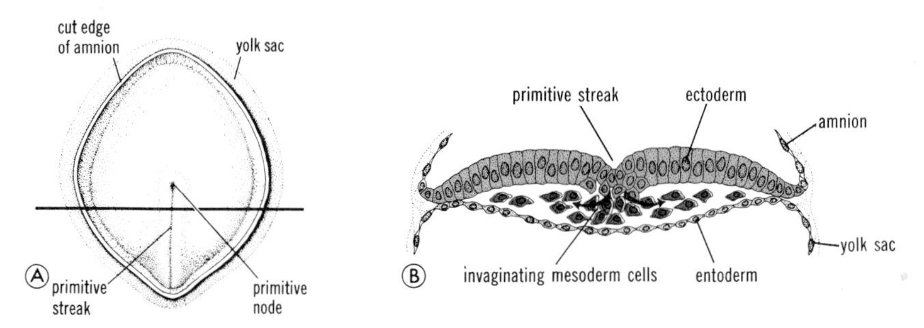

Fig. 5-5. (A) Dorsal view of the embryonic disc showing formation of the primitive streak in the caudal region; (B) transverse section of the primitive streak indicated by the transverse line in A. (From J. Langman, *Medical Embryology*, Ed. 3, The Williams & Wilkins Co., Baltimore, 1975.)

portions (Fig. 5-6). The mesoderm closest to the notochord is the **paraxial mesoderm** which differentiates into a series of cube-like blocks of tissue called **somites.** These will contribute to various portions of the musculoskeletal system and will form the dermis of the skin in some regions of the body. Just lateral to the somites is the **intermediate mesoderm** which will develop into embryonic kidneys, and lateral to the intermediate mesoderm is the **lateral plate mesoderm.** At first the lateral plate mesoderm is a solid mass of cells, but eventually cavities develop within it and coalesce to form the **intraembryonic coelom,** much like the formation of the extraembryonic coelom. Thus, the intraembryonic coelom splits the lateral plate mesoderm into a **somatic layer** which lies in contact with the surface ectoderm and a **splanchnic layer** in contact with the endoderm of the yolk sac. For a very brief period of time the intraembryonic coelom and extraembryonic coelom communicate with each other, but the communication is lost when the lateral and ventral walls of the embryonic body become apparent.

The ectoderm, endoderm, and mesoderm are known as **germ layers,** and various portions of the embryonic organs will be derived from these three layers. These derivatives may be summarized as follows. The **ectoderm** is involved in the formation of the nervous system and epidermis of the skin. The **endoderm** contributes to much of the inner linings of the digestive system and respiratory system, as well as part of the urinary system and of some endocrine glands. The **mesoderm** develops into musculoskeletal structures, the cardiovascular system, much of the reproductive and urinary systems, and connective tissues, including the dermis of the skin. During early stages of development most of the mesoderm consists of loosely arranged **mesenchyme cells** which will eventually develop into the more highly differentiated cells characteristic of the adult mesodermal derivatives.

DEVELOPMENT OF BODY FORM

Near the end of the 3rd week the flattened embryonic disc is transformed into the cylindrical body of the early embryo by a series of folds. The first of these occurs in the cranial region of the disc and is termed the **head fold** (Fig. 5-7). Somewhat later a **tail fold** occurs in the caudal region near the connecting stalk. At the same time the lateral portions of the embryonic disc become folded under as **lateral body folds** so that the entire embryo begins to lift upward from the surface of the yolk sac. In the cranial and caudal regions of the embryo, the folding results in the formation of the **foregut** and **hindgut** portions of the endodermally lined **primitive gut.** The yolk sac soon collapses but remains in communication with the **midgut** portion by means of the **vitelline duct.** A small balloon-like diverticulum also develops from the caudal region of the gut (hindgut) and is known as the **allantois.** In some animals the

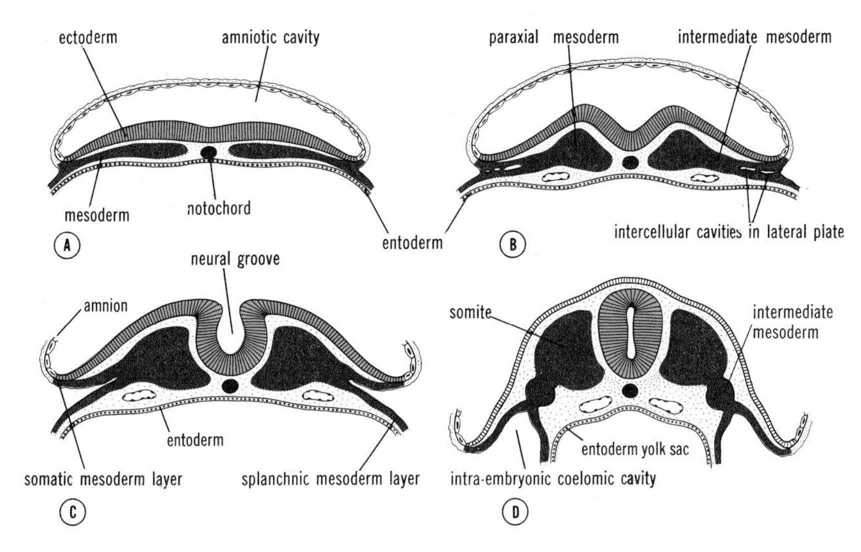

Fig. 5-6. Transverse sections through a series of embryos showing development of the intraembryonic mesoderm. (A) 17-day embryo. The notochord as well as three germ layers are present: ectoderm, mesoderm, and endoderm (entoderm). (B) 19-day embryo. Note differentiation of the mesoderm into three parts. (C) 20-day embryo. The lateral plate mesoderm splits into somatic and splanchnic layers. (D) 21-day embryo. The intraembryonic coelomic cavity is well defined, and somites have developed from the paraxial mesoderm. (From J. Langman, *Medical Embryology,* Ed. 3, The Williams & Wilkins Co., Baltimore, 1975.)

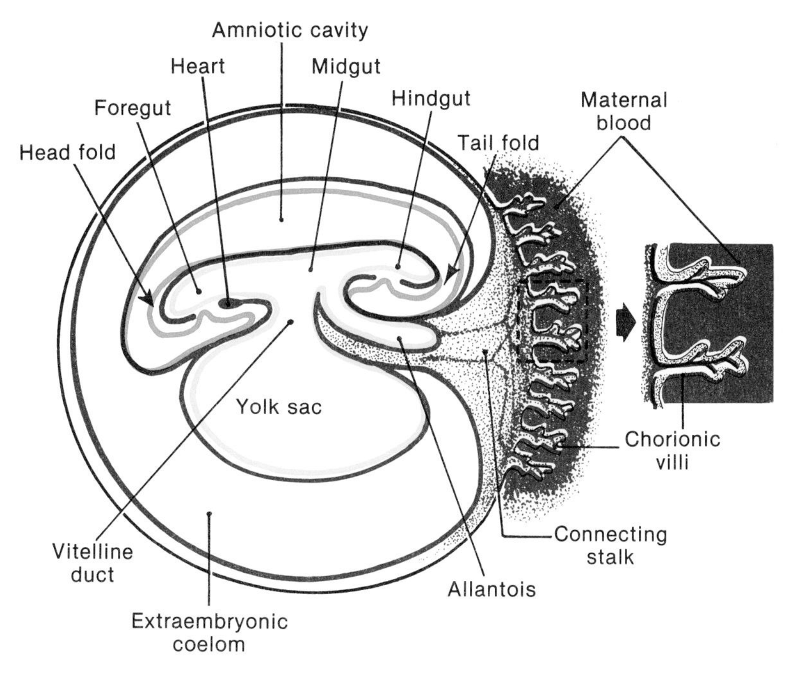

Fig. 5-7. Diagram of a sagittal section through an early embryo showing formation of the head fold and tail fold. The amniotic cavity is expanding in all directions. The chorionic villi and adjacent maternal blood and tissues comprise the placenta, a portion of which is enclosed in the box and shown in higher magnification at right.

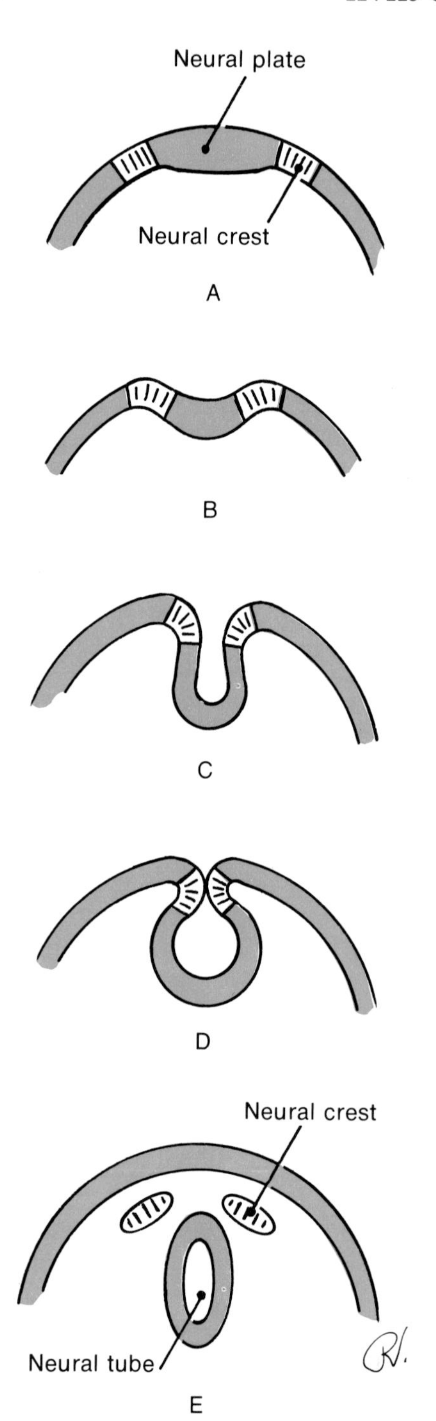

Fig. 5-8. Transverse sections showing formation of the neural tube. (A) Surface ectoderm cells thicken to form the neural plate; (B, C) neural folds elevate; (D) neural folds pinch off from surface ectoderm; (E) neural tube closes and is flanked on each side by neural crest cells.

yolk sac is nutritive, and the allantois serves a respiratory and excretory function; in higher mammals these functions are performed by the placenta, and so the yolk sac and allantois are poorly developed. As the body folds develop, the amniotic cavity simultaneously expands cranially, caudally, and laterally so as to envelop the embryo.

EARLY DEVELOPMENT OF ORGAN SYSTEMS

In addition to the primitive gut, other organ systems make their appearance during these early stages of development. During the 3rd week of gestation, the nervous system begins to develop from the surface ectodermal cells which become thickened in the midline to form the **neural plate.** At the edges of the neural plate are a group of **neural crest cells.** The neural plate then becomes elevated in the form of two neural folds which fuse dorsally so as to form a hollow longitudinal **neural tube** (Fig. 5-8). The neural tube pinches off from the overlying ectoderm, which becomes the epidermis of the skin. The neural folds close first in the cervical region, from which point the closure then proceeds cranially and caudally (Fig. 5-9). The last regions to close are at the cranial and caudal tips of the neural tube (the **anterior** and **posterior neuropores**), and the tube then eventually develops into the brain and spinal cord.

As the neural tube pinches off from the surface ectoderm, the neural crest cells are left behind as a longitudinal band on each side of the neural tube (Fig. 5-8*E*). The neural crest cells are unique in that they migrate extensively throughout the body and differentiate into a variety of cell types, including nerve cells in ganglia, supporting cells of the nervous system, secretory cells in the medulla of the suprarenal (adrenal) glands, pigment cells in the skin, and even some cartilage and muscle cells in the head region.

While the nervous system is forming, a primitive **cardiovascular system** develops from splanchnic mesodermal cells and consists of a tubular heart and an interconnecting plexus of blood vessels. The heart initially develops from a condensation of splanchnic mesoderm beneath the foregut (Fig. 5-7), and is represented by two hollow tubes which eventually fuse to form a single large tube. Mesodermal cells also condense in other regions of the body and form an extensive interconnecting system of tiny hollow tubes which form blood vessels. These eventually connect with blood vessels which have formed simultaneously in the connecting stalk (Fig. 5-10). Meanwhile tiny blood vessels also develop in the extraembryonic mesoderm associated with the trophoblastic villi, and these likewise communicate with the vessels in the connecting stalk. In this manner the blood vessels begin to distribute blood throughout the body of the embryo and also out to the trophoblastic area where an exchange of gases, nutrients, and excretory products can take place with maternal tissues. By the 4th week of gestation the heart shows erratic pulsations and then gradually begins to contract more regularly in order to pro-

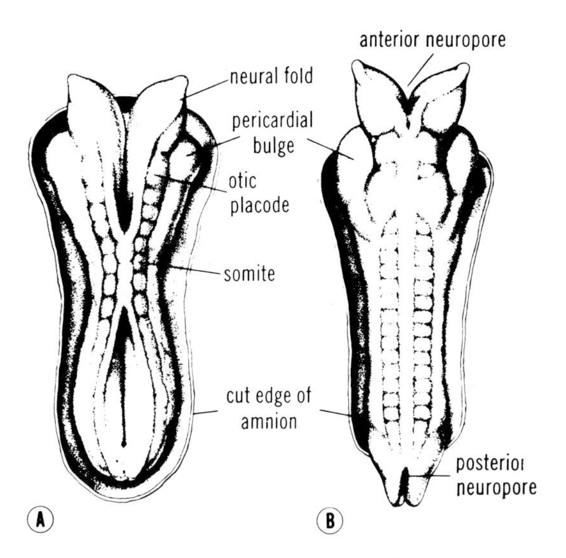

Fig. 5-9. Dorsal views of human embryos showing progressive fusion of the neural folds (A) At 22 days, (B) at 23 days. (From J. Langman, *Medical Embryology,* Ed. 3, The Williams & Wilkins Co., Baltimore, 1975).

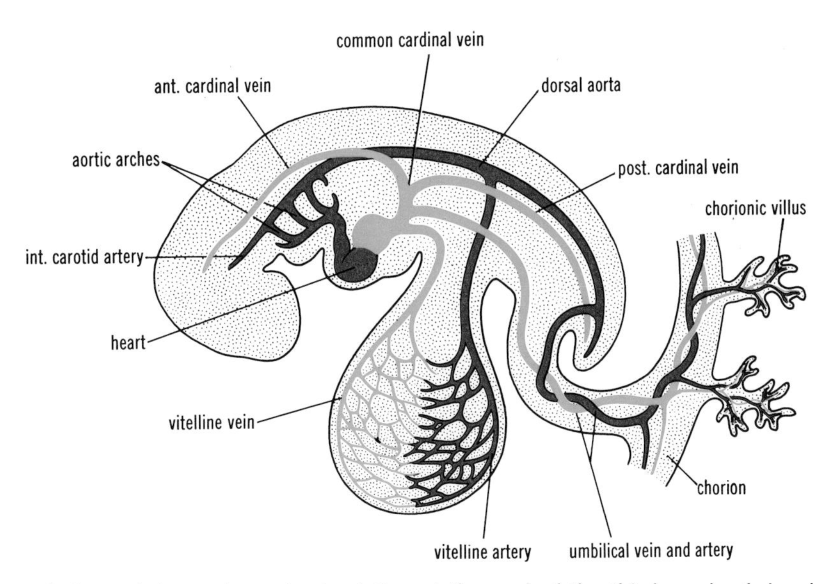

Fig. 5-10. Lateral view of the embryonic circulation at the end of the third week of development. The arteries are in red; veins in blue. (Modified from J. Langman, *Medical Embryology,* Ed. 3, The Williams & Wilkins Co., Baltimore, 1975.)

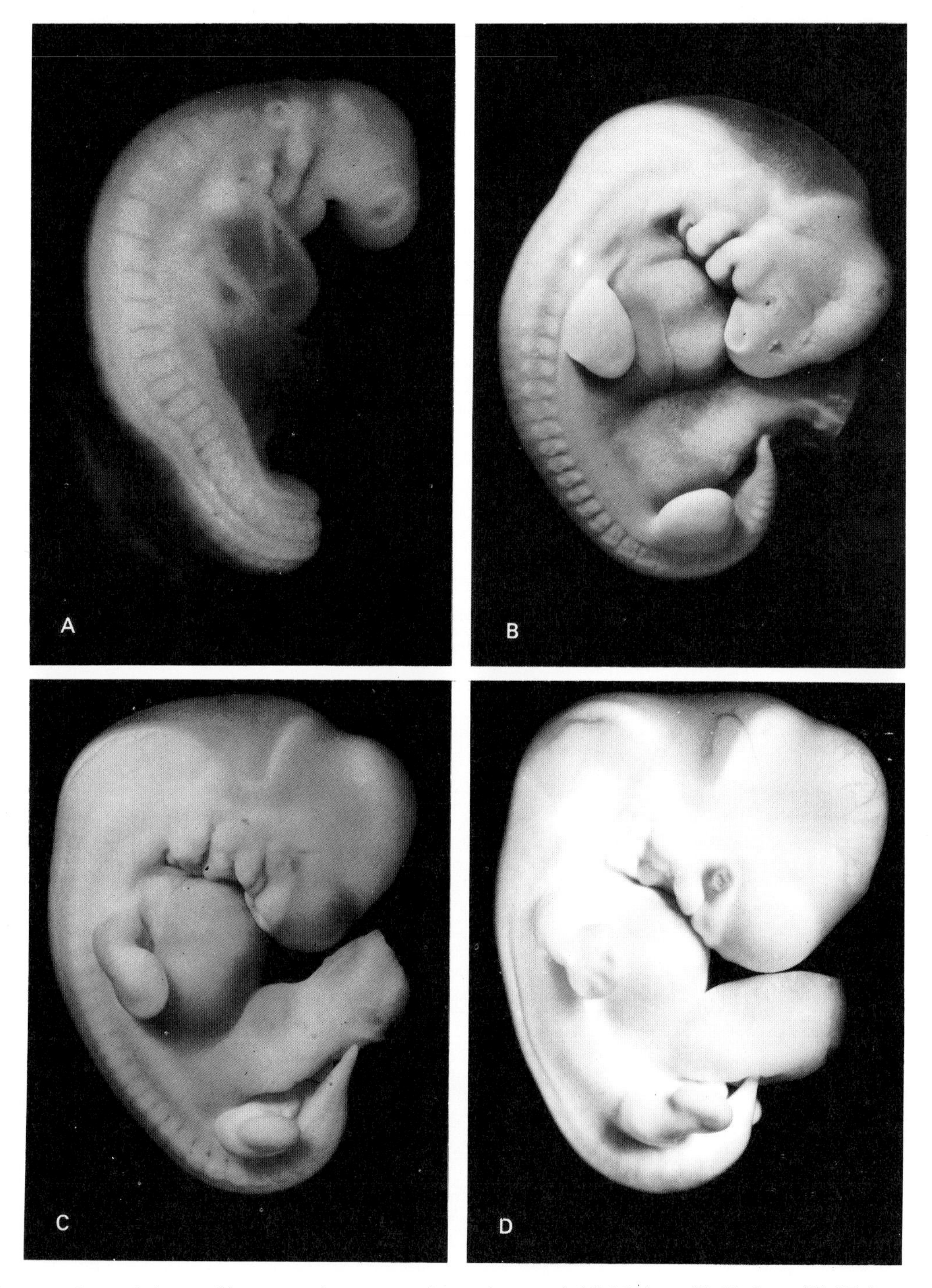

Fig. 5-11. Lateral views of human embryos at estimated ages of: (A) 26 days, (B) 32 days, (C) 37 days, and (D) 41 days. (Courtesy of the Carnegie Institution of Washington, Department of Embryology, Davis Division.)

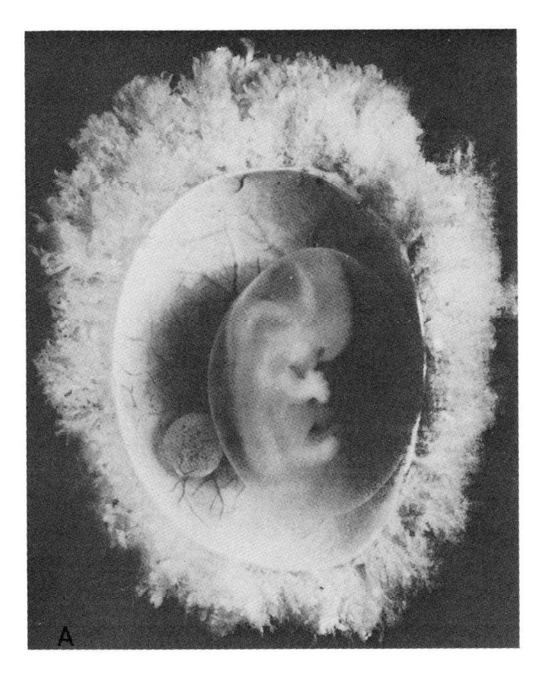

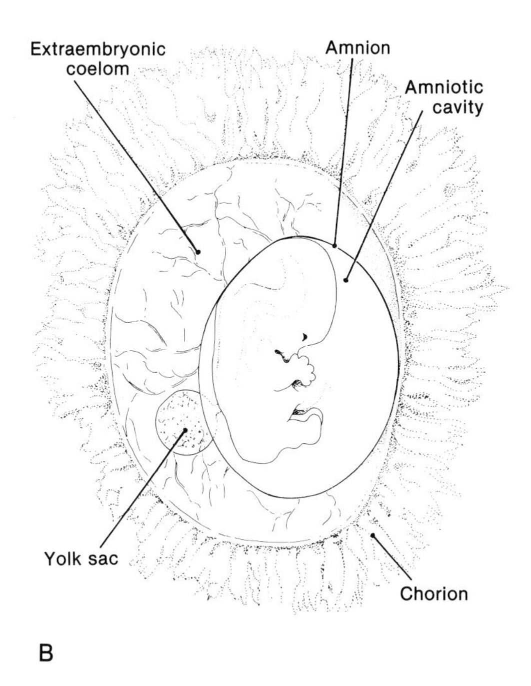

Fig. 5-12. (A) Lateral view of human embryo at approximately 48 days of gestation shown enclosed within its amnion and other extraembryonic membranes. (Courtesy of the Carnegie Institution of Washington, Department of Embryology, Davis Division.) (B) Sketch of embryo and membranes shown in A.

vide the propulsive force for the embryonic circulation.

GROWTH OF THE EMBRYO

During the 1st month of gestation, the body of the embryo gradually takes form and assumes a C-shaped appearance (Fig. 5-11). Limb buds appear at the end of the 1st month and continue to increase in size, with the upper limbs being slightly more advanced than the lower limbs during these early stages of development. Meanwhile, the brain enlarges considerably during the 2nd month (Figs. 5-12 and 5-13). By the end of the 8th week the embryo has begun to assume a more human appearance and is arbitrarily referred to as a **fetus** during its subsequent stages of development.

GROWTH OF THE EXTRAEMBRYONIC MEMBRANES

During the first 2 months of gestation the connecting stalk becomes transformed into the **umbilical cord,** which eventually assumes a more ventral attachment in the caudal region of the embryo. The amniotic cavity continues to expand and envelop the embryo with fluid secreted by the cells of the amnion (Fig. 5-12). The progressive expansion of the amniotic cavity results in a gradual obliteration of the extraembryonic coelom. The trophoblast cells and the extraembryonic mesoderm are together termed the **chorion,** which becomes highly developed near the peripheral attachment of the original connecting stalk (Fig. 5-7). This region of the chorion as well as the nearby uterine tissues of the mother constitute the **pla-**

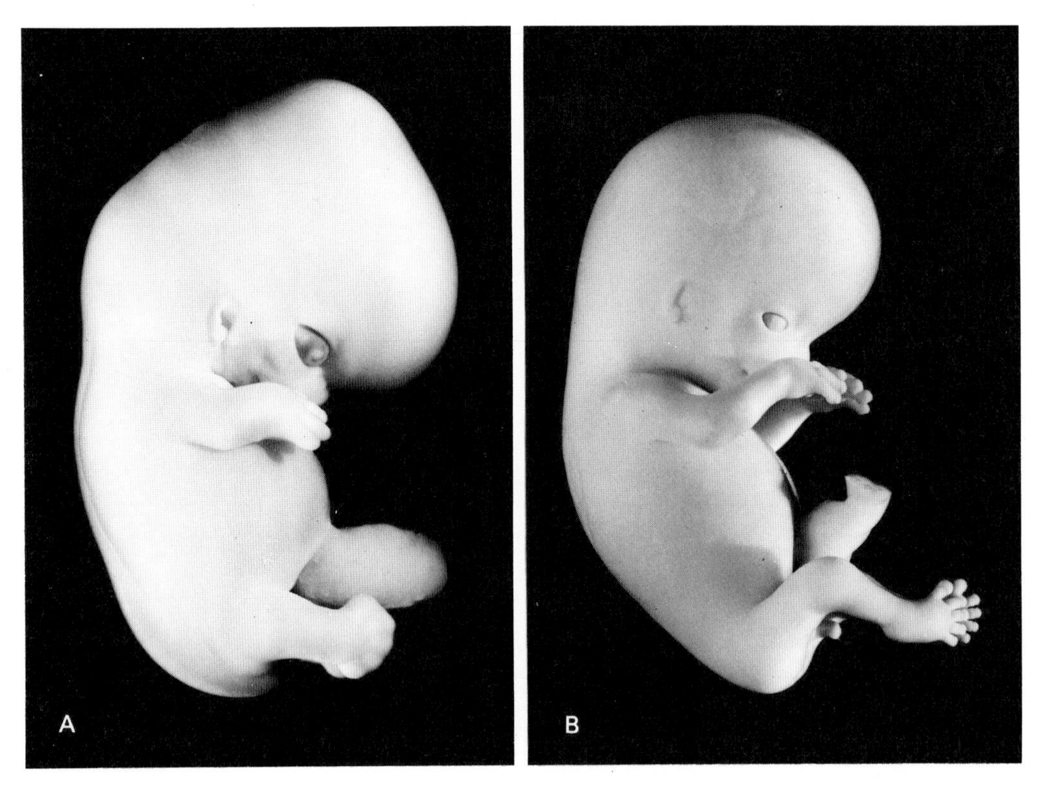

Fig. 5-13. Lateral views of human embryos at estimated ages of: (A) 51 days, (B) 57 days. (Courtesy of The Carnegie Institution of Washington, Department of Embryology, Davis Division.)

centa, which in human embryos is disc-shaped. At the time of birth the placenta and much of the uterine lining will be shed as the "**after-birth.**"

In some instances the trophoblast cells of the chorion produce an enormous mass of large fluid-filled cysts. This is known as a "**hydatidiform mole**" which prevents the placenta from functioning properly in exchanging nutrients and waste products and ultimately results in death of the embryo. The chorionic cells occasionally may also transform into a malignancy known as a **choriocarcinoma.**

II

SYSTEMIC ANATOMY

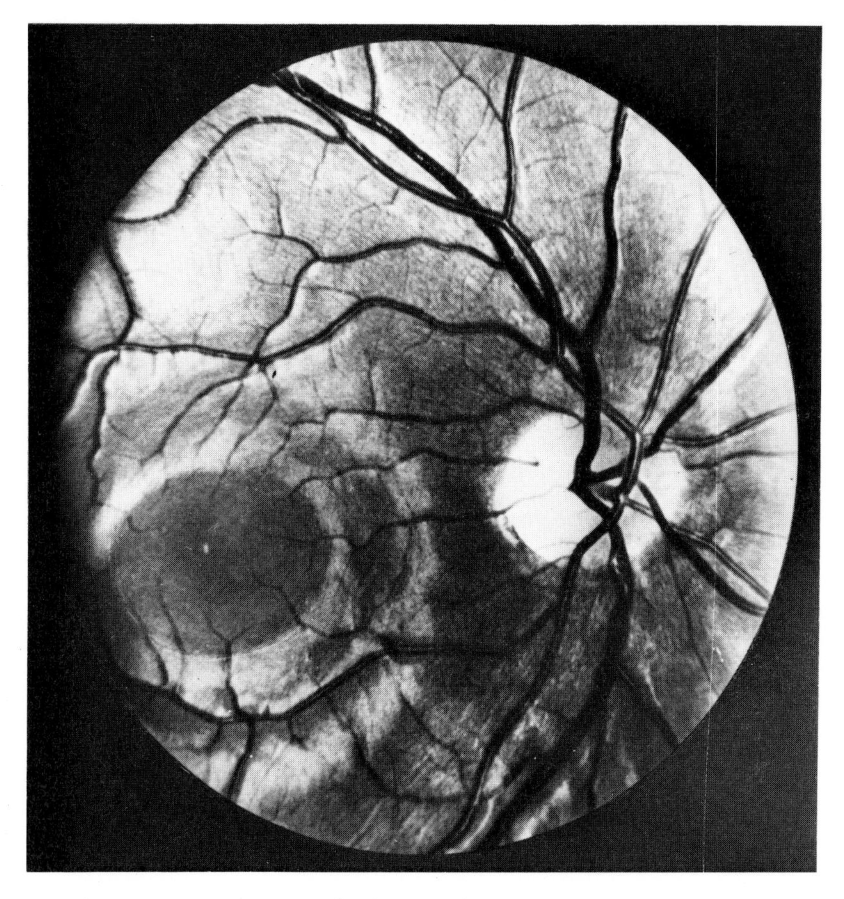

This section integrates the basic information presented in Part I into a study of each major organ system. The organs of each system will be approached from a structural and functional point of view with an emphasis on their gross, microscopic, developmental, and clinical anatomy.

6

The Integumentary System

The integumentary system consists of the skin and its accessory structures such as hair, nails, sweat glands, and sebaceous glands. The integument is a relatively waterproof covering which protects the deeper tissues of the body by keeping out foreign material including microorganisms. It also prevents loss of body fluids, helps to regulate body temperature, and provides an extensive area for receiving sensory input such as pain, temperature, and touch. The integument acts as an excretory organ whereby sweat and sebaceous glands discharge their products onto the surface of the body. It also serves as a site for synthesis of vitamin D under the influence of ultraviolet rays from the sun. The loss of many of these vital functions can be lethal in cases of severe burns where extensive areas of the integument are damaged.

SKIN

The skin is composed of a superficial epithelial portion, the **epidermis,** and a deeper connective tissue portion, the **dermis** (corium) (Fig. 6-1). The thickness of the epidermis and dermis varies in different parts of the body. For example, the epidermis is thicker on the palms of the hands and soles of the feet than it is in other regions of the body, whereas the dermis is thicker in the back region than elsewhere. Beneath the dermis is the **subcutaneous layer (superficial fascia)** which anchors the skin to deep fascia which in turn is continuous with muscles and bones. The surface of the skin shows tiny ridges and grooves. These are particularly well developed on the palmar surfaces of the fingers and provide the friction needed to grasp objects more readily. The pattern of these ridges is unique for each individual and represents one's "fingerprints."

Epidermis

The epidermis is a stratified squamous epithelium which contains the protein **keratin** in its upper layers and is thus said to be cornified. This serves as an added barrier between the external and internal environments.

Five layers can be identified in the epidermis, the lowermost being the **stratum basale** (Fig. 6-2). This is an irregular, wavy layer of columnar cells which are separated from the underlying connective tissue of the dermis by a thin basement membrane. The stratum basale is the site where most mitotic activity occurs in the epidermis. Cells are generated in this layer and pass upward into progressively more superficial layers of the skin.

The **stratum spinosum** lies above the stratum basale and is several layers thick. It consists of irregularly shaped cells, some of which may also undergo mitosis. For this reason the stratum basale and the stratum spinosum are sometimes referred to as the **stratum germinati-**

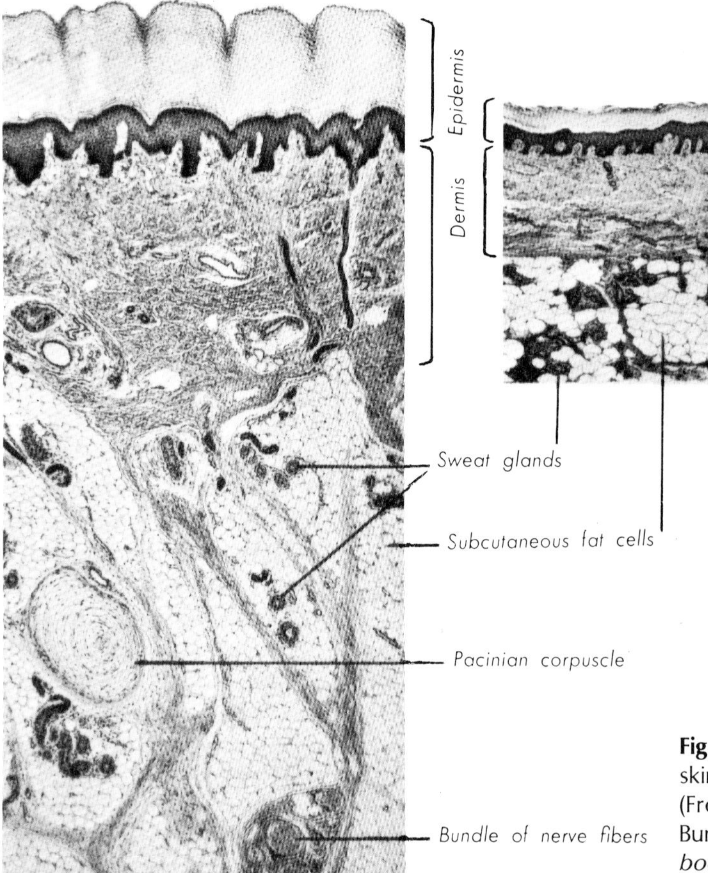

Fig. 6-1. Microscopic sections of thick skin *(left)* and thinner skin *(right)*. (From W. M. Copenhaver, R. P. Bunge, and M. B. Bunge, *Bailey's Textbook of Histology*, Ed. 16; The Williams & Wilkins Co., Baltimore, 1971).

vum (Malpighian layer). The stratum basale and stratum spinosum contain specialized pigment-producing cells called **melanoblasts** whose long slender branches extend into upper layers of the epidermis. These cells manufacture the pigment **melanin** in response to an individual's genetic background, thereby producing darker or lighter skin. Environmental factors also affect melanin production. For example, exposure to ultraviolet light increases the amount of melanin and results in a suntan. Unfortunately, melanin-producing cells may also become transformed into malignant **melanomas.**

The **stratum granulosum** lies just above the stratum spinosum and contains 2–5 layers of slightly flattened cells. These cells contain keratohyalin granules which are precursors of the keratin fibers occurring in the uppermost layers. These granules stain brightly with basic dyes and are not related to melanin pigment.

The **stratum lucidum** is a clear narrow layer found only in thickened areas of the epidermis. By the time the cells reach this layer they are in various stages of degeneration.

The **stratum corneum** consists of keratinized flattened cells which are dead and in the process of being cast off. The thickness of this layer varies according to its location in the body. The palms and soles have a thick stratum corneum to withstand abrasions and are thus designated as thick skin. Corns and callouses are mechanically induced thickenings of the stratum corneum.

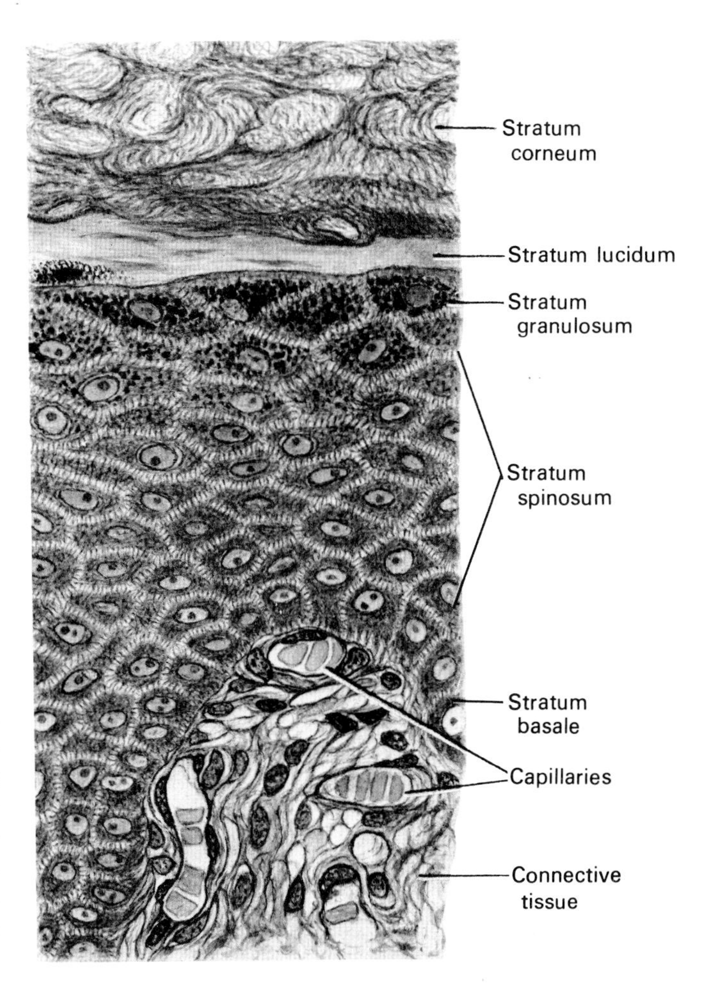

Fig. 6-2. High magnification of a microscopic section through the epidermis of thick skin, as well as connective tissue and capillaries in the upper portion of the dermis. (From W. M. Copenhaver, R. P. Bunge, and M. B. Bunge, *Bailey's Textbook of Histology*, Ed. 16, The Williams & Wilkins Co., Baltimore, 1971.)

Dermis

The dermis lies beneath the epidermis and consists of dense irregular connective tissue (Figs. 6-1 and 6-3). The blood vessels in the dermis do not penetrate the epidermis, which must depend on the process of diffusion to receive nutrients. Hence, the lowermost layers of the epidermis contain healthy, actively dividing cells, whereas the cells begin to degenerate as they move upwards into more distant layers.

The dermis is composed of two regions, of which the most superficial is called the **papillary layer** because of the fingerlike papillae which project upward beneath the epidermis. These papillae contain blood vessels and special sensory receptors for the sense of touch, especially in the finger tips (see Chapter 12: The Nervous System). The lower region of the dermis is the **reticular layer** composed of coarse collagenous and elastic fibers, the majority of which are arranged parallel to the surface. Some skeletal muscles, such as the muscles of facial expression, insert into this region of the dermis.

Subcutaneous Layer (Superficial Fascia)

This layer consists of loose connective tissue which blends above with the reticular layer of the dermis. A fair amount of fat occurs in the subcutaneous layer, especially in such regions as the abdomen. The subcutaneous layer also contains sensory receptors known as **Pacinian**

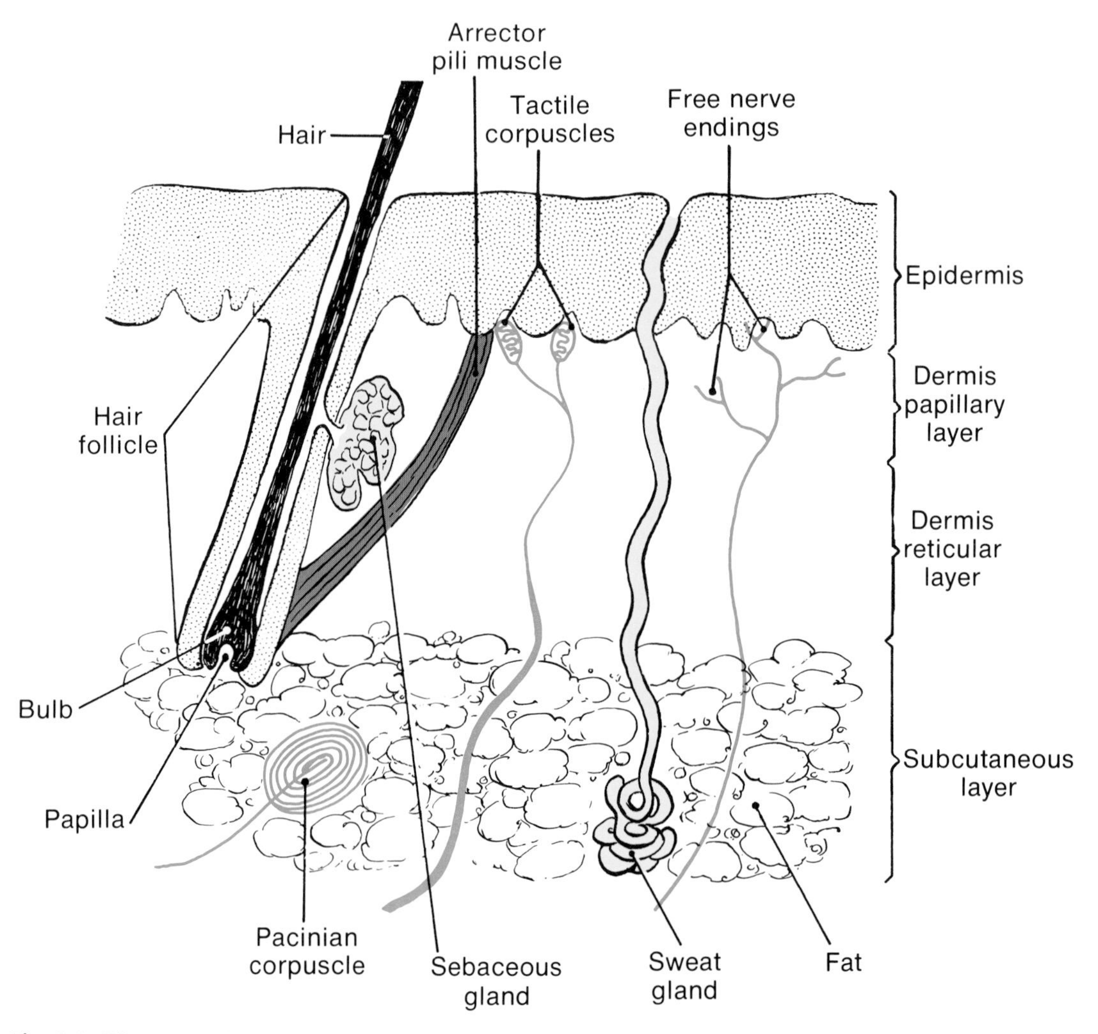

Fig. 6-3. Diagrammatic section of the skin and subcutaneous layer. (The sensory nerve endings are indicated in blue, the sebaceous and sweat glands in yellow, and the arrector pili muscle in red.)

corpuscles (Figs. 6-1 and 6-3). Although the subcutaneous tissue attaches the skin to deeper structures, it also allows a considerable degree of mobility, except in the palms and soles where it is more dense. In most regions of the body the elasticity of the skin and subcutaneous layer decreases with age.

HAIR

Hairs are present over the entire surface of the skin except on the palms, soles, and at various body orifices such as the lips. Hairs vary in thickness and number per unit area. They act as a protection, in regulating body temperature, and for sensory reception such as the sense of touch. Each hair is composed of an outer **cuticle** of scaly degenerate cells, an inner **cortex** of keratinized cells with variable amounts of pigment, and in some hairs a central **core (medulla)** of softer keratinized cells. Hair color depends on the amount and kind of pigment present in the cortex and the amount of air space between the cells. Hair whitens when pigment formation stops.

Each hair consists of a **shaft** above the surface of the epidermis and a **root** which extends downward into the dermis and even into the subcutaneous layer. The root is enclosed within a tubelike hair **follicle** lined by epidermal cells (Fig. 6-3). The follicle is usually slanted, and the lower end of the root is expanded into a **bulb.** The bulb contains cells which constantly proliferate and move upward, thereby causing the hair to grow. The bulb is invaginated below by a **papilla** containing vessels and nerves.

Hairs are continually being lost and replaced. With increasing age, some hair follicles on the head may degenerate, resulting in varying degrees of baldness. Baldness is more common in males, and its pattern and extent often reflect hereditary factors.

Associated with each hair follicle is a thin band of smooth muscle extending from the upper part of the dermis to the root. This is the **arrector pili muscle** which contracts and causes the hair and surrounding tissue to elevate, particularly in response to cold, resulting in "goose pimples." The muscle also compresses the sebaceous gland located within the angle formed by the arrector pili muscle and the root of the hair.

GLANDS

Sebaceous Glands

The sebaceous glands are situated in the dermis and consist of sacs whose ducts usually open into hair follicles (Fig. 6-3). The glands secrete **sebum,** an oily material composed of fats and of cast-off epithelial cells from the gland. Sebum lubricates the skin.

Sweat (Sudoriferous) Glands

These glands are widely distributed in the skin and are particularly numerous (several hundred per square centimeter) in the palms and soles. The secretory part of each gland is coiled and often lies in the subcutaneous layer (Fig. 6-3). This leads upward into a straight duct passing through the dermis and epidermis and eventually emptying onto the surface of the skin via a tiny pore. The watery secretion has a cooling effect on the body and also serves as a means for excreting waste products.

Modifications of sweat glands occur in various regions of the body. Among these are the **ceruminous glands** of the external ear. These glands secrete a waxy substance into the external acoustic (auditory) meatus (the canal leading from the external flap of the ear to the eardrum). The **mammary glands** are also considered to be highly modified derivatives of sweat glands.

NAILS

Nails are derivatives of the skin and consist of a cornified **nail plate** (composed of the highly modified stratum corneum and stratum lucidum) overlying a specialized region of the skin termed a **nail bed** (composed of the germinative layer of the epidermis and the upper part of the dermis). Nails function mainly for protection of the upper surfaces of the digits, as an aid in picking up objects, and as a means for scratching.

Each nail consists of a proximal hidden part (the **root**) and a distal exposed part (the **body**) (Fig. 6-4). The root is covered by a curved fold of skin called the **eponychium** (cuticle). The body of the nail is a hard layer of keratinized epidermal cells which are transparent and thin. The pinkish color is due to blood vessels situated in the dermis of the nail bed. The opaque moon-shaped area is the whitish **lunula** just beyond the eponychium (Fig. 6-4). The proximal part of the nail bed lies beneath the root and consists of a thick **matrix** where the germinative layer of the epidermis produces keratinized cells resulting in the growth of the nail plate. The distal part of the nail bed does not contribute very much to nail growth. The dermis portion of the nail bed attaches directly to underlying bony structures, since a subcutaneous layer is lacking in the region of the nails. Beneath the distal free edge of the nail the outer layers of the epidermis are thickened to form the **hyponychium,** which is attached to the underside of the nail.

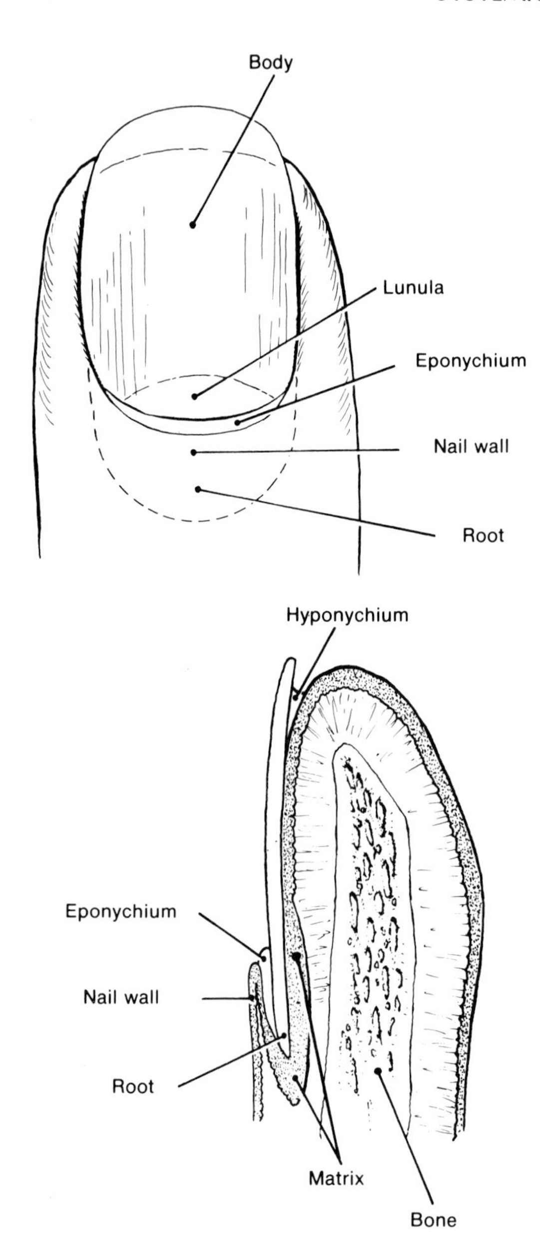

Fig. 6-4. Fingernail. *(Top)* Dorsal view, *(bottom)* longitudinal section.

DEVELOPMENTAL AND CLINICAL ANATOMY

The epidermis of the skin is derived from embryonic ectoderm; the dermis develops from the underlying mesoderm. Downy hairs first appear on the face of the fetus and eventually can be seen on other regions of the body. Each hair develops as a downward solid growth of epidermal cells into the dermis. The epidermal mass then transforms into a hollow tubelike follicle, the lower end of which becomes invaginated by a dermal papilla. The sebaceous and sweat glands likewise develop from epidermal thickenings.

By the time of birth the hair on the head has become more dense than that on other parts of the body. With the approach of adolescence (puberty) increasing amounts of the sex hormones cause a coarsening of the hair in the pubic and axillary (arm pit) regions of both sexes. In males a beard also develops.

If the skin is burned, the capillaries in the dermis dilate (causing redness), and blood plasma may even escape from the capillaries and collect between the dermis and epidermis. This results in a **blister.** Severely damaged epithelium can be replaced by regeneration from the epithelium lining the hair follicles. However, if the burn is deep enough to destroy the epithelium in the follicles, then replacement of epithelial cells can occur only from the periphery of the burned area. Since this requires a long period of time, particularly in the case of extensive burns, skin grafts are used to promote healing and to help protect the dermis from infection and inflammation.

7

The Skeletal System

GENERAL FEATURES

The skeletal system consists of bones, cartilages, and joints. These structures protect vital organs (such as the brain, heart, and lungs), support various regions of the body and the body as a whole, and serve as a point of attachment for skeletal muscles. In addition, certain regions of bones are sites where blood formation takes place. Bones also act as reservoirs for calcium which can be mobilized to meet the needs of other tissues and organs.

Bones

Bones can be classified on the basis of shape (Fig. 7-1). **Long bones** possess an elongated shaft or **diaphysis,** two slightly expanded ends or **epiphyses** (singular: epiphysis), and a transitional area between the diaphysis and each epiphysis known as the **metaphyses** (singular: metaphysis). **Short bones** are shaped like cubes, whereas **flat bones** are thin and slightly curved. **Irregular bones** show a variety of shapes and do not fit any of the above categories. In addition, some short bones are embedded in tendons and are called **sesamoid bones.**

Cartilages

Cartilages often occur where bones meet one another, as in joints. They also provide a framework for highly pliable portions of the skeletal system as in the nasal region and external ears. Cartilages lend support to some of the respiratory organs and also are important during development of the fetal and immature skeleton before it is replaced by bone.

Joints

A joint or articulation is a region where bones are joined to one another. **Arthrology** is the study of the structure and function of these articulations. Although joints can be classified in a number of ways, one useful classification places them into three groups on the basis of the nature of the material between the bones: fibrous, cartilaginous, and synovial.

Fibrous joints contain a variable amount of fibrous connective tissue. If the bones articulate closely and there is only a small amount of connective tissue between them, the joint is considered to be a **suture,** and little or no movement is possible (Fig. 7-2*A*). A larger amount of fibrous connective tissue is found in a **syndesmosis** which thus allows greater mobility.

A **cartilaginous joint** is characterized by fibrocartilage or hyaline cartilage, which is situated between the articular surfaces of the bones (Fig. 7-2*B*). A fibrocartilaginous joint is called a **symphysis** and is capable of a slight amount of movement. A hyaline cartilage joint

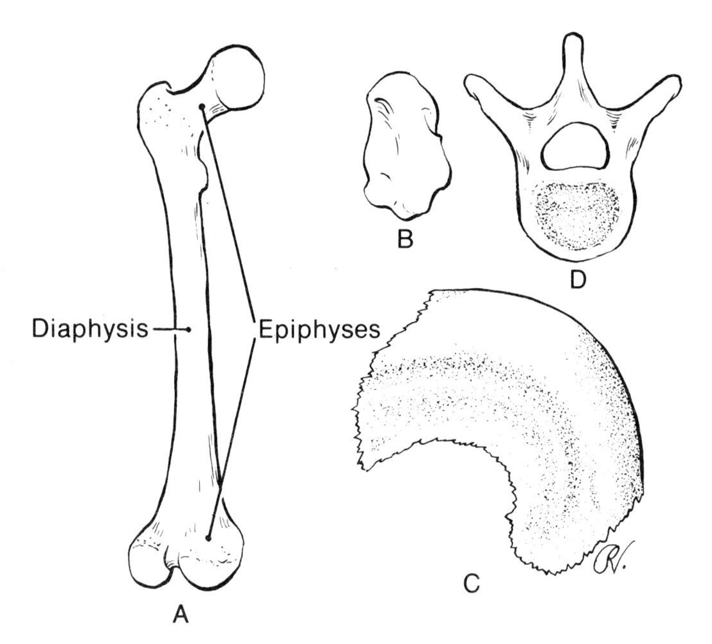

Fig. 7-1. Types of bones based on shape (not drawn to scale). (A) Long bone (femur), (B) short bone (carpal), (C) flat bone (parietal), (D) irregular bone (vertebra).

is called a **synchondrosis** and is virtually immovable.

A **synovial joint** consists of a fluid filled **synovial cavity** which allows considerable freedom of movement between the bones (Fig. 7-2*C*). Synovial joints are surrounded by a **joint capsule** consisting of fibrous connective tissue lined internally by a **synovial membrane,** which secretes a thick synovial fluid to lubricate the joint. The capsule is reinforced externally by ligaments. The articular ends of the bones are covered with hyaline cartilage which helps to prevent shearing of the bones. Some synovial joint cavities also contain fibrocartilaginous discs which serve as shock absorbers.

Synovial joints are often classified according to their type of movement (Fig. 7-2*D*):

Hinge joints allow movements in only one plane (flexion and extension) just as hinges on a door allow it only to be opened and closed. The humeroulnar joint at the elbow is a hinge joint.

Pivot joints move around a single axis, so that one bone moves or rotates around another, as when the head rotates from side to side.

Condylar joints are similar to hinge joints but show movement in two planes. The knee joint is often classified as a condylar joint.

Plane (gliding) joints allow one bone to slide over another in several directions, as occurs at the tarsometatarsal joints.

Ball and socket joints are characterized by a rounded end of one bone fitting into a socket of the other, thereby allowing a wide range of movement. The shoulder is a ball and socket joint.

Saddle joints involve two bones which are saddle-shaped with reciprocal surfaces allowing movement in two planes. The joint at the base of the thumb is a saddle joint.

GROSS ANATOMY

There are approximately 206 bones which comprise the skeleton of the human body (Fig. 7-3). These bones can be classified into two groups: the axial skeleton, and the appendicular skeleton. The **axial skeleton** is concerned with the support, protection, and movement of the head, neck, and trunk. It consists of the skull, the vertebral column, and the thoracic cage. The **appendicular skeleton** functions

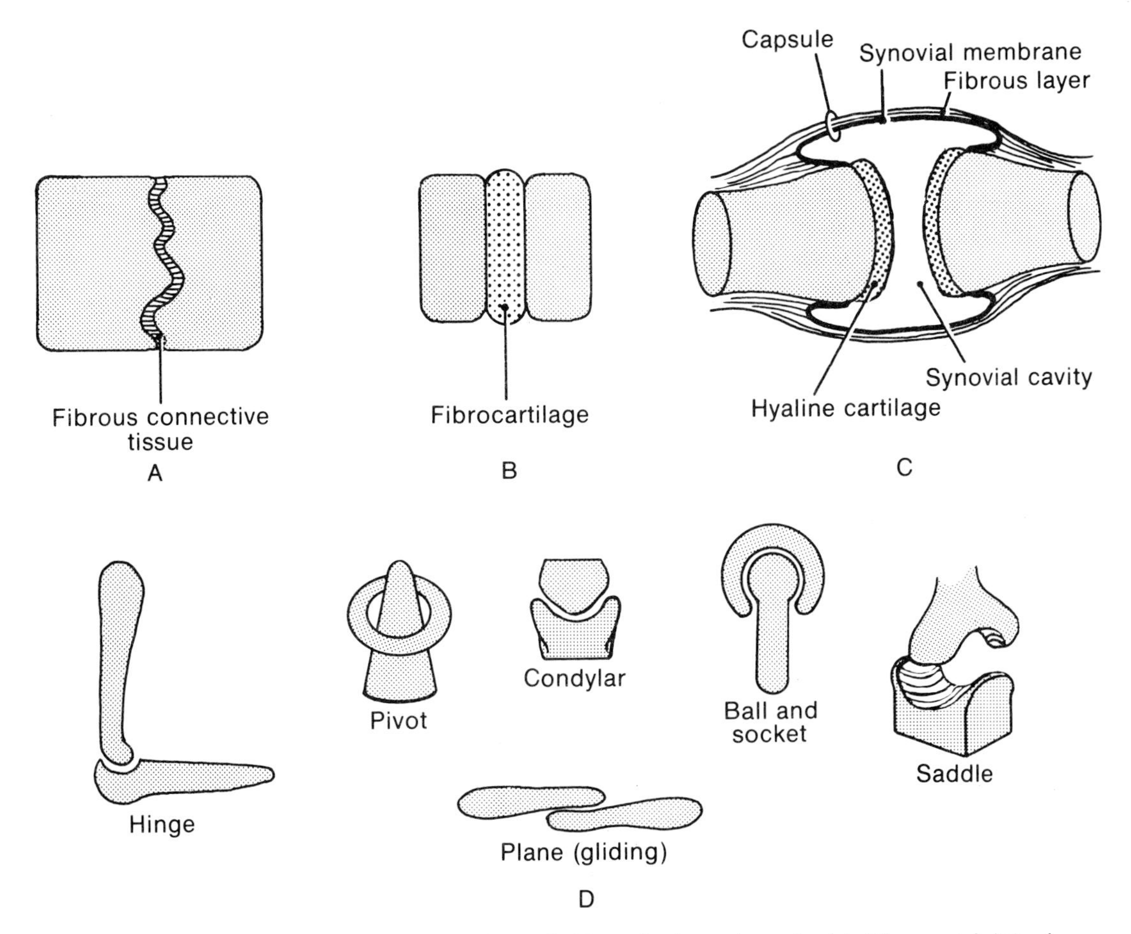

Fig. 7-2. Classification of joints. (A) Fibrous (suture), (B) cartilaginous (symphysis), (C) synovial, (D) scheme of synovial joints based on range of movement.

primarily in limb movement and includes the shoulder (pectoral) girdle, the hip (pelvic) girdle, and the bones of the upper and lower limbs.

Axial Skeleton: Skull

The skull is an impressive structure consisting of 29 bones perched on top of the vertebral column. The bones which make up the skull show a variety of shapes, interlocking closely with one another like pieces in a jigsaw puzzle. Adjacent skull bones articulate with one another by means of sutures, and there is little or no movement between the bones. This feature is important in lending stability and strength to the skull, especially that portion which houses the brain.

The skull consists of two groups of bones: the cranium and the facial bones. The **cranium** protects the brain and contains holes called **foramina** (singular: **foramen**) which allow nerves and blood vessels to enter and exit from the cranial cavity. The floor of the cranium is thicker and more substantial than the thin bony plates which arch upward to form the walls and roof (calvaria) of the cranial cavity. Ordinarily most of the cranial cavity is occupied by a sizeable organ, the brain. However, if a major portion of the brain is lacking, as occurs in the

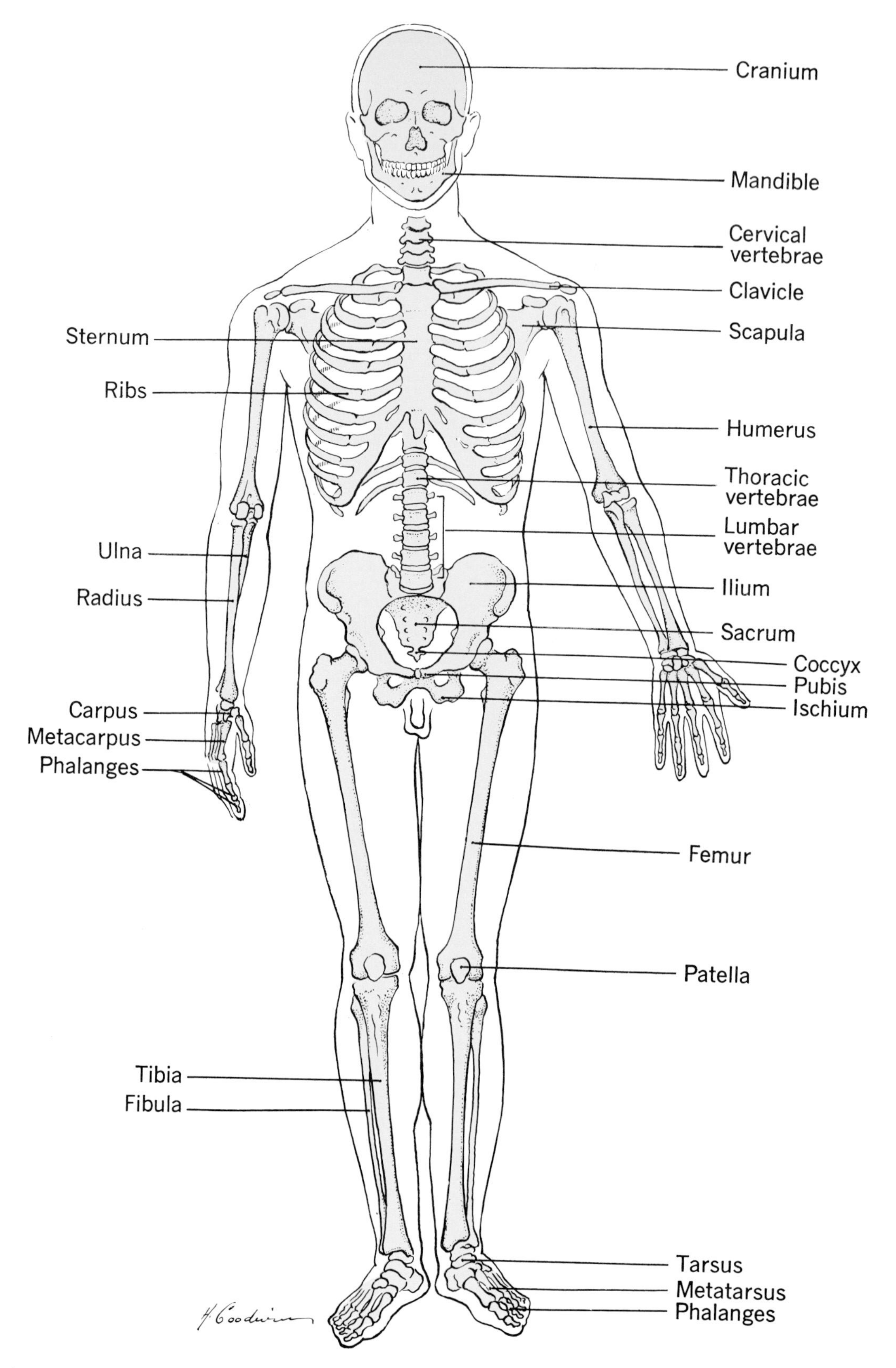

Fig. 7-3. The skeleton, anterior view. (From *Stedman's Medical Dictionary,* Ed. 23, The Williams & Wilkins Co., Baltimore, 1976.)

congenital anomaly known as **hydranencephaly,** the cranial cavity consists of a large fluid-filled space.

The **facial bones** surround the mouth, nasal openings, and lower portions of the orbits (the sockets containing the eyeballs). In addition to the facial bones, the facial skeleton includes cartilages which project outward from the face and constitute "the nose" as we see it externally. The upper portion of the nose, however, is bony. Cartilage also contributes to the nasal septum which subdivides the nasal cavity internally into right and left passageways.

Skull—Superior Aspect. Four skull bones can be easily seen from above: a single **frontal bone** in the anterior region, two **parietal bones** occupying the middle region, and a small portion of a single **occipital bone** in the posterior region (Fig. 7-4). The **coronal suture** connects the frontal bone with the two parietal bones; thus the coronal (frontal) plane passes parallel to this suture. The **sagittal suture** unites the two parietal bones in the midline (indicating the direction of the sagittal plane), and the **lambdoid suture** connects the occipital bone with the two parietal bones. (The lambdoid suture lies in the coronal plane, there being no lambdoidal plane.)

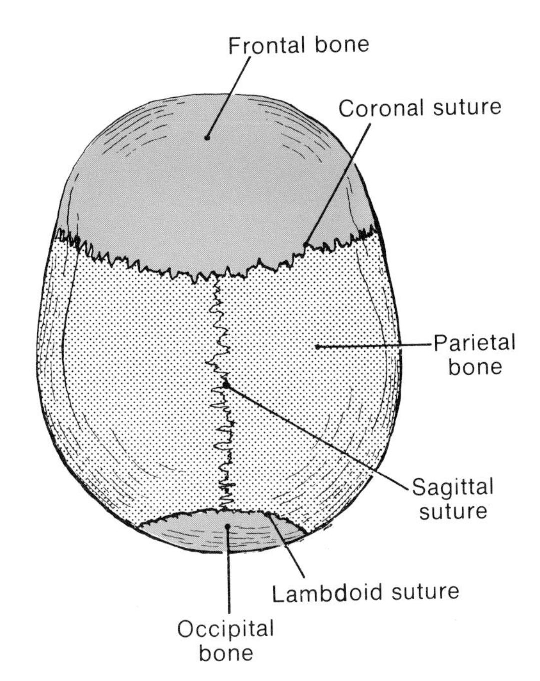

Fig. 7-4. Superior aspect of the skull.

In a newborn infant these sutures are incomplete, particularly where the coronal and sagittal sutures meet one another, and this large gap is known as the **anterior fontanelle** or **bregma** (Fig. 7-5). A second less prominent gap occurs at the junction of the sagittal and lambdoid sutures **(posterior fontanelle).** Several other fontanelles occur in lateral regions of the skull. The fontanelles and incomplete sutures lend the considerable amount of flexibility which is necessary as the head of the infant passes through the vagina at the time of birth. They also allow the brain to grow and expand during the first two years after birth.

Skull—Anterior and Lateral Aspects. In an anterior view the skull is dominated by the forehead, two large orbits (sockets for the eyeballs), nasal cavities, and the upper and lower jaws which contain the teeth (Fig. 7-6). The forehead consists of the anterior portion of the

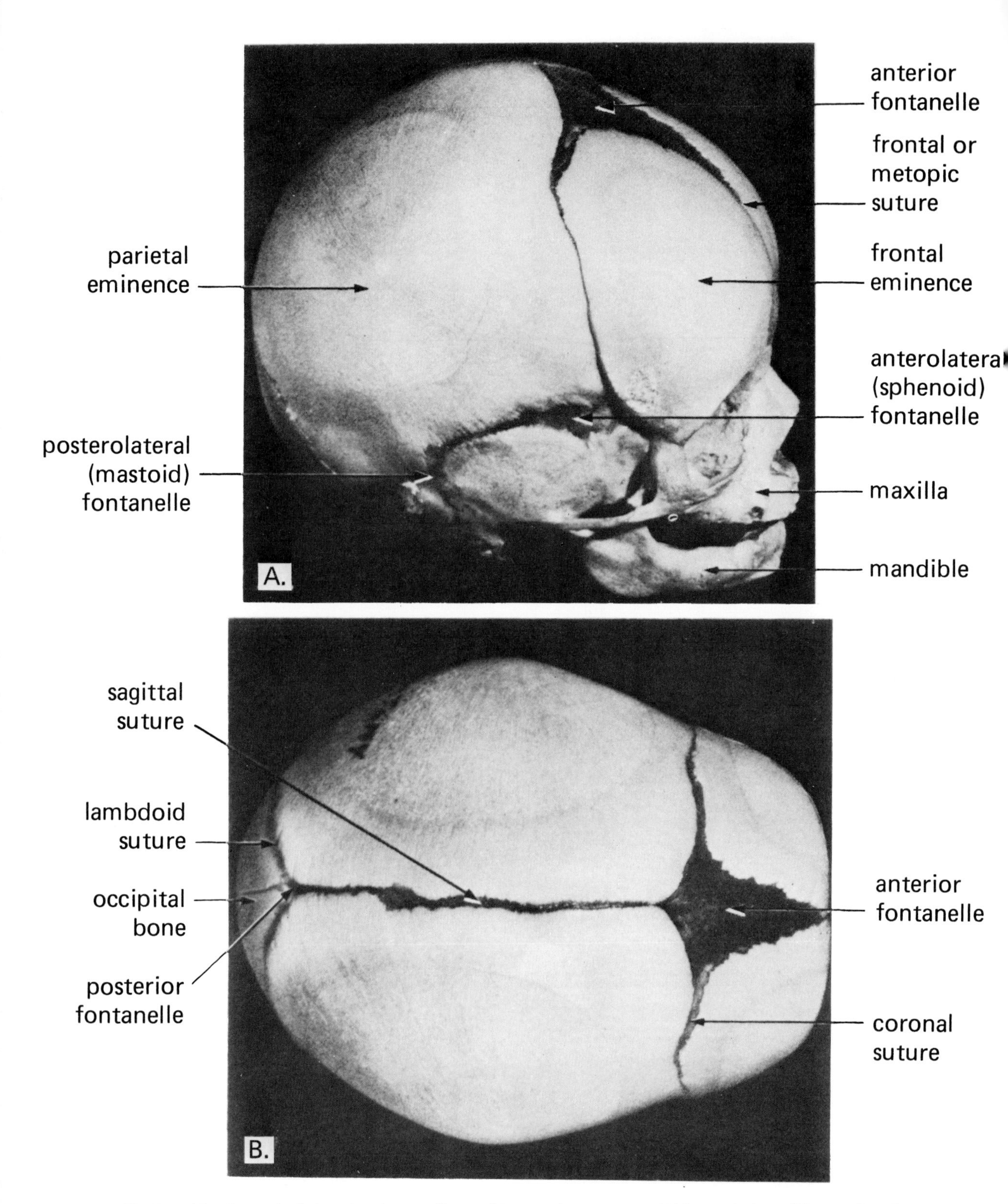

Fig. 7-5. Newborn skull showing fontanelles and incomplete sutures. (A) Lateral view, (B) superior view. (From K. L. Moore, *The Developing Human,* Ed. 2, W. B. Saunders Co., Philadelphia, 1977.)

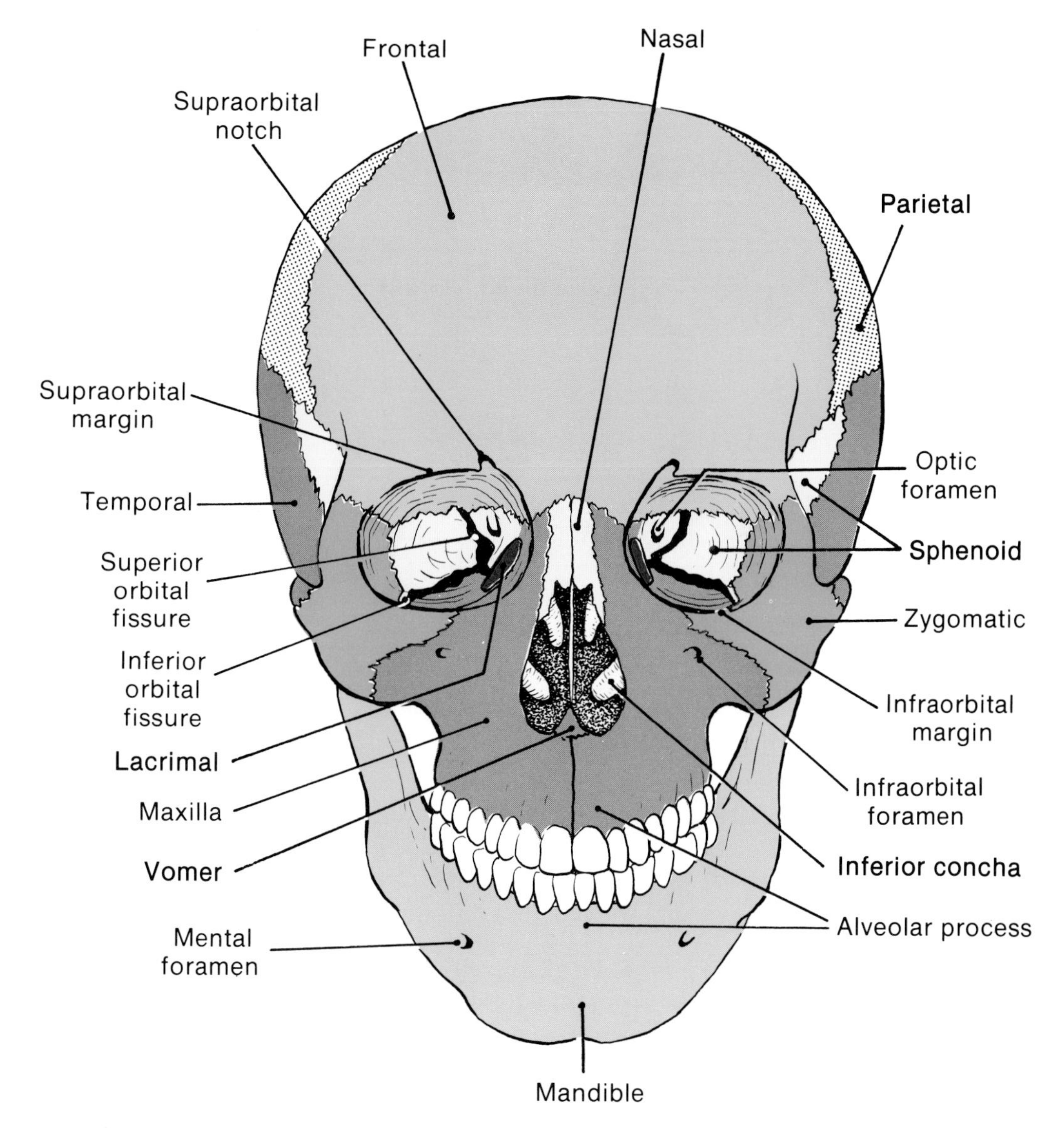

Fig. 7-6. Bones of the skull, anterior view. (Modified after *Stedman's Medical Dictionary.*)

frontal bone, which also extends backward to form the roof of the orbits. The upper border of each orbit is known as the **supraorbital margin** and is indented medially by a **supraorbital notch** (transmitting the supraorbital nerve and blood vessels from the orbit to the forehead and anterior portions of the scalp). The supraorbital notch often occurs in the form of a **supraorbital foramen.**

At the medial aspect of each orbit the frontal bone articulates with a pair of small **lacrimal bones** most easily seen in a lateral view of the skull (Fig. 7-7). The frontal bone also articulates medially with the two **maxillae** (singular: maxilla) and with two slender **nasal bones** situated on each side of the midline.

At the lateral aspects of the orbits the frontal bone articulates with the zygomatic bones. Each **zygomatic bone** is responsible for producing a lateral bulge and is commonly re-

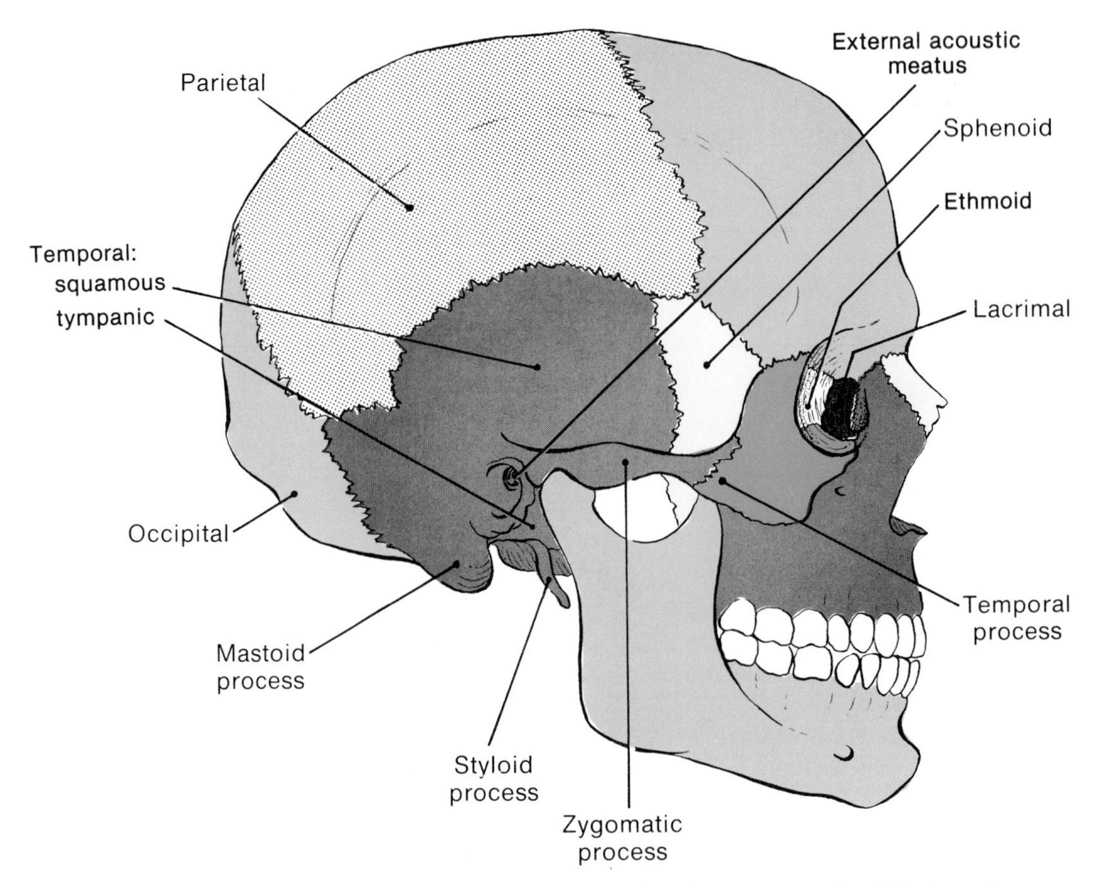

Fig. 7-7. Bones of the skull, lateral view. (Modified after *Stedman's Medical Dictionary*.)

ferred to as the "cheek bone." This bone also forms portions of the lateral wall and floor of the orbit.

Each **maxilla** articulates superiorly with the frontal bone and contributes to the medial wall and most of the floor of the orbit. The inferior margin of the orbit **(infraorbital margin)** is thus formed in large part by the maxilla. A prominent **infraorbital foramen** is situated in the maxilla below the orbit and transmits the infraorbital nerve and blood vessels to the face. The maxilla articulates laterally with the zygomatic bone and medially with the nasal bone. The maxilla also forms a portion of the lateral wall of the nasal cavity.

The inferior border of each maxilla is termed the **alveolar process (border)** because of the bony sockets (alveoli) for the upper teeth. These sockets can be seen and felt as ridges along the alveolar process. Projecting horizontally and inward from the alveolar process is the **palatine process of the maxilla** (best seen in an inferior view of the skull, Fig. 7-10) which forms most of the hard palate in the roof of the mouth. An **incisive fossa** (containing several incisive foramina) occurs anteriorly between the two palatine processes and transmits the nasopalatine nerves and vessels.

The **mandible** is a single bone and is unique with respect to other skull bones in that it has two articulations which allow it to swing freely in a variety of movements, particularly during the act of chewing (mastication). The mandible consists of a body with a ramus from each end projecting upward toward the base of the skull. The **body** contains an alveolar process similar in form and function to that in the maxillae. Two **mental foramina** are located anteriorly on the surface of the body and transmit mental nerves and vessels which supply superficial structures of the chin.

The **ramus** of the mandible can be easily seen in a lateral view since it projects upward from the posterior portion of the body (Figs. 7-7 and 7-8). The inferior portion of the ramus forms the **angle** of the mandible, while the superior portion of the ramus bifurcates into two projections: the **condylar process** (containing a head and neck) which articulates with the temporal bone at the **temporomandibular joint,** and the **coronoid process** which serves as a point of attachment for one of the muscles of mastication (temporalis muscle). The concave indentation between these two processes is the **mandibular notch.** The inner (medial) aspect of each ramus contains a **mandibular foramen** through which pass inferior alveolar nerves and vessels to enter the **mandibular canal** in the interior of the bone (Fig. 7-8). The mandibular canal ends anteriorly at the mental foramen.

The **temporal bone** is best observed from the lateral aspect of the skull and exhibits several general regions (Fig. 7-7). The flat **squamous** portion articulates with the parietal bone and with the sphenoid bone. A projection, the **zygomatic process,** extends forward from the squamous part of the temporal bone and articulates with a **temporal process** projecting backward from the zygomatic bone. The zygomatic process and temporal process together constitute the **zygomatic arch** which can be palpated externally as it extends backward from the zygomatic bone toward the ear. The zygomatic arch bridges a shallow depression along the lateral aspect of the skull. That portion superior to the arch is the **temporal fossa,** while that inferior to the arch is the **infratemporal fossa.** The temporal fossa and infratemporal fossa communicate with one another deep to the zygomatic arch.

The temporal bone also contains a **tympanic** portion which includes two parts of the ear: the external acoustic meatus and tympanic cavity. The **external acoustic (auditory) mea-**

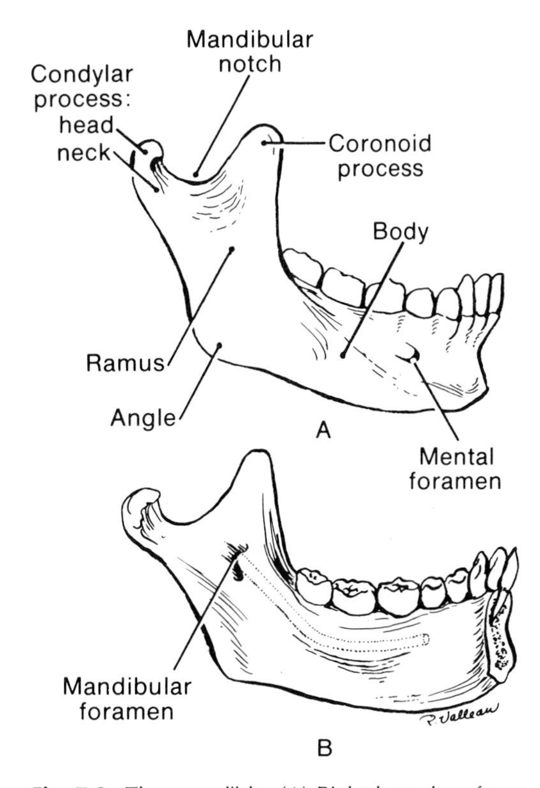

Fig. 7-8. The mandible. (A) Right lateral surface, (B) left medial surface. *Dotted lines* indicate course of mandibular canal starting at mandibular foramen and ending at mental foramen.

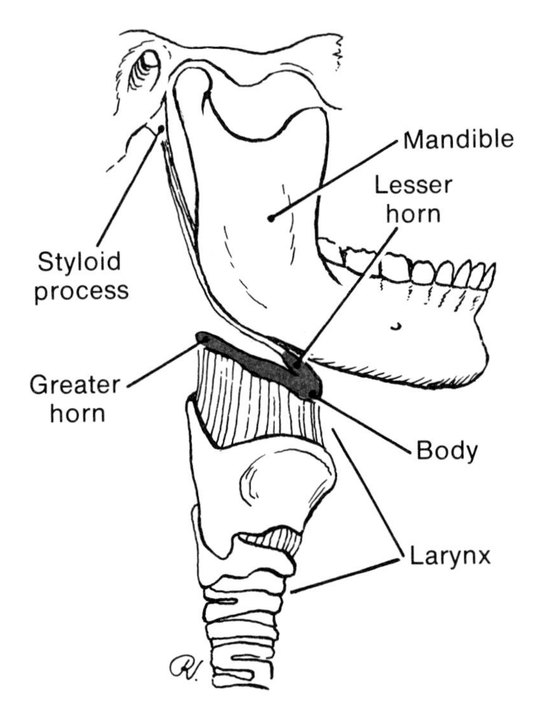

Fig. 7-9. Lateral view of the hyoid bone (red) and its relationships.

tus is an oblique passageway which begins just posterior to the point where the head of the mandible articulates with the temporal bone. The meatus extends inward to the **tympanic cavity**, where three small bones (ossicles) are lodged: the malleus, incus, and stapes. A slender **styloid process** projects inferiorly from the tympanic region and is important as a point from which a ligament (the stylohyoid ligament) suspends the hyoid bone.

The **mastoid** portion of the temporal bone is located behind the external acoustic meatus and projects inferiorly as the **mastoid process.** This region contains numerous cavities called **air spaces** which are often prone to infection (mastoiditis), especially in young children. The **petrous** portion of the temporal bone contributes to the floor of the cranial cavity and houses the inner ear. It is more easily understood when viewed from within the cranial cavity.

A portion of the **sphenoid bone** can be identified in a lateral view of the skull, although much of the bone is hidden by the coronoid process of the mandible and the zygomatic arch. The remainder of this bone is best studied from an inferior view of the skull.

The unpaired **hyoid bone** is included with the skull bones, although it is more closely associated with the larynx (Fig. 7-9). The hyoid contains a middle portion (the **body**) from which a **greater horn** (cornu) and **lesser horn** project on each side.

Skull—Inferior Aspect. The inferior aspect of the skull is most easily viewed when the mandible is removed (Fig. 7-10). The hard palate is situated anteriorly and forms part of the roof of the mouth. The hard palate consists of contributions from two bones: the **palatine processes** of the **maxillae** (already described), and the **horizontal plates** of the two **palatine bones.** At the lateral border of each horizontal plate is a **greater palatine foramen,** with a **lesser palatine foramen** located nearby through which pass greater and lesser palatine nerves and vessels, respectively. In addition to the horizontal plates, each palatine bone possesses a perpendicular plate projecting superiorly in the sagittal plane; however, because of

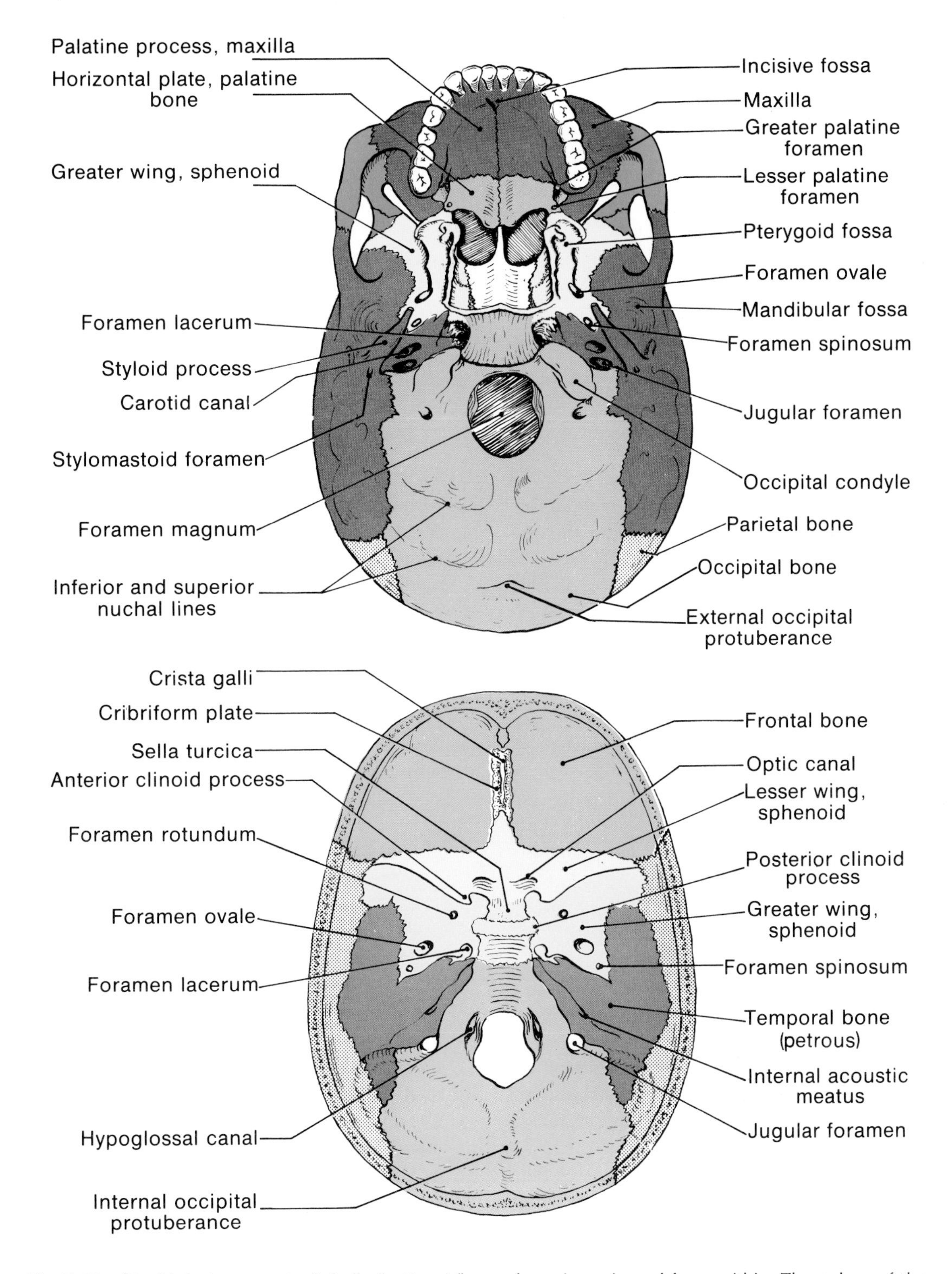

Fig. 7-10. *(Top)* Inferior aspect of skull, *(bottom)* floor of cranium viewed from within. The colors of the bones are the same as those used in Figures 7-6 and 7-7. (Modified after *Stedman's Medical Dictionary.*)

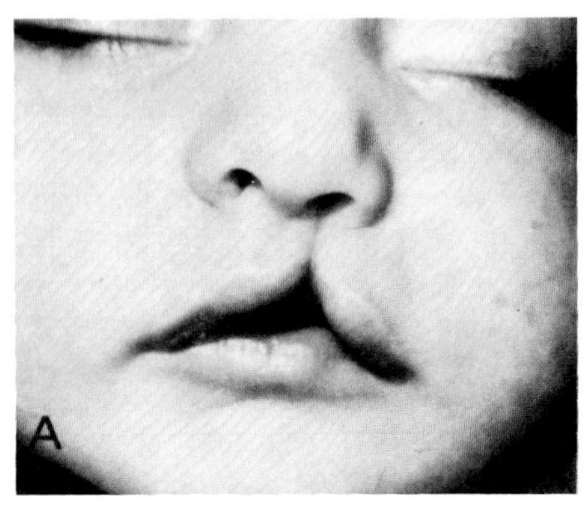

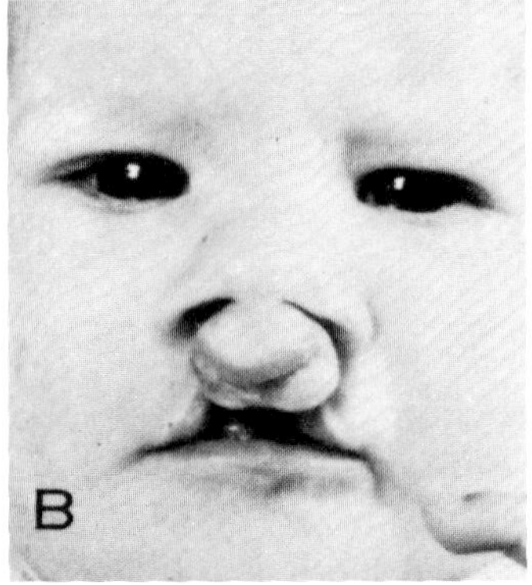

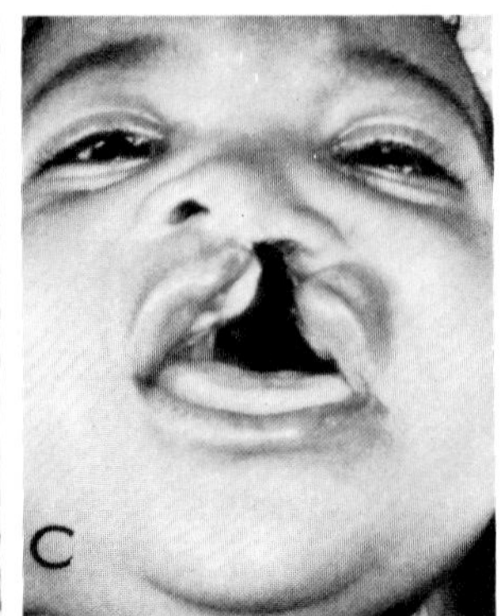

Fig. 7-11. Photographs of cleft lip and cleft palate. (A, B) Cleft lip, (C) cleft lip and cleft palate. (Courtesy of Dr. M. Edgerton, Department of Plastic Surgery, University of Virginia, from J. Langman, *Medical Embryology,* Ed. 3, The Williams & Wilkins Co., Baltimore, 1975).

its deep location the perpendicular plate of the palatine bone cannot be viewed from the anterior or inferior aspects of the skull.

Suture lines are usually detectable in the midline between the two palatine processes of the maxillae and the two horizontal plates of the palatine bones. If these bones fail to unite during embryonic development, a **cleft palate** results (Fig. 7-11) in which case food may pass from the mouth upward into the nasal cavities. A cleft palate can also interfere with speech.

Several portions of the **sphenoid bone** can also be seen from an inferior view of the skull (Fig. 7-10). The **greater wings** flare laterally and superiorly from the **body** of the sphenoid bone which arches across the midline and articulates posteriorly with the base of the occipital bone. Projecting inferiorly on each side is a pair of **pterygoid processes** between which is the **pterygoid fossa.** The pterygoid processes and fossae serve as points of attachment for important muscles associated with mastication and swallowing. The **lesser wings** of the sphenoid can best be seen from within the cranial cavity (Fig. 7-10).

The **occipital bone** is located at the posterior pole of the skull, and is characterized by a large foramen, the **foramen magnum,** through which the brain becomes continuous with the spinal cord. On each side of the foramen magnum are rounded prominences known as **occipital condyles.** These condyles articulate with the first cervical vertebra and help to support the skull as well as to allow for its movement. The occipital bone is also marked by a median crest extending posteriorly from the foramen magnum to a projection, the **external occipital protuberance.** Extending laterally from the crest and protuberance are **inferior** and **superior nuchal lines.** These surface markings indicate points of attachment for ligaments and posterior neck muscles involved in support and movements of the head.

Various parts of the temporal bone can also be seen from below, in particular the **mandibular fossa** on each side indicating the region where the ramus of the mandible articulates with the squamous portion of the temporal bone.

In contrast to the superior aspect of the skull, the inferior aspect is riddled with foramina. This is because most cranial nerves and blood vessels tend to leave and enter the cranium from below. Some of the foramina are relatively unimportant and only transmit small blood vessels such as emissary veins leaving the cranial cavity. Other foramina, however, serve as exits for important cranial nerves and as entrances and exits for major blood vessels. The principal foramina are: 1) the **foramen ovale** for the mandibular division of the trigeminal nerve, 2) the **carotid canal** for the internal carotid artery, 3) the **foramen lacerum,** a jagged aperture which is normally covered with car-

Table 7-1. Major Foramina of the Skull

NAME	BONE	STRUCTURES PASSING THROUGH
Carotid (canal)	Temporal	Internal carotid artery
Greater palatine	Between maxilla and palatine	Greater palatine nerve and vessels
Hypoglossal	Occipital	Hypoglossal nerve (XII)
Incisive (fossa)	Maxilla	Nasopalatine nerves and vessels
Inferior orbital fissure	Between maxilla and sphenoid	Maxillary division of trigeminal nerve (V); infraorbital vessels
Infraorbital	Maxilla	Infraorbital nerve & vessels
Jugular	Between petrous temporal and occipital	Glossopharyngeal (IX), vagus (X), and accessory (XI) nerves; internal jugular vein
Lesser palatine	Palatine	Lesser palatine nerves and vessels
Magnum	Occipital	Medulla oblongata and membranes, accessory nerves (XI), vertebral and spinal arteries
Mandibular	Mandible	Inferior alveolar nerve and vessels
Mental	Mandible	Mental nerve and vessels
"Olfactory" (apertures in cribriform plate)	Ethmoid	Olfactory nerve (I)
Optic	Sphenoid	Optic nerve (II) and ophthalmic artery
Ovale	Sphenoid	Mandibular division of trigeminal nerve (V)
Rotundum	Sphenoid	Maxillary division of trigeminal nerve (V)
Spinosum	Sphenoid	Middle meningeal artery
Stylomastoid	Temporal	Facial nerve (VII)
Superior orbital fissure	Sphenoid	Oculomotor (III) trochlear (IV), and abducens (VI) nerves, and ophthalmic division of trigeminal nerve (V)
Supraorbital (notch)	Frontal	Supraorbital nerve and vessels

tilage and which does not actually transmit structures of any importance, 4) the **stylomastoid foramen** through which the facial nerve emerges from the skull, 5) the **jugular foramen** transmitting the internal jugular vein, vagus, glossopharyngeal, and accessory nerves, 6) the **foramen spinosum** for the middle meningeal artery, 7) the **hypoglossal canal** (passing horizontally above the occipital condyles) which transmits the hypoglossal nerve, and 8) the **foramen magnum,** at which point the brain merges with the spinal cord.

Interior of the Skull. The internal aspect of the base of the skull is irregular because of a series of ridges, projections, deep depressions, and foramina. Three distinct fossae can be identified, and these are (from anterior to posterior): the anterior cranial fossa, middle cranial fossa, and posterior cranial fossa.

The **anterior cranial fossa** cradles portions of the cerebral hemispheres which rest upon the orbital plates of the frontal bone. These plates form most of the floor of the anterior fossa as well as the roof of the orbits. Small portions of the **ethmoid bone** can be seen where the orbital plates briefly part. These portions are the **crista galli** projecting upwards in the midline and the **cribriform plate** (Fig. 7-10). The cribriform plate lies horizontally and is perforated by numerous small apertures ("ol-

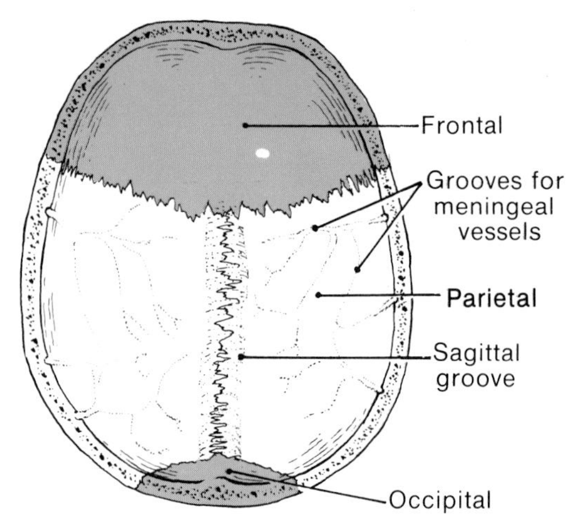

Fig. 7-12. Internal aspect of the calvaria.

factory" foramina) which transmit olfactory nerve fibers. The remainder of the ethmoid bone contributes to the nasal cavities and orbits and is hidden from view because it lies just inferior to the frontal bone and medial to the maxillae.

The **middle cranial fossa** houses portions of the cerebral hemispheres and the pituitary gland. The sphenoid and temporal bones are major contributors to the floor of this fossa. The **lesser wings** of the sphenoid represent the anterior boundary of the middle fossa as they flare anterolaterally to articulate with the orbital plates of the frontal bone. Each lesser wing of the sphenoid also contains an **optic foramen (canal)** which transmits an optic nerve and ophthalmic artery to the orbit. Caudally the lesser wings present a pair of sharp projections, the **anterior clinoid processes.** Just caudal to the anterior clinoid processes the body of the sphenoid contains a saddle-shaped depression, the **sella turcica,** in which the pituitary gland sits. **Posterior clinoid processes** project from the posterior border of the sella turcica.

Hidden from view between the lesser and greater wings of the sphenoid are the **superior orbital fissures** through which pass nerves and vessels supplying various orbital structures. (The superior orbital fissures, as well as **inferior orbital fissures** in the floor of the maxilla, can be better seen anteriorly in the orbits Figs. 7-6 and 7-14.)

Each greater wing of the sphenoid presents three foramina: 1) the **foramen rotundum** which transmits the maxillary division of the trigeminal nerve, 2) the **foramen ovale** for the mandibular division of the trigeminal nerve, and 3) the **foramen spinosum** (spinous foramen) through which passes the middle meningeal artery (Fig. 7-10). (These foramina are listed along with the other major foramina of the skull in Table 7-1.) The **petrous** (petrosal) **part** of the temporal bone contains structures of the middle and inner ear, and the summit of this region marks the division between the middle and posterior cranial fossae.

The **posterior cranial fossa** cradles the pons, medulla, and cerebellum of the brain.

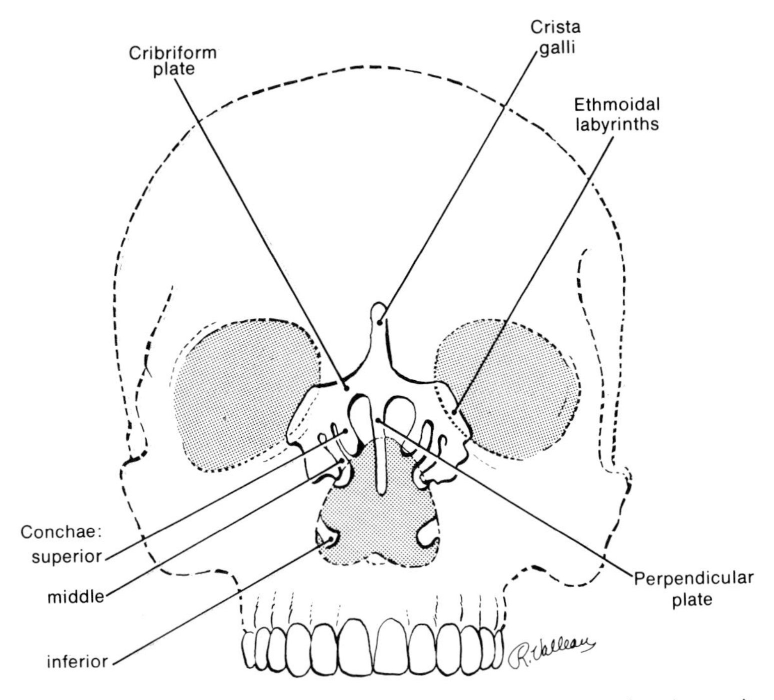

Fig. 7-13. The ethmoid bone *(solid lines)* and its position in the skull *(broken lines),* anterior view.

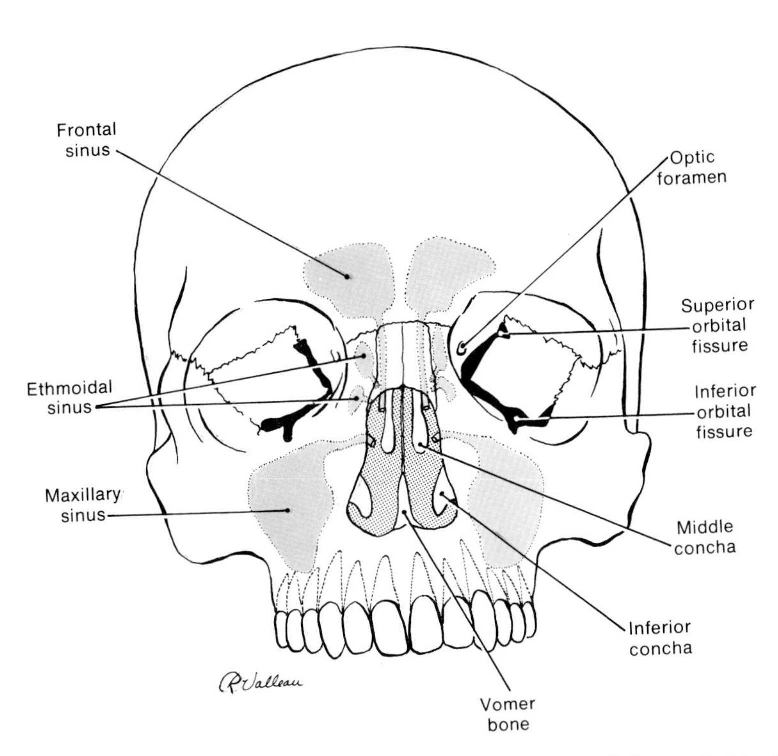

Fig. 7-14. Anterior view of the orbital fossae, nasal cavities, and paranasal sinuses (in blue), except for the sphenoidal sinus which is located in the body of the sphenoid bone.

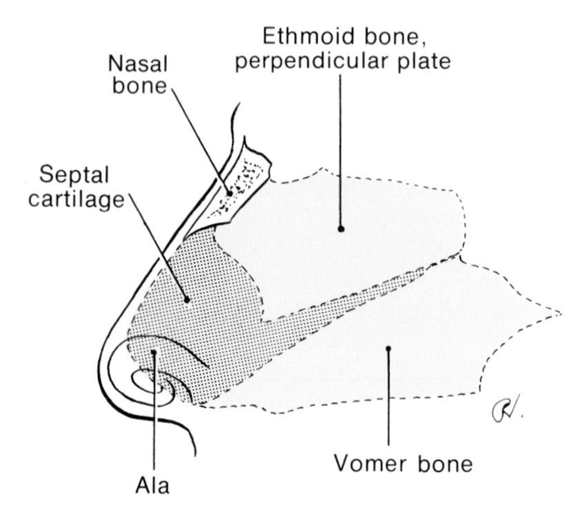

Fig.7-15. Lateral view of the nasal septum indicated in yellow, of which the cartilaginous portion is stippled.

The occipital bone contributes to most of the floor of the fossa, in the center of which is the foramen magnum noted previously. The **internal occipital protuberance** occupies a position similar to that of its counterpart on the external surface of the occipital bone. The opening of the **internal acoustic (auditory) meatus** occurs medially near the posterior aspect of the petrous portion of the temporal bone. This meatus serves as a passageway for the facial and vestibulocochlear (auditory) nerves and internal auditory vessels.

In contrast to the base of the skull, the internal surface of the **calvaria** or skull cap is relatively smooth, except for a series of grooves in which are lodged the meningeal vessels. A shallow depression, the **sagittal groove,** runs along the midline and contains the superior sagittal sinus, a venous structure carrying blood from the brain and cranial cavity (Fig. 7-12).

The Orbital Fossae and Nasal Cavities. The bony sockets for the eyeballs are composed of contributions from several bones (including the frontal, ethmoid, lacrimal, maxillary, zygomatic, sphenoid, and palatine bones). The medial wall is quite thin and thus more easily damaged than is the lateral wall, which is stronger and can withstand blows against the side of the head. Each orbit contains an **optic foramen, superior orbital fissure,** and **inferior orbital fissure** for the entrance and exit of nerves (Fig. 7-6).

The walls of the nasal cavities likewise are represented by several bones (the ethmoid, frontal, sphenoid, lacrimal, maxillary, vomer, and palatine bones). Of these, the **ethmoid bone** plays a major role. The cribriform plate of the ethmoid lies horizontally, with the **crista galli** projecting upward into the anterior cranial fossa (Figs. 7-10 and 7-13). The **perpendicular plate** of the ethmoid contributes to the upper part of the nasal septum, whereas the **ethmoidal labyrinths** form the upper lateral walls of the nasal cavities as well as the medial walls of the orbits (Fig. 7-13). From the medial aspect of each labyrinth, two scroll-like bony processes project into each nasal cavity. These are the **superior** and **middle conchae.** In con-

The Upper Limb

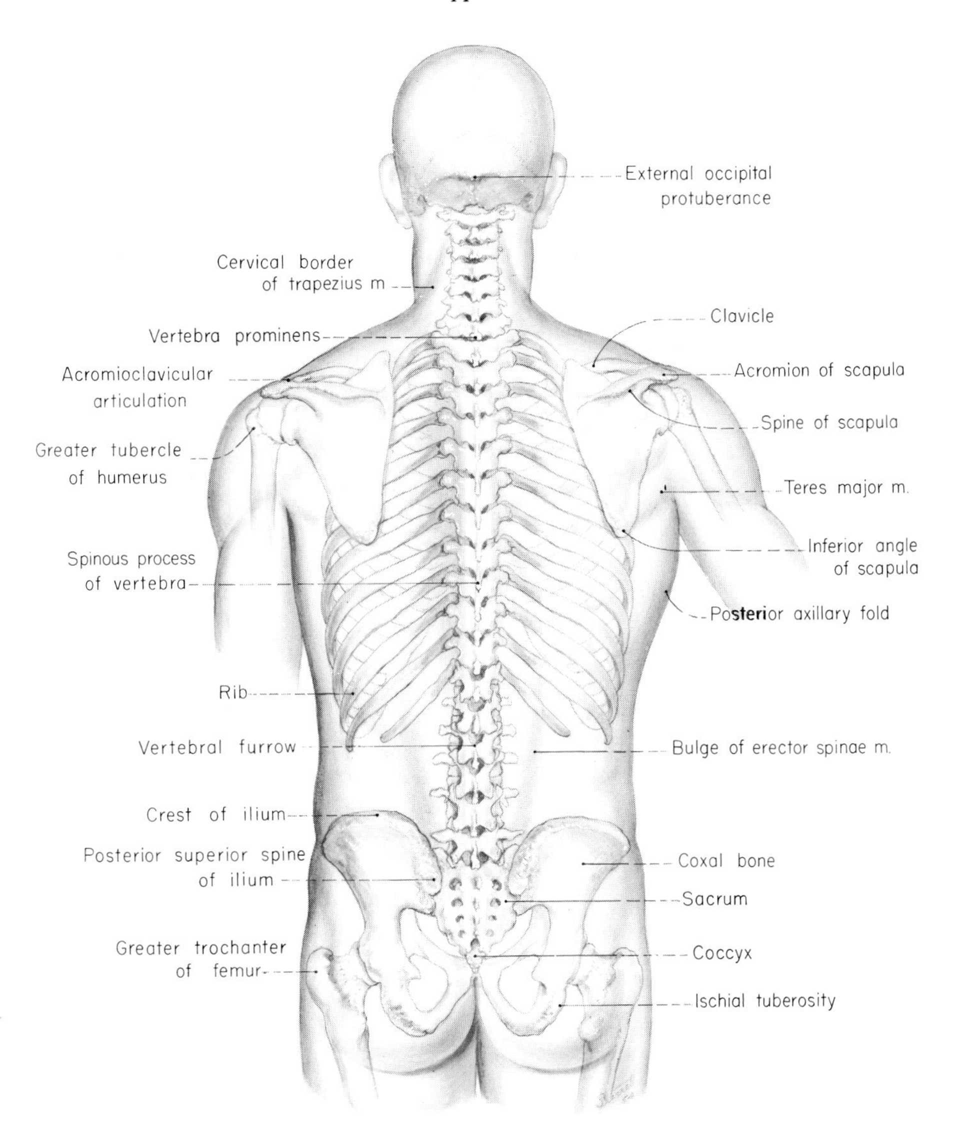

Fig. 7-16. Surface anatomy of the vertebral column and associated bones of the back. (From *Essentials of Human Anatomy,* Sixth Edition, by Russell T. Woodburne. Copyright © 1957, 1961, 1965, 1968, 1973, 1978 by Oxford University Press, Inc. Reprinted by permission.)

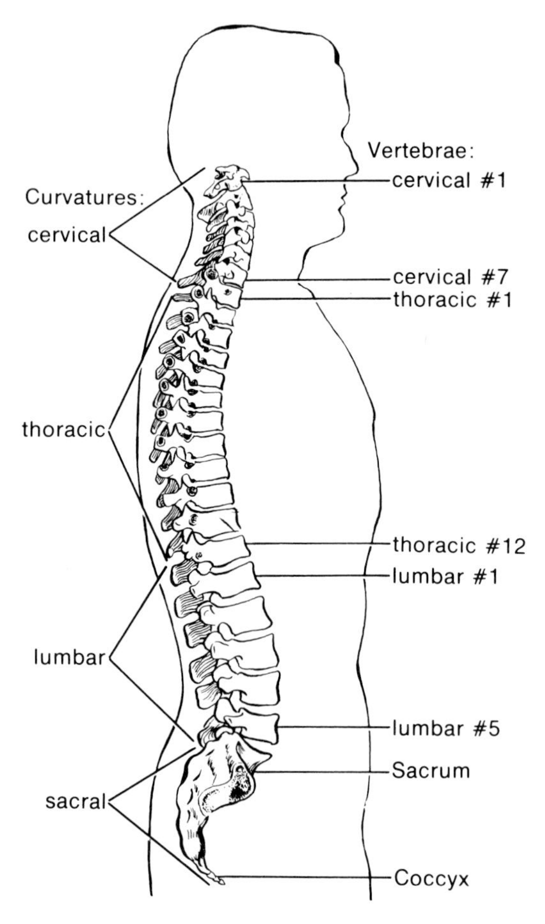

Fig. 7-17. Vertebral column, lateral view.

trast, the **inferior conchae** occur as separate bones attached to the lateral walls of the nasal cavities. The ethmoidal labyrinths and the conchae contain air spaces similar to those in the mastoid portion of the temporal bone.

The **nasal cavity** is subdivided into two nasal passages by means of the nasal septum. The **nasal septum** is a median structure composed anteriorly of cartilage and posteriorly of bone. The inferior portion of the bony part is the **vomer,** a single bone which slopes upward and backward (Figs. 7-14 and 7-15). The nasal region is described in greater detail with respect to the respiratory system.

Paranasal Sinuses. The paranasal sinuses consist of air spaces whose function is obscure; however, they may serve to lighten the skull, to provide insulation around the nasal cavities, or to assist in resonation during speaking. There are four pairs of sinuses: maxillary, frontal, ethmoidal, and sphenoidal. The **maxillary sinuses** are the largest and occupy a central position in each maxilla (Fig. 7-14). Because of the close relationship with the upper teeth, infections in a maxillary sinus often can produce toothaches; conversely, abscesses deep in the roots of the upper teeth can spread to the maxillary sinuses. The **frontal sinuses** are found in the frontal bones at variable distances above the supraorbital margins. The **ethmoidal sinuses** occur in the ethmoidal labyrinths, the **sphenoidal sinuses** within the body of the sphenoid bone. All of these sinuses communicate with the nasal cavities by means of one or more tiny apertures and are in indirect communication with one another; hence, an infection in one sinus, or in the nose itself, can easily spread to other sinuses, and occasionally even to the orbits and anterior cranial fossa. Also, skull fractures may involve the paranasal sinuses, and blood from damaged vessels may then ooze into the mouth, orbits, or nose.

Axial Skeleton: Vertebral Column

The vertebral column consists of a series of bones called **vertebrae** which provide rigid support for the head, neck, and trunk, as well as flexibility for movement in these regions. The vertebral column also serves as a protective passageway for the spinal cord and as a point of direct attachment for the ribs and pelvic girdle (Fig. 7-16). (The pectoral girdle is only indirectly associated with the vertebral column.) There are normally 26 vertebrae which are grouped and named as follows (Fig. 7-17). The upper 7 are **cervical vertebrae** which support the head and neck. The next 12 are **thoracic vertebrae** to which the 12 pairs of ribs are attached. The lower 5 are massive **lumbar vertebrae** which support the thorax. Below the fifth lumbar vertebra is the **sacrum,** composed actually of 5 vertebrae fused into a single bone. At the lowermost end of the vertebral column is the **coccyx** ("tailbone") consisting of a variable number of small rudimentary bones (usually 4) partially fused and showing little mobility.

Within each regional group, the vertebrae are numbered consecutively from superior to inferior; thus lumbar vertebra 1 is inferior to thoracic vertebra 12 and superior to lumbar vertebra 2. The vertebral column is often used as a point of reference for describing the position of other structures of the body. For example, the large artery known as the abdominal aorta bifurcates into two vessels at the level of lumbar vertebra 4.

The adult vertebral column shows four curves, of which two are concave posteriorly (in the cervical and lumbar regions), and two are convex posteriorly (in the thoracic and sacral regions) (Fig. 7-17). At the time of birth the vertebral column shows only a slight thoracic curvature and a prominent sacral curvature, after which the two concave curves in the cervical and lumbar regions become prominent as one acquires the ability to support the head and to sit and stand upright (Fig. 7-18). An abnormal accentuation of the thoracic curvature results in **kyphosis** (hunchback); an exaggerated lumbar curvature results in **lordosis** (swayback), while a deviation of the vertebral column in the lateral plane is termed **scoliosis** (Fig. 7-19).

The Typical Vertebra. Although the vertebrae possess special features relative to their

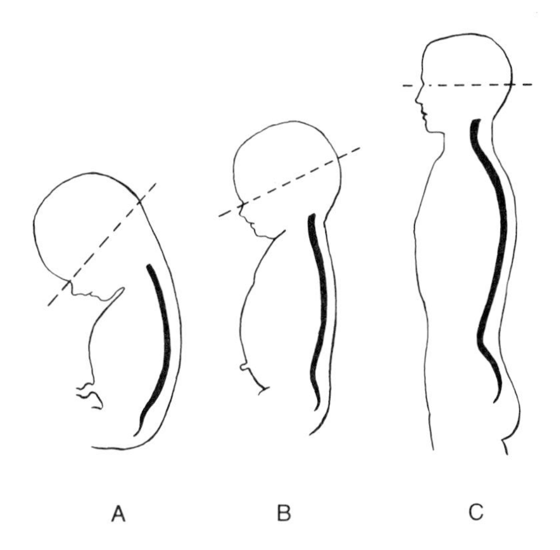

Fig. 7-18. Schematic view of changes in the curvatures of the vertebral column. (A) In the midterm fetus, (B) at birth, (C) in the adult. (Modified from *Grant's Method.*)

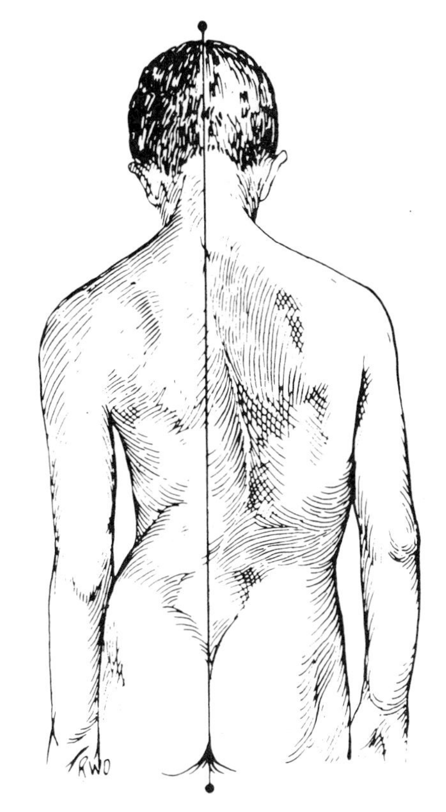

Fig. 7-19. Scoliosis, a lateral deviation of the vertebral column. (From *Stedman's Medical Dictionary,* Ed. 23, The Williams & Wilkins Co., Baltimore, 1976.)

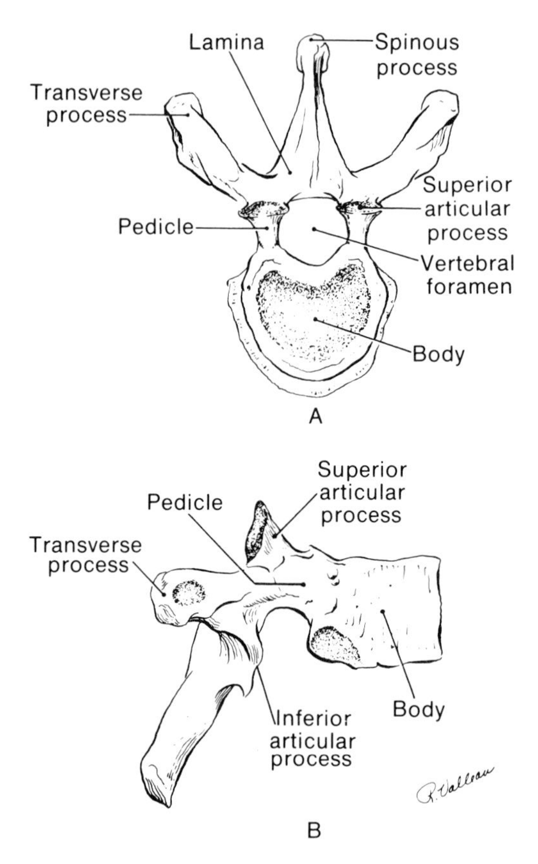

Fig. 7-20. A typical vertebra. (A) Superior view, (B) lateral view.

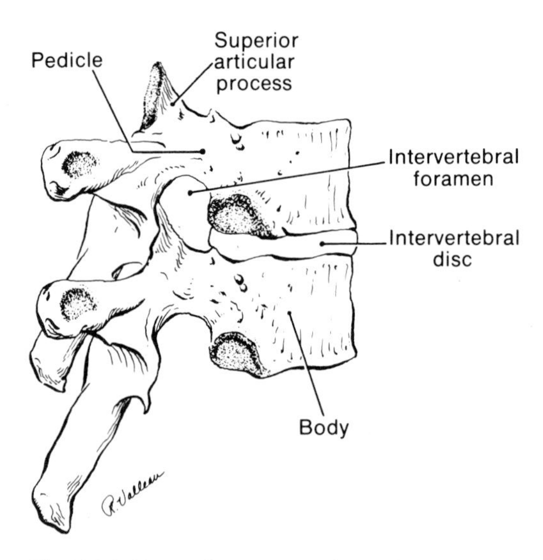

Fig. 7-21. Two adjacent vertebrae, lateral view.

location in the vertebral column, certain characteristics are shared in common. Most vertebrae contain a body, an arch, and various processes or projections (Fig. 7-20). In the anatomical position the **body** projects anteriorly as a solid flattened disc. It is separated from the body of an adjacent vertebra by a fibrocartilaginous **intervertebral disc** (Fig. 7-21). Extending posteriorly from the body of the vertebra is the **vertebral arch** consisting of right and left **pedicles** which attach it to the body, and right and left **laminae** (singular: lamina) uniting in the midline, at which point a **spinous process** projects posteriorly. The spinous process is the only portion of the vertebra capable of being palpated externally from the body surface. Each vertebral arch encloses a cavity known as the **vertebral foramen.** The series of vertebral foramina formed by adjacent vertebrae constitutes the **vertebral canal** through which passes the spinal cord.

A **transverse process** projects laterally at the junction of the lamina and pedicle. The laminae of adjacent vertebrae tend to overlap slightly, and each vertebra articulates with the vertebra above and below by means of facets located on **superior** and **inferior articular processes,** respectively (Fig. 7-21). Gaps occur between adjacent pedicles and represent **intervertebral foramina** through which the spinal nerves and vessels can pass to and from the vertebral canal (Fig. 7-26).

Regional differences occur among the vertebrae and suggest functional attributes. For example the first two cervical vertebrae are adapted to allow movement of the head at the summit of the vertebral column, whereas the thoracic vertebrae show specializations for the attachments of the ribs. As one progresses down the vertebral column the vertebrae become larger since more weight must be borne. In general there is a gradual transition in features between each region so that the lowermost cervical vertebra and uppermost thoracic vertebra resemble one another, as do the lowermost thoracic and uppermost lumbar vertebrae.

Cervical Vertebrae. Of the seven cervical

vertebrae the first two (atlas and axis) show a unique form and are important for various skull movements. The **atlas** is so named because it supports the heavy skull (much as the Greek mythological Atlas supported the world on his shoulders). The superior aspect of the atlas contains two concave **superior articular facets** which articulate with the occipital condyles of the skull and enable the skull to nod forward and backward (Fig. 7-22). The atlas lacks a body and spine, but it has an **anterior arch,** a **posterior arch,** and two transverse processes. Each transverse process contains a **transverse foramen.**

The second vertebra, or **axis,** contains a **body** with a pair of **superior articular facets,** a spinous process (referred to as being **bifid** because it bifurcates distally), and two transverse processes, each with a transverse foramen (Fig. 7-23). The most distinctive feature of the axis is the **dens (odontoid process)** which projects forward to articulate against the anterior arch of the atlas, thereby allowing the skull to turn from side to side (Figs. 7-24 and 7-25).

Cervical vertebrae 3 through 6 show characteristics typical of most vertebrae, except that they contain transverse foramina and bifid spinous processes. In the articulated vertebral column, the transverse foramina of cervical vertebrae 1–6 form a canal which transmits the vertebral artery, vein, and nerve plexus upward to the cranial cavity (Fig. 7-25). The 7th cervical vertebra is characterized by a long prominent spine which is not bifid. Although this vertebra shows a transverse process with a small transverse foramen, it does not transmit the vertebral vessels and nerve plexus. The 7th vertebra may occasionally possess a rudimentary rib, in which case difficulties can arise if it compresses blood vessels or nerves in the cervical area.

Thoracic Vertebrae. The 12 thoracic vertebrae are unique in that they possess facets for articulation with the ribs (Fig. 7-26). Also, the spinous processes of most thoracic vertebrae are relatively long and thin, and those of thoracic vertebrae 2–10 tend to slope posteriorly and inferiorly. The spinous process on the first thoracic vertebra is thick and prominent. The

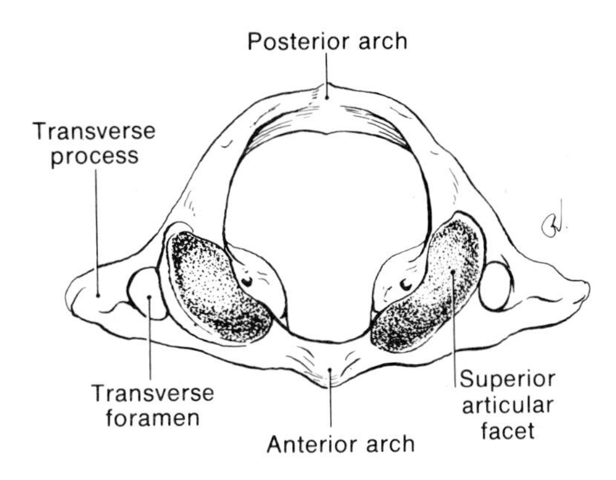

Fig. 7-22. Atlas, superior view.

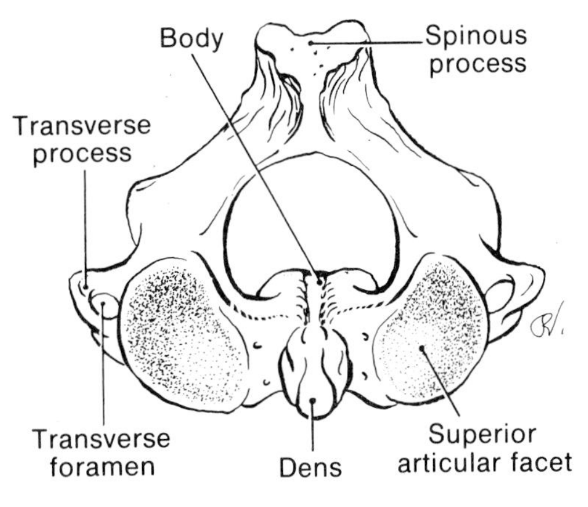

Fig. 7-23. Axis, superior view and tilted slightly forward to show the dens.

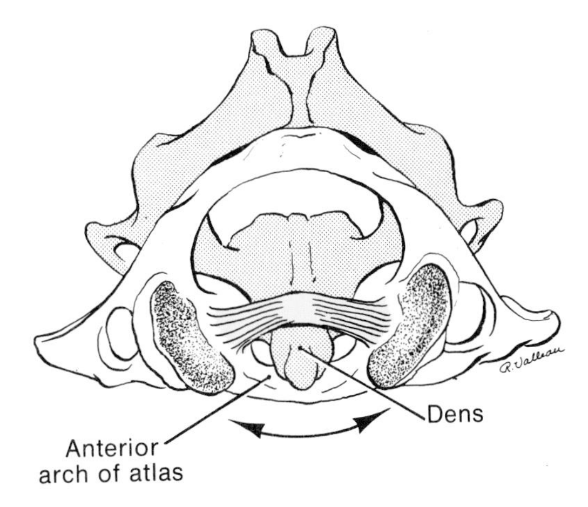

Fig. 7-24. Superior view of atlas and axis (gray stippled) in articulation and tilted slightly forward. *Arrow* indicates direction of movement taken by the atlas around the axis. The ligament (yellow) of the atlas keeps the dens in place against the anterior arch of the atlas.

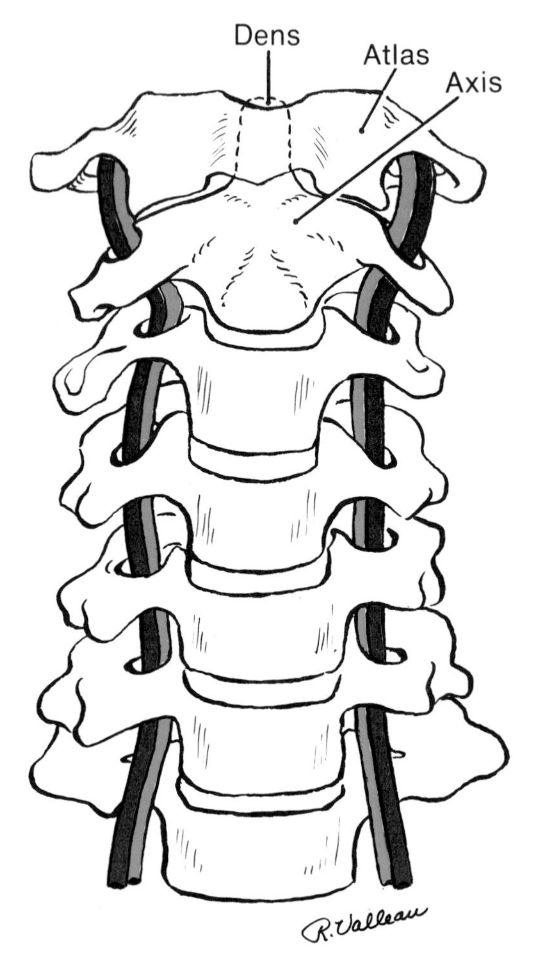

Fig. 7-25. Anterior view of articulated cervical vertebrae in the anatomical position. (Intervertebral discs not shown.) A portion of the dens from the axis is shown in *broken line* to illustrate its position behind the anterior arch of the atlas. The vertebral arteries and veins pass upward within the transverse foramina of the first six vertebrae.

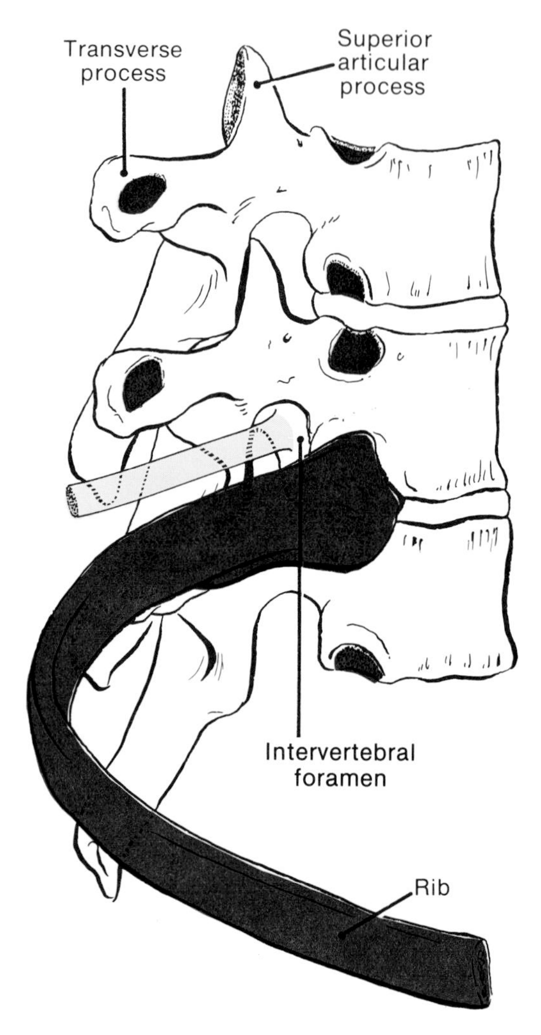

Fig. 7-26. Lateral view of three thoracic vertebrae showing facets (red) for articulation with ribs, one of which is indicated in red. The intervertebral foramen is the site where a spinal nerve (yellow) exits from the vertebral canal.

eleventh and twelfth vertebrae exhibit shorter spinous processes which do not slope very much, and the larger bodies of these vertebrae resemble those of lumbar vertebrae.

Lumbar Vertebrae. The lumbar vertebrae are characterized by massive thick bodies, short and flat spinous processes, and large transverse processes which do not bear ribs (Fig. 7-27). The fifth lumbar vertebra is generally the largest.

Sacrum. The sacrum consists of five sacral vertebrae and their intervening intervertebral discs which in the adult have all fused into a single triangular bone (Fig. 7-28). The posterior surface of the sacrum shows a convex curve from which projects a median crest represent-

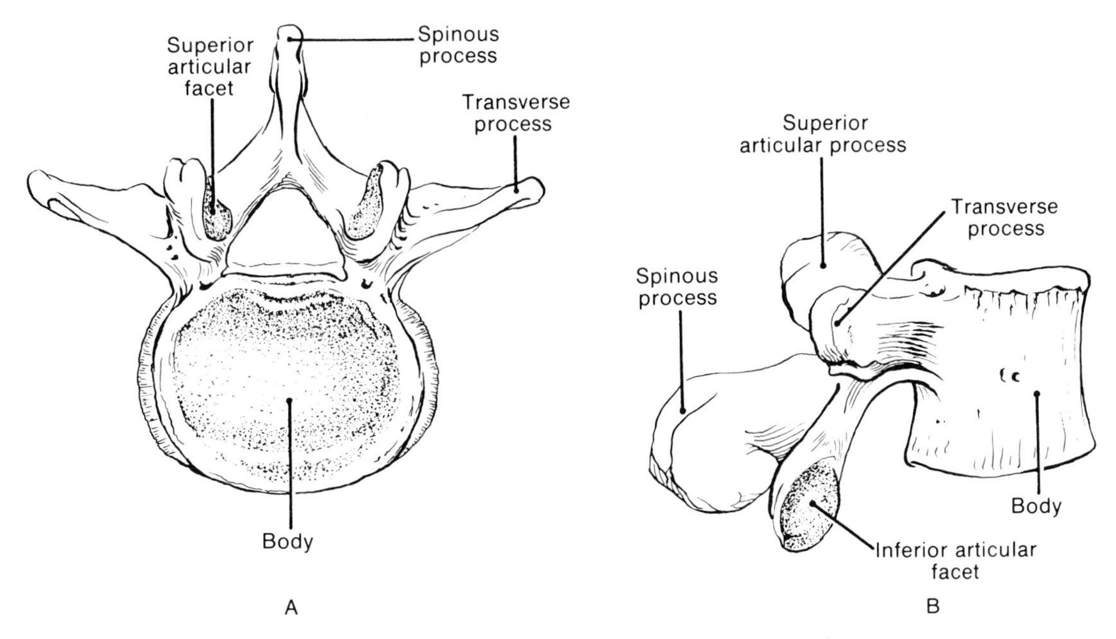

Fig. 7-27. Lumbar vertebra. (A) Superior view, (B) lateral view.

ing the fused spinous processes. The laminae are likewise fused, and beyond them are four pairs of **posterior sacral foramina.** Anteriorly, a series of transverse ridges marks the region at which the adjacent vertebral bodies and intervertebral discs have fused. Just lateral to the fused bodies are four pairs of **anterior sacral foramina.** (The anterior and posterior foramina transmit anterior and posterior divisions of the sacral nerves, respectively.) The vertebral foramina form the **sacral canal.**

Projecting laterally from the superior region of the sacrum is a pair of wing-shaped expansions, or **alae,** (singular: **ala**) which articulate with the pelvic girdle. The **sacral promontory** is a liplike ridge projecting anteriorly from the body of the 1st sacral vertebra.

Coccyx. The inferior end of the vertebral column is represented by a series of rudimentary and partially fused vertebrae collectively termed the coccyx (Fig. 7-28). It is usually difficult to identify typical vertebral features, although the first coccygeal vertebra shows reduced transverse processes. Slight mobility does exist between various portions of the coccyx, and this plays an important role in females during childbirth when the coccyx can be pushed posteriorly as the head of the infant passes along the birth canal.

Joints and Movements of the Vertebral Column

The degree of movement permitted in each region of the vertebral column depends on a variety of factors, including the types of joints, size and shape of the vertebrae and intervertebral discs, and the vertebral ligaments. The cervical and lumbar regions of the vertebral column show greater mobility than does the thoracic region, which is somewhat limited by the overlapping spinous processes and laminae.

The joint between the atlas and skull is the **atlanto-occipital joint** and enables one to move the head forward and backward, as in nodding "yes." The opposite movement of shaking the head "no" involves side-to-side movement at the **atlanto-axial joint** between the atlas and axis. The dens of the axis is held

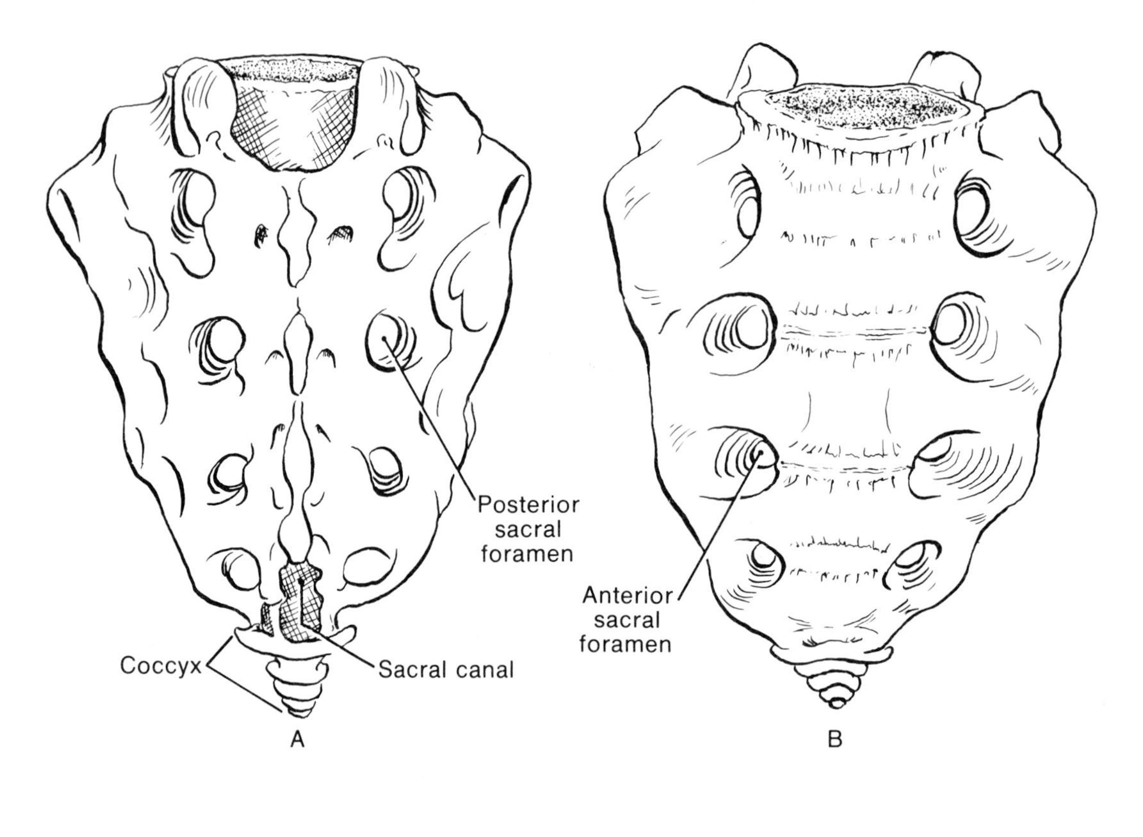

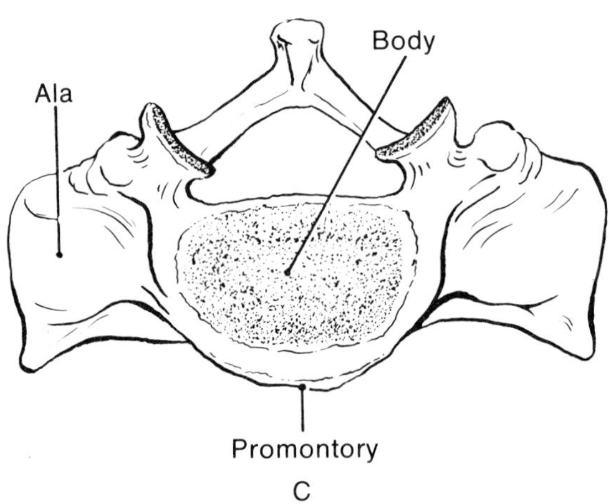

Fig. 7-28. Sacrum and coccyx. (A) Posterior view, (B) anterior view, (C) superior view of sacrum.

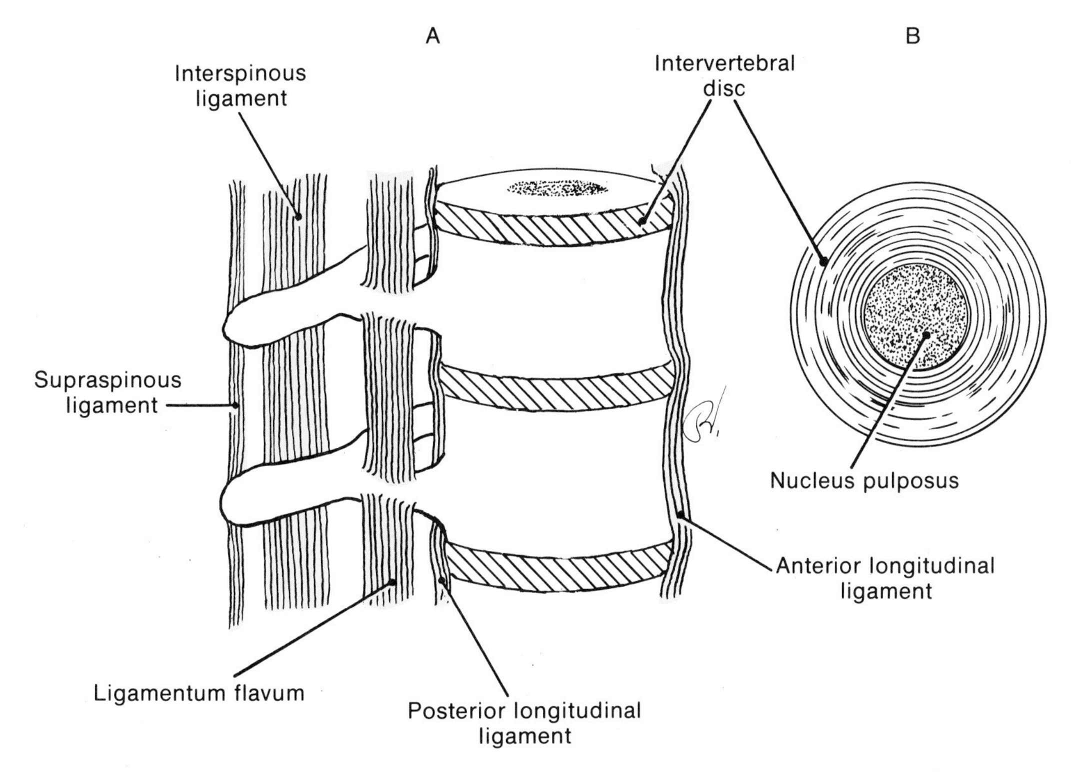

Fig. 7-29. (A) Ligaments of the vertebral column. (The ligamentum flavum is paired but is shown on one side only. Transverse processes of vertebrae are not shown.) (B) Intervertebral disc showing nucleus pulposus.

in place against the anterior arch of the atlas by means of the **transverse ligament** of the atlas (Fig. 7-24.).

The joints between the vertebral bodies are classified as symphyses, since an **intervertebral disc** of fibrocartilage occurs between two adjacent bodies. These joints allow the movements of flexion and extension. They are stabilized by **longitudinal ligaments** (**anterior** and **posterior**) which connect two adjacent vertebral bodies (Fig. 7-29). In the center of each intervertebral disc is a mass of spongy material called the **nucleus pulposus,** which represents a remnant of the notochord of the embryo. If a disc ruptures, the nucleus pulposus oozes outward, and considerable pain can occur from irritation of nearby nerves. The discs in the thoracic region are thin and do not allow as much movement between thoracic vertebral bodies as do the thicker discs in the cervical and lumbar regions.

The small joints which occur between adjacent laminae are synovial in nature and tend to allow slight rotation movements. Adjacent laminae are connected by ligaments termed the **ligamenta flava,** (singular: **ligamentum flavum,** meaning "yellow ligament" composed of yellow elastic tissue), while **supraspinous ligaments** and **interspinous ligaments** bridge several of the spinous processes. In the cervical region the supraspinous ligament is prominent and is called the **ligamentum nuchae** and is particularly well-developed in four-footed animals in order to help support the heavy skull.

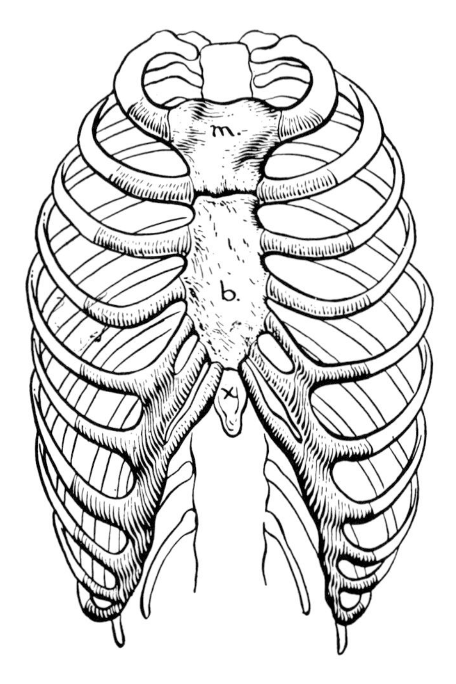

Fig. 7-30. The thoracic cage. Portions of the sternum are designated as m, manubrium; b, body; x, xiphoid process. (From J. V. Basmajian, *Primary Anatomy,* Ed. 7, The Williams & Wilkins Co., Baltimore, 1976.)

Axial Skeleton: Thoracic Cage

The thoracic cage is considered a part of the axial skeleton and functions during respiration as well as in protecting vital organs such as the heart and lungs. The ribs, costal cartilages, sternum, thoracic vertebrae, and thoracic intervertebral discs comprise the thoracic cage. The upper part of the cage is dome-shaped and is slightly narrower than the lower part (Fig. 7-30).

The thorax shows a surprising degree of mobility despite its rather sturdy, immovable appearance. This mobility is imparted particularly by the costal cartilages and by synovial joints between the ribs and vertebrae.

Ribs. The 12 pairs of ribs articulate posteriorly with the 12 thoracic vertebrae. Anteriorly each rib joins a bar of hyaline cartilage, the **costal cartilage.** The ribs may be classified as true, false, and floating on the basis of what happens to the costal cartilages anteriorly. Thus, ribs 1–7 are termed **true (vertebrosternal) ribs** because the costal cartilage of each rib articulates directly with the sternum, the elongate flattened bone lying anteriorly in the midline. Ribs 8–12 are the **false ribs** because their costal cartilages do not articulate directly with the sternum. The costal cartilages of ribs 8–10 join the next adjacent cartilage superiorly and thus the ribs are termed **vertebrochondral** because they articulate only indirectly with the sternum via costal cartilage 7. The two oblique arches formed by these lower cartilages on each side are the **costal margins** (Fig. 7-31). The costal cartilages at the tips of ribs 11 and 12 fail to join adjacent cartilages. Since they end freely, ribs 11 and 12 are termed **floating** (or **vertebral**) **ribs** (Fig. 7-30).

Each rib consists of a head, neck, and shaft (Fig. 7-32). The **head** shows two articular facets, one of which articulates with the body of the thoracic vertebra bearing the same number as the rib, and the other articulates with the body of the vertebra above (Fig. 7-26). (The portion of the head between the two facets lies directly against the intervertebral disc.) The

neck of the rib curves slightly posteriorly and ends in a **tubercle** containing a facet for articulating with the transverse process of the corresponding thoracic vertebra. The **shaft** is the remainder of the rib and slopes posteriorly and inferiorly before turning forward at the **angle** of the rib. The shaft then continues anteriorly and inferiorly and unites with its costal cartilage. Along the lower inner aspect of each shaft is the **costal groove** carrying intercostal vessels and nerves.

Sternum. The sternum consists of three segments: the manubrium, body, and xiphoid process (Fig. 7-31). The **manubrium** is the uppermost wedge-shaped portion and is characterized by a concave superior border, the **jugular notch,** which can be easily palpated. The two clavicles of the pectoral girdle articulate with the manubrium at the **sternoclavicular** joints, below which the costal cartilages of the first pair of ribs also join the manubrium. The manubrium in turn articulates below with the body of the sternum, at which point a slight anteroposterior angle occurs. This is known as the **sternal angle** and serves as an important bony landmark, since the second costal cartilages also join the sternum at this point. Deeper structures of the thorax can be located relative to the sternal angle, and the angle itself lies on approximately the same horizontal plane as the intervertebral disc between the 4th and 5th thoracic vertebrae.

The **body** of the sternum is characterized by three transverse lines which mark the junctions of what were separate segments during embryonic development. Indeed, the union of these segments is still incomplete in children. The costal cartilages of ribs 3, 4, and 5 articulate with the sternum at the lateral borders of the transverse lines. The costal cartilages of ribs 6 and 7 articulate at the lower lateral border of the body.

Near the junctions of the 7th costal cartilage, the body of the sternum articulates with the **xiphoid process,** a slender variable structure consisting of cartilage and bone. The xiphoid process can seldom be palpated, but it proj-

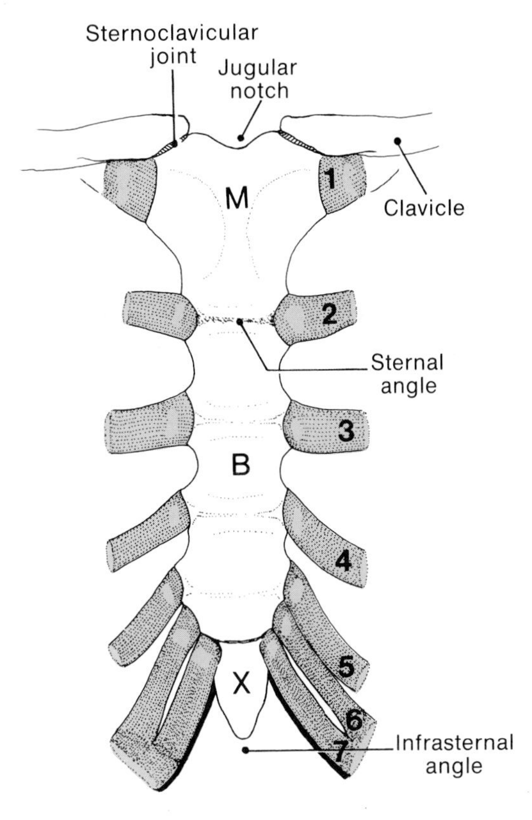

Fig. 7-31 Anterior view of sternum showing articulations with costal cartilages (blue) and clavicles. M, manubrium; B, body; X, xiphoid process. The dark black line indicates the costal margins.

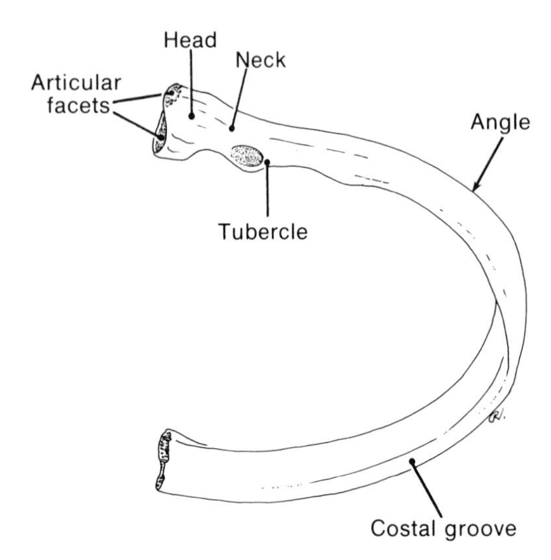

Fig. 7-32. Posterior view of a typical rib.

ects downward into the apex of the **infrasternal angle** formed between the cartilaginous **costal margins** as they pass obliquely upward to join the body of the sternum.

Because of its superficial location, the sternum is often the site where bone marrow can be sampled by means of needle puncture and aspiration. Since the heart lies deep to the sternum, strong rhythmic pressure against the sternum can actually compress the heart chambers and help to propel blood out of the heart. This maneuver is widely used as an emergency procedure during a cardiac arrest.

Appendicular Skeleton

The appendicular skeleton consists of the shoulder and pelvic girdles and the bones of the upper and lower limbs.

Shoulder (Pectoral) Girdle

The shoulder (pectoral) girdle contains two pairs of bones, the scapula and clavicle, which are closely associated with the upper portion of the thoracic cage (Fig. 7-3).

Scapula. The **scapula** is a flat triangular-shaped bone overlying the posterior portions of the upper 2–7 ribs. The scapula presents three borders: a long **medial (vertebral) border** which extends parallel to the vertebral column, a short **superior border** which slopes laterally out to the tip of the shoulder, and an oblique **lateral border** which completes the third side of the triangle (Fig. 7-33). The junction between the medial and lateral borders is the **inferior angle** of the scapula which is easily palpated and moves freely as the arm moves. At the junction between the superior and lateral borders is the concave **glenoid cavity** which is rimmed with fibrocartilage, the **glenoid labrum.** This serves to deepen the glenoid cavity so that it can articulate more closely with the humerus of the arm. The superior border of the scapula contains the **scapular notch** (through which passes the suprascapular nerve) and a hook-shaped projection, the **coracoid process** which serves as a point of attachment for some muscles.

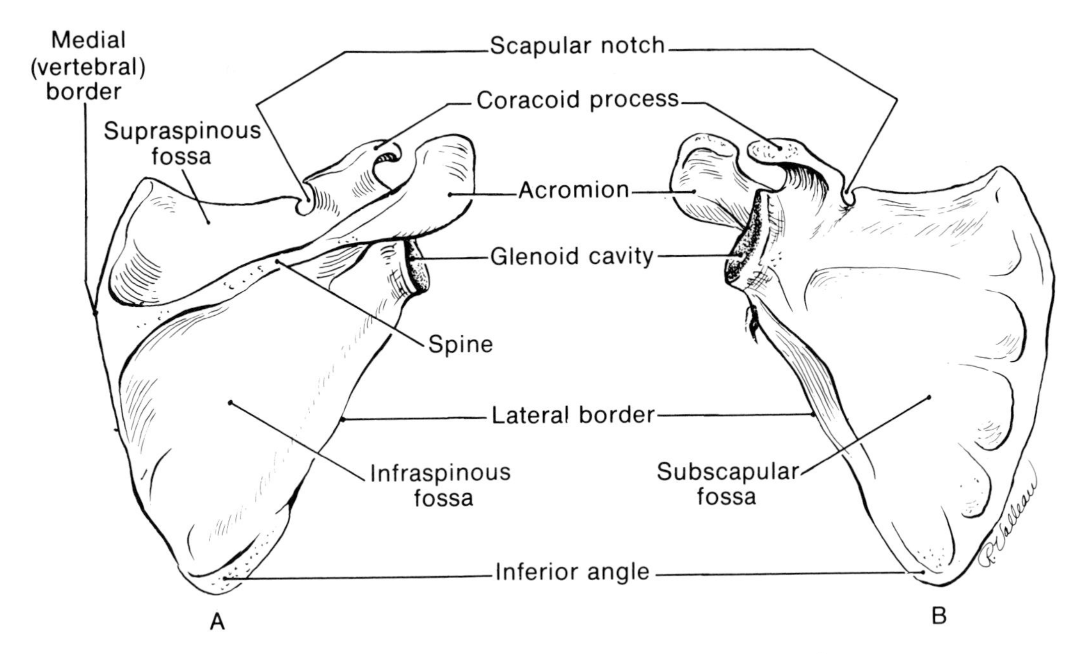

Fig. 7-33. Right scapula. (A) Posterior view, (B) anterior view.

The posterior surface of the scapula is slightly convex posteriorly and presents a prominent ridge, the **spine** of the scapula, which begins near the upper third of the medial border and slopes laterally and superiorly out to the tip of the shoulder. At this point the spine expands and ends as the **acromion.** On the posterior surface of the scapula a **supraspinous fossa** occurs superior to the spine; inferior to the spine is the **infraspinous fossa.**

The anterior or costal surface of the scapula is smooth and slightly concave and thus fits easily over the posterior curvatures of the ribs. The concavity of this surface is the **subscapular fossa.** The subscapular, supraspinous, and infraspinous fossae contain muscles which act on the upper limb and which are named the subscapular, supraspinatus, and infraspinatus muscles, respectively.

Clavicle. The **clavicle** ("collarbone") is an S-shaped bone which articulates laterally with the acromion of the scapula **(acromioclavicular joint)** and medially with the manubrium of the sternum **(sternoclavicular joint)** (Fig. 7-34). It thus provides a bony attachment between the shoulder girdle and thoracic cage, in contrast to the muscular attachment which exists between the scapula and the upper ribs. The medial two-thirds of the clavicle is convex anteriorly, whereas the lateral one-third is concave. These curvatures are easily palpable, as are the movements of the clavicle when the arm and scapula move.

The clavicle serves as a point of attachment for certain muscles of the neck, thorax, back, and arm. It also is important in bracing the scapula and pushing it backward, thereby holding the shoulder outward so as to allow the upper limb to swing freely away from the body. The clavicle is easily broken because of

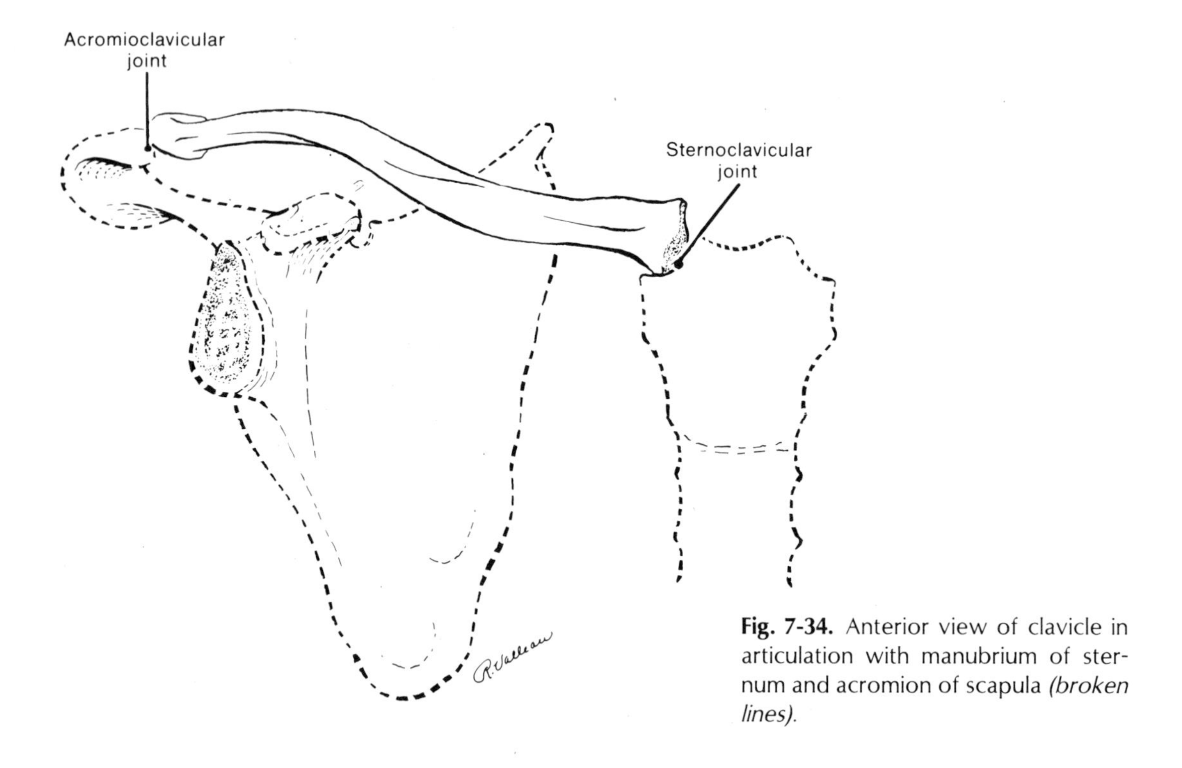

Fig. 7-34. Anterior view of clavicle in articulation with manubrium of sternum and acromion of scapula *(broken lines)*.

its superficial position and because it bears the brunt of forces against the out-stretched upper limb. The ligaments surrounding the acromioclavicular joint may become stretched and weakened, in which case the clavicle may separate from the acromion (a "shoulder separation").

Upper Limb

The upper limb consists of the **arm** extending from the shoulder to the elbow, the **forearm** from elbow to wrist, and the **hand.** In order to avoid confusion with directional terms, keep in mind the anatomical position which arbitrarily places the hand and forearm in the supinated position with the thumb facing laterally.

Arm. The arm or brachial region contains a single long bone, the **humerus** (Fig. 7-35). The rounded **head** of the humerus articulates with the glenoid cavity of the scapula. Just inferior to the head is a slightly narrower region called the **anatomical neck,** below which the **shaft** (body) extends distally. Near the upper end of the shaft are two elevations for muscle attachments: the **greater tubercle** laterally and the **lesser tubercle** anteriorly. The **intertubercular** or **bicipital groove** lies between the two tubercles and transmits the tendon of the long head of the biceps muscle. The shaft of the humerus narrows just inferior to the tubercles, and this region is referred to as the **surgical neck** because the humerus tends to fracture at this site.

Midway down the shaft of the humerus there is a roughened area, the **deltoid tuberosity,** projecting laterally and serving as a point of insertion for the deltoid muscle. The distal end of the shaft contains **medial** and **lateral epicondyles** for the attachment of several fore-

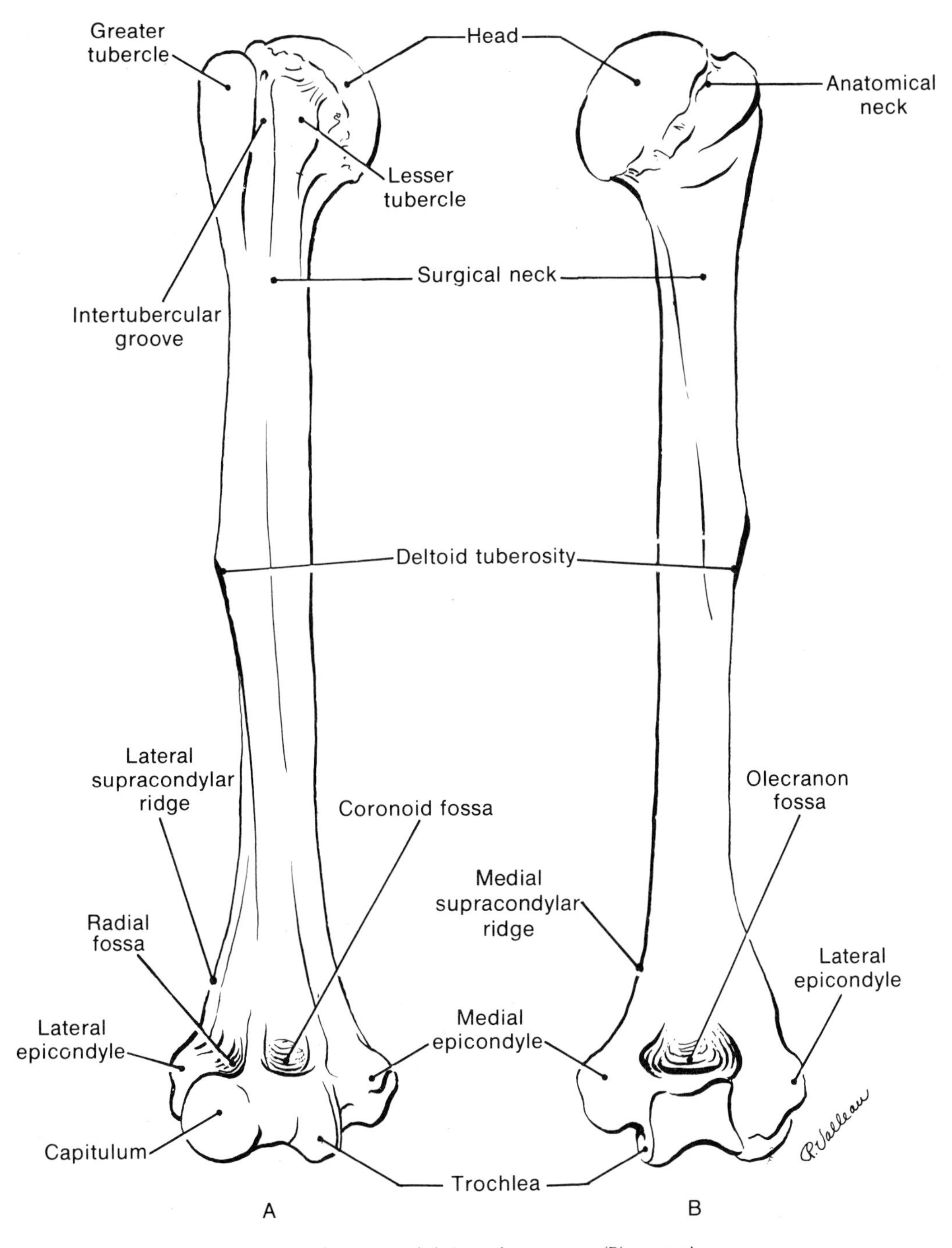

Fig. 7-35. Right humerus. (A) Anterior aspect, (B) posterior aspect.

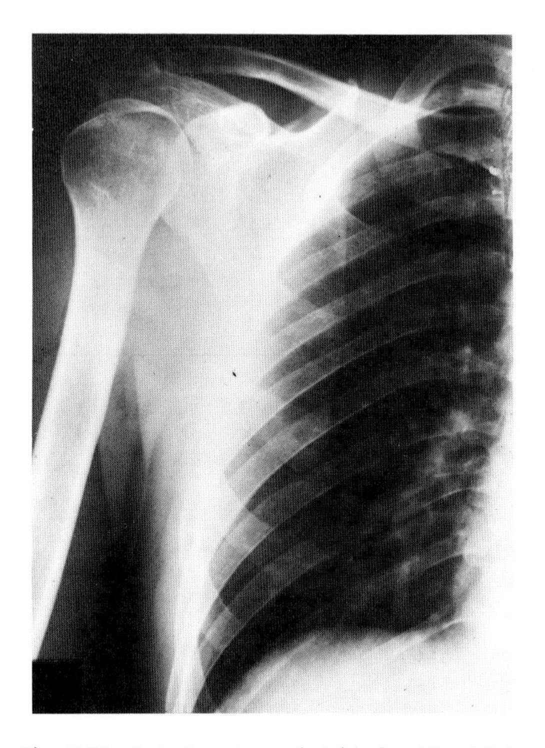

Fig. 7-36. Anterior view of right shoulder joint and right side of thoracic cage, as seen on X-ray. See also Figure 7-37. (From E. D. Gardner, D. J. Gray, and R. O'Rahilly, *Anatomy*, Ed. 4, W. B. Saunders Co., Philadelphia, 1975.)

arm muscles. Just superior to the medial epicondyle is a **medial supracondylar ridge;** inferior to the medial epicondyle is the **trochlea** which projects forward to articulate with the ulna of the forearm. A depression, the **coronoid fossa,** occurs anteriorly just above the trochlea, while a deeper **olecranon fossa** occurs posteriorly. Both fossae articulate with projections from the ulna. Superior to the lateral epicondyle is the **lateral supracondylar ridge;** inferior to the lateral epicondyle is the **capitulum,** a rounded prominence articulating with the radius of the forearm. Immediately above the capitulum is the **radial fossa** into which a portion of the radius fits when the forearm is flexed.

Shoulder Joint. This is a weak but highly mobile ball-and-socket joint. The head of the humerus articulates with the glenoid cavity of the scapula. Although the fibrocartilaginous glenoid labrum deepens the glenoid cavity, only a small portion of the head of the humerus is contained within the socket (Fig. 7-36). The fibrous joint capsule is lined by synovial membrane and extends from the glenoid labrum to the anatomical neck (Fig. 7-37). Several bursae occur among the muscles and bones at the shoulder, and these bursae can communicate with the synovial cavity of the shoulder joint. Although the bursae help to facilitate movements in this region, an inflammation can result in **bursitis** which may eventually spread into the joint cavity itself.

The joint capsule is partially strengthened by ligaments (glenohumeral passing from glenoid cavity to humerus, and coracohumeral from coracoid process to humerus). The remainder of the capsule, particularly the posterior aspect, is strengthened by a musculotendinous cuff of surrounding muscles. Despite this cuff, the shoulder joint is particularly susceptible to dislocation whereby the head of the humerus pulls out from the glenoid cavity.

Forearm. The forearm contains the radius laterally and the ulna medially. These two long bones articulate with one another at their proximal and distal ends, while the gap between the remainder of the two bones is bridged by an **interosseous membrane** (Fig. 7-38).

The **radius** is shorter than the ulna and is tapered proximally and expanded distally (Fig. 7-38). The proximal end consists of a flattened **head** articulating superiorly with the capitulum of the humerus and medially with a notch (the radial notch) of the ulna. Projecting medially from the upper part of the radius is the **radial tuberosity** for the insertion of the biceps muscle. Distally the radius expands to articulate directly with the lateral wrist bones. The medial surface of the distal radius contains an **ulnar notch** for articulation with the head of the ulna; laterally a long **styloid process** projects inferiorly and serves as an attachment for a wrist ligament.

The **ulna** is longer than the radius and shows an expanded proximal portion containing the **olecranon,** which can be palpated as the sharp point of the elbow. The tip of the olecranon fits into the olecranon fossa of the humerus; the anterior surface of the olecranon **(trochlear notch)** articulates with the trochlea of the humerus. Anteriorly the proximal end of the ulna presents a sharp ridge, the **coronoid process** which, not surprisingly, fits into the coronoid fossa of the humerus when the ulna is flexed. This region of the ulna also contains a **radial notch** into which fits the head of the radius. The ulna tapers distally and ends as the **head** with its short **styloid process.** The head articulates indirectly with the wrist bones by means of a fibrous articular disc.

Elbow Joint. This is a complex joint consisting of articulations between the trochlea of the humerus and trochlear notch of the ulna, the capitulum of the humerus and the head of the radius, and the head of the radius and radial notch of the ulna (Figs. 7-39 and 7-40). All three articulations share a common joint capsule which extends above from the top of the coronoid, radial, and olecranon fossae of the humerus to the borders of the trochlear notch of the ulna below. The capsule is strengthened laterally and medially by **radial** and **ulnar collateral ligaments,** respectively. The articulation between humerus and ulna is basically of the hinge type, whereas that between ulna and radius (called the **proximal radioulnar joint**) is a pivot type enabling the two bones to rotate

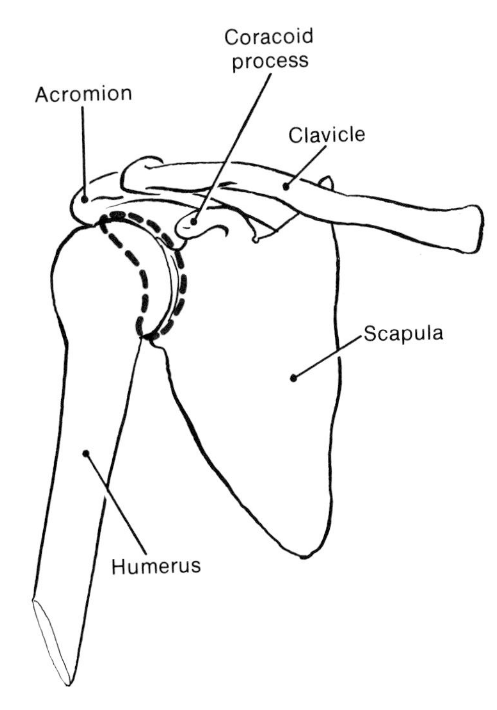

Fig. 7-37. Sketch of right shoulder joint depicted in Figure 7-36. *Broken red line* indicates the extent of the joint cavity. (Modified after Gardner, Gray, and O'Rahilly.)

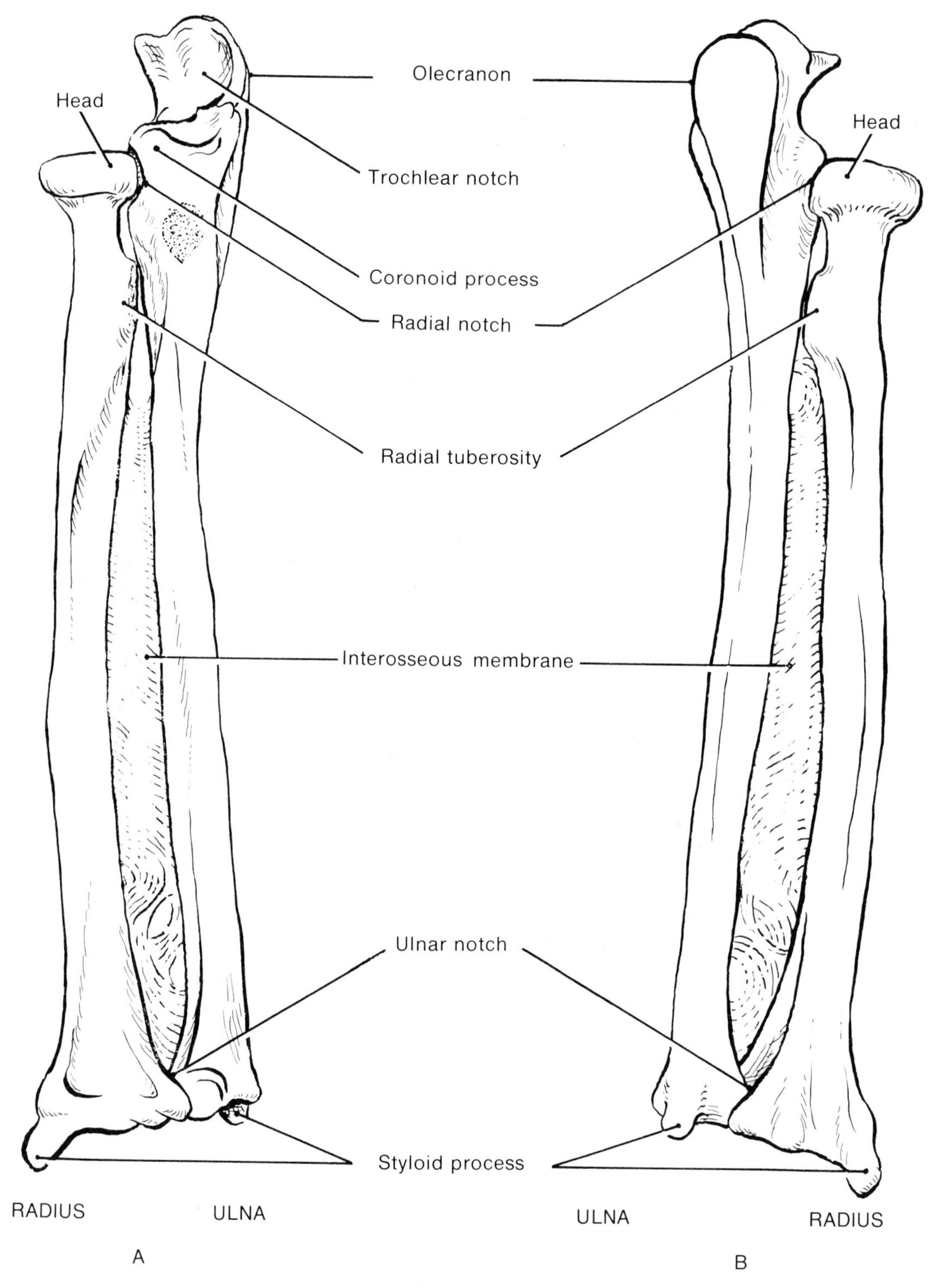

Fig. 7-38. Right ulna and right radius. (A) Anterior view, (B) posterior view.

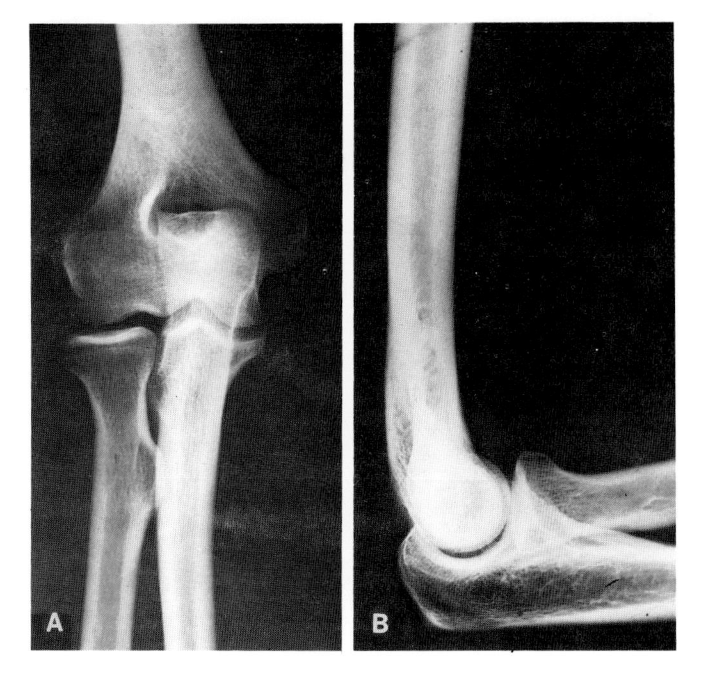

Fig. 7-39. X-rays of elbow joint. (A) Anterior view with forearm supinated, (B) lateral view. (Courtesy of Sir Thomas Lodge, The Royal Hospital, Sheffield, England. From E. D. Gardner, D. J. Gray, and R. O'Rahilly, *Anatomy,* Ed. 4, W. B. Saunders Co., Philadelphia, 1975.)

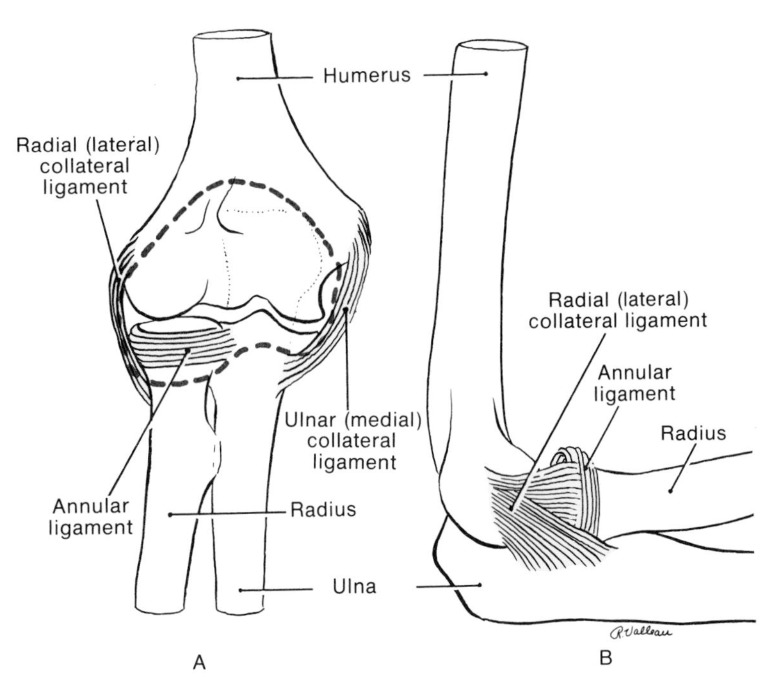

Fig. 7-40. Sketch of the elbow joint shown in the X-ray in Figure 7-39. Ligaments have been added in yellow. (A) Anterior view. The *broken red line* represents the extent of the joint capsule. (B) Lateral view. The radial collateral ligament blends with the annular ligament. (Modified after Gardner, Gray, and O'Rahilly.)

over one another to turn the palm of the hand anteriorly (supination) or posteriorly (pronation). An **annular ligament** surrounds the head of the radius and is important in keeping it in contact with the ulna. This ligament is not particularly strong in children; hence jerking a child's hand or forearm can dislocate the head of the radius downward.

Distal and Intermediate Radioulnar Joints. The distal radioulnar joint permits the distal ends of the ulna and radius to participate in pronation and supination, much like the proximal radioulnar joint at the elbow. As mentioned above, an interosseous membrane passes between the shafts of the ulna and radius; this membrane is sometimes designated as the intermediate radioulnar joint.

Wrist (Carpus). The wrist consists of eight carpal bones arranged in two rows, each of which contains four bones (Fig. 7-41). The four proximal bones are (from lateral to medial) the **scaphoid, lunate, triquetrum,** and **pisiform,** (the smallest and most readily palpable). These four proximal bones articulate proximally with the radius and a cartilaginous **articular disc** lying just distal to the ulna. The four distal carpal bones are the **trapezium, trapezoid, capitate,** and **hamate;** these articulate distally with the metacarpal bones of the hand. The two rows of carpal bones are arranged in a transverse arch which is concave anteriorly.

Wrist Joint. This constitutes the **radiocarpal joint** consisting basically of the articulation between the distal radius (plus articular disc) and the first three proximal bones of the carpus. With the forearm and hand maintained in the anatomical position, the radiocarpal joint permits the hand to move medially (adduction) and laterally (abduction) (Fig. 7-42). However, the degree of abduction is more limited because the styloid process on the radius is longer than that on the ulna, and this slightly impedes the movement. Although a slight degree of flexion and extension are allowed at the radiocarpal joint, these two actions occur also at the **midcarpal joint** between the proximal and distal rows of metacarpals.

Hand. The skeleton of the hand consists of 5 **metacarpal bones** (numbered 1 to 5 from lateral to medial, i.e., starting at the thumb side) and 14 **phalanges** which are the bones in the fingers (digits) and thumb (pollex) (Fig. 7-41). The proximal end or base of each metacarpal bone articulates with various bones in the distal row of carpals **(carpometacarpal joints);** the distal end or head articulates with the proximal phalanx of each finger and thumb **(metacarpophalangeal joints).** The heads of the metacarpal bones are the prominent "knuckles" at the metacarpophalangeal joints. The first carpometacarpal joint is saddle-shaped and allows more freedom of movement for the thumb than do the carpometacarpal joints for the fingers.

The **phalanges** (singular: phalanx) are short cylindrical bones which articulate with one another at **interphalangeal joints.** Each finger contains a proximal, middle, and distal phalanx, except for the pollex (thumb) which has only a proximal and distal phalanx. The distal ends or heads of the phalanges are responsible for the knuckles at the interphalangeal joints. Small bones called **sesamoids** are often variably found embedded in the tendons at the interphalangeal as well as metacarpophalangeal joints (Fig. 7-41; see also X-ray in Fig. 7-56).

Pelvic Girdle

Just as the shoulder girdle connects the upper limbs with the thorax, so the pelvic girdle serves as a connection between the lower limbs and trunk. The pelvic girdle consists of two **hip bones** which articulate with each other anteriorly at the **symphysis pubis.** Posteriorly each hip bone forms the **sacroiliac joint** with the sacrum (Fig. 7-43). This joint is strengthened by fibrous **sacroiliac ligaments** and does not allow much movement since it is important in stabilizing the lower region of the trunk when sitting or standing. Unfortunately the ligaments can become stretched and weakened, leading to joint instability and often resulting in lower back pain.

Each hip bone is composed of three portions: the ilium, ischium, and pubis (Fig. 7-44).

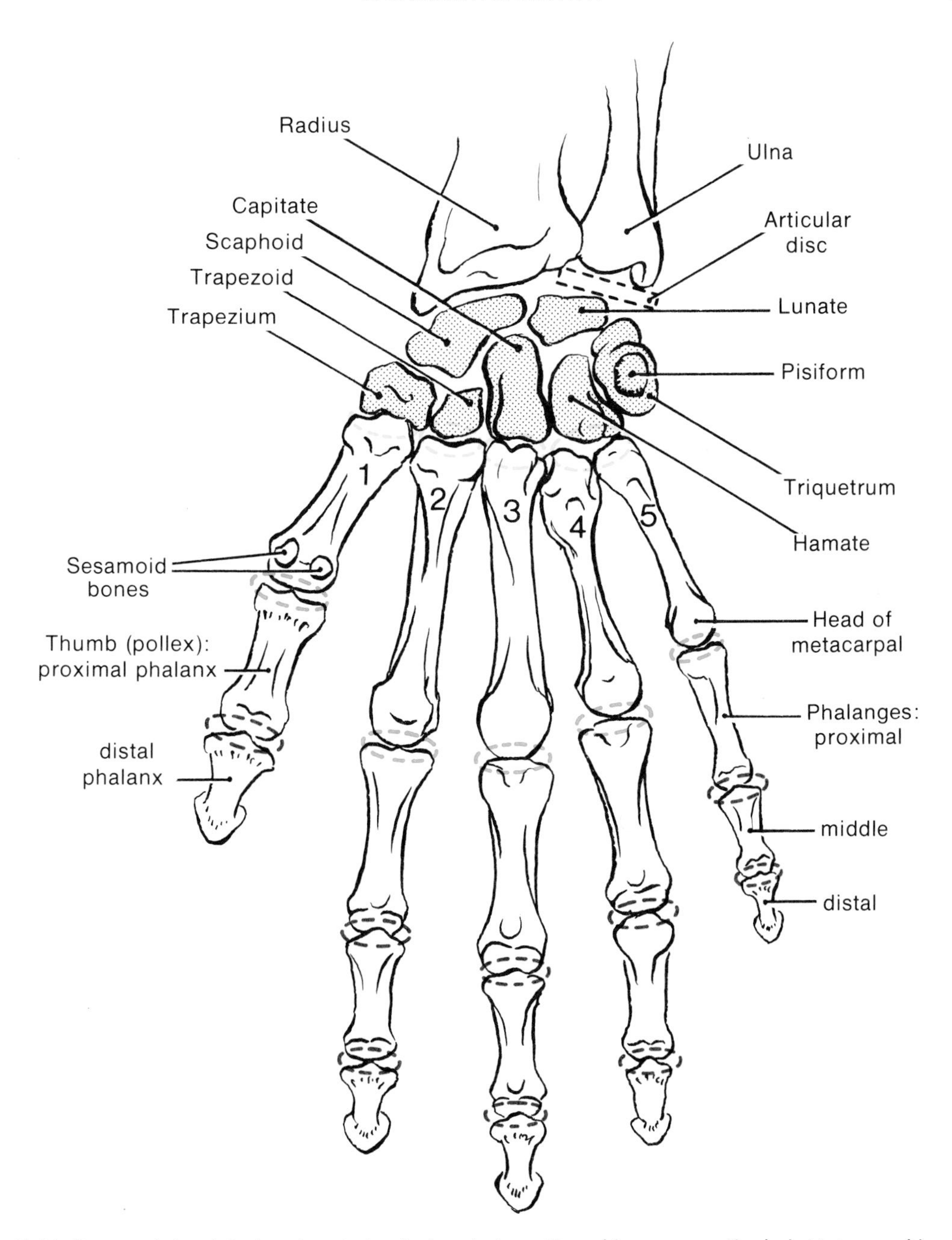

Fig. 7-41. Bones of the right hand, anterior (palmar) view. Carpal bones are stippled. Metacarpal bones are numbered 1–5. Two sesamoid bones often occur at the head of the first metacarpal. The articular disc *(broken line)* consists of a cartilaginous plate. The *dotted lines* in color indicate joints: carpometacarpal (yellow); metacarpophalangeal (blue); interphalangeal (red).

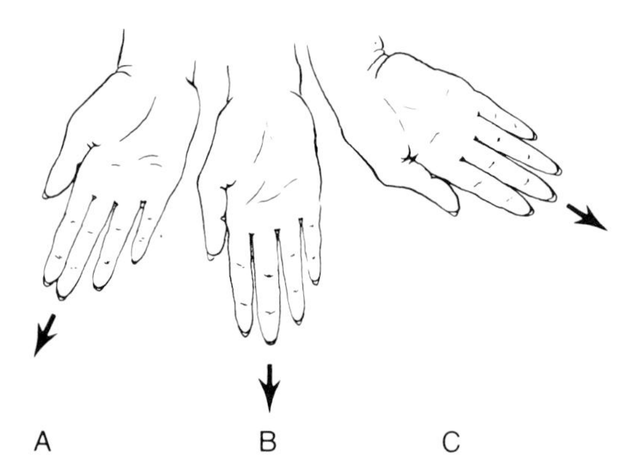

Fig. 7-42. Abduction and adduction of the right hand, anterior view. (A) Abduction, (B) straight position, (C) adduction. Note that the hand can be adducted farther than it can be abducted.

These develop embryonically as three separate bones which eventually fuse to form a single bone, but the lines of fusion are usually ill-defined. The lateral surface of the hip bone contains the **acetabulum,** a cup-shaped socket which is formed by portions of all three bones and into which the head of the femur (thigh bone) fits at the hip joint.

The ilium consists of a **body** (which joins the pubis anteriorly and the ischium posteriorly), and a fan-shaped wing (**ala**) which curves upward and whose superior border is the **iliac crest.** The crest arches between two sharp points, the **anterior superior iliac spine** and **posterior superior iliac spine,** inferior to which are the **anterior inferior** and **posterior inferior iliac spines,** respectively (Fig. 7-44). These spines serve as points of attachment for various muscles and ligaments.

The crest of the ilium can be palpated, and the site of the posterior superior iliac spines can often be seen externally as a pair of dimples in the skin. A roughened area on the inner aspect of the ilium near the posterior superior and posterior inferior spines serves as an articular surface where the ilium articulates with the sacrum at the sacroiliac joint. Just anterior to this area the concave medial surface of the ala is called the **iliac fossa** which is delimited by a thin line passing forward into the pubic region of the hip bone. A deep notch, the **greater sciatic notch,** occurs below the posterior inferior iliac spine. The lower portion of this notch is actually a part of the ischium.

The **ischium** constitutes the posterior and inferior portion of the hip bone (Fig. 7-44). As indicated previously, the lower part of the greater sciatic notch is a part of the ischium. The notch ends at the sharp **ischial spine,** inferior to which is another but shallower indentation, the **lesser sciatic notch.** Below the lesser notch the ischium shows a prominent bulge which is called the **ischial tuberosity.** This massive part of the ischium bears the body weight in the sitting position. The **ramus** of the **ischium** projects forward from the tuberosity and fuses with the inferior ramus of the pubis. Just above the two fused rami is a large opening, the **obturator foramen.**

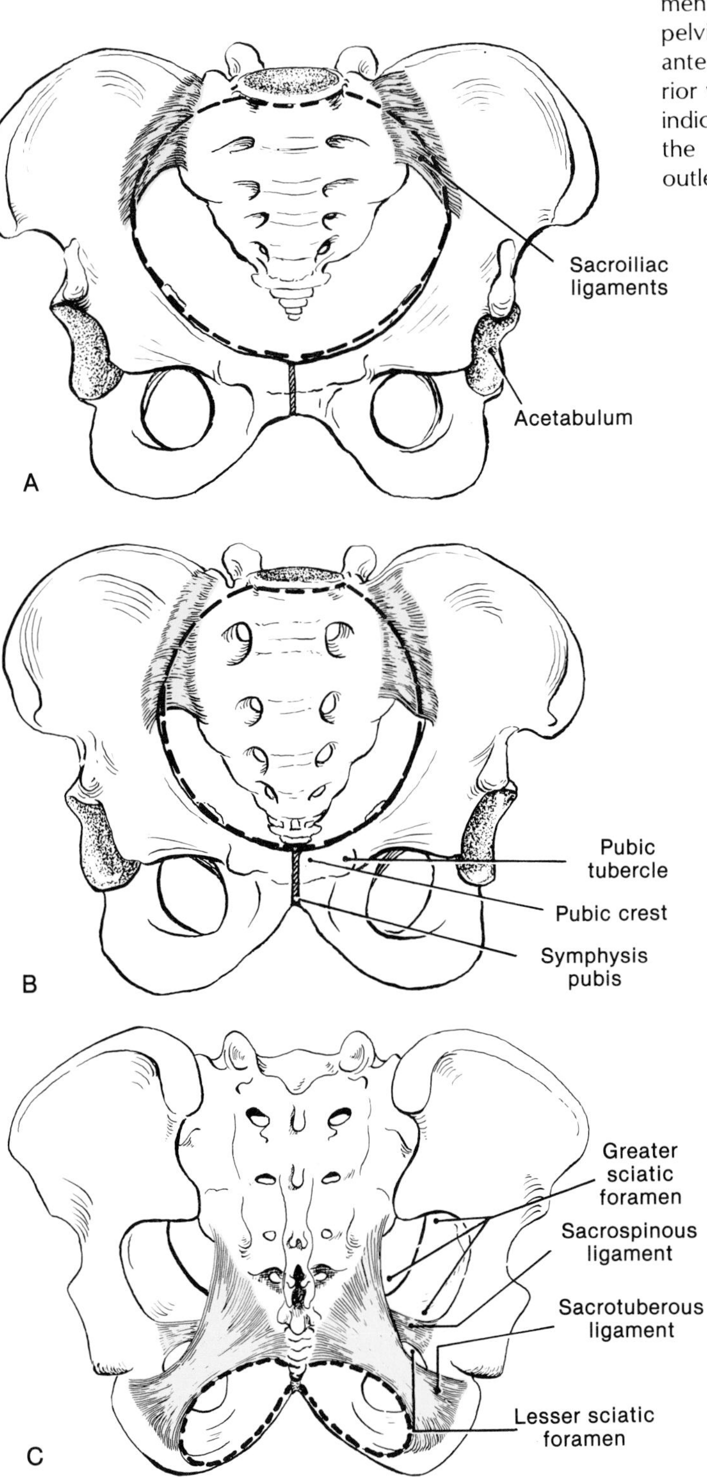

Fig. 7-43. The bony pelvis, with ligaments indicated in yellow. (A) Female pelvis, anterior view, (B) male pelvis, anterior view, (C) male pelvis, posterior view. In A and B the *broken lines* indicate the pelvic brim (inlet); in C, the *broken lines* indicate the pelvic outlet.

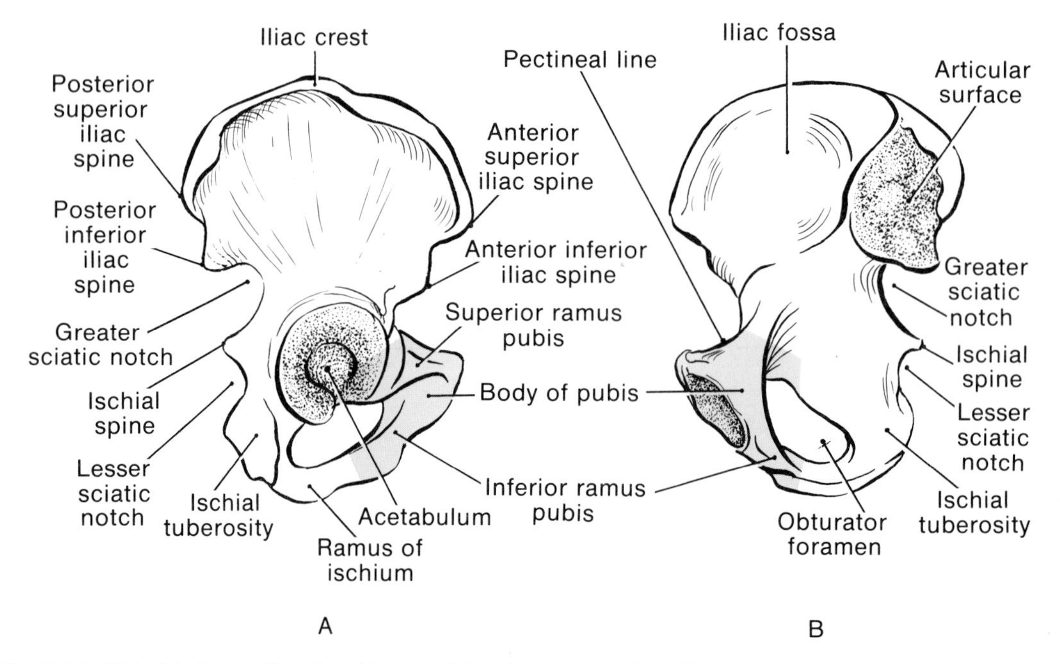

Fig. 7-44. Right hip bone. Ilium in white, pubis in blue, ischium in yellow. (A) Lateral view, (B) medial view.

The greater sciatic notch of the ilium and the lesser sciatic notch of the ischium are converted into the **greater sciatic foramen** and **lesser sciatic foramen,** respectively, by means of two ligaments (Fig. 7-43). The **sacrospinous ligament** extends between the sacrum and ischial spine; the **sacrotuberous ligament** extends between the sacrum and ischial tuberosity.

The **pubis** constitutes the anterior and inferior portion of the hip bone and consists of a body and two rami (inferior and superior). The **body** of the pubis lies medial to the two rami and unites with its counterpart from the opposite side to form the **symphysis pubis** (pubic symphysis) in the midline (Fig. 7-43). The symphysis contains fibrocartilage, which ordinarily does not allow much movement except toward the end of pregnancy when this junction becomes softened so as to facilitate passage of the infant's head through the pelvis. The short superior border of the pubic body is rough and known as the **pubic crest** which ends laterally as the **pubic tubercle** (Fig. 7-43). The latter is palpable and often used as a bony landmark. The **inferior ramus** of the pubis joins the ramus of the ischium; the **superior ramus** joins the ilium and ischium at the acetabulum. On the inner surface of the superior ramus one can trace the **pectineal line** beginning near the pubic tubercle and extending obliquely upward to meet and become continuous with a line extending downward along the inner surface of the ilium. This continuous line is the **arcuate line.**

Bony Pelvis. The two hip bones, sacrum, and coccyx make up the bony pelvis (Fig. 7-43). An important landmark is the **pelvic brim,** above which is the **greater** or **false pelvis** and below which is the **lesser** or **true pelvis.** The pelvic brim is demarcated by the sacral promontory, the arcuate line sweeping along the inner surfaces of the ilium and pubis, and the pubic crests and symphysis. The pelvic brim is often termed the **pelvic inlet,** whereas an imaginary line extending along the inferior rami of the pubis, ischial tuberosities, and inferior borders of the sacrotuberous ligaments to the tip of the coccyx is considered to be the **pelvic outlet.** The pelvic inlet is tilted slightly forward so that in the anatomical position the crests of the pubic bones lie in the same vertical plane as the anterior superior iliac spines (Fig. 7-44). The bodies of the pubic bones thus actually slope slightly backward and thereby help to support pelvic organs such as the bladder.

The bony pelvis shows a variety of shapes and sizes as well as sexual differences (Figs. 7-43 and 7-46). In general, the female pelvic inlet and outlet are wider, as is the subpubic angle (formed by the union of the two inferior pubic rami at the symphysis). The greater sciatic notch also tends to be wider. In the female, an adequate size and configuration of the pelvis are necessary to safely accommodate the head of an infant during childbirth; otherwise, a caesarian section may be necessary.

Lower Limb

The lower limb consists of the **thigh** extending from hip to knee, the **leg** from knee to ankle, and the **foot.** Because of our upright position, the lower limb and pelvis have become specialized for supporting body weight. Consequently, the lower limb does not exhibit as much mobility as does the upper limb. Also, during embryonic development the lower limbs undergo a rotation so that in the anatomical position the big toe is medial to the other toes.

Thigh. The skeleton of the thigh consists of a single bone, the **femur,** most of which cannot be palpated because it is thickly cloaked with muscles. The rounded **head** of the femur fits into the acetabulum of the hip bone and thus participates in the hip joint. Below the head is the **neck,** which slants downward and joins the **shaft** at an angle (Fig. 7-45). Near the junction of the neck and shaft are two eminences: the **greater trochanter** laterally and the **lesser trochanter** which faces medially and backward. In front, the two trochanters are connected by the **intertrochanteric line,** while posteriorly the more prominent **intertrochanteric crest** connects the two. The shaft shows a slight convexity anteriorly; posteriorly there is a prominent ridge, the **linea aspera,** for important muscle attachments.

The distal portion of the femur ends in a **lateral condyle** and **medial condyle** separated posteriorly by a deep **intercondylar fossa.** The two condyles are less distinct anteriorly where they form a large knob. **Lateral** and **medial epicondyles** project from atop the lateral and medial condyles, respectively, and serve as points of attachment for some ligaments of the knee. Just above the medial epicondyle is the prominent **adductor tubercle** for the insertion of adductor muscles.

Patella. The **patella** (knee cap) is a large sesamoid bone lodged in the tendon of a muscle (quadriceps femoris). The patella articulates posteriorly with the patellar surface of the femur (Fig. 7-45) and completes the anterior aspect of the knee joint.

Hip Joint. The hip joint is a synovial joint of the ball and socket type (Figs. 7-46 and 7-47). The rim of the acetabulum is extended by a strip of fibrocartilage **(acetabular labrum)** which deepens the acetabular fossa so as to grasp the head of the femur more efficiently. Although a narrow **round ligament** extends from the depth of the socket to the head of the femur, it does not contribute much to stabilizing the joint but instead carries nutrient vessels. The joint is surrounded by a fibrous synovial capsule lined by synovial membrane (Fig. 7-47). Externally the capsule is strengthened by ligaments extending from the ilium, ischium, and pubis to the intertrochanteric line. Although the hip joint is adapted to bear weight, it also shows a fairly wide range of movement. It can also become dislocated, in which case the head of the femur pulls out of the acetabulum. Congenital dislocation of the hip is frequently due to a poorly developed acetabulum.

Leg. The leg contains the tibia medially and the fibula laterally (Fig. 7-48). The **tibia** (shin bone) is a long bone easily palpated along its anterior and medial surfaces, but clothed posteriorly with bulky muscles commonly called the calf muscles. The upper expanded end of the tibia contains a **medial** and **lateral condyle** which articulate at the knee joint with

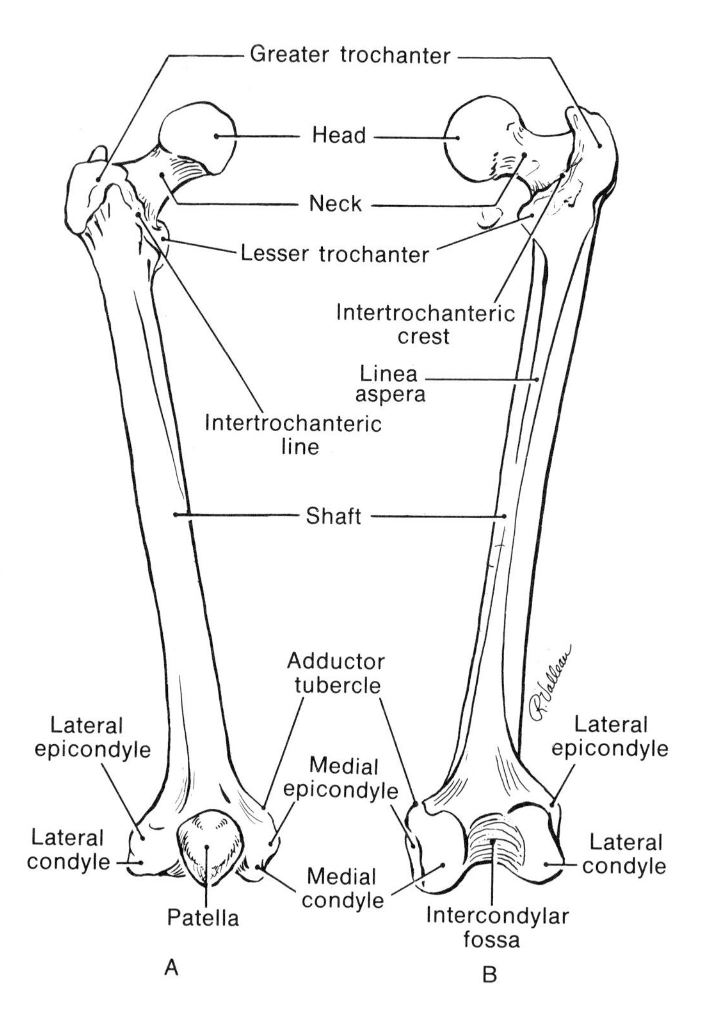

Fig. 7-45. Right femur and patella. (A) Anterior view, (B) posterior view.

the corresponding condyles of the femur. The condyles are separated from each other anteriorly and posteriorly by intercondylar depressions. At the inferior aspect of the lateral condyle is a depression for articulation with the fibula. Projecting anteriorly near the upper end of the tibia is the **tibial tuberosity,** to which is attached the patellar ligament. (The patellar ligament represents the distal part of the tendon of a massive thigh muscle, the quadriceps femoris.)

The shaft of the tibia narrows and then widens again distally. The distal end presents a medial projection, the **medial malleolus,** which is easily palpated and participates in the articulation at the ankle joint. A lateral depression articulates with the distal portion of the fibula.

The **fibula** is a long slender bone extending along the lateral aspect of the leg (Fig. 7-48). Its **head** articulates medially with the tibia but does not participate in the knee joint. The gap between the shaft of the fibula and tibia is bridged by an **interosseous membrane** similar to that described between the radius and ulna in the forearm. Distally the fibula expands to form the **lateral malleolus** which projects further inferiorly and is more prominent than the medial malleolus of the tibia.

Knee Joint. This is a complicated joint containing two fibrocartilaginous discs, the **lateral meniscus** and **medial meniscus,** associ-

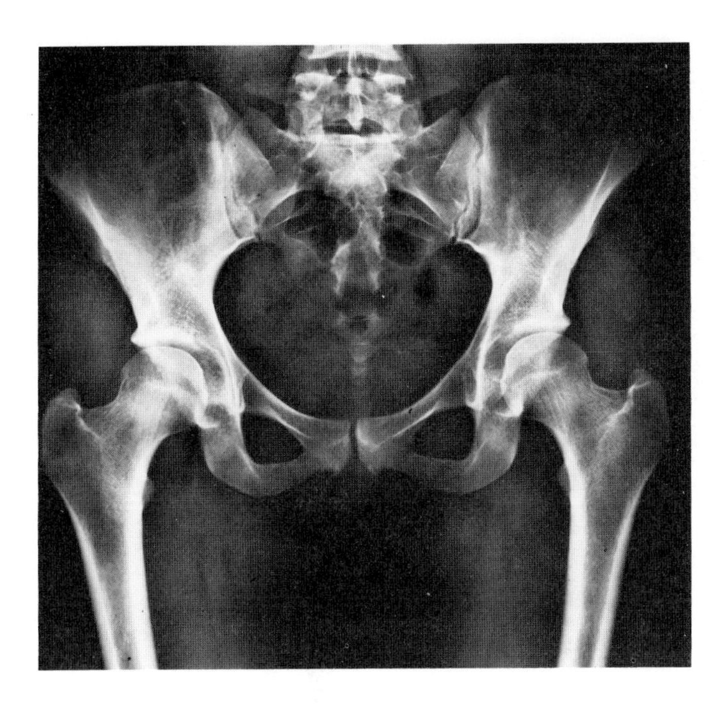

Fig. 7-46. X-ray of female pelvis showing hip joints. (From E. D. Gardner, D. J. Gray, and R. O'Rahilly, *Anatomy*, Ed. 4, W. B. Saunders Co., Philadelphia, 1975.)

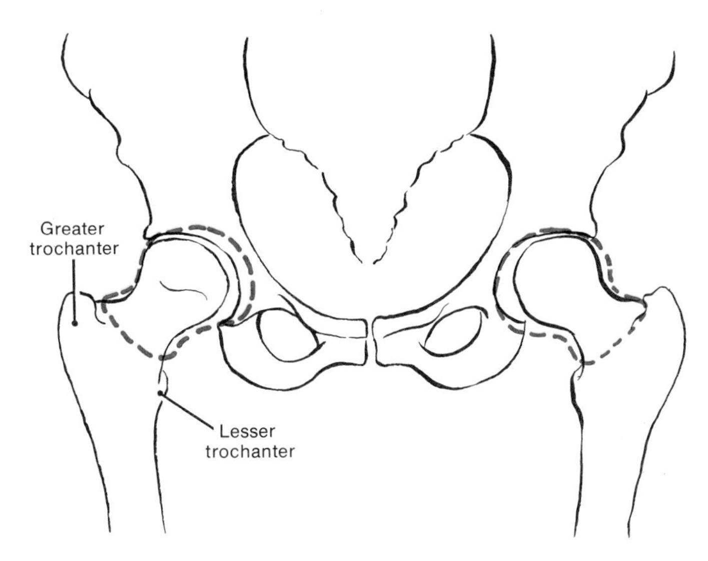

Fig. 7-47. Sketch of pelvis and hip joints depicted in Figure 7-46. *Broken red lines* indicate extent of joint cavities.

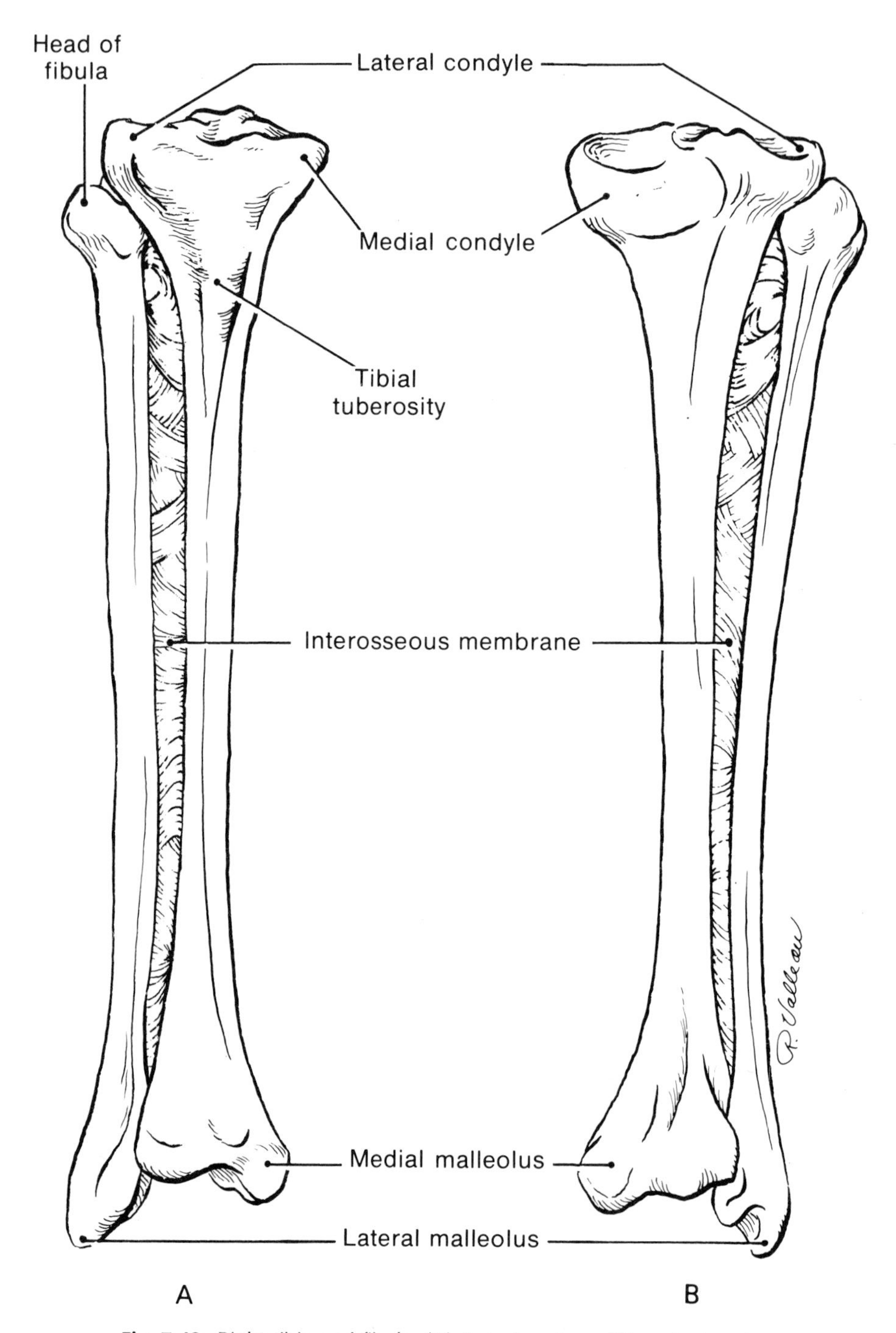

Fig. 7-48. Right tibia and fibula. (A) Anterior view, (B) posterior view.

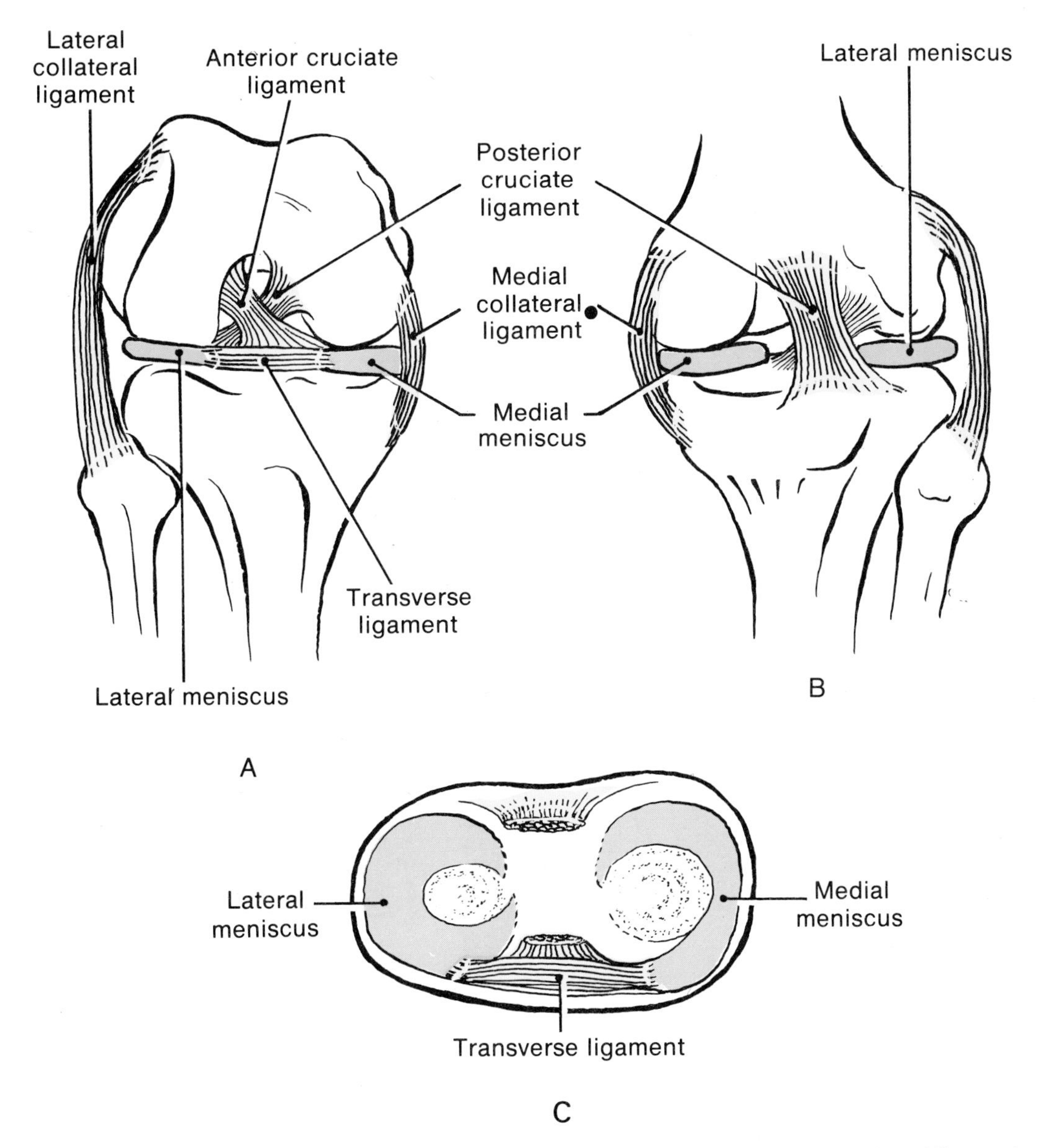

Fig. 7-49. Right knee joint. (A) Anterior view, with knee slightly flexed, (B) posterior view, (C) superior view of the tibia.

ated with the lateral and medial condyles of the tibia, respectively (Fig. 7-49). The menisci are also called **semilunar cartilages** because of their crescent shape. They are bound together anteriorly by a **transverse ligament,** and they lend stability to the joint by deepening the tibial articular surfaces with which the condyles of the femur articulate. The menisci also aid as shock absorbers and help to lubricate the joint. An **anterior cruciate ligament** passes backward through the joint from the anterior rim of the tibia to the intercondylar fossa of the femur. A **posterior cruciate ligament** passes from the posterior surface of the tibia to the

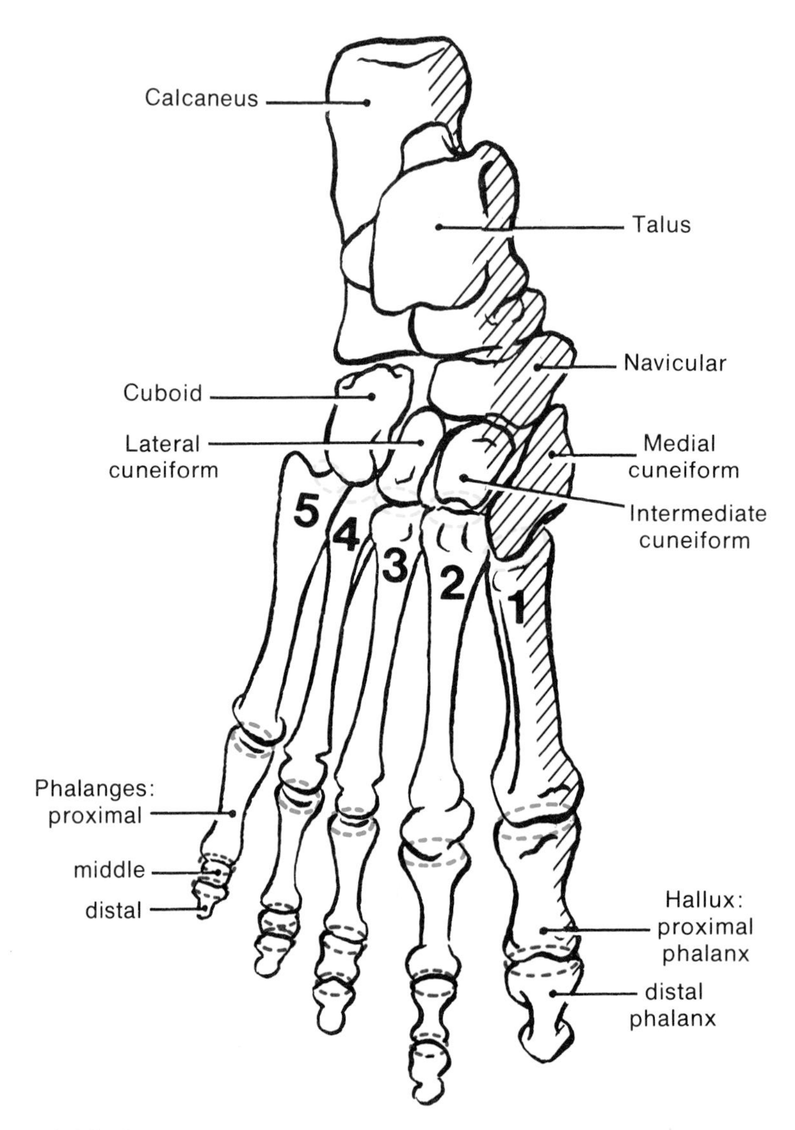

Fig. 7-50. Bones of right foot, superior view. Metatarsal bones are numbered 1–5. The dotted lines in color indicate joints: tarsometatarsal (yellow); metatarsophalangeal (blue); interphalangeal (red).

anterior aspect of the femur. These two ligaments prevent the femur and tibia from overriding one another. Hence, damage to the anterior ligament allows the tibia to slip forward in front of the femur, while damage to the posterior ligament allows the tibia to slip backward behind the femur.

The knee joint is surrounded by a fibrous capsule lined with synovial membrane. The patella and patellar ligament reinforce the capsule anteriorly. The knee is also strengthened laterally and medially by collateral ligaments. The **medial (tibial) collateral ligament** is bound to the medial meniscus whereas the **lat-**

eral (fibular) collateral ligament is only loosely associated with the lateral meniscus. Hence a sudden and severe wrenching movement at the knee is likely to tear the medial meniscus along with the medial ligament.

Various fluid-filled bursae occur at the knee and may also communicate with the synovial cavity. With injury or inflammation of these bursae the increased accumulation of fluid may result in swelling (so-called "water on the knee").

Ankle (Tarsus). The ankle consists of seven tarsal bones: the talus, calcaneus, navicular, cuboid, and three cuneiform bones (Fig. 7-50). The **talus** projects upward so as to be gripped between the medial malleolus of the tibia and the lateral malleolus of the fibula. The talus is supported from below by the shelflike **calcaneus** which projects backward as the heel of the foot. The **navicular** lies anterior to the talus on the medial side of the foot, while the **cuboid** lies anterior to the calcaneus on the lateral side. The **medial, intermediate,** and **lateral cuneiform bones** are arranged distal to the navicular bone and, along with the cuboid, articulate with the metatarsal bones of the foot.

Ankle Joint. This is a typical hinge joint formed by the medial and lateral malleoli of the tibia and fibula, respectively, and by the talus which is gripped between them (Fig. 7-51). The fibrous joint capsule is reinforced medially by the fan-shaped **deltoid ligament** passing from medial malleolus to calcaneus, talus, and navicular. Laterally, ligaments also pass between the fibula, talus, and calcaneus. Although the medial and lateral ligaments are rugged, the anterior and posterior aspects of the joint are weak, thereby allowing the hinge movement of dorsiflexion (upward movement of foot) and plantar flexion (downward movement).

Foot. The skeleton of the foot contains 5 **metatarsal bones** (numbered 1 to 5 from medial to lateral, i.e. starting at the big toe) and 14 **phalanges** (Fig. 7-50). The expanded **bases** (proximal ends) of the metatarsals articulate with the distal tarsal bones **(tarsometatarsal joints);** the **heads** (distal ends) articulate with

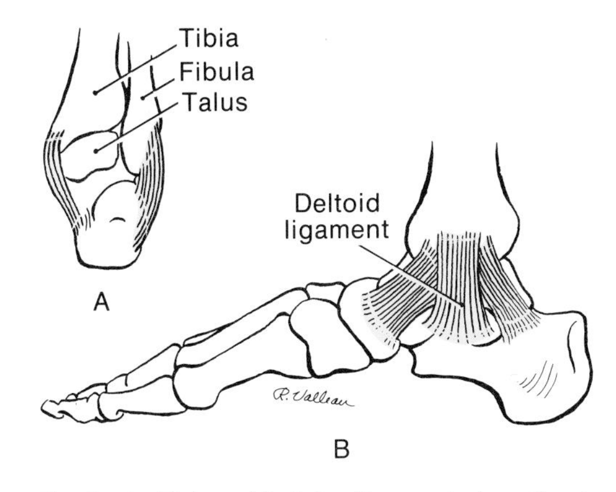

Fig. 7-51. Right ankle joint (ligaments in yellow). (A) Posterior view, (B) medial view.

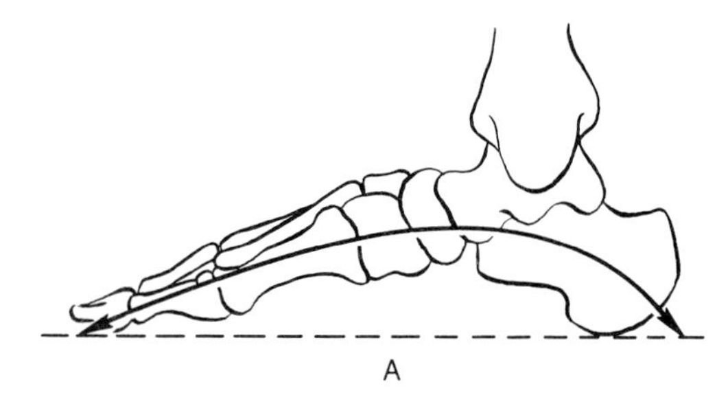

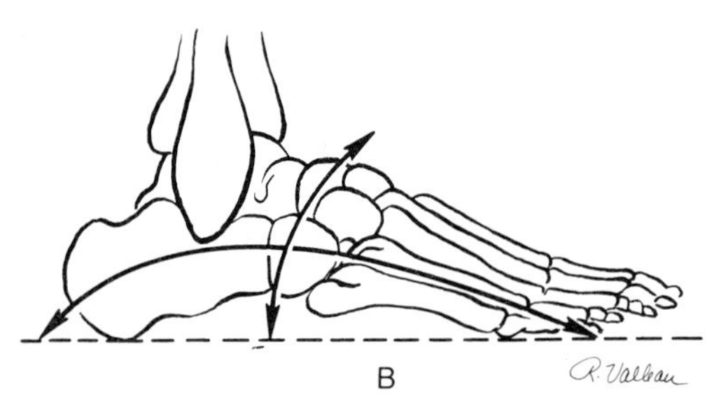

Fig. 7-52. Arches of the right foot. (A) Medial view. *Arrow* depicts medial longitudinal arch. (B) Lateral view. *Long arrow* indicates lateral longitudinal arch; *short arrow* represents transverse arch.

the proximal phalanges of the toes **(metatarsophalangeal joints).** The tarsometatarsal articulation for the big toe (hallux) shows more mobility than do the other tarsometatarsal joints; however, this mobility is not as great as that for the thumb, at least in man.

Phalanges. The 14 phalanges in the foot correspond to those in the hand. The big toe contains a **proximal** and **distal phalanx,** whereas the remaining toes contain **proximal, middle,** and **distal phalanges.** A pair of sesamoid bones often occurs at the metatarsophalangeal joint of the big toe.

Arches of the Foot. The tarsal and metatarsal bones are arranged in three arches which lend strength to the foot (Fig. 7-52). The **medial longitudinal arch** involves the calcaneus, talus, navicular, 3 cuneiforms, and first 3 metatarsals. A less prominent **lateral longitudinal arch** involves the calcaneus, cuboid, and the 2 lateral metatarsals. A **transverse arch** occurs perpendicular to the longitudinal arch. All three arches are strengthened by ligaments, although a weakening may result in "flat feet" or "fallen" arches. As one walks, the calcaneus is the first to receive the thrust of the body's weight. The weight then is rolled forward along the lateral aspect of the foot and eventually distributed to the heads of the 5 metatarsals as the foot pushes off from the ground.

MICROSCOPIC ANATOMY

Bone is a special form of connective tissue in which the dense intercellular matrix becomes mineralized (see Chapter 4). Despite a significant amount of inorganic material, bone is a dynamic and ever-changing tissue, richly supplied with vessels and nerves. Adult bones contain two forms of bone tissue: compact and spongy. **Compact bone** is characterized by dense layers **(lamellae)** of bone often arranged in concentric cylinders. **Spongy (cancellous) bone** contains an interconnecting network of rods or spicules interspersed with marrow cavities (described below).

An adult bone is composed primarily of bone tissue, with small amounts of other types of connective tissues present. Compact bone is situated peripherally in the outer portion of the bone, whereas spongy bone occurs in the interior (Fig. 7-53). Spongy bone is abundant in the ends **(epiphyses)** of long bones and in the center of short, flat, and irregular bones. The spongy bone of flat bones (such as those of the skull) is often given the special name **diploë** and occurs between outer and inner "tables" of compact bone.

Compact bone is covered by a dense layer of fibrous connective tissue, the **periosteum,** except at articular surfaces where there are plates of hyaline cartilage. Muscles attach to bone by means of the dense fibrous connective tissue of tendons. This tissue becomes continuous with the periosteum, which in turn is anchored to the compact bone via collagenous fibers called **Sharpey's fibers.** These prevent the periosteum from being stripped off the bone as the tendons pull on it. The inner aspect of compact bone is lined by a comparable but less conspicuous layer of connective tissue termed the **endosteum.**

Spongy bone contains cavities known as the bone **marrow.** There are two types of marrow: **red marrow** where red blood cells and some white blood cells are formed, and **yellow marrow** which contains mainly fat.

A bone depends on an elaborate system of blood vessels and channels to serve the metabolic needs of its cells **(osteocytes),** which are trapped in the mineralized intercellular matrix. Numerous blood vessels pierce the periphery of the compact bone via transverse canals (Volkmann's canals) and then travel in the compact bone via longitudinal hollow channels running parallel to the surface (Fig. 7-53). These longitudinal channels are called **Haversian canals,** each of which serves as an axis around which are situated concentric cylinders of bony tissue. Each Haversian canal and its concentric lamellae constitute a **Haversian system.** The Haversian canals and their vessels communicate with one another via a network of smaller channels and vessels. The bony channels eventually join extremely small slits known as **canaliculi** (Fig. 7-53). The latter emanate from tiny cavities called **lacunae,** which house the osteocytes, each of which sends out minute cytoplasmic processes into the canaliculi.

The canaliculi from one lacuna join those from nearby lacunae as well as the larger channels of the Haversian system; an interconnecting network thus exists to bring nutrients to the osteocytes. Since even the smallest blood vessels are too large to travel into the canaliculi, an exchange of materials takes place between the blood vessels and the tissue fluid in the network of larger channels, and this fluid then flows through the canaliculi to the cytoplasmic processes of the osteocytes, thus serving as a means for metabolic exchange. Well organized Haversian systems do not exist in spongy bone, although there are some channels whereby blood vessels from the marrow cavities can enter the bony spicules.

In addition to the numerous small periosteal blood vessels penetrating the compact bone externally, most bones receive a large **nutrient vessel** which passes via a **nutrient foramen** and **canal** directly to the marrow cavity. Here the blood flows through the spaces of the spongy bone and then into perforating vessels which pass outward to join the network of vessels in the compact bone.

Nerve fibers accompany the blood vessels in bone, and the periosteum is also well supplied with fibers. For this reason diseases such as bone cancer can be quite painful, as are bone fractures.

DEVELOPMENTAL AND CLINICAL ANATOMY

Bones develop from embryonic mesenchyme (connective tissue) in one of two ways. If the bone ossifies directly from a condensation of mesenchyme cells, the process is called **intramembranous** bone formation. Many of the flat bones in the skull develop in this manner. A second and more common method of bone formation is termed **endochondral,** whereby the mesenchyme develops first into a cartilaginous model which later is replaced by bone. Since cartilage can grow internally, endochondral

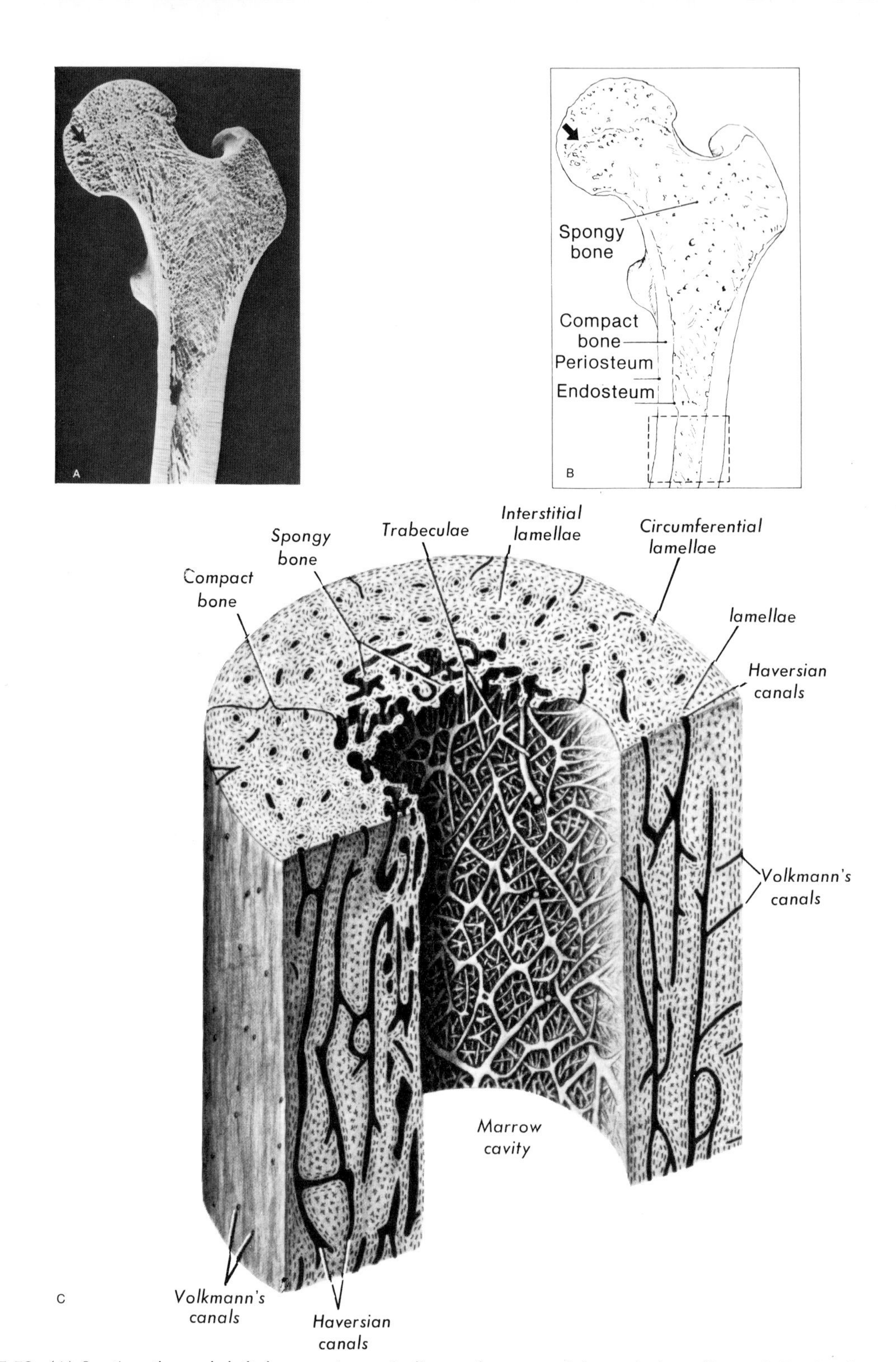

Fig. 7-53. (A) Section through left femur. *Arrow* indicates former epiphyseal plate. (From E. D. Gardner, D. J. Gray, and R. O'Rahilly, *Anatomy,* Ed. 4, W. B. Saunders Co., Philadelphia, 1975.) (B) Sketch of bone section in A. The area enclosed by the rectangle is shown three-dimensionally in C. (C) Diagram of a shaft of a bone after much of the marrow has been removed. (From W. M. Copenhaver, R. P. Bunge, and M. B. Bunge, *Bailey's Textbook of Histology,* Ed. 16, The Williams & Wilkins Co., Baltimore, 1971.)

bone shows great capacity to increase in size as an individual grows.

Intramembranous Development

In regions where this type of development occurs, some of the mesenchyme cells differentiate into a cluster of bone cell precursors, the **osteoblasts.** The osteoblasts produce various fiber types (particularly collagenous fibers) which, along with the intercellular ground substance, constitute the organic component of the intercellular matrix. Ossification eventually begins when various mineral salts (calcium phosphate and calcium carbonate) are precipitated in the matrix, thereby trapping the osteoblasts in spaces (lacunae). The osteoblasts are then called **osteocytes,** and the plate of bony tissue constitutes a bone **spicule** (Fig. 7-54). Along the outside of the spicule, the mesenchyme cells continue to produce osteoblasts, and in this manner the spicule increases in size. Note, however, that this type of growth occurs from the outside and that neither the osteoblasts nor osteocytes show mitotic activity. This external laying down of bone is called **appositional growth.**

The bony spicule eventually unites with other spicules to form a network of spongy bone. This network is surrounded by a dense fibrous periosteum whose mesenchyme cells continue to differentiate into osteoblasts; the periosteum is thus said to be osteogenic. The bone produced by the periosteum forms a solid thin layer of compact bone around the periphery, while spongy bone remains inside. As the compact bone continues to grow by direct apposition from the periosteum, it is constantly eroded from the inside so that the extent of spongy bone can keep pace from within. This erosion of bone is carried out by special multinucleated cells called **osteoclasts.**

Endochondral Development

Endochondral bones begin as condensations of mesenchyme cells which differentiate into **chondroblasts.** The chondroblasts lay down collagenous and elastic fibers, as well as an intercellular matrix rich in chondroitin sulfate, and the chondroblasts transform into **chondro-**

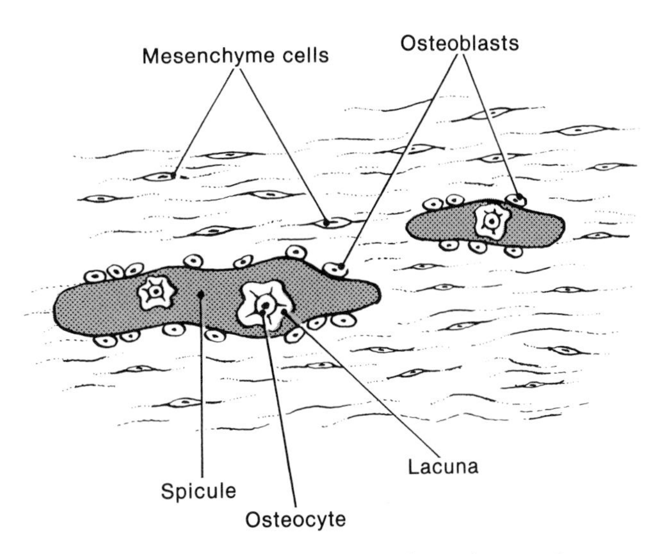

Fig. 7-54. Diagrammatic view of two bone spicules formed during intramembranous development of bone.

cytes as they become trapped in the matrix. A cartilaginous model thus develops in the shape of the adult bone (Fig. 7-55). The model is initially covered by a **perichondrium** consisting of dense fibrous connective tissue. The perichondrium is chondrogenic and produces new chondroblasts whereby the cartilage model can grow externally by apposition. The model can also grow internally, since the chondrocytes can multiply by cell division. This is known as **interstitial growth.**

In order for ossification to occur, the cartilage eventually must be removed and replaced by bone tissue. This process usually begins at the center of the bone and spreads peripherally. The chondrocytes proliferate and enlarge (hypertrophy), and the intercellular cartilaginous matrix becomes calcified with inorganic salts. Since the matrix no longer allows nutrients to reach the chondrocytes, they begin to die, leaving behind only the spicules of calcified matrix. Meanwhile the perichondrium around the shaft of the bone becomes transformed into a periosteum and begins producing osteoblasts. The osteoblasts proceed to deposit bone on the surface of the shaft, and a bone collar of **periosteal bone** is produced. This serves as a splint for the shaft and develops into compact bone which gradually extends toward the ends of the bone.

The periosteal bone is penetrated by **periosteal buds** consisting of blood vessels, osteoblasts, and osteoclasts which pass into the central region of degenerating cartilage cells. The osteoblasts use the remaining spicules of calcified cartilage as a framework on which to lay down bone, and the calcified cartilage eventually degenerates and disappears, leaving behind only the spicules of newly formed bone. The osteoclasts break down the bone tissue from the inner aspect of the periosteal bone so as to prevent it from becoming too thick.

Ossification begins before birth in the cartilage models at sites known as **primary centers** of ossification. **Secondary centers** begin usually in the ends **(epiphyses)** of the models after birth, but the process of ossification is essentially the same as that in the primary center. As the primary and secondary centers approach one another a plate of hyaline cartilage is retained between the shaft **(diaphysis)** and epiphysis at each end of the bone. These are known as **epiphyseal plates (discs),** in which the cartilage shows four zones (resting or reserve, proliferating, maturing or hypertrophy, and calcifying). The zone of proliferating cartilage allows the disc to grow interstitially and thus provide a means whereby the bone can grow in length (Figs. 7-55 and 7-56). (Growth in width continues appositionally from the periosteal bone.) The epiphyseal plates are gradually replaced by bone, at which time growth ceases. This usually occurs in the late teens, but generally one or two years earlier in females. By this time cartilage has disappeared from all regions of the bone except its ends, where it remains on the surface as the articular cartilage.

Bone Fractures and Repair

Trauma to a bone may cause it to break. Such a fracture can be complete or partial. If the fracture also breaks through the skin it is called a **compound fracture,** in contrast to a **simple fracture** which remains covered by skin. A particular danger with fractures comes from possible damage to the surrounding tissues and structures such as blood vessels and nerves. Indeed, the sharp ends of a broken rib can create serious damage to a lung should they perforate into the pleural cavity or lung tissue.

In order for a fracture to heal properly the broken ends must first be reapposed to fit properly again. This is known as "reduction." The bone is then immobilized, usually by a cast, so as to prevent muscles from pulling at the broken pieces until the bone is reconstituted.

The events which take place during bone formation also take place in modified form after a bone is damaged. Connective tissue elements such as fibroblasts and chondroblasts invade the area and form a temporary fibrocartilaginous mass called a **callus.** The periosteum once again produces osteoblasts which begin to lay down new bone around the callus. As in endochondral development, the callus becomes calcified, is resorbed, and replaced by bone.

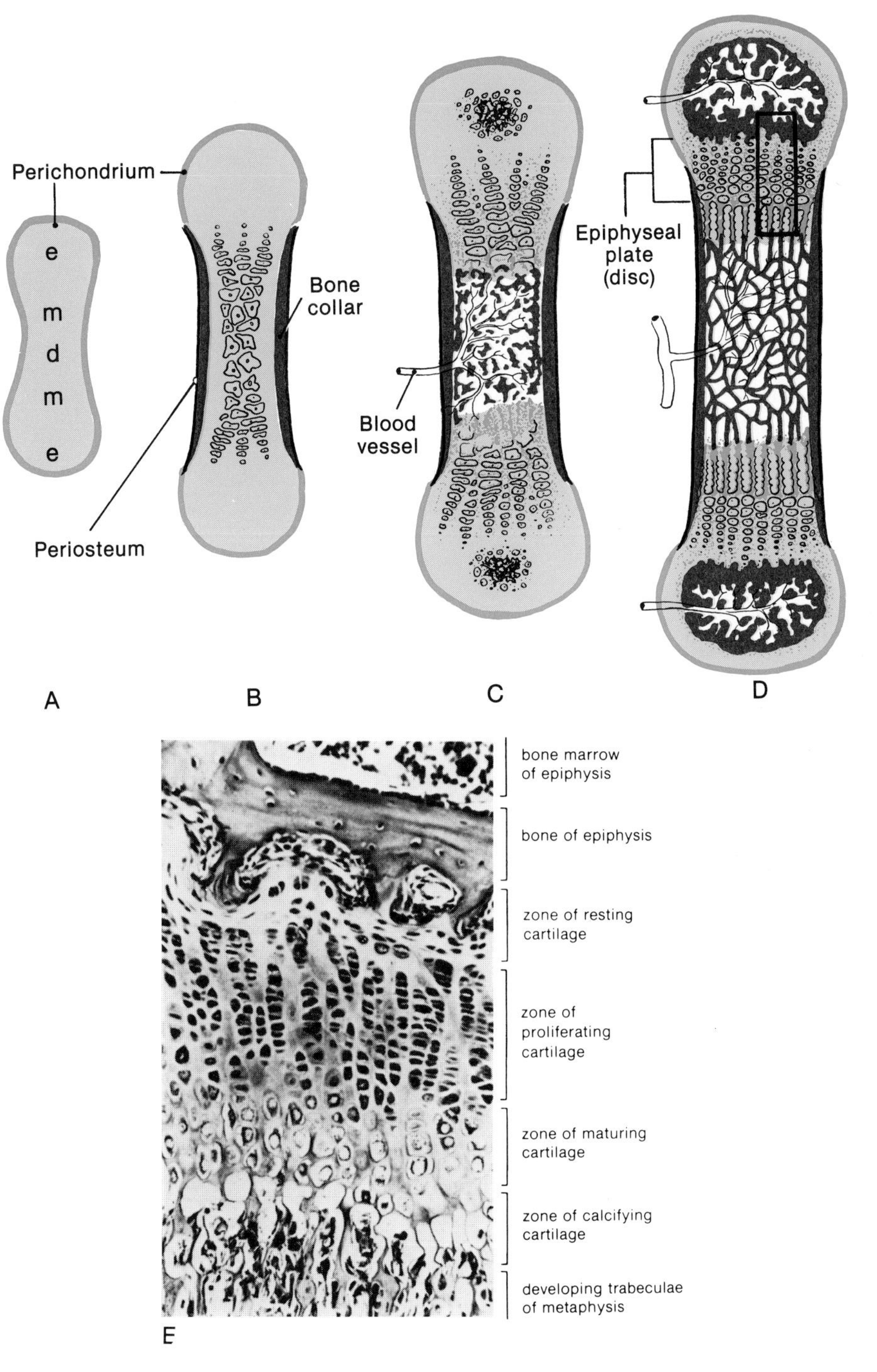

Fig. 7-55. Endochondral bone development. (A) The cartilaginous model is surrounded by perichondrium; e, epiphysis, d, diaphysis, m, metaphysis. (B) A bone collar (red) forms around the diaphysis, and metaphyses. (C) The diaphysis is penetrated by blood vessels, and bone is deposited in the ossification center. Ossification centers also begin to develop in one or both epiphyses. (D) The epiphyseal centers are penetrated by blood vessels, and bone is deposited. The remaining cartilage between the diaphyseal center and epiphyseal centers represents the epiphyseal plates (discs). The area delimited by the rectangle is shown in E. (E) Photomicrograph of a portion of a developing bone showing the four zones of cartilage which occur in an epiphyseal plate. (From A. W. Ham and D. H. Cormack, *Histology,* Ed. 8, J. B. Lippincott Co., Philadelphia, 1979.)

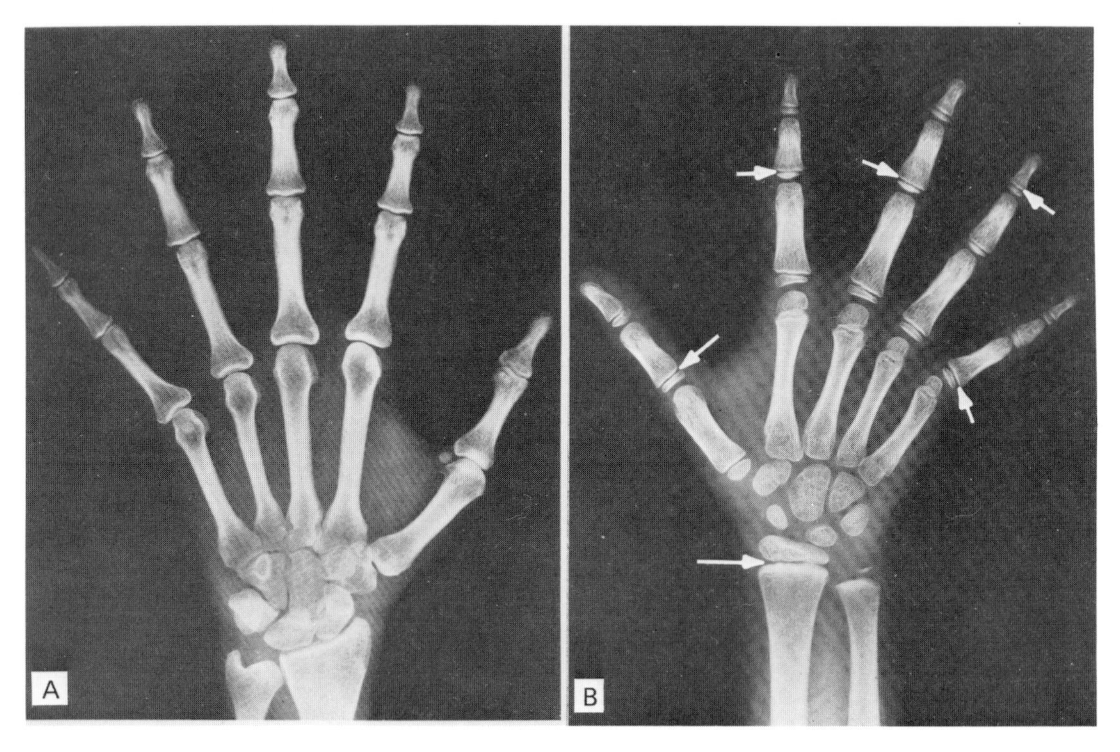

Fig. 7-56. A comparison of X-rays of (A) an adult hand and (B) a child's hand. The *arrows* indicate the epiphyseal plates which are composed of cartilage and thus appear as gaps in the bones. (Modified from E. D. Gardner, D. J. Gray, and R. O'Rahilly, *Anatomy,* Ed. 4, W. B. Saunders Co., Philadelphia, 1975.)

Bone Physiology

Although bone may give an impression of being somewhat inert, it actually is a dynamic tissue which is constantly being laid down, resorbed, and reconstituted. The calcium salts, in particular, are released into the blood stream when bone is resorbed, and this provides the calcium ions essential for the maintenance and activities of other tissues such as muscles and nerves. (A severe depletion of calcium ions can result in a form of tetany whereby the muscles go into a continuous state of contraction.)

The process of bone resorption and the release of calcium into the blood stream is under hormonal control. Excessive resorption occurs in some diseases, such as **hyperparathyroidism,** in which case the bones become demineralized. Also, during pregnancy, the maternal bones are susceptible to calcium depletion to meet the needs of the developing fetus, should there be insufficient intake of calcium in the diet. Calcium depletion from bones can also occur from disuse, as in bedridden patients.

8

The Muscular System

The muscular system is responsible for movement. This movement may be performed by **skeletal muscle** which moves bones, or by **smooth muscle** which propels substances through visceral organs, or by **cardiac muscle** which pumps blood. The muscular system gives form and shape to the body and is also important as a source of heat to help maintain body temperature. The microscopic anatomy of skeletal, smooth, and cardiac muscle is presented in Chapter 4. Since special characteristics of smooth and cardiac muscle are discussed with respect to various organ systems in later chapters, the present chapter will be devoted solely to skeletal muscle.

There are over 600 skeletal muscles in the body, and the total muscle mass makes up at least 30–40% of the body weight. Muscles are usually attached at one end to a relatively fixed point called the **origin,** and at the other end to a relatively movable point called the **insertion.** The fleshy portion of a muscle between its origin and insertion is the **belly** of the muscle. When a muscle contracts and shortens, the insertion moves toward the origin. However, this movement may be reversed in some muscles when the insertion becomes fixed in position, and then the origin may move toward the insertion during contraction. The origin and insertion are on different bones, and muscle contraction results in an action across the joint between the bones.

A muscle attaches to a bone by means of a fibrous band of connective tissue known as a **tendon.** The connective tissue of the tendon blends with the periosteum of the bone. In some regions, tendons are surrounded by collapsed, fluid-filled sacs called **bursae** which help to lubricate the tendon as it slides back and forth. If the tendon is a flattened sheet it is called an **aponeurosis.**

The names of muscles may reflect their shape (trapezius), size (minimus), action (extensor), location (tibialis anterior), number of heads (triceps), or bony points of attachment (sternohyoid). An understanding of the principles of muscle action can help one ascertain what a muscle does on the basis of its origin and insertion. Conversely, the action of some muscles (as reflected by their names) can enable one to determine their origins and insertions.

Certain muscles are antagonistic to one another. When one muscle (called the **prime mover**) contracts, the **antagonist** relaxes. Other muscles act together to assist one another as **synergists.** Muscles may also act as **fixators** in stabilizing a joint so that other muscles can act on the joint as prime movers. Muscle movements rarely can be simplified into a single action, but instead consist of complex interactions among these prime movers, antagonists, synergists, and fixators.

Each muscle is enveloped by the **deep fascia,** a tough dense connective tissue which helps to support the muscle. This deep fascia blends with a thinner layer of connective tissue called the **epimysium** lying on the surface of the muscle (Fig. 8-1). The epimysium sends connective tissue partitions inward into the muscle, and these form the **perimysium** which ensheaths a bundle (or fasciculus) of muscle fibers. The perimysium in turn sends inward a thin layer of connective tissue which surrounds each individual muscle fiber and is called the **endomysium.** It is important to keep in mind that these connective tissues form a network which binds together the muscle fibers and which also serves as a pathway for the blood vessels and nerves supplying the fibers.

Each muscle fiber is a single cell containing numerous myofibrils, each of which is composed of myofilaments (Fig. 8-1). The fine structure and function of skeletal muscle fibers are discussed in greater detail in Chapter 4.

Muscles depend upon a rich supply of blood vessels and on nerves carrying the impulses for contraction. If a muscle is deprived of its innervation, it is said to be denervated and eventually will **atrophy** as each muscle fiber decreases in size. A muscle can also **hypertrophy** from constant use, in which case the muscle fibers increase in size, but the number of fibers and fibrils remains the same.

As we proceed to study the gross anatomy of skeletal muscles, it is worthwhile to keep in mind that interactions occur among muscles, bones, cartilages, joints, ligaments, tendons, and nerves. In fact, muscles and bones are often considered together as one large system: the musculoskeletal system. Also, muscles are more easily learned and remembered if they are grouped together according to location or action.

Table 8-1 has been provided at the end of this chapter as a quick reference and review of the major named muscles. The innervation of each muscle is also listed.

MUSCLES OF THE HEAD

Muscles of Facial Expression

The most superficial muscles of the head are the muscles of facial expression. Most of these muscles originate from facial bones, insert into the skin, and are extremely delicate. As a person ages and the skin loses its resiliency, ridges occur in the skin perpendicular to the direction of the facial muscle fibers.

The facial muscles are responsible for the wide range of expression by which emotions are communicated to others. Some of these muscles, particularly those associated with the lips, are also important in speech. Some are poorly developed, such as the muscles which wiggle the ears (anterior, superior, and posterior **auricularis muscles**), and few people have developed the ability to contract these muscles.

The **epicranius** is a sheet of muscular and fibrous tissue which consists of a muscle mass (the **frontalis** muscle) on the forehead connected by the fibrous **galea aponeurotica** (**epicranial aponeurosis**) to a smaller muscle mass at the base of the scalp (the **occipitalis** muscle) (Fig. 8-2). The frontalis muscle can raise the eyebrows and is better developed than the occipitalis, which pulls the scalp backward.

Each orbit is encircled by an **orbicularis oculi** muscle which passes also into the upper and lower eyelids and forcefully closes the eye. The antagonists of the orbicularis oculi muscles are the **levator palpebrae superioris** muscles (to be described with the eye muscles), and to some extent the frontalis muscles.

A large group of muscles is associated with the mouth. The **orbicularis oris** surrounds the mouth and is involved in closing the lips. A series of **levator** and **depressor** muscles also inserts here and is responsible for elevating and depressing the lips, respectively. The levator muscles include: **zygomaticus** (**major** and **minor**) and **levator labii superioris**; the depressor muscles include: **depressor anguli oris, depressor labii inferioris,** and **mentalis.** In addition, the **risorius** muscle retracts the angle of the mouth.

A deeper muscle is the **buccinator** which originates laterally from the mandible and maxilla and from a fibrous band (the pterygomandibular raphe). The buccinator inserts into the side of the mouth (Fig. 8-2). This muscle serves an important function in compressing

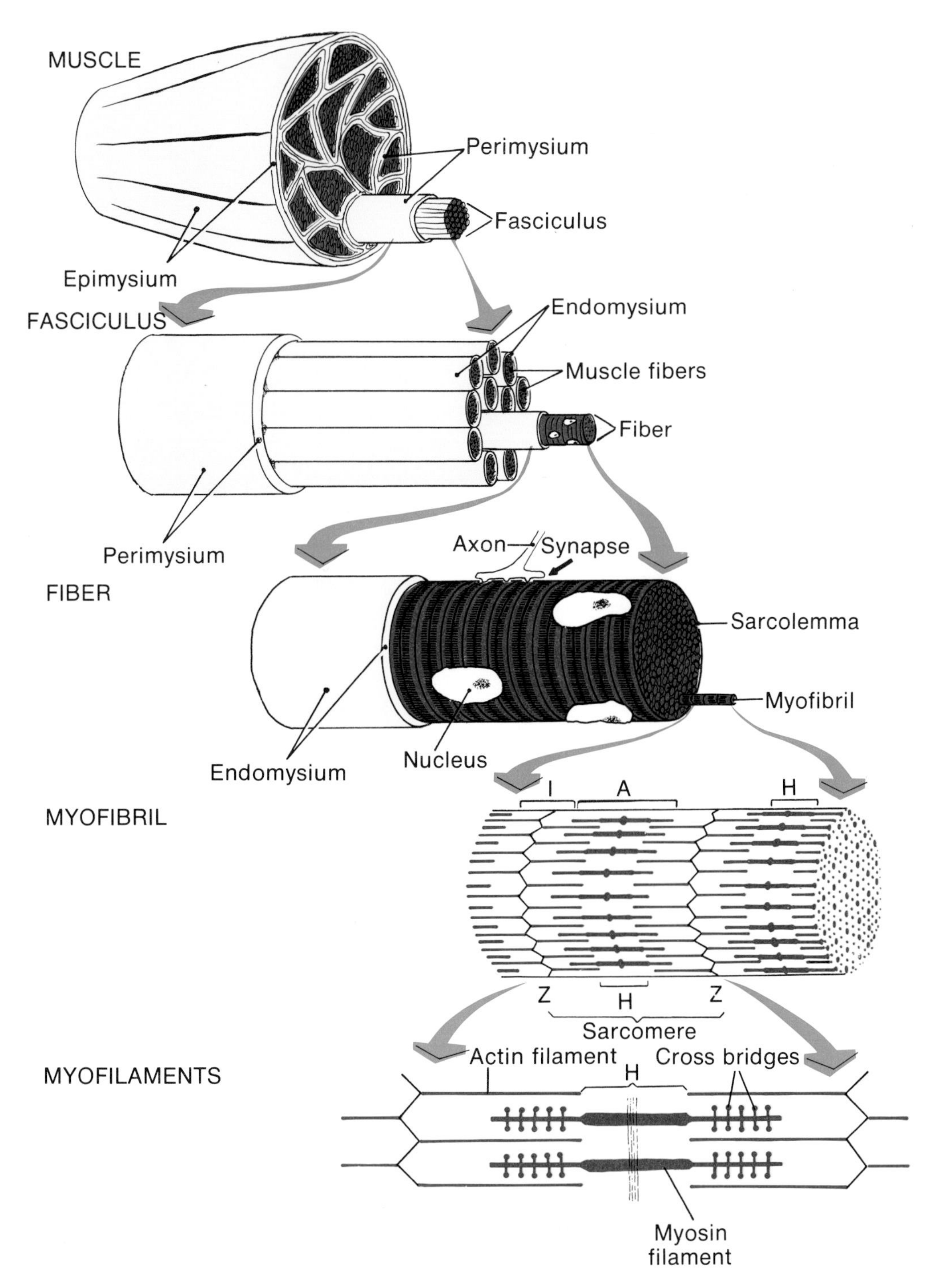

Fig. 8-1. Organization of skeletal muscle.

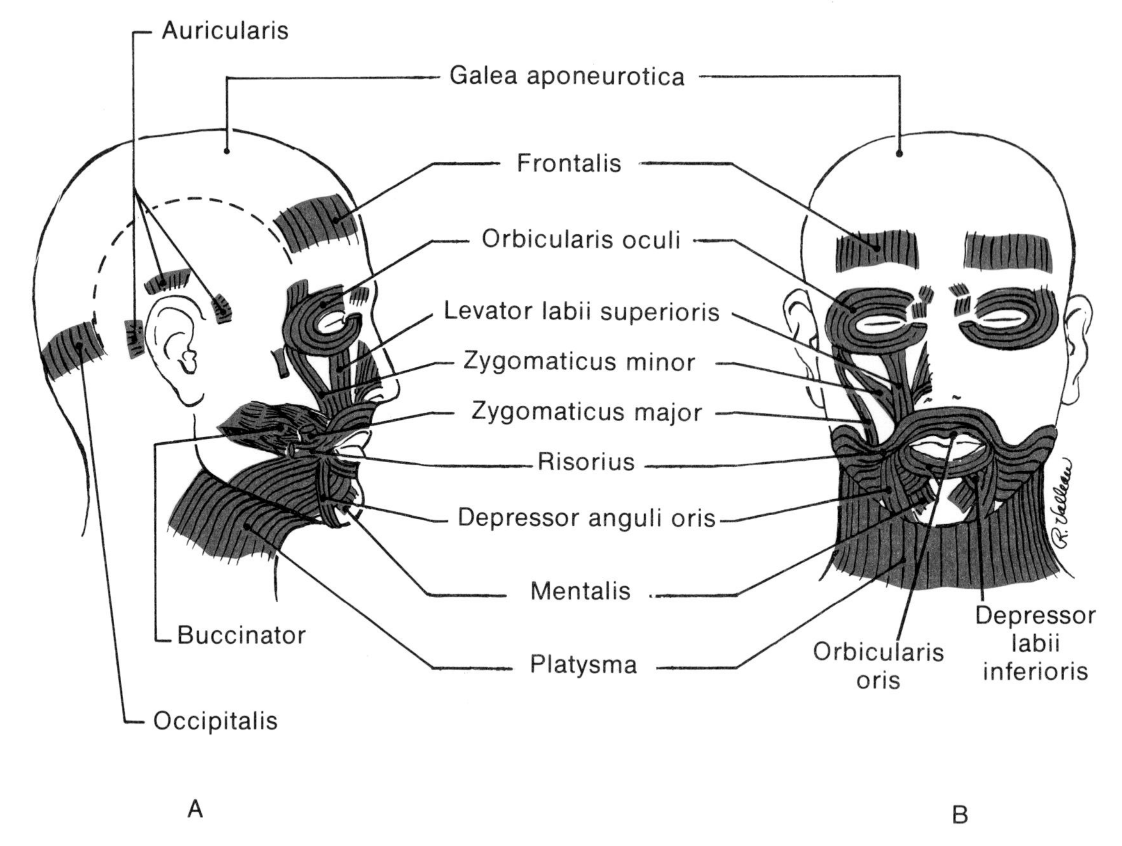

Fig. 8-2. Muscles of facial expression. (A) Lateral view. (The zygomaticus major and risorius have been cut to show the deeper lying buccinator muscle.) (B) Anterior view.

the cheeks so as to prevent food from accumulating between the teeth and cheeks during chewing. It also plays a role in blowing air out from the mouth as in whistling.

Finally, the **platysma** muscle is also included as a muscle of facial expression even though it lies superficially on the anterior aspect of the neck. It originates from fascia in the upper thoracic region and passes obliquely upward to insert into the mandible and corner of the mouth, which it depresses.

Muscles of Mastication

There are four pairs of muscles which are concerned with chewing (mastication): the masseter, temporalis, medial pterygoid, and lateral pterygoid muscles. The **masseter** passes from the zygomatic arch to the lateral surface of the ramus of the mandible and thus elevates the mandible (Fig. 8-3). The **temporalis** is a fan-shaped muscle which occupies and originates from the temporal fossa and inserts on the coronoid process of the mandible and likewise elevates the mandible. The **medial pterygoid** and **lateral pterygoid** muscles originate from the medial and lateral surfaces of the lateral pterygoid plate of the sphenoid bone, respectively. The medial pterygoid inserts on the medial surface of the ramus of the mandible and, like the masseter and temporalis, elevates the mandible and thereby closes the mouth. The lateral pterygoid, however, passes posteriorly and inserts into the capsule of the temporomandibular joint. Contraction of this muscle moves the mandible forward (protrudes the jaw). The lateral pterygoid may also aid

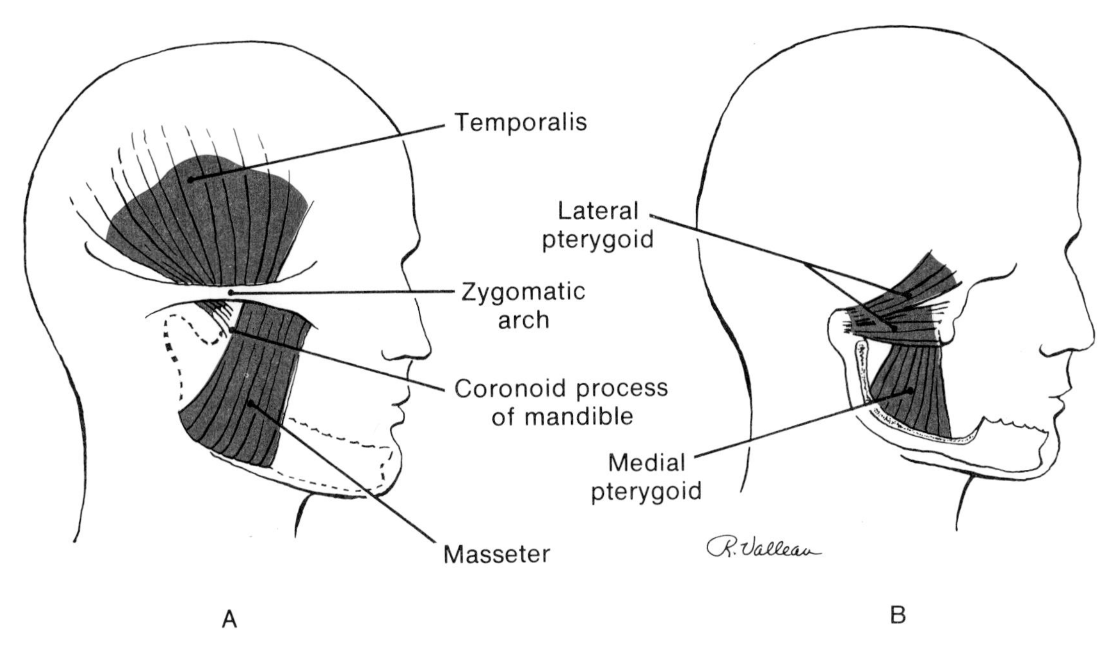

Fig. 8-3. Muscles of mastication. (A) Masseter and temporalis muscles, (B) lateral and medial pterygoid muscles. (Masseter and temporalis muscles have been removed, along with the zygomatic arch and a portion of the mandible.)

slightly in opening the mouth, although it is believed that the pull of gravity is largely responsible for depressing (lowering) the mandible when the three other muscles of mastication (masseter, temporalis, and medial pterygoid) are relaxed.

Tongue Muscles

The muscles within the tongue are termed **intrinsic** muscles and pass in three different planes. **Extrinsic** muscles **(genioglossus, hyoglossus, styloglossus,** and **palatoglossus)** originate outside the tongue and insert into its base (Fig. 8-4). The extrinsic and intrinsic muscles provide a considerable range of movement for speaking, chewing, and deglutition (swallowing).

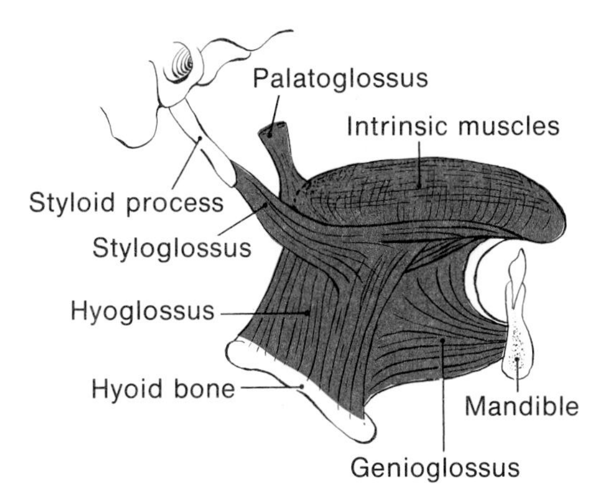

Fig. 8-4. Extrinsic and intrinsic muscles of the tongue.

Eye Muscles

Each eyeball is moved by six **extrinsic eye** muscles. These muscles originate from the bony orbit and insert into the outermost covering of the eyeball. In addition, the upper eyelid contains the **levator palpebrae superioris**

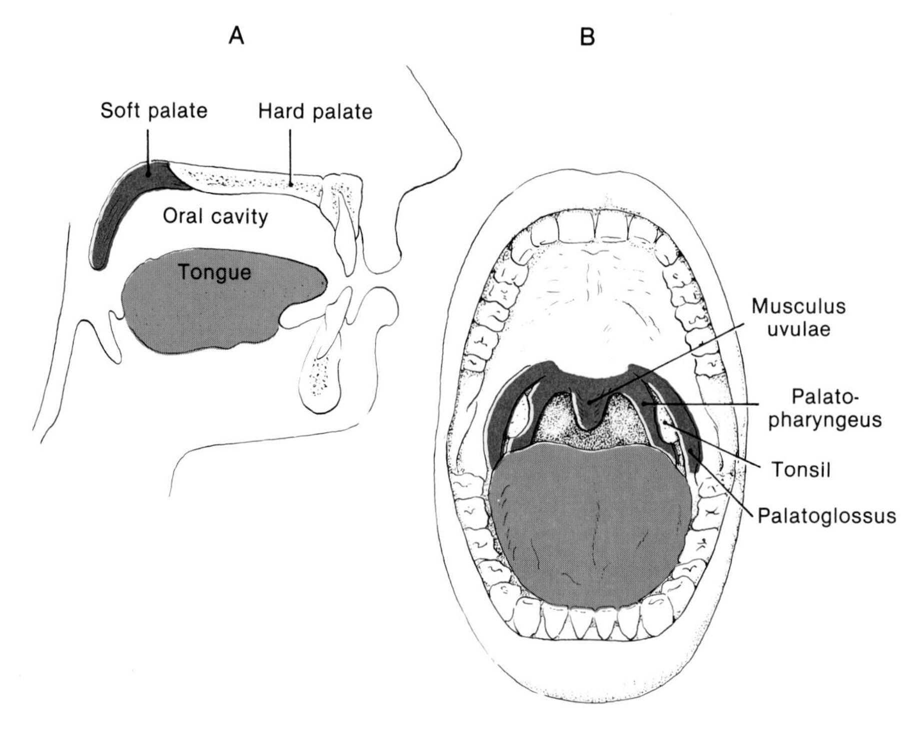

Fig. 8-5. (A) The hard and soft palate as seen in a sagittal section through the head, (B) anterior view of the mouth showing muscles of the soft palate.

muscle which raises the upper lid and keeps the eye open. (The **orbicularis oculi** muscles in the upper and lower eyelids close the eye.) The interactions of these muscles are discussed in relation to the eye (Chapter 12).

Muscles of the Palate

The **hard palate** is a bony shelf consisting of the palatine processes of the maxillae and the horizontal portions of the palatine bones. It forms the roof of the mouth and separates the oral cavity from the nasal cavity. The **soft palate** is composed of muscular tissue which hangs backward and downward from the posterior border of the hard palate (Fig. 8-5). During swallowing the soft palate is pulled upward so as to prevent food and liquid from passing into the nasal region known as the nasopharynx.

The free edge of the soft palate shows a median projection, the **uvula** which contains a small unpaired muscle, the **musculus uvulae** (Fig. 8-5.) Laterally the soft palate continues into two folds of muscle: the **palatoglossus** to the base of the tongue, and the **palatopharyngeus** to the pharyngeal region. In children, the tonsils can be seen situated between these two folds. (Two other muscles, the **levator** and **tensor veli palatini** help to pull the soft palate upward and backward.)

Although the palatal muscles are associated with the pharyngeal muscles, the latter extend deeply into the neck region and will be discussed later.

MUSCLES OF THE NECK

Anterior Muscles

The anterior surface of the neck consists of several layers of muscles, the most superficial one being the **platysma** which was included with the muscles of facial expression. Just deep to the platysma is a large prominent muscle, the **sternomastoid,** or **sternocleidomastoid** muscle, so named because of its origin from the

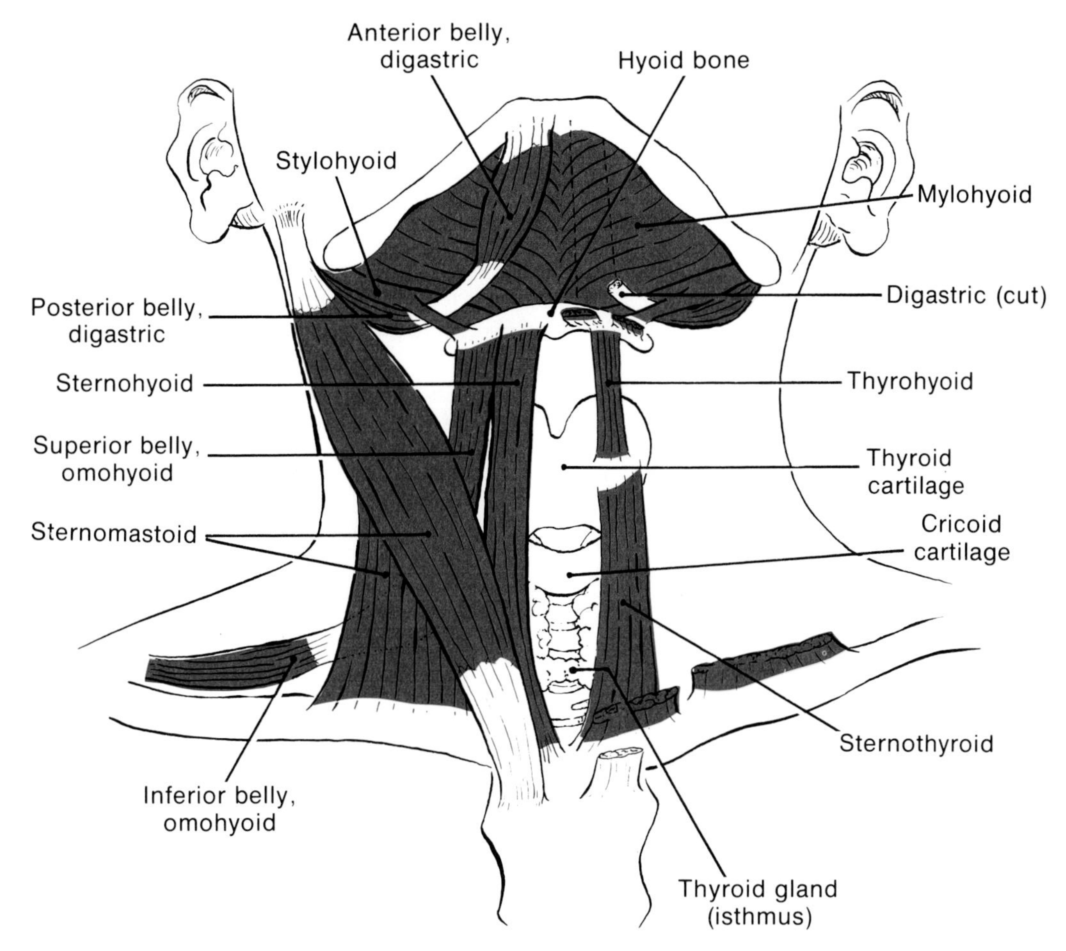

Fig. 8-6. Infrahyoid and suprahyoid muscles. The left sternomastoid, omohyoid, and sternohyoid muscles have been removed so as to expose the deeper lying sternothyroid and thyrohyoid muscles. The left digastric anterior belly has also been cut and removed, and the broken lines indicate the outline of the left geniohyoid muscle lying deep to the mylohyoid muscle.

sternum ("sterno") and clavicle ("cleido") and its insertion on the mastoid portion of the temporal bone (Fig. 8-6). When the two sternomastoid muscles contract together, they flex the head forward. Acting alone, each muscle brings the head closer to the shoulder of the same side and rotates the face to the opposite side.

Infrahyoid Muscles

Deep to the sternomastoid muscles is a group of four long flat infrahyoid muscles (sometimes called the "strap" muscles) of which two are more superficially placed (sternohyoid and omohyoid), and two are deep (sternothyroid and thyrohyoid). The **sternohyoid** originates from the sternum and passes upward to insert on the hyoid bone (Fig. 8-6). The **omohyoid** is composed of an **inferior belly** passing from the scapula to an intermediate tendon bound to the clavicle, and a **superior belly** extending obliquely from the clavicle upward to the hyoid bone. Deep to the sternohyoid muscle are the **sternothyroid** which passes from sternum to thyroid cartilage of the larynx, and the **thyrohyoid** from thyroid cartilage to hyoid bone. These four infrahyoid muscles depress the hyoid bone and larynx.

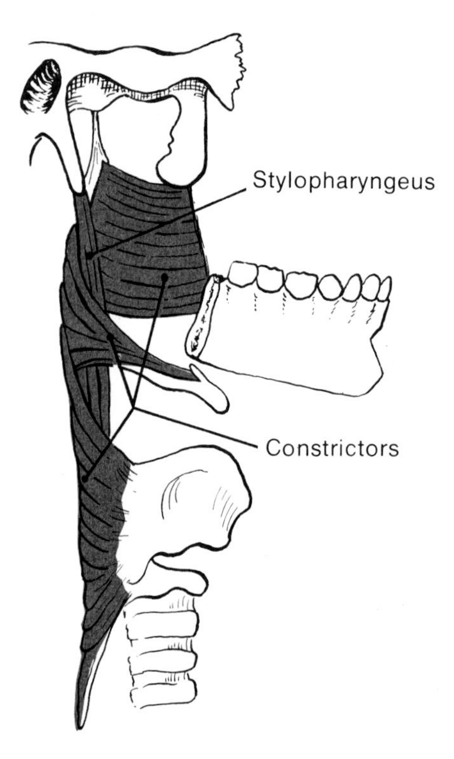

Fig. 8-7. Pharyngeal muscles, lateral view. Of the longitudinal muscles, only the stylopharyngeus is depicted.

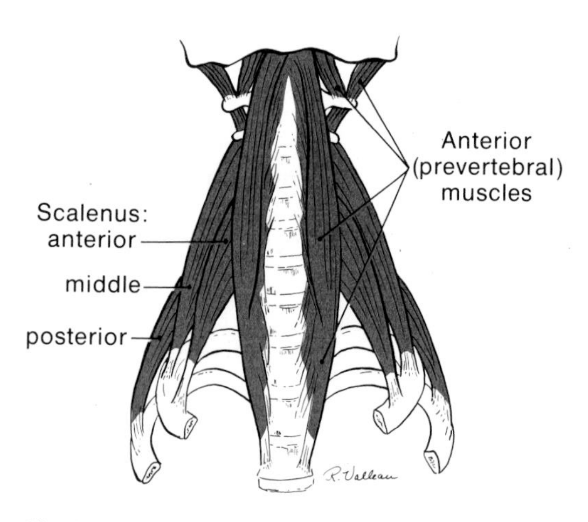

Fig. 8-8. Anterior and lateral vertebral muscles of the neck, anterior view.

Suprahyoid Muscles

The suprahyoid muscles are situated above the hyoid bone and consist of muscles which elevate the hyoid bone (and larynx) during deglutition (swallowing), as well as some muscles which form the floor of the mouth.

The **digastric** muscle consists of a **posterior belly** passing from the mastoid region of the temporal bone to an intermediate tendon bound to the hyoid bone, and an **anterior belly** from the tendon to the tip of the mandible (Fig. 8-6). The digastric not only elevates the hyoid but also can depress the mandible. A slender **stylohyoid** muscle runs along with the posterior belly of the digastric and inserts on the hyoid bone.

The **mylohyoid** muscle lies deep to the anterior belly of the digastric and contributes to the floor of the mouth. It originates from the inner aspect of the mandible and passes medially to insert along with its counterpart from the opposite side into a median strip of connective tissue. (The posterior border of the muscle inserts into the hyoid bone.) Above the mylohyoid is the narrow **geniohyoid** muscle whose fibers extend from the tip of the mandible to the hyoid bone, thereby contributing to the floor of the mouth. Two other muscles in this region (the genioglossus and hyoglossus) have already been described with the extrinsic muscles of the tongue.

Pharyngeal Muscles

The pharyngeal muscles form a muscular tube located deep within the head and neck. These muscles consist of the **pharyngeal constrictors (superior, middle,** and **inferior)** arranged as circular and overlapping tubes, and a set of deeper and more slender muscles **(stylopharyngeus, palatopharyngeus,** and **salpingopharyngeus)** arranged longitudinally (Fig. 8-7). The pharyngeal muscles are particularly important during swallowing when they squeeze food downward along the pharynx.

Laryngeal Muscles

Intrinsic as well as extrinsic muscles are associated with the larynx. The **intrinsic laryn-**

geal muscles function in speech (phonation) by regulating the position and tension of the vocal cords. The **extrinsic laryngeal** muscles include the suprahyoid and infrahyoid muscles and are concerned with movement of the larynx during deglutition. The interrelationships and actions of these muscles will be discussed more fully with the respiratory system (Chapter 11).

Anterior and Lateral Vertebral Muscles

These muscles occur along the anterior and lateral surfaces of the cervical vertebral column (Fig. 8-8). The anterior (prevertebral) muscles work together to flex the head, or by acting singly they can turn or bend the head laterally. The lateral vertebral muscles consist of three **scalenus** muscles **(anterior, middle,** and **posterior)**. The scalenus muscles originate from the transverse processes of the 2nd to 6th cervical vertebrae and insert onto the first 2 ribs. They elevate the ribs and enable one to inhale deeply especially during forced breathing.

Posterior Muscles

The most superficial muscle on the posterior surface of the neck is the **trapezius** muscle, which also extends down the upper portion of the back (Fig. 8-9). This large muscle originates from the occipital bone, from a ligament **(ligamentum nuchae)** along the spines of the cervical vertebrae, and from the spines of the thoracic vertebrae. Depending on the level of their origins, the trapezius fibers pass either obliquely downward or upward to insert on the spine and acromion of the scapula and the clavicle. The trapezius provides the natural line of slope from head to shoulder, and the actions of this muscle are extensive and varied including elevation, depression, rotation, and retraction of the scapula.

Deep to the trapezius is the **splenius** muscle which originates from the lower portion of the ligamentum nuchae and from spines of the upper thoracic vertebrae (Fig. 8-10). The splenius extends upward and laterally to insert onto the transverse processes of the upper cervical vertebrae and mastoid process and occipital bone of the skull.

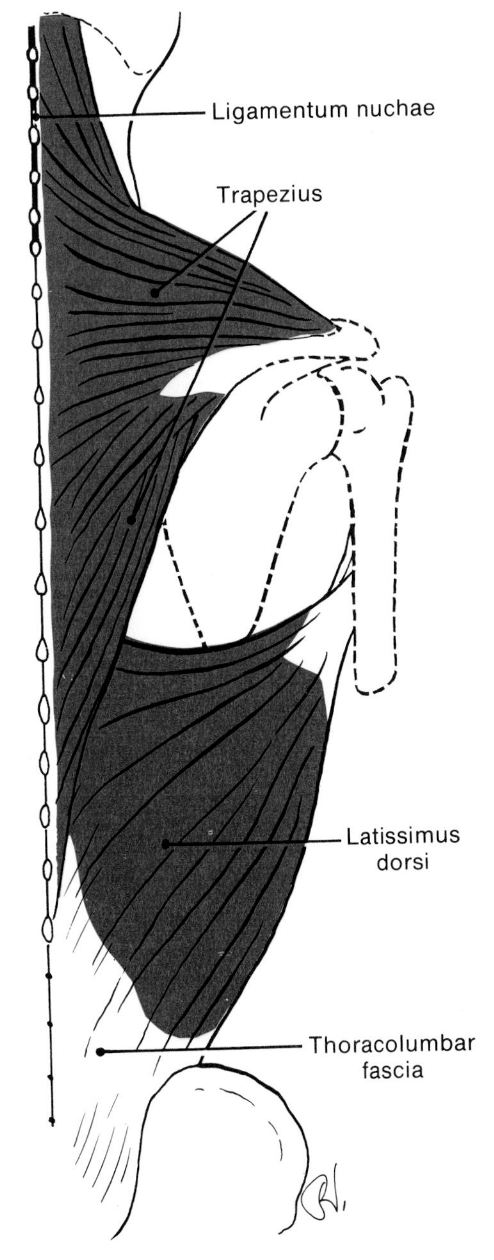

Fig. 8-9. Superficial muscles on the posterior surface of the neck and back, right side.

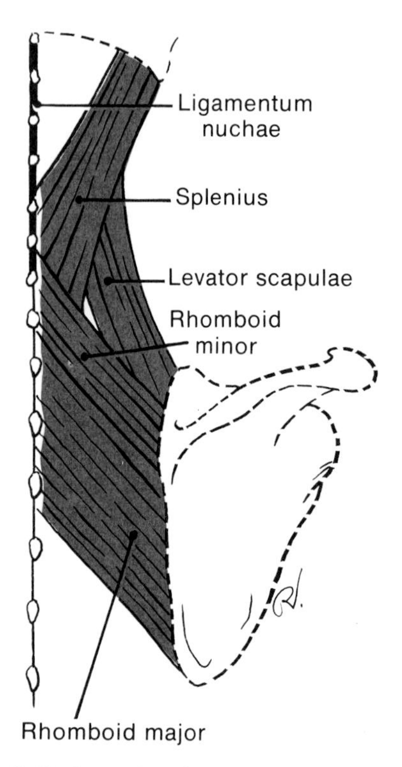

Fig. 8-10. Posterior deep muscles of the neck and upper back, right side. (The trapezius muscle has been removed.)

The splenius, as well as deeper muscles of the neck, are often grouped together as **posterior vertebral** muscles and are responsible for extending the neck and head and thus counteracting the action of the anterior vertebral group of muscles. Many of the posterior muscles correspond in form and function to deep muscles of the back, and thus will be alluded to again with the musculature of the trunk. In addition, several small **suboccipital** muscles serve a special function in moving the atlas around the dens of the axis, thereby rotating the head from side to side (as in shaking the head "no").

MUSCLES OF THE TRUNK

Posterior Muscles

The posterior trunk muscles act on the axial skeleton, including the vertebral column, ribs, and skull, and on the shoulder girdle and humerus of the appendicular skeleton. The superficial layer consists of two large muscles: the trapezius and the latissimus dorsi. The upper portion of the **trapezius** has already been described along with muscles of the posterior surface of the neck, and it helps to elevate the scapula. The lower portion of the trapezius extends from the vertebral column superficially across the upper thoracic region to insert on the spine of the scapula (Fig. 8-9). These lower fibers of the trapezius adduct (retract) the scapula. As mentioned previously, the trapezius is also important in rotating the scapula.

The **latissimus dorsi** is a large broad muscle which originates from the iliac crest, from dense fascia **(thoracolumbar fascia)** in the lower region of the back, from the spines of the lower thoracic vertebrae, and from the lower ribs (Fig. 8-9). The latissimus dorsi extends upward and laterally, crosses the inferior angle of the scapula, and inserts anteriorly on the upper end of the humerus. The muscle acts primarily as an extensor, adductor, and medial rotator of the arm, although it may also help to keep the inferior angle of the scapula flat against the thoracic cage.

Deep to the trapezius muscle is a group of

muscles which act on the scapula. The **levator scapulae** originates from the transverse processes of the upper cervical vertebrae and inserts on the upper medial border of the scapula; it thus elevates the scapula (Fig. 8-10). The **rhomboid minor** passes from the seventh cervical and first thoracic vertebrae to the base of the spine of the scapula. The **rhomboid major** originates from the upper thoracic vertebrae and inserts on the lower medial border of the scapula below the base of its spine. The two rhomboids together adduct (retract) the scapula and help to brace it in place.

Deep to the rhomboids and latissimus dorsi are two thin and poorly developed muscles: the **serratus posterior superior** and **inferior** (Fig. 8-11). These muscles may aid in elevating and depressing the ribs during inspiration and expiration, respectively.

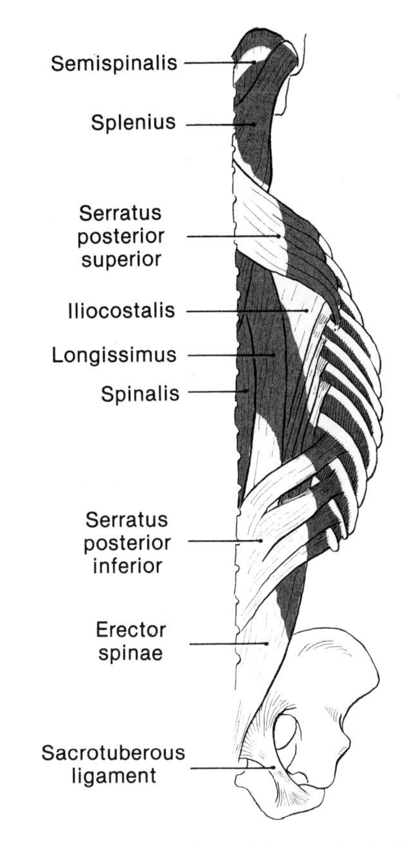

Fig. 8-11. Deep muscles of the back, including the erector spinae muscles (spinalis, longissimus, and iliocostalis). (Modified after Basmajian.)

Deep Muscles of the Trunk

The deep muscles of the back (and neck) are often referred to as the **posterior vertebral** or **postural muscles** and are responsible for maintaining the erect position of the trunk. They are grouped together as the **erector spinae** muscles, and they extend from the sacrum upward along the back and neck to the base of the skull. The muscles are arranged in bundles which originate at different levels of the vertebral column and insert as they pass upward onto ribs and higher levels of the vertebral column and skull.

There are three longitudinal divisions of the erector spinae muscles (Fig. 8-11). The most medial one is the **spinalis** which extends for varying distances along the spines of the vertebrae. The intermediate division of the erector spinae is the **longissimus** which is larger and extends along the ribs and transverse processes of the vertebrae. The lateralmost division is the **iliocostalis** and passes upward along the angles of the ribs. Specific regions of the spinalis, longissimus, and iliocostalis are often designated on the basis of the level at which the muscle bundles occur; thus, the iliocostalis thoracis is that portion of the iliocostalis

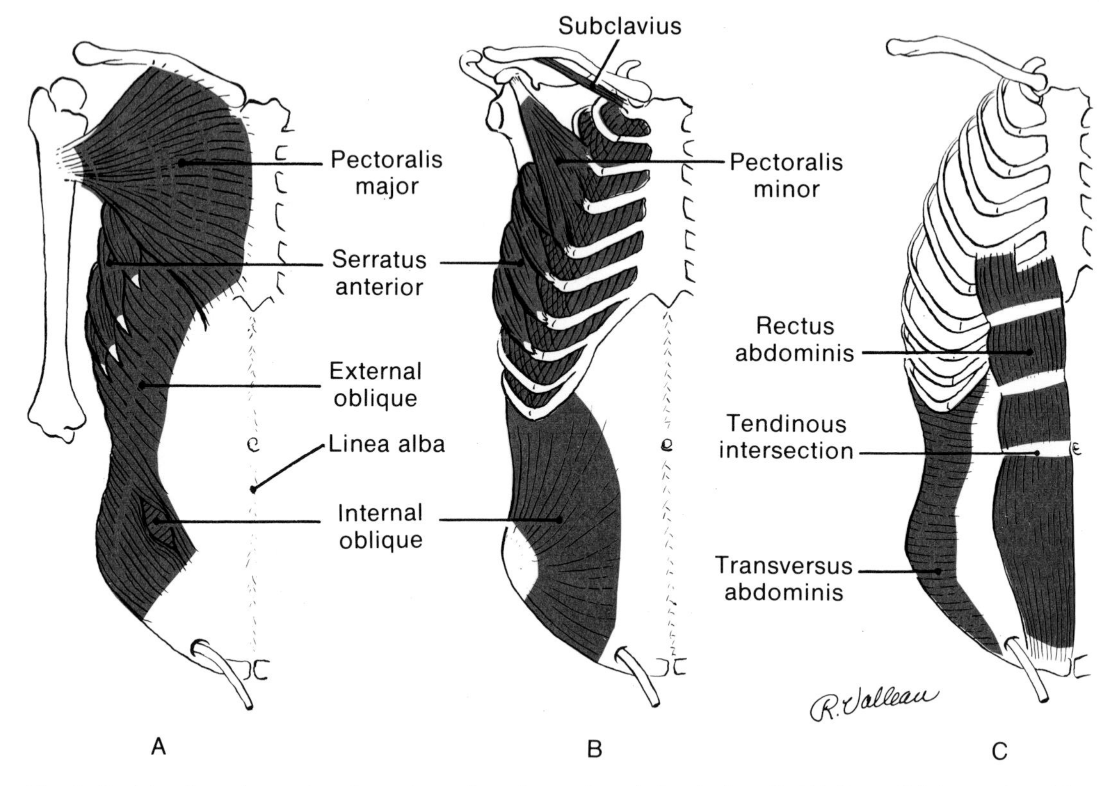

Fig. 8-12. Muscles of anterior thoracic wall and anterior abdominal wall. (A) Superficial muscles. (The lower fibers of the external oblique have been slit and spread apart to show the deeper lying internal oblique muscle.) (B) Deeper muscles, with pectoralis major and external oblique muscles removed. (C) The thoracic muscles, external oblique, and internal oblique muscles as well as their aponeuroses have been removed to show the transversus abdominis and rectus abdominis muscles.

which is found in the thoracic region, whereas the iliocostalis cervicis is located in the cervical region.

There is another set of smaller back muscles deep to the erector spinae. These are collectively termed the **transversospinal** muscles, and they pass obliquely upward and medially from the transverse processes of the vertebrae to the spinous processes. (In the neck region, some of these form the semispinalis cervicis muscle.) Many of these deeper muscles help to rotate the trunk around the longitudinal axis. Also sometimes included with these muscles are the **levatores costarum** which pass from vertebrae to ribs and help to elevate the ribs during respiration.

It should be obvious that the erector spinae and transversospinalis muscles are difficult to distinguish from one another and that they show extremely complex interactions and anatomical relationships. This can also pose a problem clinically, since it is often difficult to diagnose and treat injuries or disease which may affect one or more of these muscles. Moreover, back pain may result not only from muscular disorders, but also from involvement of the bones, joints, and ligaments of the vertebral column, as well as from injuries to nerves in the area.

Beneath the deep muscles of the back are muscles of the posterior thoracic and abdominal walls. These muscles will be discussed later in relation to the anterior and anterolateral thoracic and abdominal musculature.

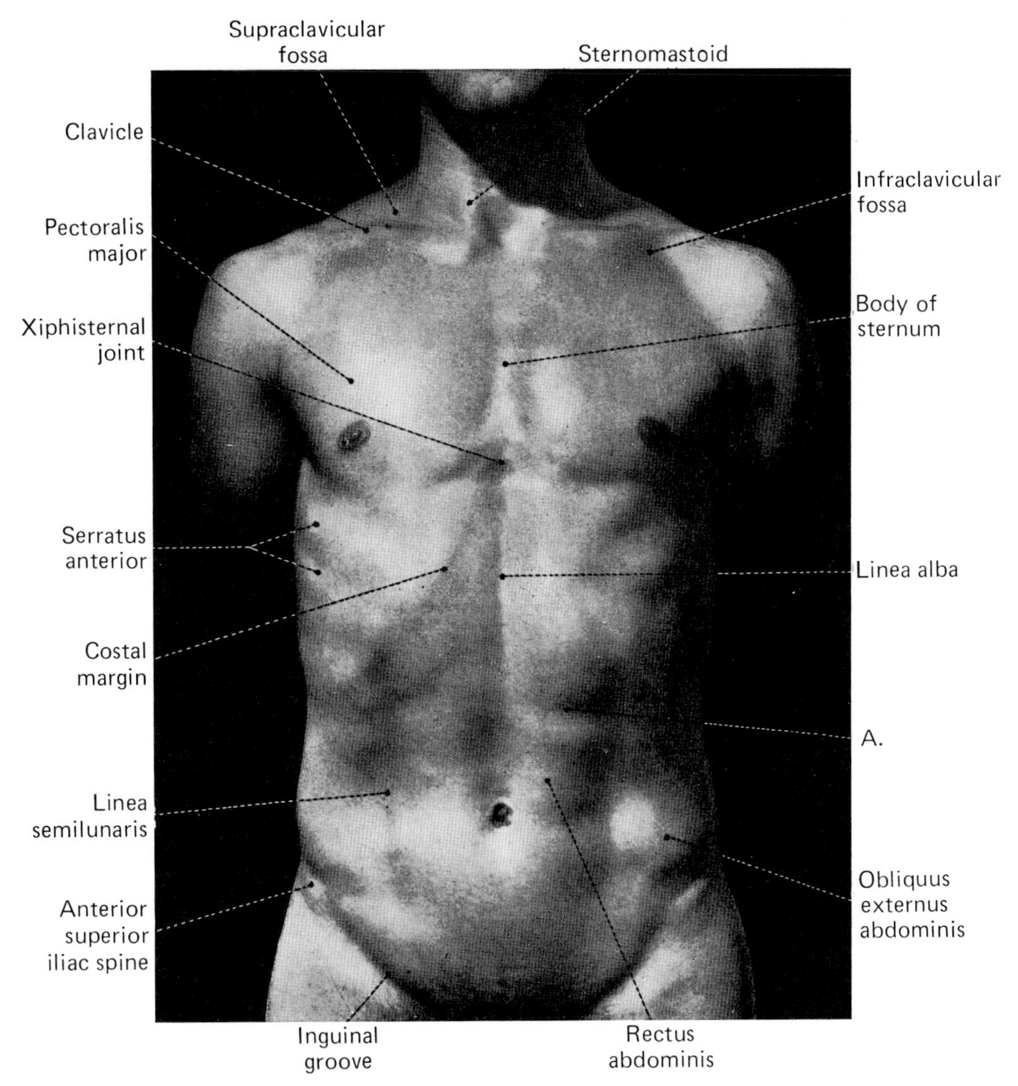

Fig. 8-13. Surface anatomy of the anterior thoracic wall and anterior abdominal wall. A, tendinous intersection. (From W. J. Hamilton, G. Simon, and S. G. I. Hamilton, *Surface and Radiological Anatomy,* Ed. 5, The Macmillan Press, London, 1971.)

Anterior Muscles of the Thorax

The anterior region of the thorax contains groups of muscles which act on the ribs, shoulder girdle, and humerus. Some of these muscles originate from bones of the axial skeleton and insert on appendicular bones, while other muscles both originate and insert on axial bones.

The **pectoralis major** is a large fanshaped muscle which takes origin from the sternum, ribs, and medial portion of the clavicle (Figs. 8-12 and 8-13). It passes across the upper anterior surface of the chest and inserts on the upper end of the humerus. It is a strong adductor of the arm.

The **pectoralis minor** is a smaller fan-shaped muscle which lies deep to the pectoralis major and which passes from the ribs upward

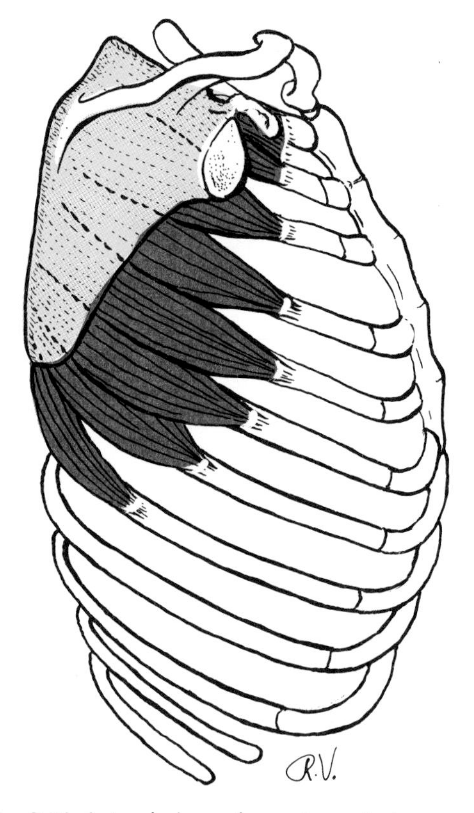

Fig. 8-14. Lateral view of serratus anterior muscle. The muscle fibers pass beneath the scapula to insert on its medial (vertebral) border. (Modified after *Grant's Method.*)

to insert on the coracoid process of the scapula. Another small muscle, the **subclavius** extends from the first rib to the inferior surface of the clavicle. The actions of these two muscles are not clear, although they most likely depress the tip of the shoulder and lateral region of the clavicle, respectively. In addition, the subclavius also may protect underlying vessels such as the subclavian vein.

The **serratus anterior** originates by slips of muscle from the upper eight ribs, extends laterally and posteriorly in close contact with the lateral surface of the thoracic cage, and passes under the anterior surface of the scapula to insert on its medial border (Fig. 8-14). It thus pulls the scapula laterally (abduction, protraction), an action which is important in order for the arm to be elevated.

Intercostal Muscles

The intercostal muscles are located between the ribs in the posterior, lateral, and anterior regions of the thoracic cage. The intercostals are arranged in three layers: external, internal and innermost. Each **external intercostal** muscle originates from the rib above and inserts on the rib below (Fig. 8-15). In the anterior region of the thorax, the external intercostal fibers slant downward and medially; at the junction of the ribs with the costal cartilages, the external intercostal muscle fibers become continuous with a membranous sheet of connective tissue which extends medially to the sternum. In the posterior region the external intercostal muscles slant downward and laterally. The external intercostals elevate the ribs.

The fibers of the **internal intercostal** muscles lie deep and perpendicular to those of the external intercostals. Thus the internal intercostal muscles originate from the rib above and slant downward and laterally in the anterior region of the thorax and downward and medially in the posterior region. Posteriorly at the angles of the ribs the internal intercostal muscles become continuous with a membranous sheet of connective tissue extending to the vertebrae.

The **innermost intercostal** muscles actually constitute the deep portion of the internal intercostals since their fibers pass in the same direction. Intercostal blood vessels and nerves pass between the internal and innermost intercostals, and both muscle groups are involved in expiration, although their exact action is unclear. Anteriorly the innermost intercostals are absent from the medial region of the thorax where they are replaced by a group of **transversus thoracis** muscles passing from the inner aspect of the sternum upward and laterally to span several ribs above. A comparable group termed the **subcostal** muscles occurs near the angles of the ribs in the posteromedial region of the thorax. The transversus thoracis and subcostal muscles most likely act to depress and draw the ribs together, respectively. **Levatores costarum** muscles also occur posteriorly and slant downward from the thoracic vertebrae to the next rib below. They elevate the ribs.

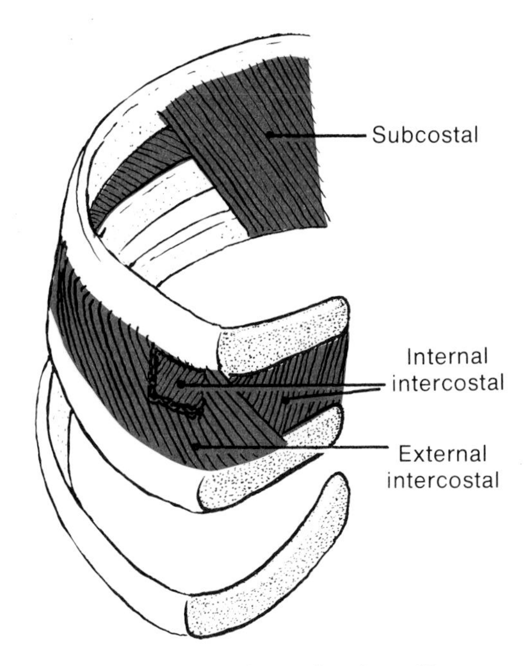

Fig. 8-15. Anterior and superior view of intercostal muscles in one intercostal space. A portion of the external intercostal muscle has been removed to show the underlying internal intercostal muscle. Posteriorly a subcostal muscle can be seen spanning one rib.

Anterior Muscles of the Abdomen

The muscles which comprise the anterior and anterolateral abdominal wall show similarities to the intercostal muscles of the thorax. In fact the intercostal, serratus anterior, and upper abdominal muscles interdigitate and overlap with one another so closely that it is often difficult to separate these groups. Much of the anterior abdominal wall consists of dense fibrous connective tissue in the form of **aponeuroses.** The aponeuroses, as well as the muscles, serve to compress the abdomen. The muscles also rotate and flex the vertebral column.

The outermost layer of abdominal muscles is the **external oblique** muscle which originates from the lateral portion of the lower eight ribs and slants downward and medially (Fig. 8-12). Some of the fibers insert on the iliac crest, while others insert by means of the fibrous **external oblique aponeurosis** into a median band of connective tissue called the **linea alba** (white line).

The middle layer of abdominal muscles is the **internal oblique** which originates from the iliac crest, inguinal ligament (see below), and a mass of dense connective tissue **(thoraco-**

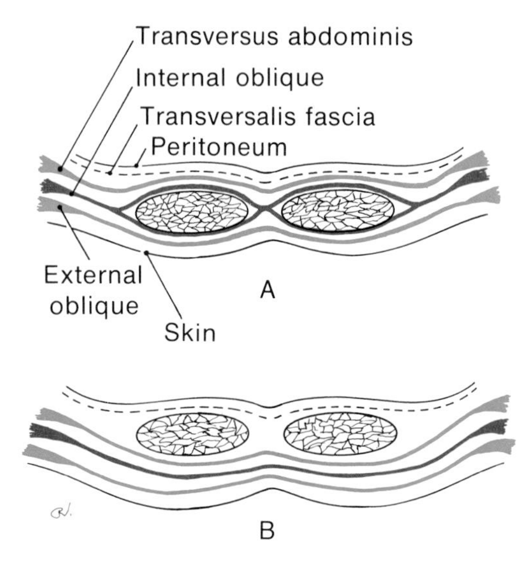

Fig. 8-16. Cross sections of both rectus abdominis muscles and their sheaths at two levels: (A) above the umbilicus, (B) at a variable distance below the umbilicus.

lumbar fascia) on the back of the trunk. The internal oblique fibers pass upward and forward around the side of the trunk and then upward and medially to insert on the lower ribs and on the linea alba by means of an **internal oblique aponeurosis.**

The innermost layer is the **transversus abdominis** muscle originating mainly from the iliac crest and thoracolumbar fascia. The transversus fibers pass forward and medially in primarily a horizontal plane and insert into the linea alba by means of a **transversus aponeurosis.** The inner surface of the transversus abdominis muscle is lined by a sheet of dense fascia termed the **transversalis fascia,** which lies between the muscle and the mesothelial lining (parietal peritoneum) of the abdominal cavity.

The **rectus abdominis** is a long, straight muscle which lies alongside the linea alba and extends from the symphysis pubis and pubic crest upward to insert on the xiphoid process of the sternum and the lower costal cartilages (Figs. 8-12 and 8-13). Contraction of the rectus causes the trunk to flex at the hips, as in sitting up from the recumbent position. The rectus is characterized by three or more cross-bands of connective tissue termed **tendinous intersections** which reflect the segmental development of this muscle.

The rectus abdominis is enclosed by a **rectus sheath** composed of dense fibrous connective tissue from the aponeuroses of the anterior abdominal muscles (Fig. 8-16). Above the level of the umbilicus the dense sheath passes in front and behind the rectus muscle; at a variable distance below the umbilicus the posterior wall of the sheath is quite thin and consists only of transversalis fascia and the peritoneum of the abdominal cavity.

The inguinal region of the anterior abdominal wall deserves special attention because of its predisposition to hernias. The inferior border of the external oblique aponeurosis forms a thickened band of connective tissue, the **inguinal ligament,** which passes from the anterior superior iliac spine to the pubic tubercle (Fig. 8-17). Just above and parallel to the ligament is the **inguinal canal** which in males

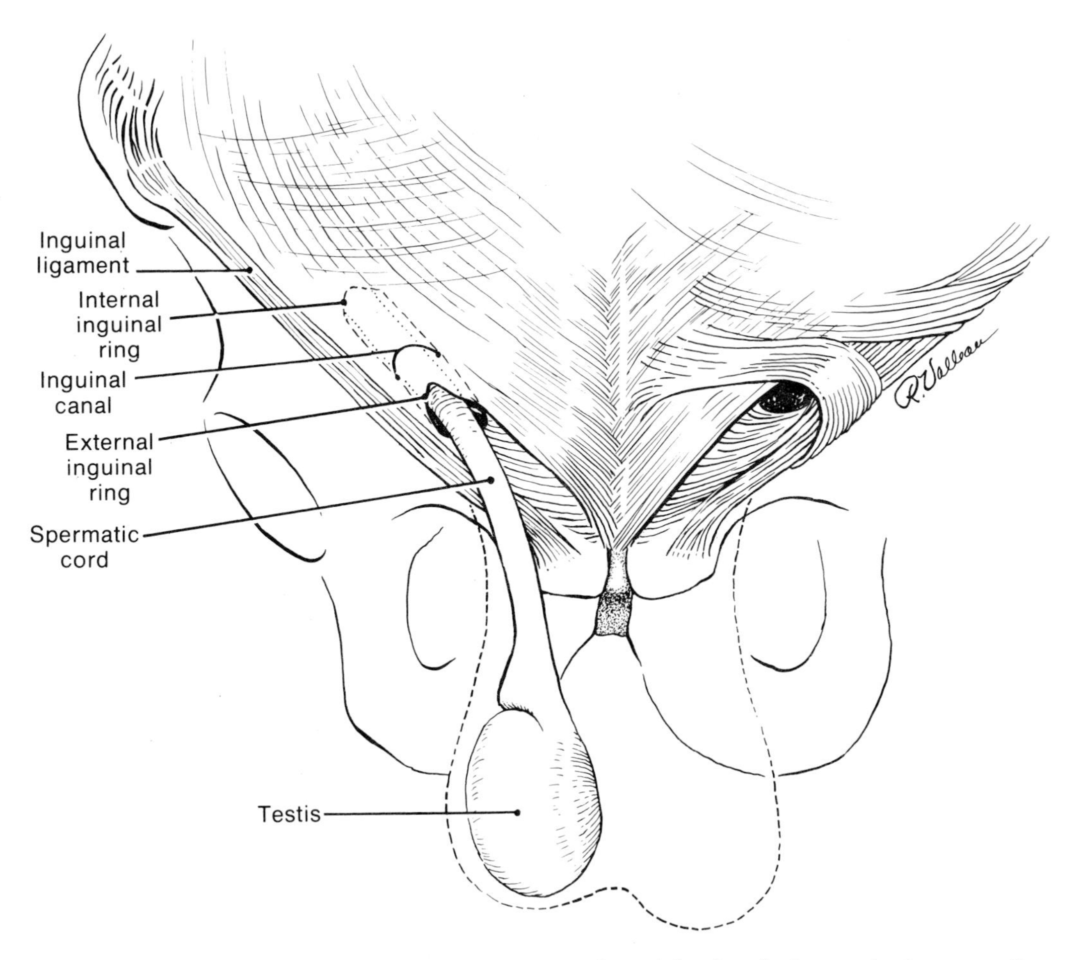

Fig. 8-17. The inguinal region, anterior view. The inguinal canal *(broken line)* transmits the spermatic cord from the scrotum to the abdominal cavity. On the left side of the body the spermatic cord and testis have been removed.

transmits the **spermatic cord** (ductus deferens and blood vessels) from the testis in the scrotum to the abdominal cavity. In the female the inguinal canal transmits a thin fibrous band of connective tissue (the **round ligament**). The opening of the inguinal canal into the abdomen is termed the **internal inguinal ring**, whereas the opening nearer to the scrotum (or its female counterpart, the labium majus) is the **external inguinal ring.**

During embryonic development the inguinal canal serves as a broad pathway along which the testis descends from the abdominal cavity to the scrotum. After the testis completes its descent, the canal narrows and becomes occluded, so that only the spermatic cord is transmitted along its wall. However, the canal may reopen, particularly after severe straining, and portions of abdominal organs such as the intestine may be pushed downward into the canal. This is known as an **inguinal hernia.** The inguinal canal in females is much narrower, since the ovaries do not descend along it; inguinal hernias are less common in females.

As the testis descends, it and the spermatic cord acquire a thin layer of skeletal muscle fibers from the internal oblique muscle. These fibers constitute the **cremaster** muscle, which enables the testis to be drawn upward reflexively to a higher position within the scrotum.

Posterior Abdominal Wall

The posterior wall of the abdominal cavity contains the following muscles: psoas major and minor, iliacus, quadratus lumborum, and portions of the diaphragm (Fig. 8-18). The psoas major, minor, and the iliacus are often grouped together as a single **iliopsoas** muscle which flexes the thigh and trunk. The **psoas major** originates from the lumbar vertebrae and slants downward and laterally beneath the inguinal ligament to insert onto the lesser trochanter of the femur. (The **psoas minor** is a small variable muscle lying on the anterior surface of the psoas major, inserting on the pubic bone, and probably acting along with the psoas major to flex the trunk.) The **iliacus** originates from the ilium and sacrum and covers much of the inner surface of the ilium. It inserts into the tendon of the psoas major and thus on the lesser trochanter.

The **quadratus lumborum** is located lateral to the psoas major and passes upward from the iliac crest and lumbar vertebrae to the twelfth rib. (The erector spinae muscles lie posterior to the quadratus, and the internal oblique and transversus abdominis muscles originate along its lateral edge.) When the quadratus lumborum muscles of both sides act together, they help to fix and steady the last rib. Acting alone, each muscle can flex the trunk laterally.

Diaphragm

The **diaphragm** is an important skeletal muscle concerned with respiratory movements. It is a dome-shaped mass which separates the thoracic and abdominal cavities. Anteriorly and laterally the diaphragm originates from the inner surfaces of the sternum, costal cartilages, and ribs. Posteriorly the origin is from the upper lumbar vertebrae in the form of two muscular **crura** (**right crus** and **left crus**) which arch upward to form the openings for the aorta and esophagus (Fig. 8-18). Lateral to each crus the diaphragm also originates from the **medial** and **lateral arcuate ligaments,** which arch over the upper parts of the psoas major and quadratus lumborum muscles, respectively.

The diaphragmatic muscle fibers insert centrally in the **central tendon,** which is interrupted by an opening for the inferior vena cava, the large vein passing from abdomen to thorax. Although the diaphragm appears to function as a single muscle, it actually consists of right and left halves innervated by the right and left phrenic nerves, respectively. Thus, damage to one nerve will paralyze one half of the diaphragm but will not affect the other half. When the diaphragm contracts, its central portion moves downward, thereby increasing the size of the thorax and decreasing the size of the abdominal cavity. In addition to its role in respiration, the diaphragm also acts during bowel movements (defecation), urination (micturition), and childbirth (parturition) by increasing intra-abdominal pressure.

In the embryo, the diaphragm develops from a variety of components. Because of its complex development, congenital defects or gaps may occur in the diaphragm and may allow abdominal organs to push upward into the thoracic cavity, resulting in a **diaphragmatic** hernia. Such hernias may also be acquired later in life and are particularly common at the esophageal opening.

Pelvic Diaphragm

The pelvic cavity is bounded below by two muscles, the large **levator ani** muscle and the rather insignificant **coccygeus,** which together form the horizontal muscular sheet known as the **pelvic diaphragm** (Fig. 8-19). The levator ani originates from the inner surface of the lateral wall of the pelvis and slopes slightly downward to insert in the midline along with its counterpart from the opposite side. In the male two gaps occur in the midline for passage of the rectum and urethra; in the female three gaps occur in the midline for the rectum, vagina,

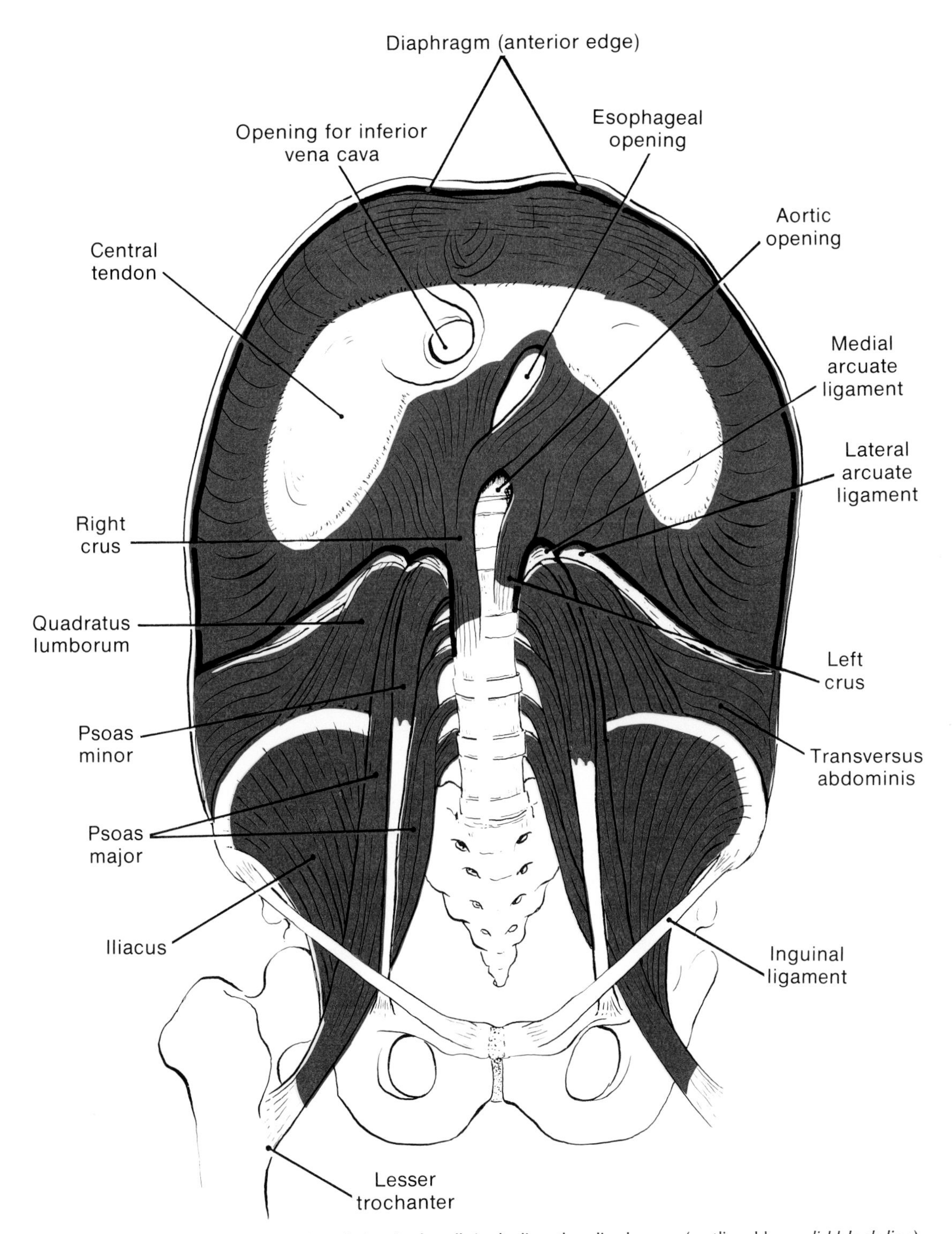

Fig. 8-18. Muscles of the posterior abdominal wall, including the diaphragm (outlined by *solid black line*). The anterior edge of the diaphragm has been lifted upward and backward so as to show the inferior surface.

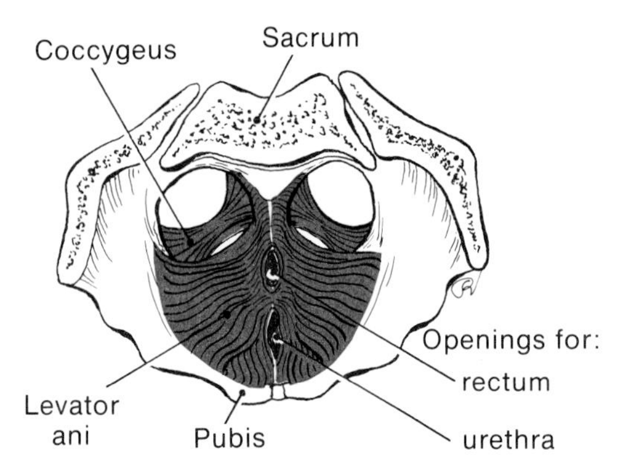

Fig. 8-19. The pelvic diaphragm viewed from above (male).

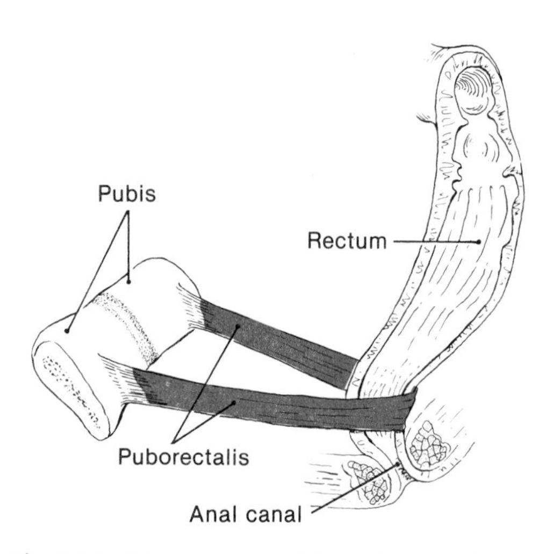

Fig. 8-20. A lateral view of the puborectalis portion of the levator ani muscle, forming a sling to keep the rectum bent forward. (Modified after Gardner, Gray, and O'Rahilly).

and urethra. In both sexes a special portion of the levator ani (the **puborectalis**) forms a sling passing from the pubis posteriorly behind the rectum, keeping the latter bent forward and preventing loss of feces (Fig. 8-20). During a bowel movement the sling relaxes and allows the rectum to straighten out, thereby facilitating passage of the feces. The coccygeus consists of some delicate muscle strands passing from the spine of the ischium to the sacrum and coccyx. The pelvic diaphragm acts as a support for the pelvic viscera as well as a means for controlling urination and defecation.

Perineal Muscles

The perineal muscles lie below the pelvic diaphragm and consist of superficial muscles associated with the external genital organs and deeper perineal muscles comprising the urogenital diaphragm. The superficial perineal muscles are the **ischiocavernosus, bulbospongiosus** (**bulbocavernosus**), and **superficial transversus perinei** muscles which are arranged in the form of a triangle and which are involved in maintaining erection of the penis or clitoris (Fig. 8-21). The **urogenital diaphragm** lies superior to the superficial perineal muscles and just below the anterior part of the pelvic diaphragm. It consists of the **sphincter urethrae** and **deep transversus perinei** muscles (Fig. 8-21) which aid the pelvic diaphragm during urination.

MUSCLES OF THE UPPER LIMB

As we have seen, some of the muscles which move the shoulder girdle and humerus are located on the anterior and posterior surfaces of the neck and thorax. These muscles will be briefly reviewed before proceeding to other muscles of the upper limb (Figs. 8-9, 8-10, and 8-12).

The **trapezius** arises from the vertebral column, inserts on the spine of the scapula, and can elevate, depress, and rotate the inferior

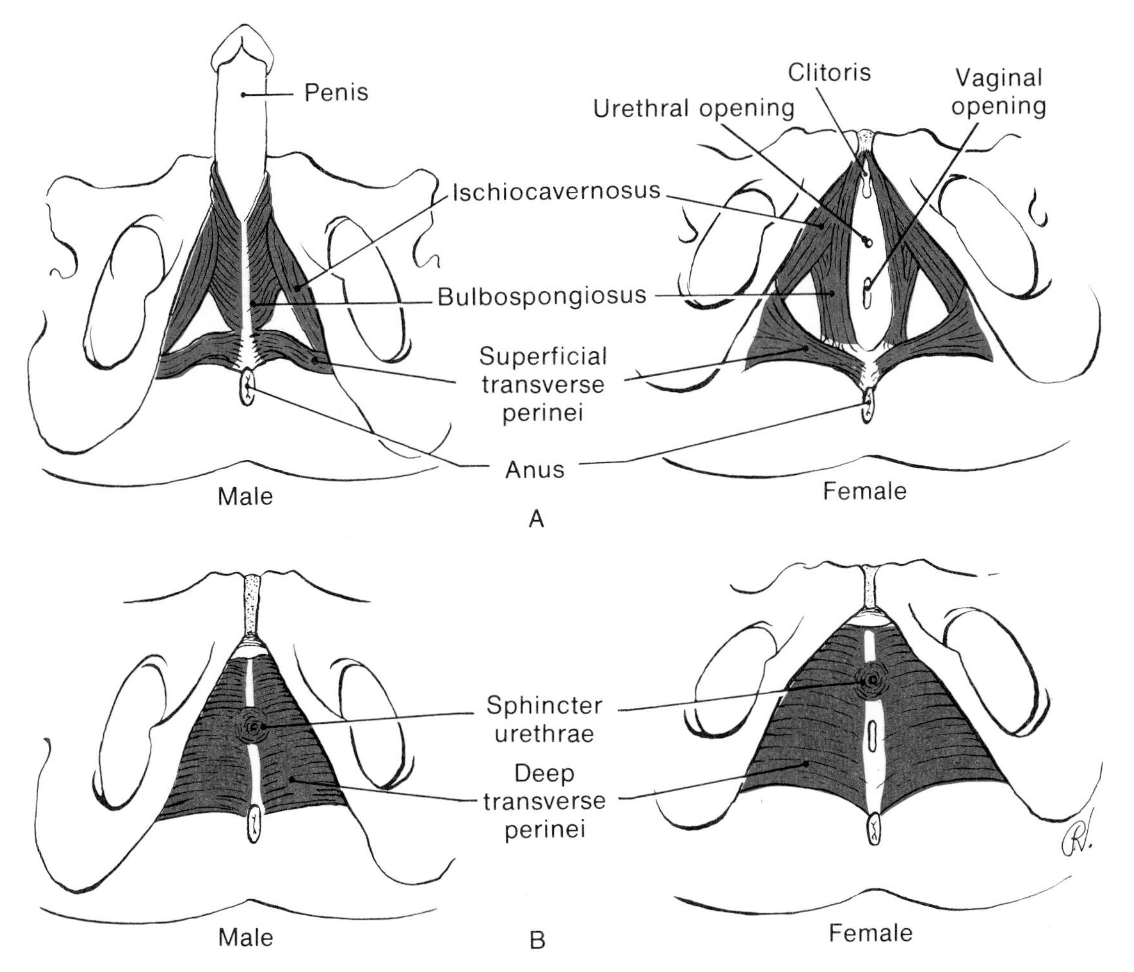

Fig. 8-21. Perineal muscles, inferior view. (A) Superficial muscles, (B) deep muscles representing the urogenital diaphragm. (Superficial muscles have been removed.) (Modified after Gardner, Gray, and O'Rahilly).

angle of the scapula upward. The **levator scapulae, rhomboid major,** and **rhomboid minor** muscles pass from the vertebral column to the medial border of the scapula and adduct (retract) the scapula. The **serratus anterior** originates from the anterolateral surfaces of the ribs and passes backward to insert on the medial border of the scapula, thereby abducting (protracting) it. The **pectoralis minor** and **subclavius** depress the tip of the shoulder.

The **pectoralis major** originates from the anterior surfaces of the ribs, sternum, and clavicle, inserts on the upper end of the humerus, and thus is an important adductor of the humerus (Fig. 8-12). The **latissimus dorsi** likewise adducts the humerus, since this muscle passes from the posterior surface of the back and inserts on the humerus near the insertion of the pectoralis major. The latissimus dorsi also extends the humerus (brings it backward in the sagittal plane).

The muscle giving the shoulder its rounded shape is the **deltoid** which originates from the lateral portion of the clavicle, acromion, and

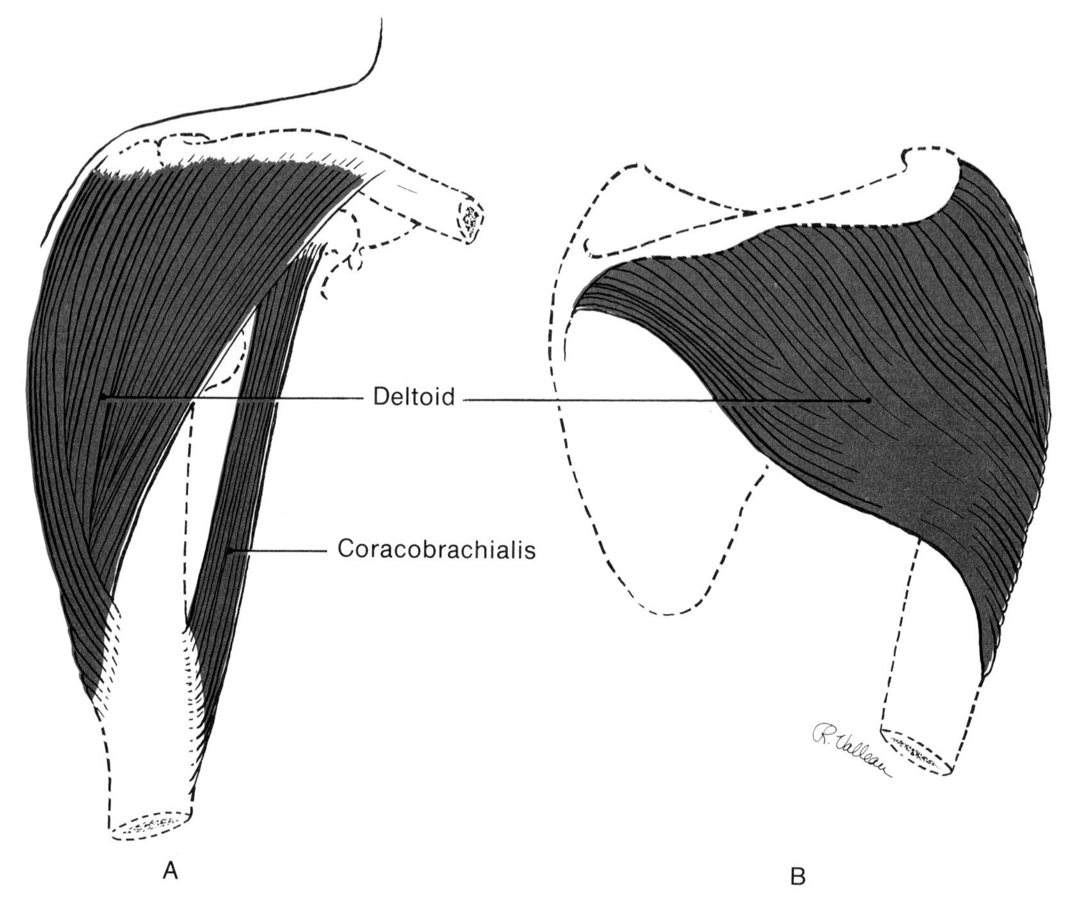

Fig. 8-22. (A) Right deltoid muscle and coracobrachialis muscle, anterior view; (B) right deltoid muscle, posterior view.

spine of the scapula and inserts on the lateral surface of the humerus (Fig. 8-22). Because of its extensive origin, the deltoid muscle has three different actions: the anterior fibers from the clavicle flex the humerus (i.e., bring it forward in the sagittal plane), the middle fibers from the acromion abduct the humerus, and the posterior fibers from the spine of the scapula extend the humerus. The humerus can also be weakly flexed by the slender **coracobrachialis** muscle originating anteriorly from the coracoid process of the scapula and passing down along the upper arm to insert in the middle of the medial aspect of the humerus.

In addition to the movements of flexion, extension, abduction, and adduction, the humerus can also be medially and laterally rotated. The muscles largely responsible for rotation are the subscapularis, teres major, supraspinatus, infraspinatus, and teres minor. The **subscapularis** originates anteriorly from the subscapular fossa on the anterior surface of the scapula and passes forward in front of the shoulder joint to insert on the lesser tubercle of the humerus (Fig. 8-23). The **teres major** originates posteriorly from the inferior angle of the scapula and passes upward and forward to insert on the humerus just below the insertion of the subscapularis (Figs. 8-23 and 8-24). These two muscles medially rotate the humerus; the teres major also adducts the arm.

The **supraspinatus** and **infraspinatus**

muscles arise posteriorly from the supraspinous and infraspinous fossae, respectively, and pass posterior to the shoulder joint to insert on the greater tubercle of the humerus (Fig. 8-24). The **teres minor** is often continuous with the medial portion of the infraspinatus muscle and inserts just below it on the greater tubercle. The supraspinatus, infraspinatus, and teres minor are all lateral rotators of the humerus.

The tendons of the medial and lateral rotators of the humerus form a musculotendinous **rotator cuff** around the articular capsule of the shoulder joint and thus strengthen it and help to keep the head of the humerus in contact with the glenoid cavity.

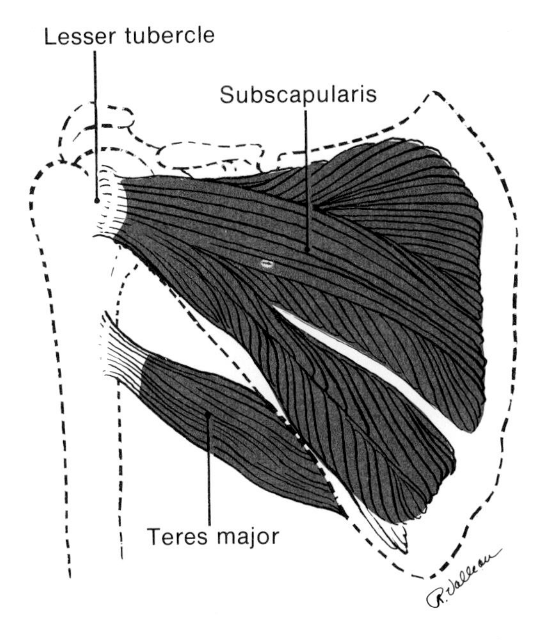

Fig. 8-23. Right subscapularis muscle, anterior view. A portion of the teres major is also shown.

Muscles of the Arm

Most of the muscles of the arm act across the elbow joint to produce flexion, extension, or supination of the forearm. These muscles include the biceps brachii, brachialis, and triceps brachii. Although the coracobrachialis (described above) occupies the upper anterior aspect of the humerus, it can only weakly flex the humerus and does not act on the forearm.

The **biceps brachii** originates by means of a short head from the coracoid process of the scapula and a long head which arises from a long tendon attached to the upper rim of the glenoid cavity (Fig. 8-25). A portion of the tendon is included in the shoulder joint and passes downward along the intertubercular groove of the humerus. This tendon is subject to considerable wear and damage and is frequently the source of shoulder pain. The two bellies of the biceps muscle insert by a common tendon which passes anteriorly across the elbow joint to the tuberosity of the radius. (An expansion of connective tissue known as the **bicipital aponeurosis** extends medially from the tendon and merges with the deep fascia of the forearm.) The biceps is a flexor of the forearm and, because of its origin from the scapula, it can also weakly flex the humerus. Another important function is supination of the forearm (rotating the radius from a medial to lateral position).

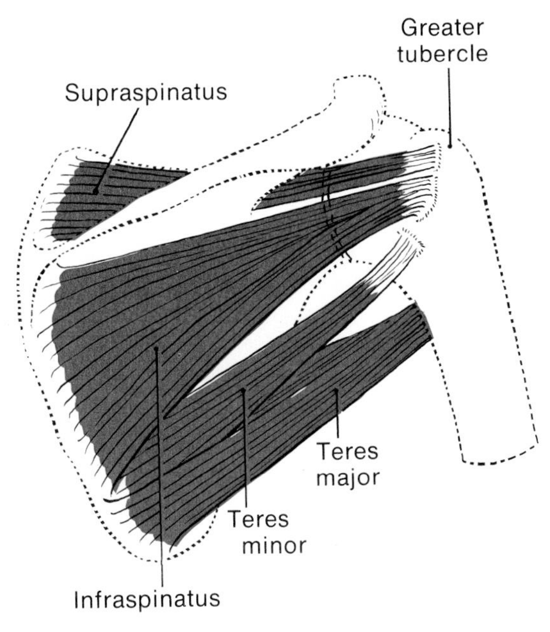

Fig. 8-24. Muscles of the posterior surface of the scapula. The teres minor has been separated and pulled downward from the infraspinatus muscle.

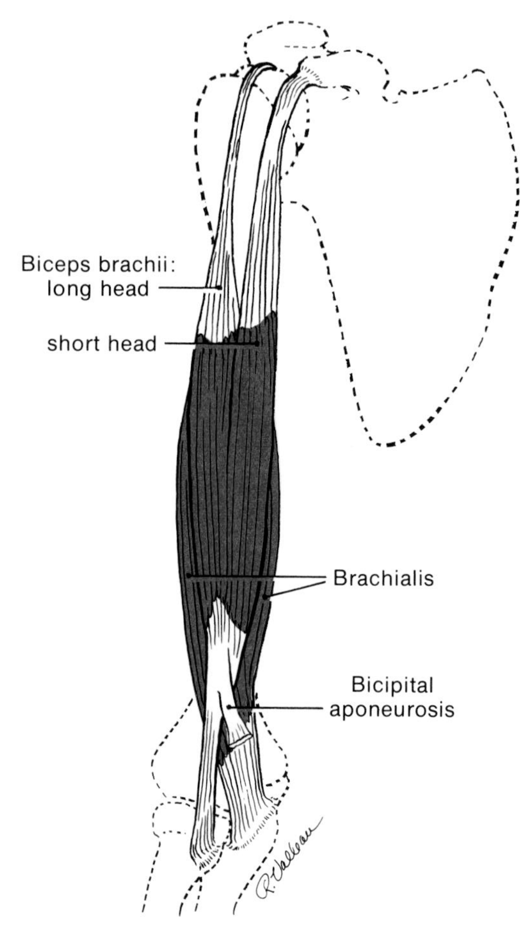

Fig. 8-25. Right biceps brachii and brachialis muscles, anterior view. The bicipital aponeurosis has been cut.

The **brachialis** originates from the middle of the humerus deep to the biceps, inserts on the coronoid process of the ulna, and is a strong flexor of the forearm.

The **triceps brachii** is a large muscle lying on the posterior surface of the arm and originating from three heads: a long head from the inferior rim of the glenoid cavity, a lateral head from the upper end of the humerus, and a medial head from the lower end of the humerus (Fig. 8-26). The medial head lies deep to the other two. The three heads unite to form a single tendon inserted onto the posterior aspect of the olecranon. The triceps extends the forearm, and the long head also helps in extension of the arm.

In a muscular individual, many of the muscles of the back and arm can be identified from a surface view (Fig. 8-27).

Muscles of the Forearm

Most of the forearm muscles act on the wrist joint and digits. They consist of flexors (anterior surface) and extensors (posterior surface). In addition, movements at the wrist include abduction (lateral deviation) and adduction (medial deviation). The thumb movements involve flexion, extension, abduction (bringing the thumb upward from the palm), and adduction (bringing it back) (Fig. 8-28). Finger movements include flexion, extension, abduction (movement away from an axial line through the middle finger) and adduction (movement toward the axial line). Some of the forearm muscles also produce pronation (bringing the palm to face posteriorly) and supination (bringing the palm to face anteriorly).

The most superficial muscles on the anterior surface of the forearm originate from the medial epicondyle of the humerus. They are: pronator teres, flexor carpi radialis, palmaris longus, and flexor carpi ulnaris (Fig. 8-29). The **pronator teres** is relatively short and inserts on the middle of the radius. As its name implies, it pronates the forearm. The **flexor carpi radialis** inserts at the bases of the second and third metacarpal bones and flexes the wrist.

The flexor carpi radialis tendon is often used as a guide for finding the pulse in the radial artery, which lies just lateral to the tendon (see Fig. 19-8). The **palmaris longus** is a variable muscle which inserts by means of a long tendon into a mass of dense connective tissue **(palmar aponeurosis)** lying just beneath the skin of the palm. The **flexor carpi ulnaris** inserts on the pisiform and base of the fifth metacarpal bones.

An intermediate layer of anterior muscles consists of the **flexor digitorum superficialis** which originates from the medial epicondyle, upper ulna, and radius, and sends four tendons to insert at the bases of the middle phalanges of digits 2–5 (Fig. 8-30). The deep group of anterior forearm muscles includes the **flexor digitorum profundus** originating mainly from the upper end of the ulna and sending four tendons to insert at the base of the distal phalanx of digits 2–5. Each tendon also gives origin to a small muscle termed a **lumbrical,** which is classified as an intrinsic muscle of the hand (see below). The deep forearm muscles also include the **flexor pollicis longus** from the upper radius to the base of the distal phalanx of the thumb (pollex) and the **pronator quadratus** which passes transversely between the distal ulna and distal radius. The actions of these muscles are evident from their names.

The posterior surface of the forearm contains a superficial group of extensors: extensor carpi radialis longus, extensor carpi radialis brevis, extensor digitorum, extensor digiti minimi, and extensor carpi ulnaris (Fig. 8-31). These muscles originate from a common extensor tendon on the lateral epicondyle of the humerus. The **extensor carpi radialis longus** and **brevis** pass along the posterior surface of the radius. Distally they are covered by two so-called "outcropping" muscles coming from the deep extensor group (see below). The extensor carpi radialis longus inserts on metacarpal 2, while the extensor carpi radialis brevis inserts on metacarpals 2 and 3. They extend the wrist and can act together with the flexor carpi radialis to abduct the wrist. Similarly, the **extensor carpi ulnaris** which inserts on the fifth me-

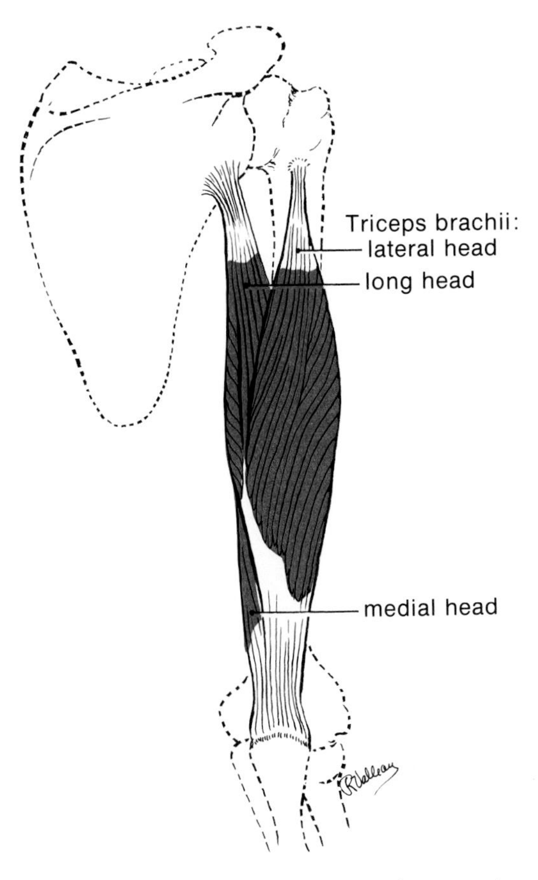

Fig. 8-26. Right triceps brachii muscle, posterior view. (Most of the medial head lies deep to the lateral and long heads.)

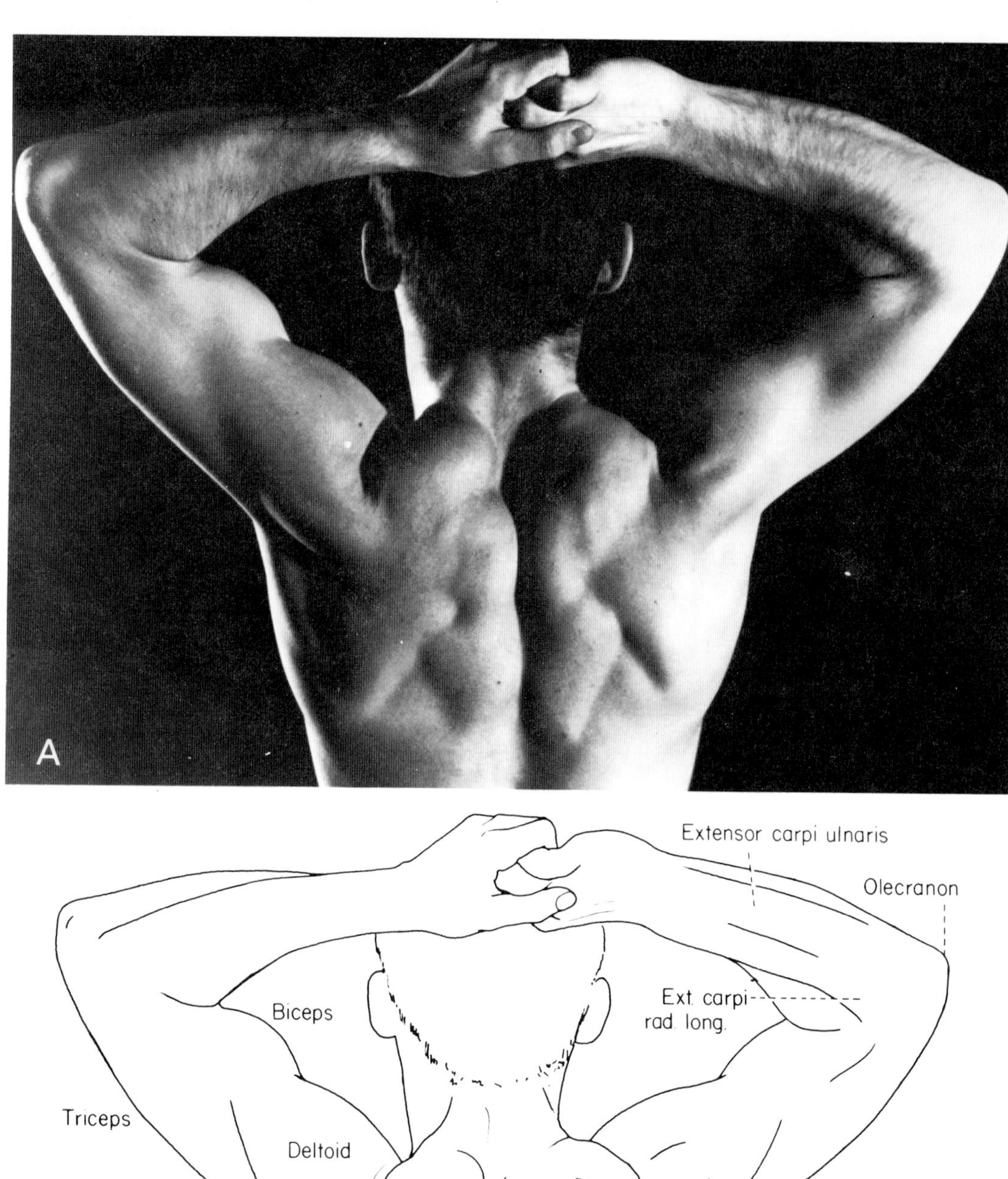

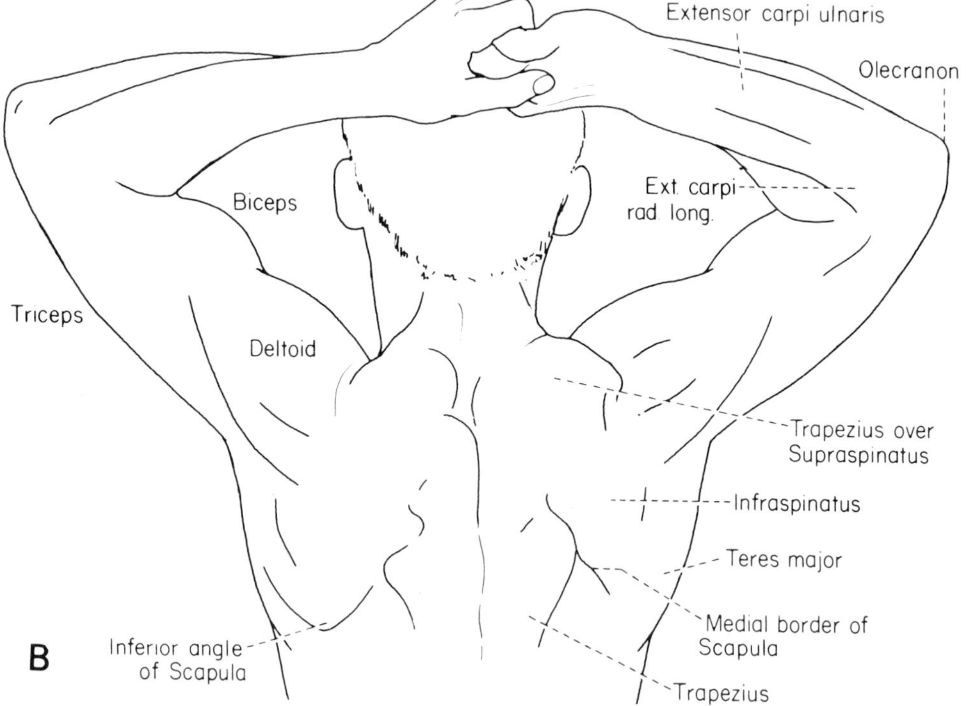

Fig. 8-27. (A) Photograph showing surface anatomy of upper back, shoulders, and upper limbs, posterior view. (B) Diagram of structures in A. (From J. Royce, *Surface Anatomy,* F. A. Davis Co., Philadelphia, 1965.)

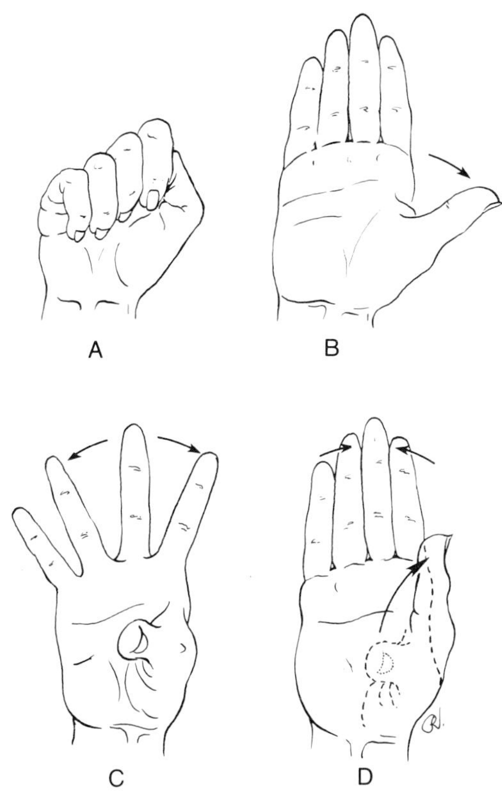

Fig. 8-28. Movements of the fingers and thumb. (A) Flexion, (B) extension, (C) abduction, (D) adduction. The axial line through the middle finger is indicated in blue. (Modified after *Grant's Method*.)

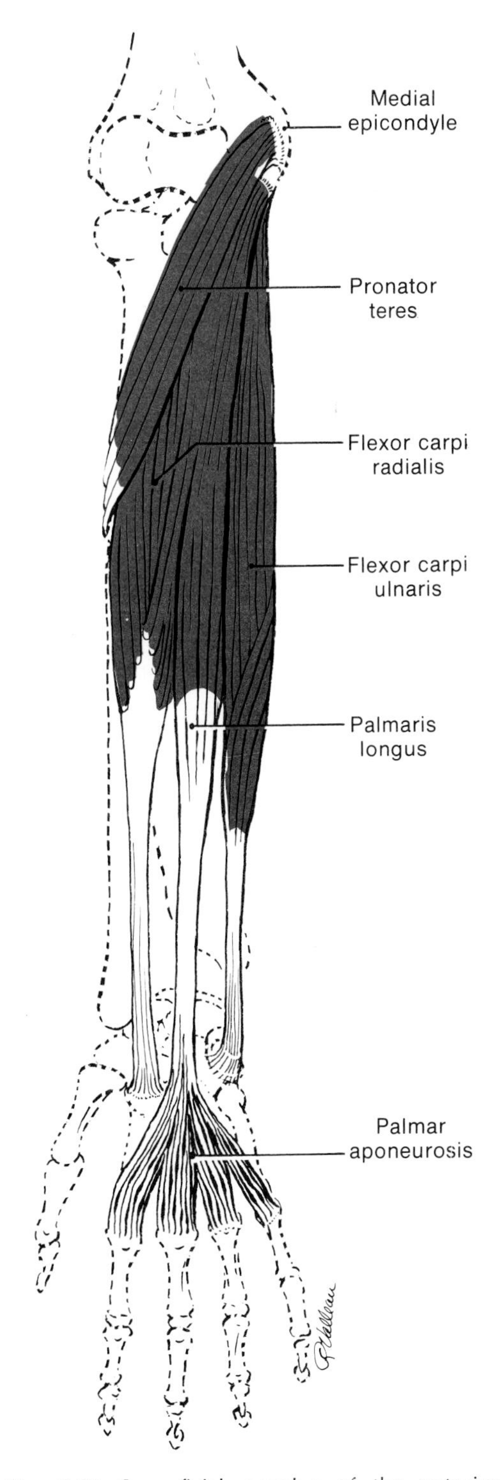

Fig. 8-29. Superficial muscles of the anterior forearm.

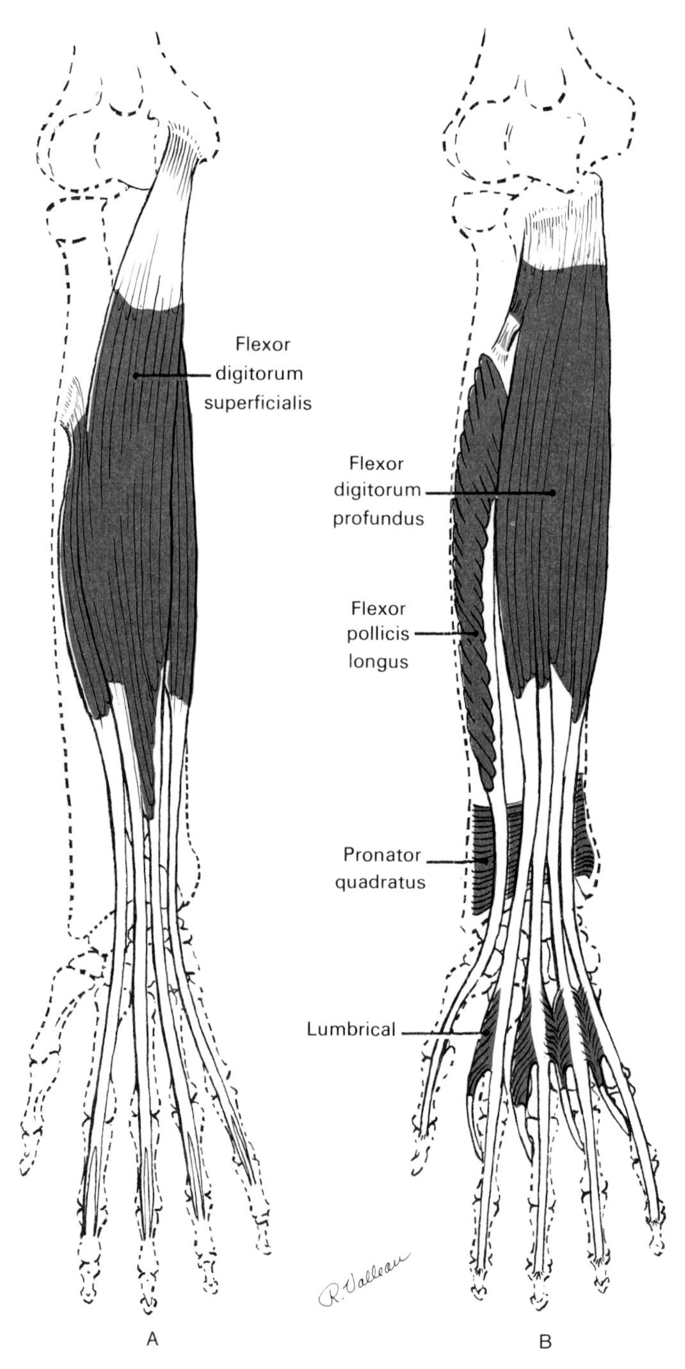

Fig. 8-30. Muscles of the anterior forearm. (A) Intermediate layer, (B) deep layer, including four lumbrical muscles from the tendons of the flexor digitorum profundus muscle and more properly classified as intrinsic muscles of the hand.

tacarpal can act together with the flexor carpi ulnaris to adduct the wrist. The **extensor digitorum** and **extensor digiti minimi** originate in common but separate distally to insert into extensor expansions on the posterior surfaces of the digits. The extensor tendons usually show interconnecting bands as they pass over the posterior aspect of the hand. For this reason it is difficult to extend individual digits without moving adjacent ones. The index finger, however, can be extended individually by means of an additional muscle of its own, the **extensor indicis,** which lies deep to the extensor digitorum muscles.

Two additional muscles originate superficially with muscles of the posterior forearm, although they are not involved in movements of the wrist or fingers. The **brachioradialis** takes origin above from the supracondylar ridge of the humerus, passes along the lateral aspect of the forearm, and inserts onto the styloid process of the radius, thereby crossing the elbow joint and flexing the forearm. The **anconeus** is a small triangular muscle which passes from the lateral epicondyle to the olecranon and probably acts in conjunction with the triceps in extending the forearm.

The deep group of muscles on the posterior surface of the forearm are: supinator, abductor pollicis longus, extensor pollicis longus, extensor pollicis brevis, and extensor indicis (Fig. 8-31). The **supinator** is relatively short, takes origin from the lateral epicondyle and ulna, and inserts on the upper radius near the insertion of its antagonist, the pronator teres. The **abductor pollicis longus** originates from the radius and ulna. It travels in close company with the **extensor pollicis brevis** originating from the radius. Both muscles produce a lateral bulge in the distal forearm, and for this reason they are often referred to as the "outcropping muscles" (Fig. 8-31). The abductor pollicis longus inserts at the base of the first metacarpal bone, while the extensor pollicis brevis travels to the proximal phalanx of the thumb. The **extensor pollicis longus** takes origin from the ulna and passes to the distal phalanx of the thumb. (When the thumb is extended, the tendons of these three muscles create a hollow depression near the wrist known as the "anatomical snuffbox.") The **extensor indicis** is a slender muscle which can extend the index finger by itself, in contrast to the extensors of digits 3–5 which tend to move together during extension because of their interconnections.

Retinacula

As the flexor and extensor tendons cross the wrist joint, they are held in place by bands of thickened fascia termed retinacula (Figs. 8-31 and 8-32). The **flexor retinaculum** helps to keep the flexor tendons from bulging outward during flexion of the wrist, and the **extensor retinaculum** serves the same purpose for the extensor tendons during extension.

Muscles of the Hand

We have already seen that many movements of the fingers are performed by muscles on the forearm. There are also intrinsic muscles of the hand which add to and refine these movements.

Thenar and Hypothenar Muscles

The fleshy mass on the lateral side of the hand is known as the **thenar eminence** and consists of three thenar muscles which act on the thumb: the **flexor pollicis brevis, abductor pollicis brevis,** and **opponens pollicis** (Fig. 8-32). The opponens pollicis lies deep to the other two thenar muscles and enables the thumb to be brought upward and medially to touch the tips of the other digits **(opposition).** In addition to the three thenar muscles, the thumb is also acted upon by the **adductor pollicis** which passes from the second and third metacarpals and carpal bones to the thumb. It can be felt externally at the base of the web between the thumb and second metacarpal.

The little finger likewise can be moved by intrinsic muscles known as **hypothenar** muscles: the **flexor digiti minimi brevis, abductor digit minimi,** and **opponens digiti minimi** (Fig. 8-32).

Lumbrical and Interosseous Muscles

The hand contains four small lumbrical muscles, each of which originates from a ten-

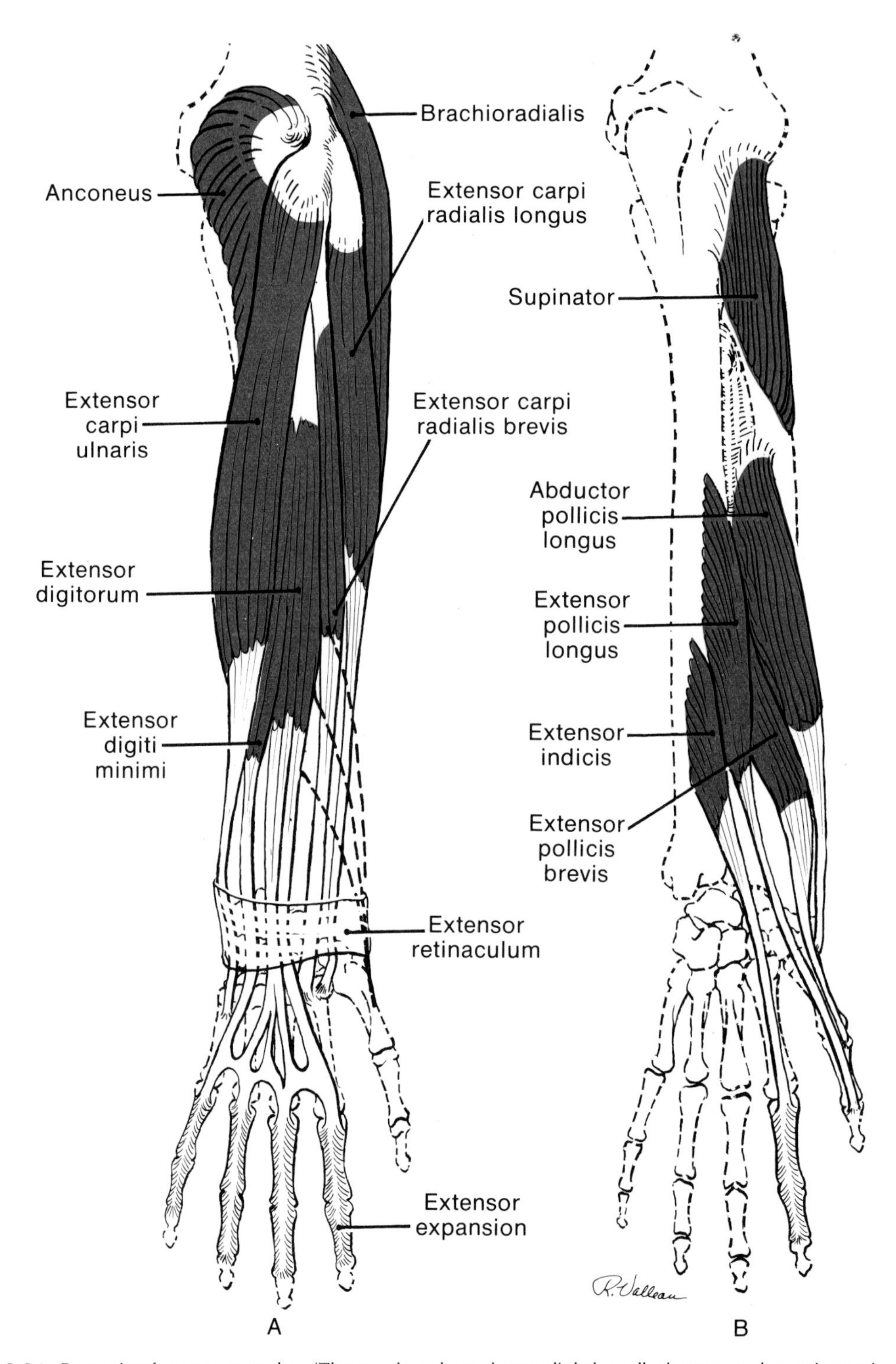

Fig. 8-31. Posterior forearm muscles. (The tendons have been slightly pulled apart at the wrist region.) (A) Superficial muscles. (*Broken lines* indicate superficial course of two deep "outcropping" muscles.) (B) Deep muscles.

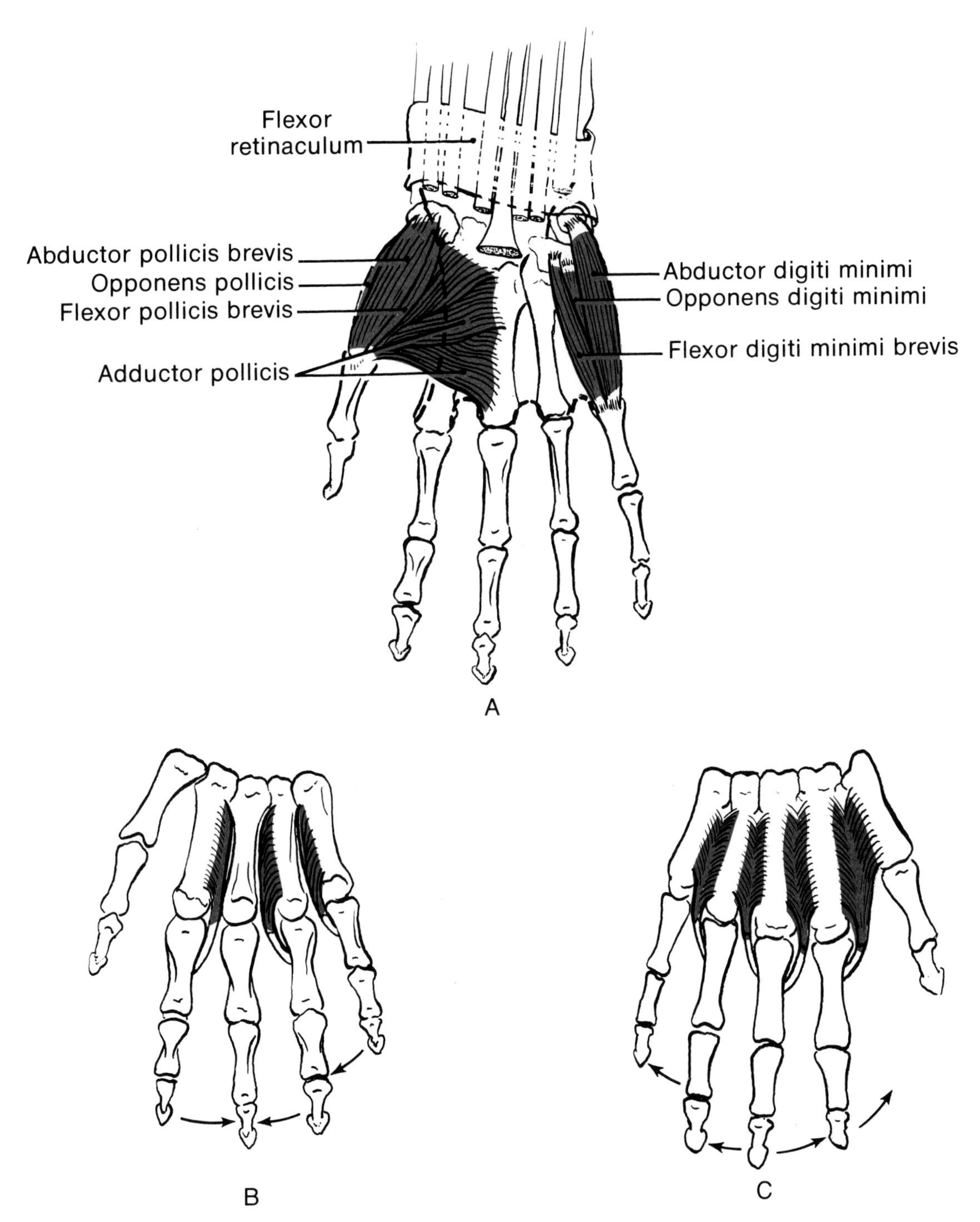

Fig. 8-32. Intrinsic muscles of the hand. (A) Thenar muscles, adductor pollicis muscle, and hypothenar muscles, anterior view. *Broken line* indicates extent of palmar aponeurosis. (B) Palmar interossei, anterior view. *Arrows* show direction of movement for adduction. (C) Dorsal interossei showing abduction, posterior view.

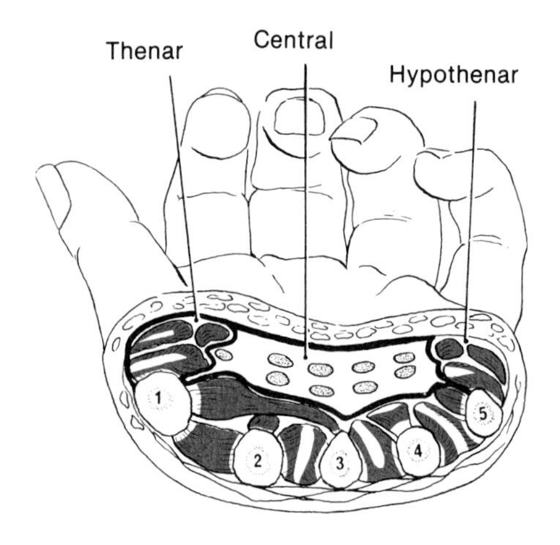

Fig. 8-33. The three major compartments of the hand as seen in a cross section through the palm. The metacarpals are numbered 1–5.

don of the flexor digitorum profundus muscle and inserts dorsally into the extensor expansions of the second to fifth fingers (Fig. 8-30). The **interosseous muscles** are arranged in palmar and dorsal layers between the metacarpal bones. The **palmar interossei** adduct the fingers toward an imaginary line through the middle finger; the **dorsal interossei** abduct the fingers away from the line. (The interossei also act along with the lumbricals to flex the metacarpophalangeal joints while extending the middle and distal phalangeal joints.)

The intrinsic muscles and the tendons of the extrinsic muscles show a complex but orderly arrangement within various fascial compartments of the hand (Fig. 8-33). These compartments often limit the spread of infection from one region of the hand to another. However, some of these compartments communicate with distal regions of the forearm, thereby allowing an infection to spread upward.

The various tendons in the palm are covered by a sheet of dense connective tissue, the **palmar aponeurosis** (Fig. 8-29). The tendon of the palmaris longus inserts into this aponeurosis, which is also anchored to the flexor retinaculum and which helps to protect the flexor tendons. The flexor tendons are enclosed by synovial sheaths, which enable them to glide easily over one another. Inflammation or infection of these sheaths can seriously reduce the wide range and complexity of movement which is characteristic of the human hand.

MUSCLES OF THE LOWER LIMB

The pelvic girdle provides stability to the lower trunk and serves also as a point of attachment for some of the muscles which move the lower limb. Because of the weight-bearing capacity of the lower limb, many movements depend on whether the limb is swinging freely or fixed in position, and some muscles appear to have quite contradictory action depending on whether one is lying, sitting, or standing. In general, the muscles which move the thigh originate on the pelvis and insert on the femur; those moving the leg originate on the femur

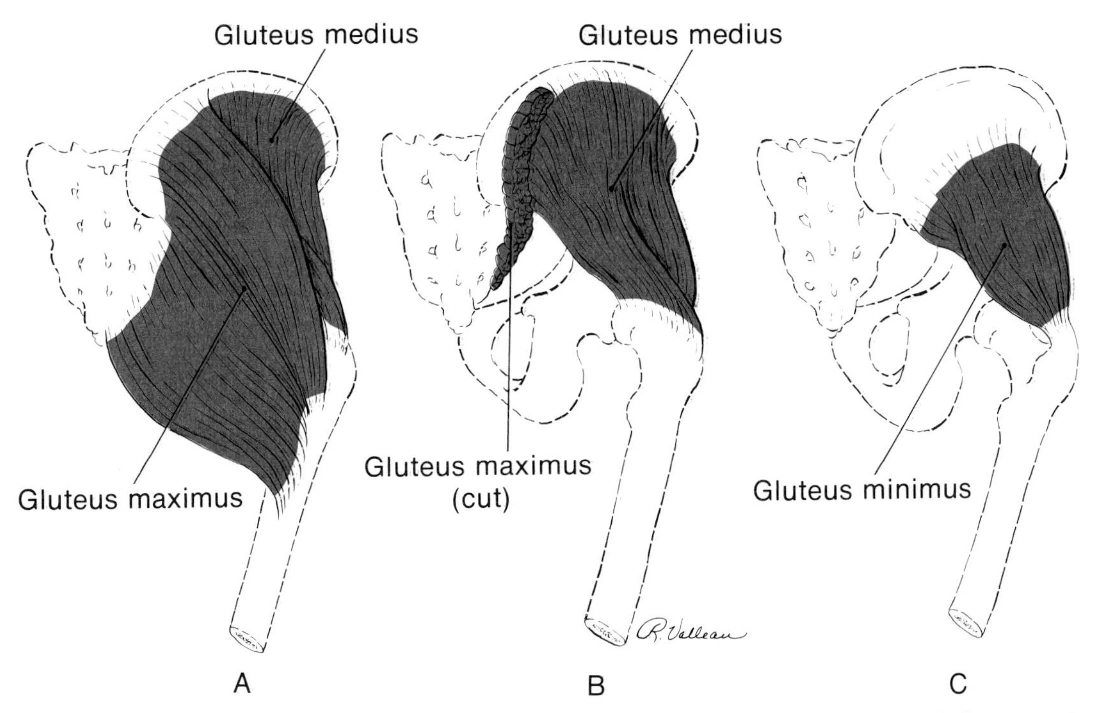

Fig. 8-34. Gluteal muscles, posterior view. (A) Gluteus maximus muscle and upper portion of gluteus medius muscle, (B) gluteus medius muscle deep to gluteus maximus, which has been cut and removed, (C) gluteus minimus muscle (gluteus maximus and medius have been removed).

and insert on the tibia and fibula. Those which move the foot and toes take origin on the tibia and fibula and insert on the tarsal, metatarsal, and phalangeal bones.

Muscles of the Hip and Thigh

The muscles overlying the hip are involved in movements of the thigh; those covering the thigh are responsible for movement of the leg. Posteriorly the muscles of the hip are termed **gluteal muscles.** The **gluteus maximus** is the largest and most superficial of these muscles and forms much of the buttocks (Fig. 8-34). It arises from the ilium, sacrum, and coccyx and inserts on the posterior surface of the femur and into a broad band of fascia (the **iliotibial tract**) along the side of the thigh. The gluteus maximus can extend the thigh or, if the lower limb is fixed, it can extend the trunk as one straightens up from a stooped position. The **gluteus medius** and **gluteus minimus** lie deep to the maximus, originate from the upper lateral surface of the ilium, and insert on lateral and anterior aspects of the greater trochanter of the femur (Fig. 8-34). They abduct and medially rotate the thigh when the lower limb swings freely. However, when the thigh is fixed, the gluteus medius and gluteus minimus pull laterally at the ilium and thus stabilize the pelvis. This action is referred to as abduction of the pelvis and is particularly important in keeping the pelvis from sagging downward from side to side as one walks (Fig. 8-35).

Six small muscles also lie deep to the gluteus maximus: the **piriformis, superior gemellus, obturator internus, inferior gemellus, quadratus femoris,** and **obturator externus** muscles (Fig. 8-36). All of these muscles are lateral rotators of the thigh.

The thigh is flexed by the **iliopsoas** muscle which has already been described with the

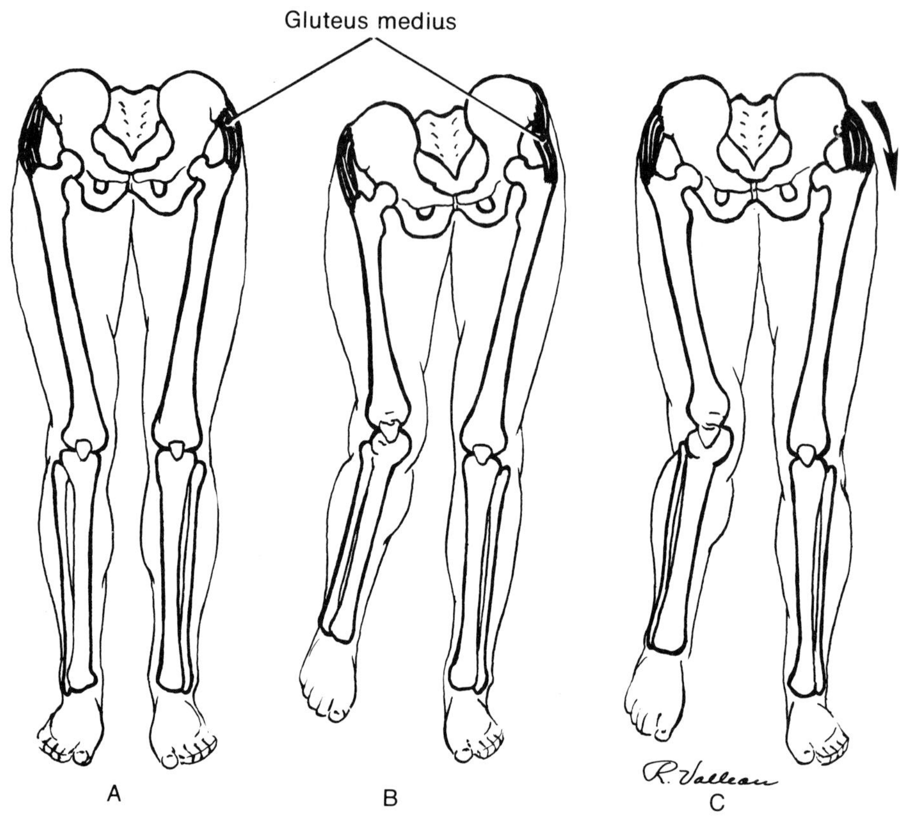

Fig. 8-35. Abduction of the hip, anterior view. (A) Standing position with both feet on the ground. (B) Tendency of right side of the pelvis to tip downward when the right foot is lifted from the ground. (C) Contraction of left gluteus medius (in the direction of the arrow) stabilizes (abducts) the left side of the pelvis and minimizes the downward tilt of the right side.

muscles of the posterior abdominal wall and pelvis. The iliopsoas inserts on the lesser trochanter and is important in flexing the thigh as one begins to take a step forward (Fig. 8-37). Another flexor of the thigh is the **tensor fasciae latae** which originates laterally from the iliac crest and anterior superior iliac spine. It inserts into the **iliotibial tract** along the side of the thigh. The tensor fasciae latae can also act along with the gluteus medius and minimus to medially rotate the thigh. In addition it acts as a fixator for other muscles to act on the hip. The iliotibial tract blends with the deep fascia of the thigh which is also known as the **fascia lata.** Still another flexor of the thigh is the **sartorius** muscle which originates from the anterior superior iliac spine and slants medially across the front of the thigh to insert on the medial aspect of the tibia. Because this muscle crosses the knee joint, it can also flex the leg.

The anterior surface of the thigh contains the **quadriceps femoris,** an important extensor of the leg (Fig. 8-38). This muscle consists of four parts: the **rectus femoris** which arises from the anterior inferior iliac spine and covers the anterior surface of the thigh, the **vastus lateralis** and **vastus medialis** which lie on the lateral and medial aspects of the femur, respectively, and the **vastus intermedius** which lies deep to the rectus femoris. These four portions insert by means of a common tendon onto the patella and the tibial tuberosity. (The patella is

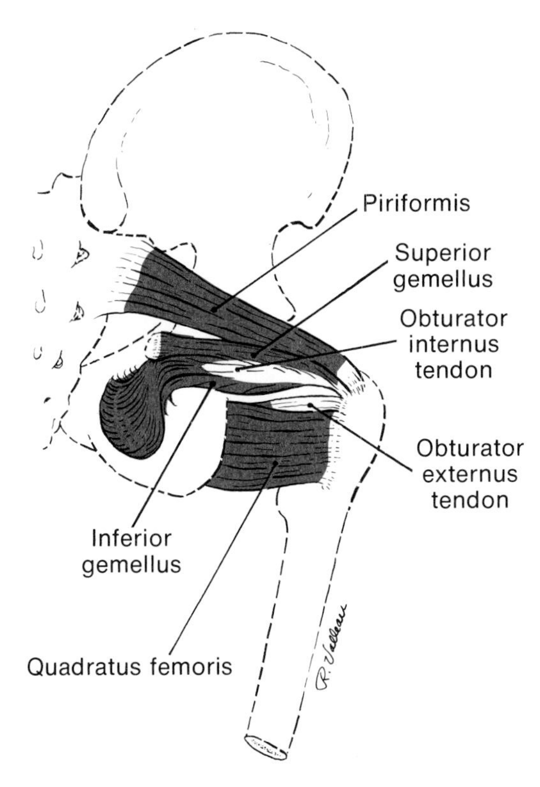

Fig. 8-36. Six lateral rotator muscles of the thigh, posterior view. (The gluteus maximus, medius, and minimus have been removed.)

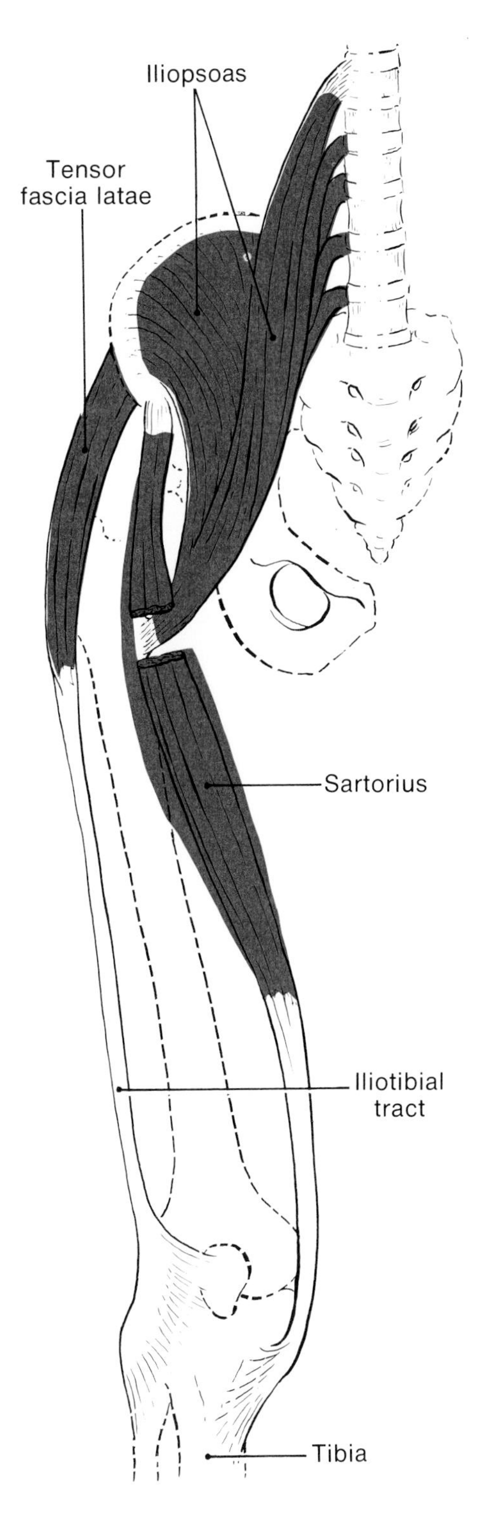

Fig. 8-37. Anterior muscles of the hip and thigh: iliopsoas, sartorius, and tensor fasciae latae. The iliotibial tract blends with the deep fascia of the thigh. A portion of the sartorius muscle has been removed to show deep insertion of iliopsoas muscle.

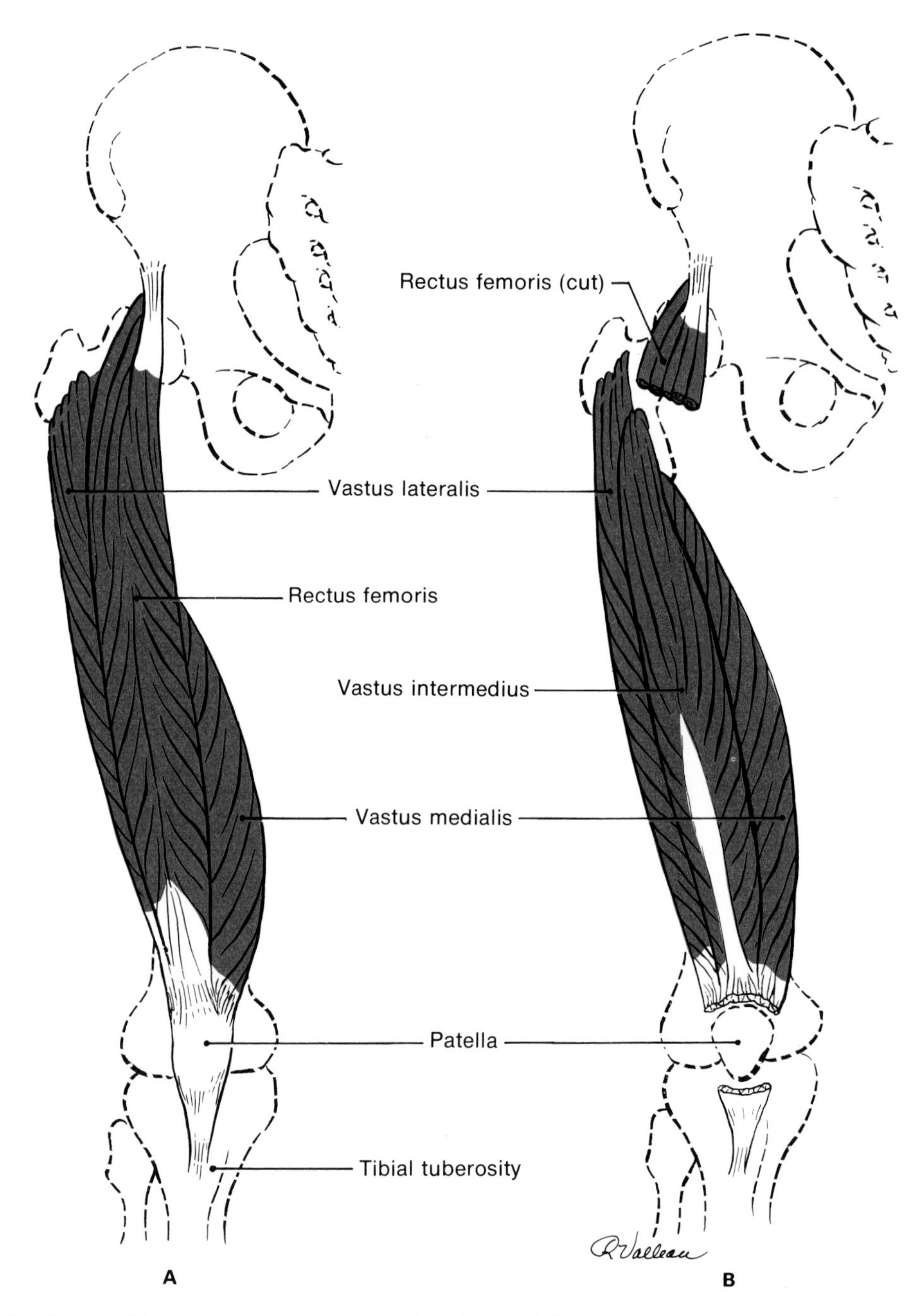

Fig. 8-38. The quadriceps femoris muscle, anterior view. (A) Rectus femoris, vastus medialis, and vastus lateralis; (B) vastus intermedius lying deep to rectus femoris, most of which has been removed. The common tendon of the quadriceps has been cut open to reveal the patella.

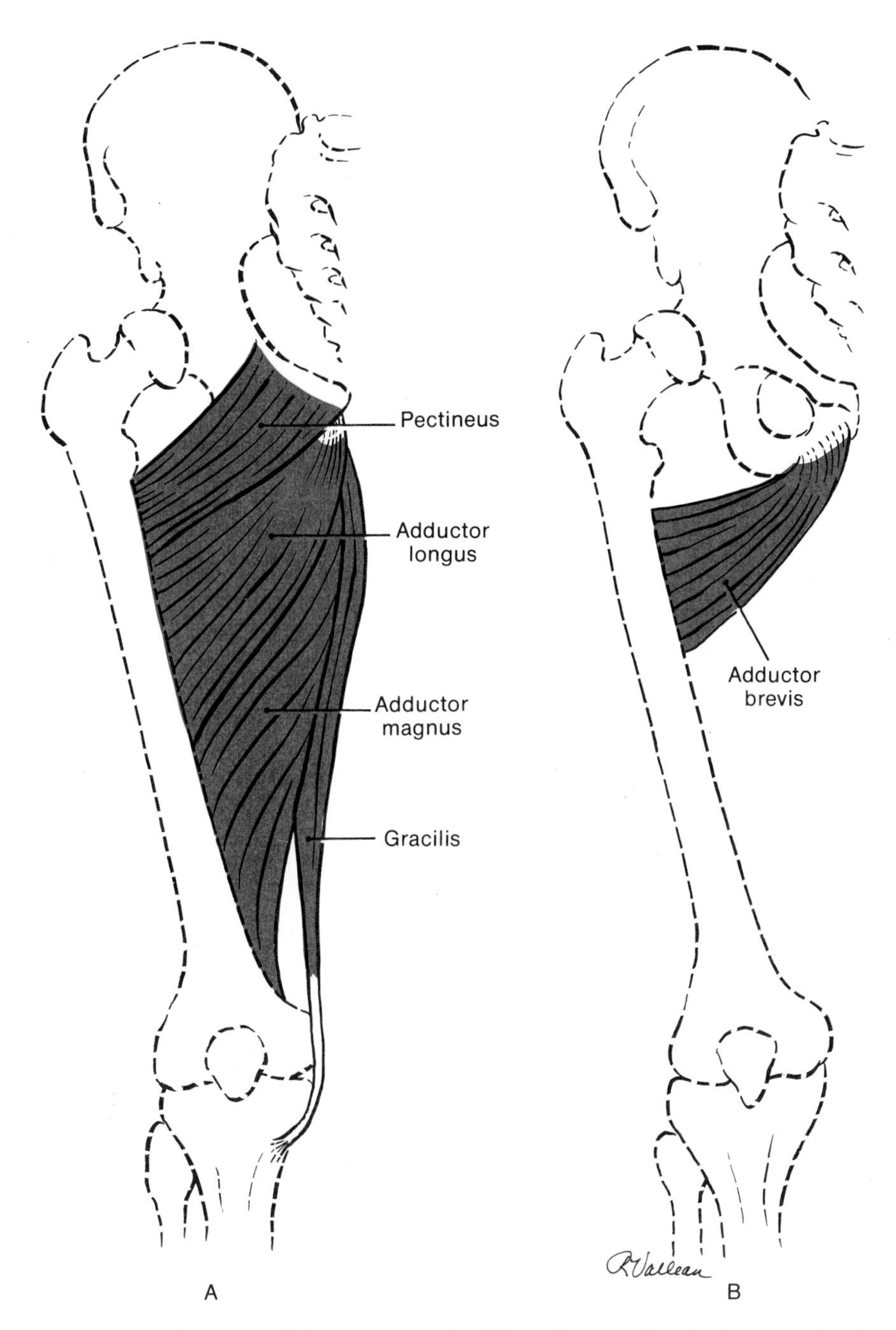

Fig. 8-39. Adductor muscles on medial aspect of thigh. (A) Pectineus, adductor longus, adductor magnus, and gracilis. (B) Muscles depicted in A have been removed to show deeper lying adductor brevis.

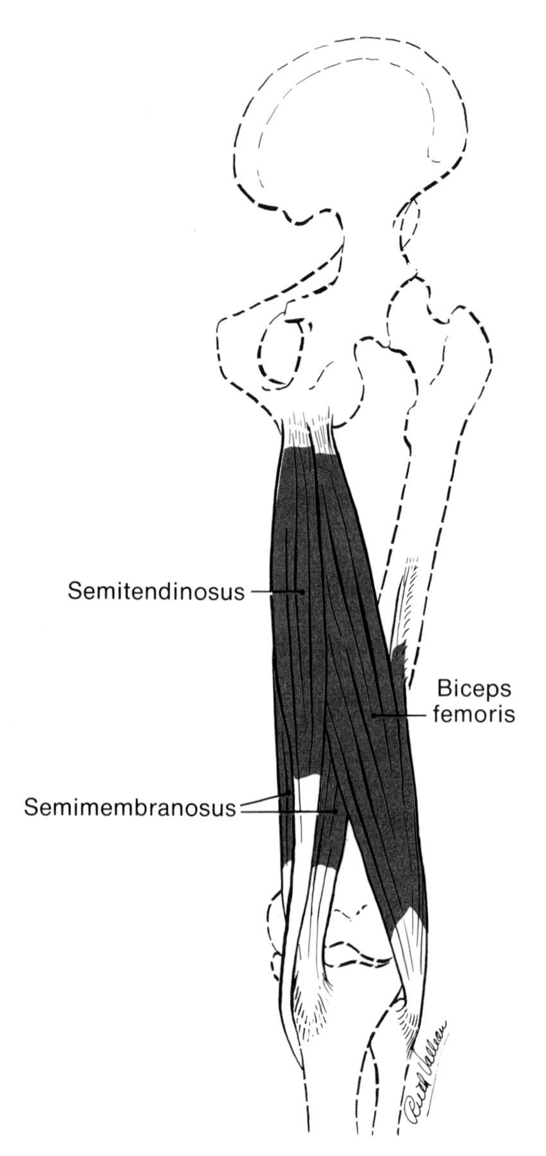

Fig. 8-40. Posterior muscles of the thigh: semitendinosus, semimembranosus, and biceps femoris. The semimembranosus lies deep to the semitendinosus.

actually a large sesamoid bone embedded in the tendon of the quadriceps muscle, and the portion of the tendon below the patella is termed the **patellar ligament.**) When the tendon is tapped the quadriceps contracts reflexively in the typical knee jerk reflex. Since the rectus femoris crosses the hip joint it is also capable of flexing the thigh, in addition to acting along with the other portions of the quadriceps in extending the leg.

The medial aspect of the femur is clothed with a group of adductor muscles: **pectineus, adductor longus, adductor brevis, adductor magnus,** and **gracilis** (Fig. 8-39). These muscles originate from the pubis and insert along the linea aspera on the posterior aspect of the femur, except for the gracilis which crosses the knee joint and inserts on the tibia. The adductors not only draw the thighs together but also act as fixator muscles. The gracilis also acts as a flexor of the leg.

The posterior surface of the thigh contains muscles collectively known as the "hamstrings." These are the **biceps femoris, semimembranosus,** and **semitendinosus** (Fig. 8-40). All three muscles originate from the ischial tuberosity, with an additional origin for the short head of the biceps from the femur. The two heads of the biceps pass laterally and insert by means of a common tendon (which can be easily palpated) onto the head of the fibula. The semimembranosus and semitendinosus insert on the medial aspect of the tibia. Since the three muscles cross both the hip joint and the knee joint they can extend the thigh as well as flex the leg. When the leg is flexed, the biceps also laterally rotates the leg, and the semitendinosus and semimembranosus medially rotate it. These muscles are subject to stretching, as occurs when you try to touch your toes without bending your knees.

Muscles of the Leg

The muscles of the leg are responsible for movements of the ankle and toes. Although many of the muscles and movements have counterparts in the forearm, the leg cannot be supinated or pronated. Moreover, the anterior surface of the leg contains extensor muscles, and the posterior surface contains flexors. Also, the movements of the foot are given special terms: **dorsiflexion** points the foot upward, **plantar flexion** points the foot downward, **eversion** rotates the foot so that the sole faces outward, and **inversion** rotates the sole inward (Fig. 8-41).

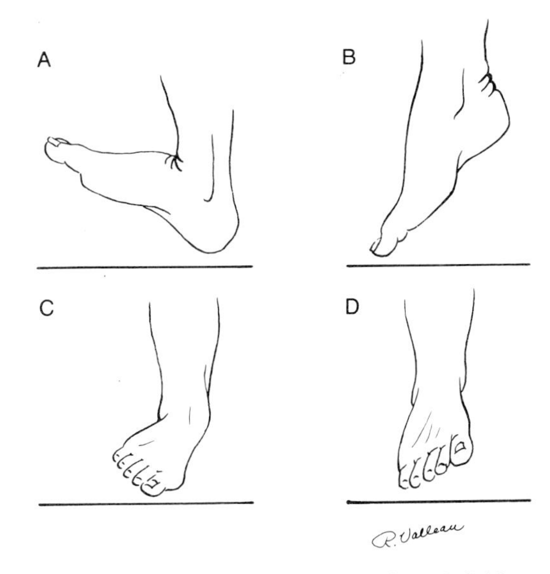

Fig. 8-41. Movements of the right foot. Solid line represents the horizontal plane, i.e., the ground. (A) Dorsiflexion (medial view), (B) plantar flexion (medial view), (C) eversion (anterior view), (D) inversion (anterior view).

The anterior leg muscles dorsiflex the foot upward and consist of the tibialis anterior, extensor digitorum longus, peroneus tertius, and extensor hallucis longus (Fig. 8-42). The **tibialis anterior** originates from the lateral aspect of the tibia and inserts on the medial cuneiform bone and base of the first metatarsal. The **extensor digitorum longus** is situated lateral to the tibialis anterior and gives rise to four tendons which pass to and extend the second to fifth toes. Although the **peroneus tertius** is partially fused with the extensor digitorum, it inserts on the fifth metatarsal and is not involved in extending the toes. The **extensor hallucis longus** lies deep to the tibialis anterior and extensor digitorum but its tendon is quite prominent as it passes on the dorsal surface of the foot to insert on the distal phalanx of the big toe.

The lateral surface of the leg contains two muscles which evert the foot: the peroneus longus and peroneus brevis (Fig. 8-43). The **peroneus longus** lies superficially along the fibula and gives rise to a prominent tendon (Fig. 8-44), which passes posterior to the lateral malleolus and curves across the sole of the foot to insert medially on the medial cuneiform and base of the first metatarsal. In addition to everting the foot the peroneus longus also plantar flexes it. The **peroneus brevis** lies under cover of the peroneus longus, and the tendons of these two muscles travel together behind the lateral malleolus, at which point the peroneus brevis tendon passes downward and forward to insert at the base of the fifth metatarsal.

The posterior leg muscles are arranged in two layers. The superficial layer consists of the gastrocnemius, soleus, and plantaris. The **gastrocnemius** has two heads which originate from the lower end of the femur (Fig. 8-45). The **soleus** is more deeply situated and origi-

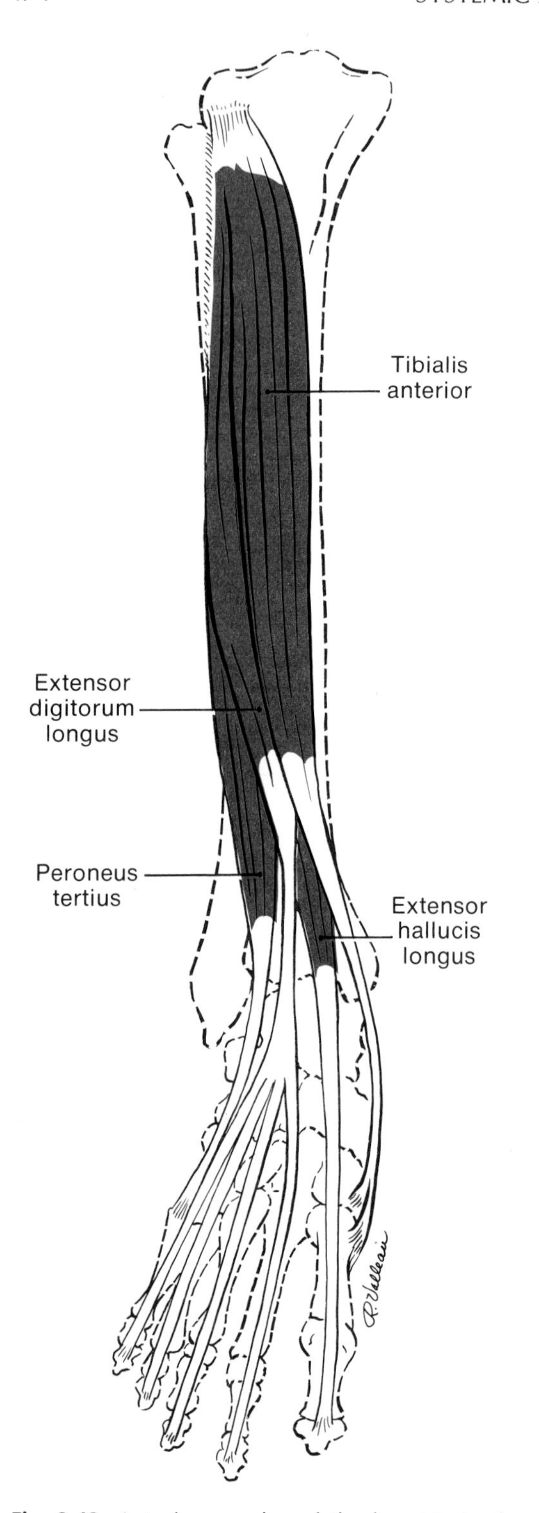

Fig. 8-42. Anterior muscles of the leg. Most of the extensor hallucis longus lies deep to the tibialis anterior and extensor digitorum longus.

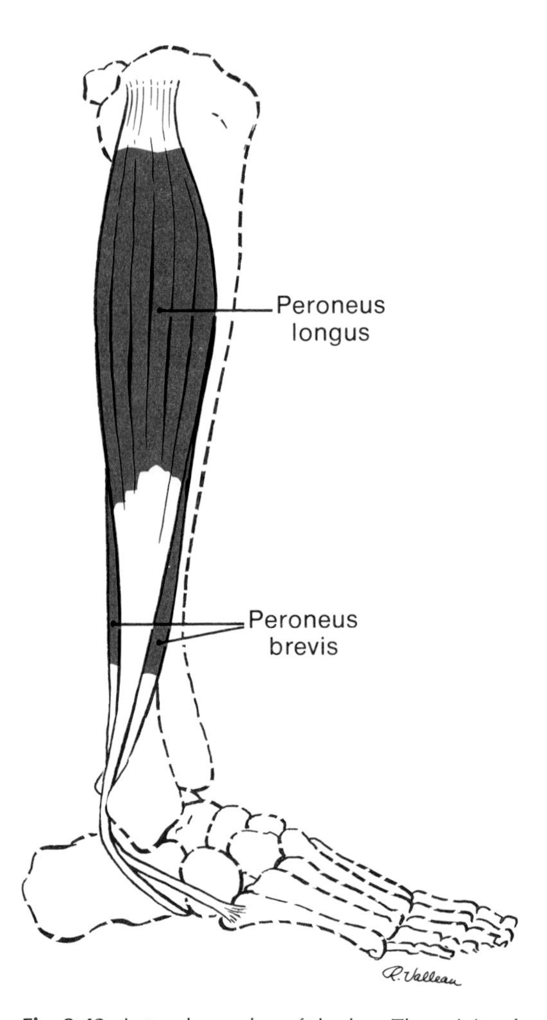

Fig. 8-43. Lateral muscles of the leg. The origin of the peroneus brevis muscle lies deep to the peroneus longus.

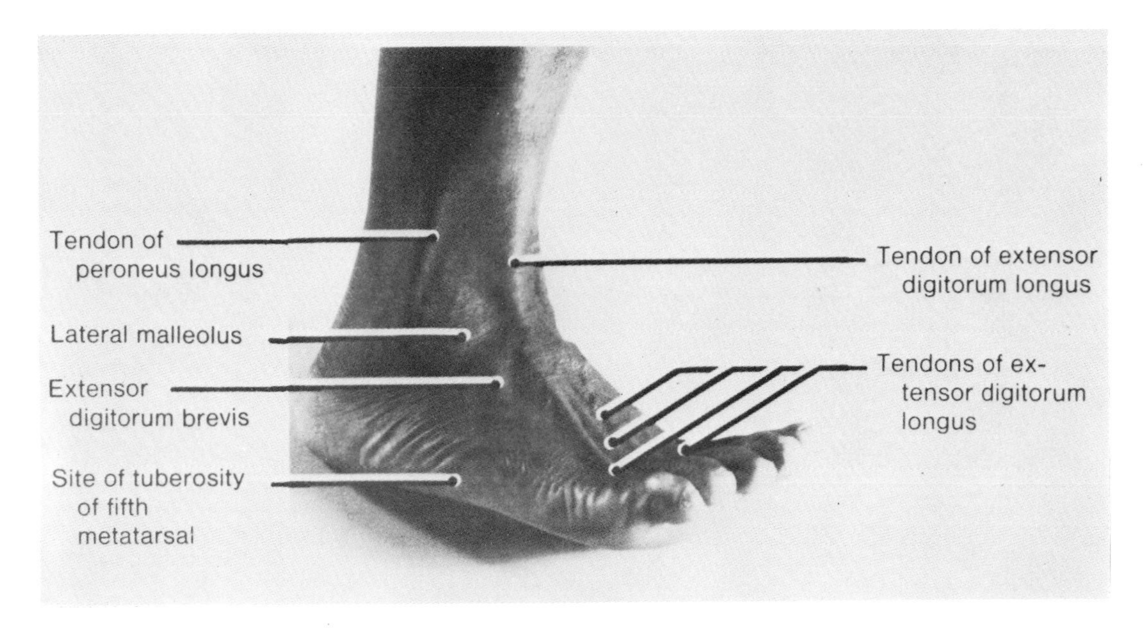

Fig. 8-44. Surface anatomy of the lateral and anterior muscles of the leg and foot. (Reproduced by permission from K. L. Moore, *Clinically Oriented Anatomy,* copyright 1980, The Williams & Wilkins Co., Baltimore.)

nates from the upper portion of the fibula and tibia. Both muscles unite to form a common tendon, the **tendo calcaneus** (calcaneal or Achilles tendon), which is easily palpated as it passes downward to insert on the calcaneus. The two heads of the gastrocnemius and the one head of the soleus together comprise the **triceps surae** ("three heads of the calf muscle") which plantar flexes the foot. Since the gastrocnemius also passes across the knee joint, it can flex the leg. (The **plantaris** is a small and variable muscle between the gastrocnemius and soleus and inserts by means of a long thin tendon into the tendo calcaneus or calcaneus.)

The two heads of the gastrocnemius and the lower ends of the biceps femoris, semimembranosus, and semitendinosus demarcate a diamond-shaped space called the **popliteal fossa** at the back of the knee (Fig. 8-45). Deep within this fossa lies the **popliteus** muscle which originates laterally from the lateral condyle of the femur and passes obliquely to insert medially on the tibia (Fig. 8-46). This muscle helps to strengthen the knee joint in the crouched position, and it also laterally rotates the femur or medially rotates the tibia depending on which bone is in the fixed position. When the knee is fully extended, medial rotation of the tibia is important in unlocking the knee so that flexion can occur.

The deep layer of posterior leg muscles contains the **flexor digitorum longus** lying medially along the tibia, the **flexor hallucis longus** along the fibula, and the **tibialis posterior** lying deep to the two flexor muscles. The tibialis posterior sends its tendon behind the medial malleolus and fans out across the sole of the foot to insert on various tarsal bones and metatarsals 2–4. It is a strong invertor of the foot.

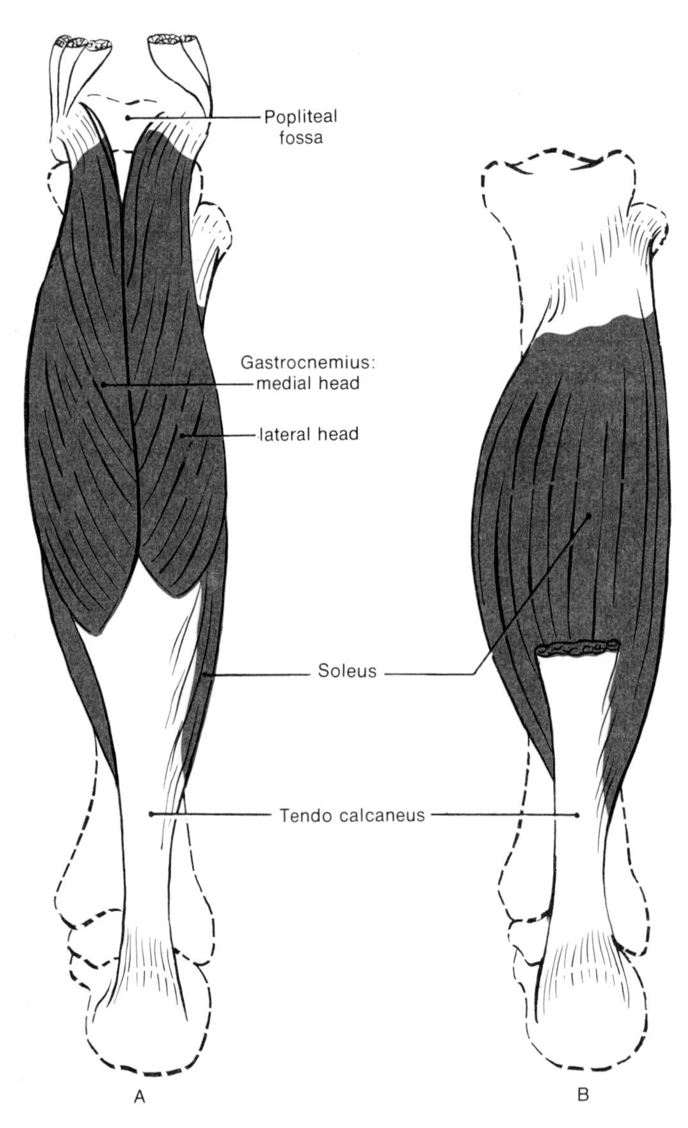

Fig. 8-45. Posterior muscles of the leg. (A) Superficial view: gastrocnemius muscle with portion of deeper lying soleus muscle apparent laterally. The two heads of the gastrocnemius form inferior boundaries of the popliteal fossa. (B) Most of the gastrocnemius muscle has been removed, revealing the soleus muscle.

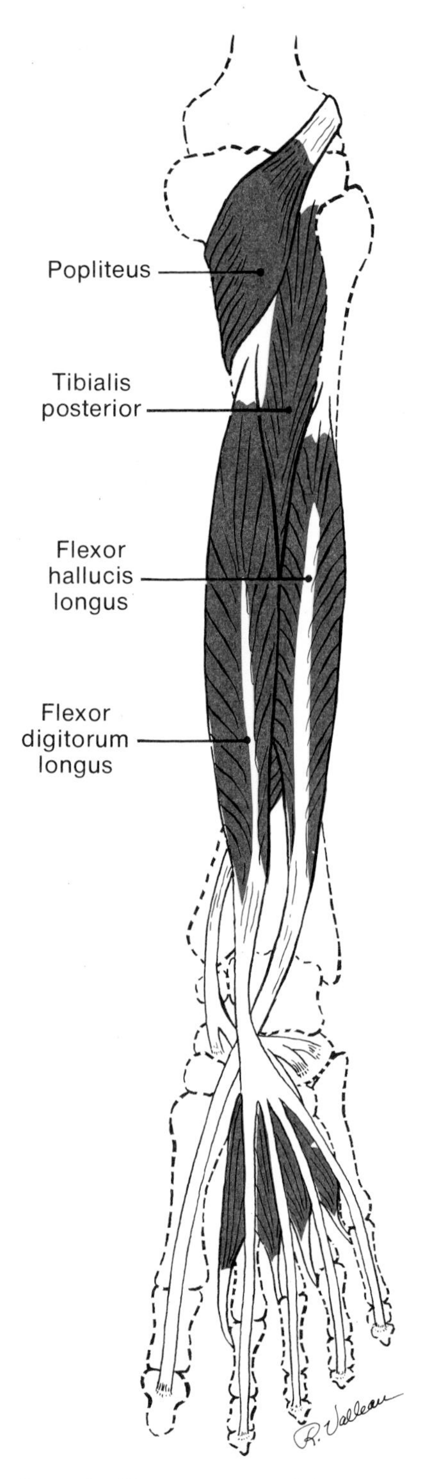

Fig. 8-46. Deep muscles of leg, posterior view. The tendons of the flexor digitorum longus give origin to the four lumbrical muscles in the sole of the foot.

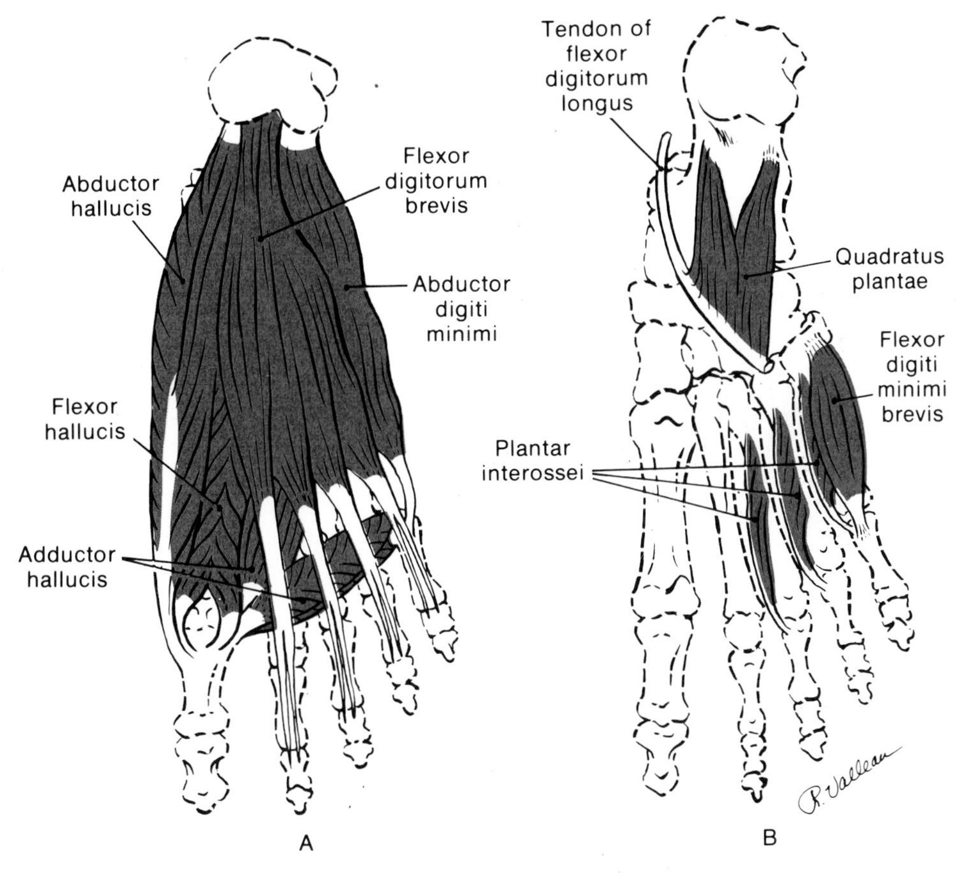

Fig. 8-47. Muscles of the plantar surface (sole) of the right foot. (A) superficial muscles, (B) deeper muscles, including quadratus plantae associated with the tendon of the flexor digitorum longus.

Muscles of the Foot

The arrangement of muscles in the foot shows many similarities to that in the hand (Figs. 8-46 and 8-48). The flexor and extensor tendons are held in place at the ankle joint by the **flexor** and **extensor retinacula,** respectively, and there is a **plantar aponeurosis** corresponding to the palmar aponeurosis. The intrinsic muscles of the foot which have counterparts in the hand are: muscles which move the big toe (**abductor hallucis, flexor hallucis brevis,** and **adductor hallucis**), those which move the little toe (**abductor digiti minimi, flexor digiti minimi brevis**), **lumbrical** muscles associated with the tendons of the flexor digitorum longus (Fig. 8-46), and **dorsal** and **plantar interossei.** (Abduction and adduction of the toes occur relative to an imaginary line passing through the second toe.) In addition, the **flexor digitorum brevis** in the sole of the foot corresponds in function to the flexor digitorum superficialis in the forearm.

The foot also shows two special muscles: the **quadratus plantae** (an accessory flexor) extending on the sole from the calcaneus to the tendon of the flexor digitorum longus (Fig. 8-47), and the **extensor digitorum brevis** ex-

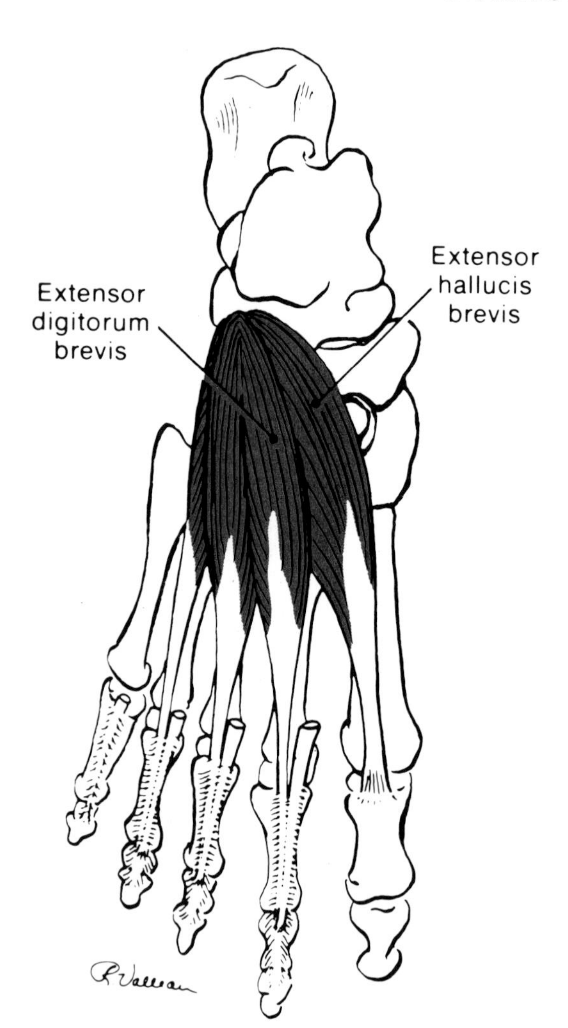

Fig. 8-48. Dorsum of right foot. The extensor digitorum brevis and extensor hallucis brevis are shown, along with cut portions of tendons of the extensor digitorum longus.

tending forward on the dorsal aspect to insert with the tendons of the extensor digitorum longus (Fig. 8-48). (The portion of the extensor digitorum brevis which passes to the big toe is often termed the **extensor hallucis brevis.**) It should be noted the foot does not have opponens muscles and that many of the intrinsic muscles do not show the range of movement characteristic of the hand. Instead, many of these muscles act to bind the foot bones together, thereby strengthening it for bearing weight and for locomotion.

Although it is useful to study muscles individually, it is also important to bear in mind the spatial and functional interrelationships among groups of muscles. Plates 1–7 (from *Stedman's Medical Dictionary*, The Williams & Wilkins Co., Baltimore, 1976) have been included for this purpose.

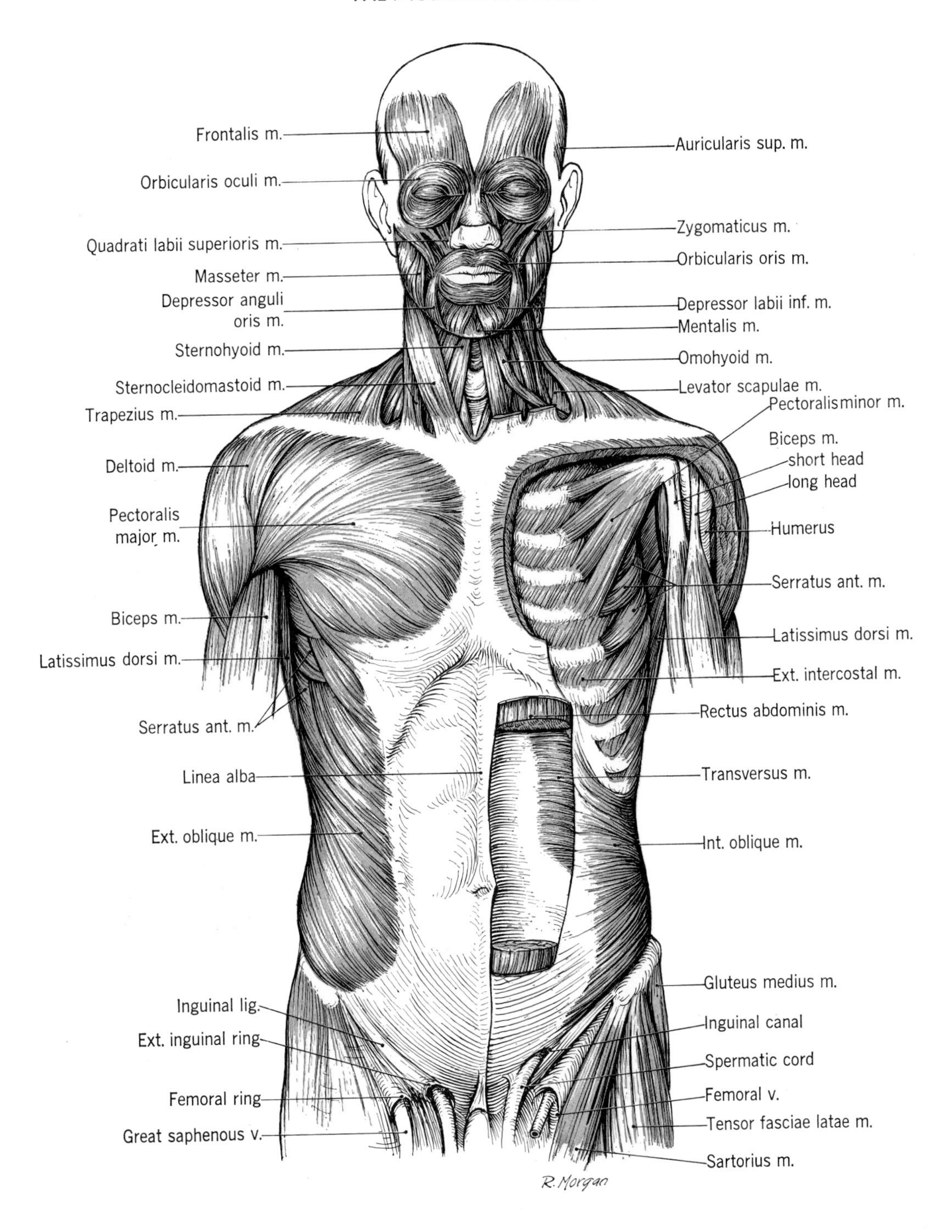

PLATE 1

Muscles of Head, Neck, and Torso, Anterior View

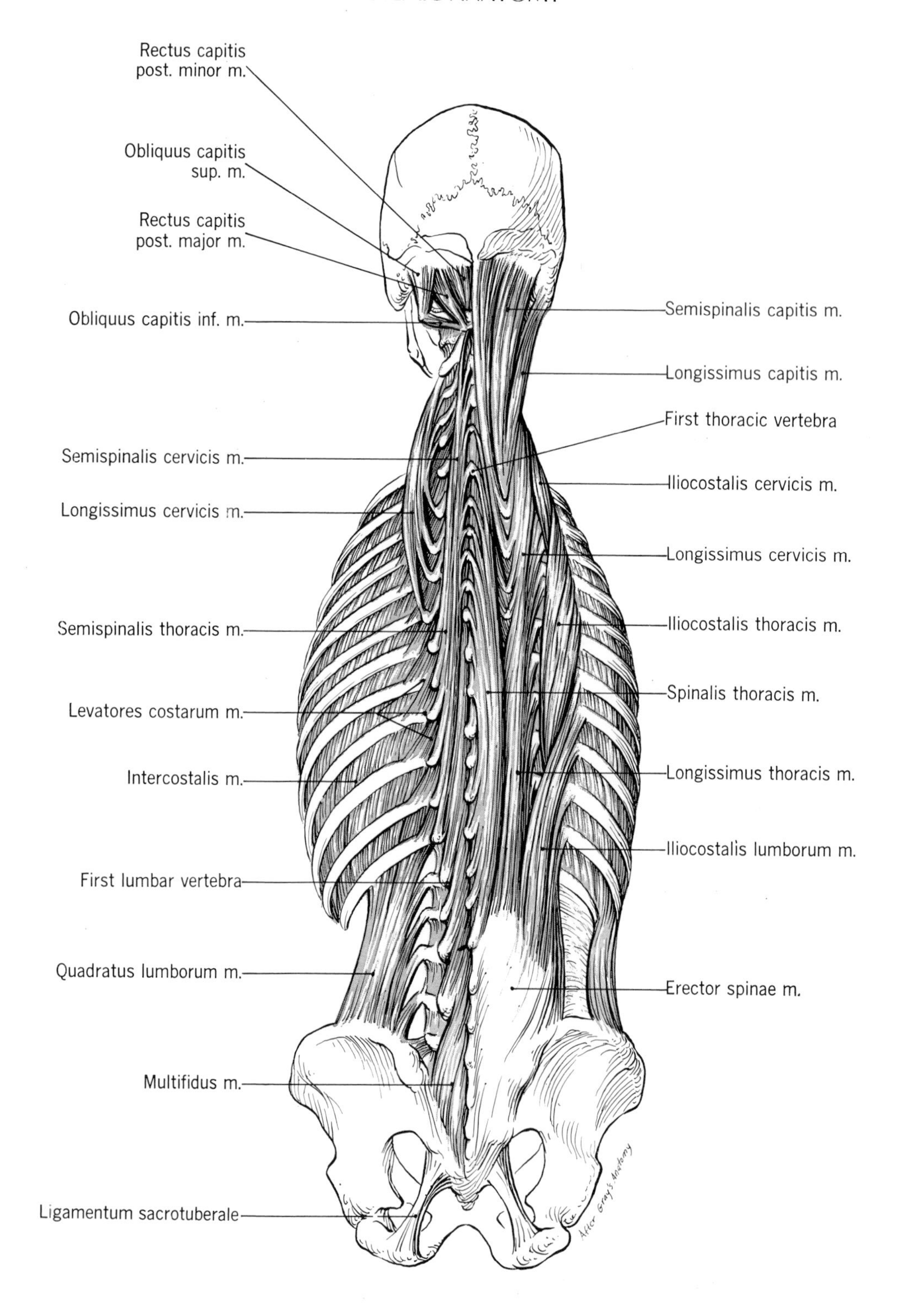

PLATE 2

Muscles of Back, Deep Dissection

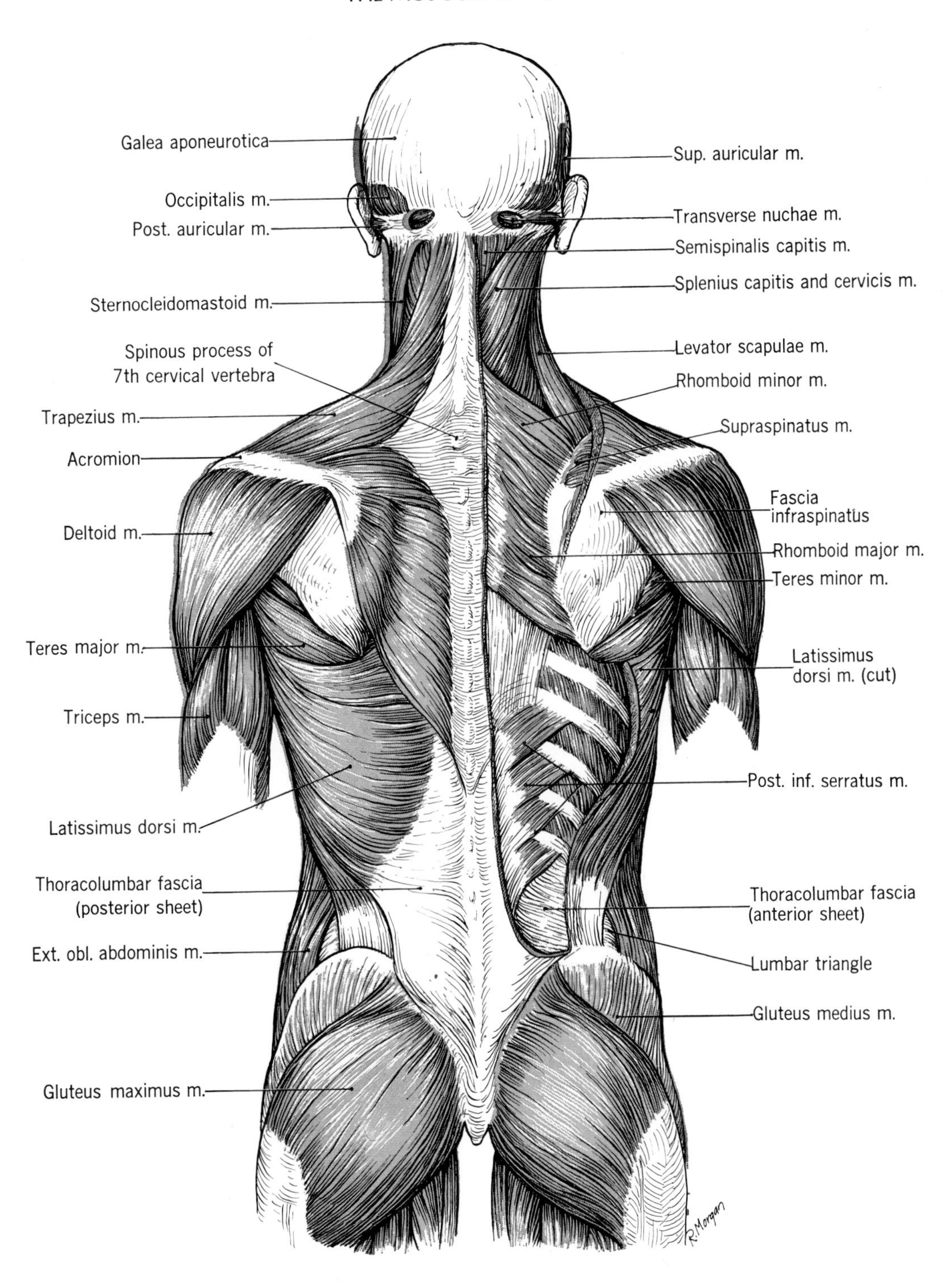

PLATE 3

Muscles of Trunk, Posterior View

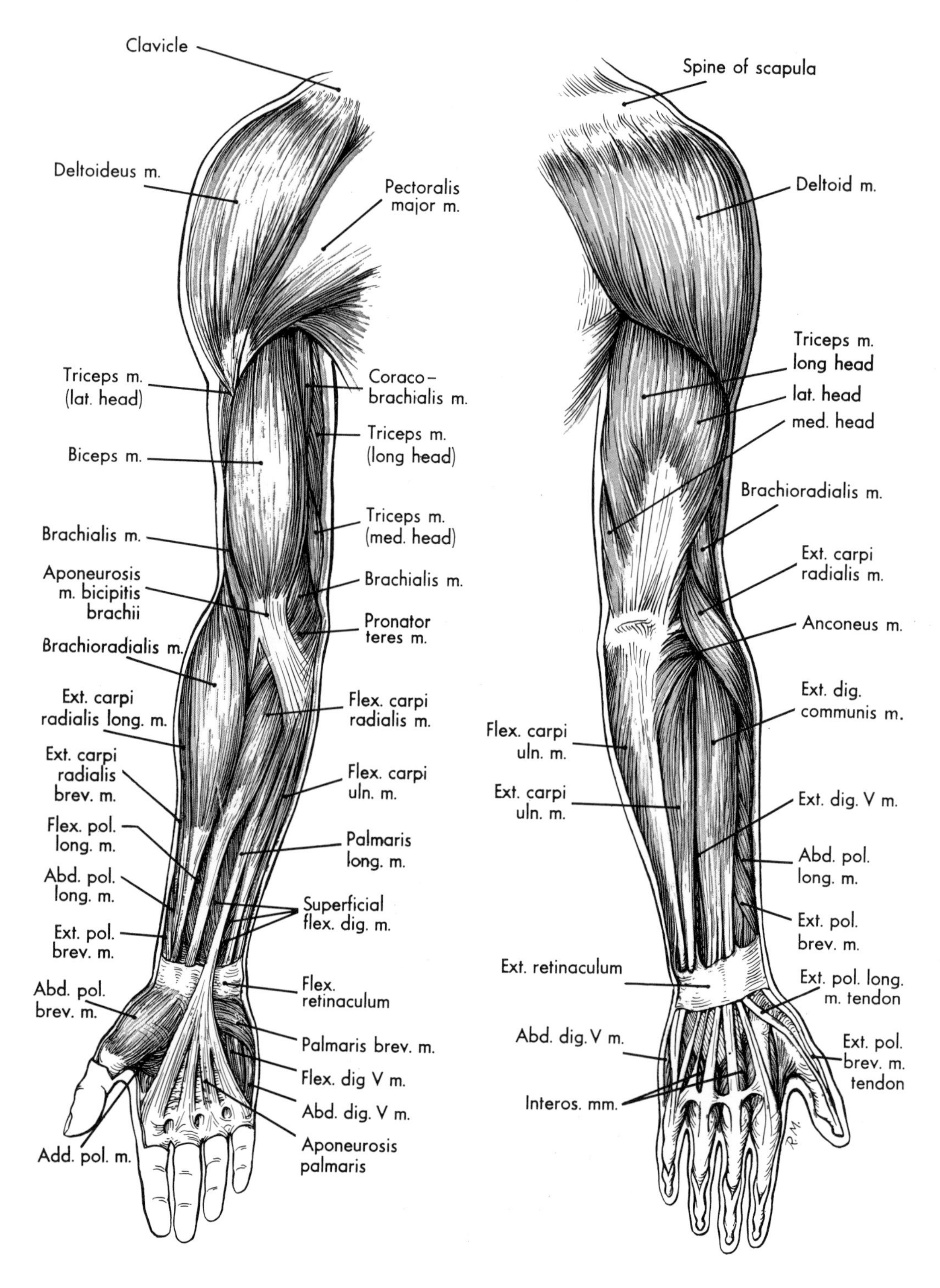

PLATE 4

Superficial Muscles of Right Upper Limb

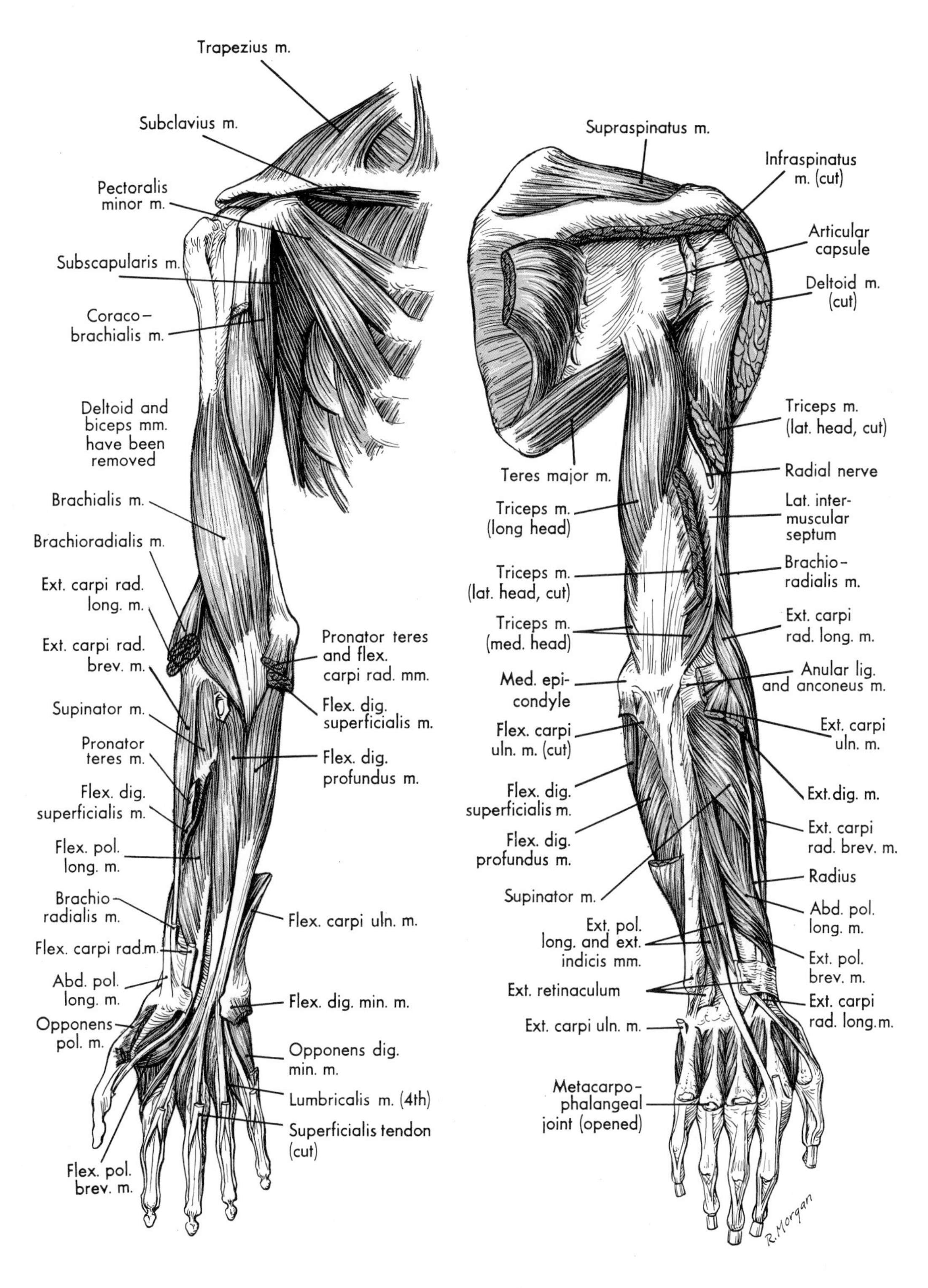

PLATE 5

Muscles of Right Upper Limb, Deep Dissection

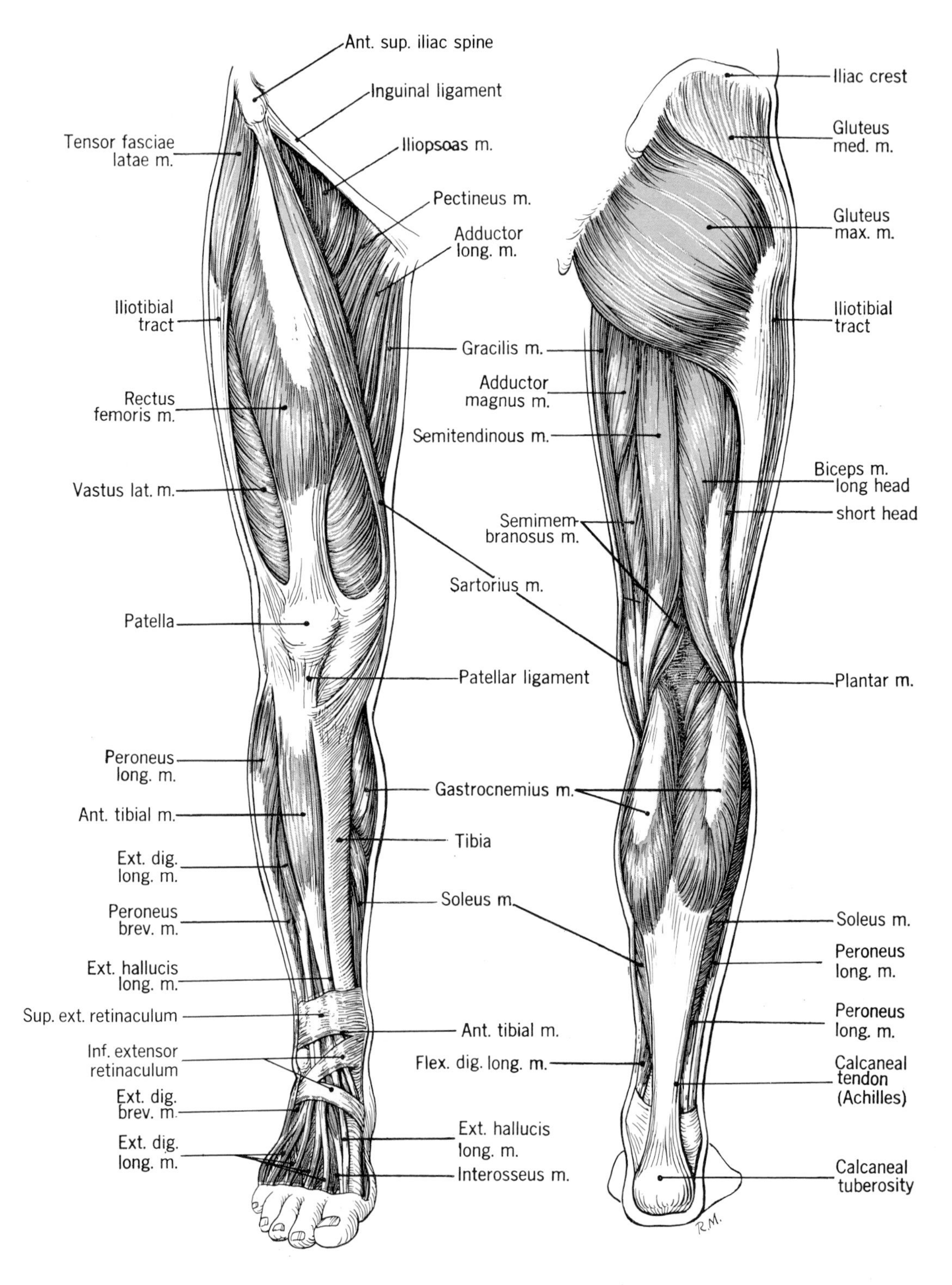

PLATE 6

Superficial Muscles of Right Lower Limb

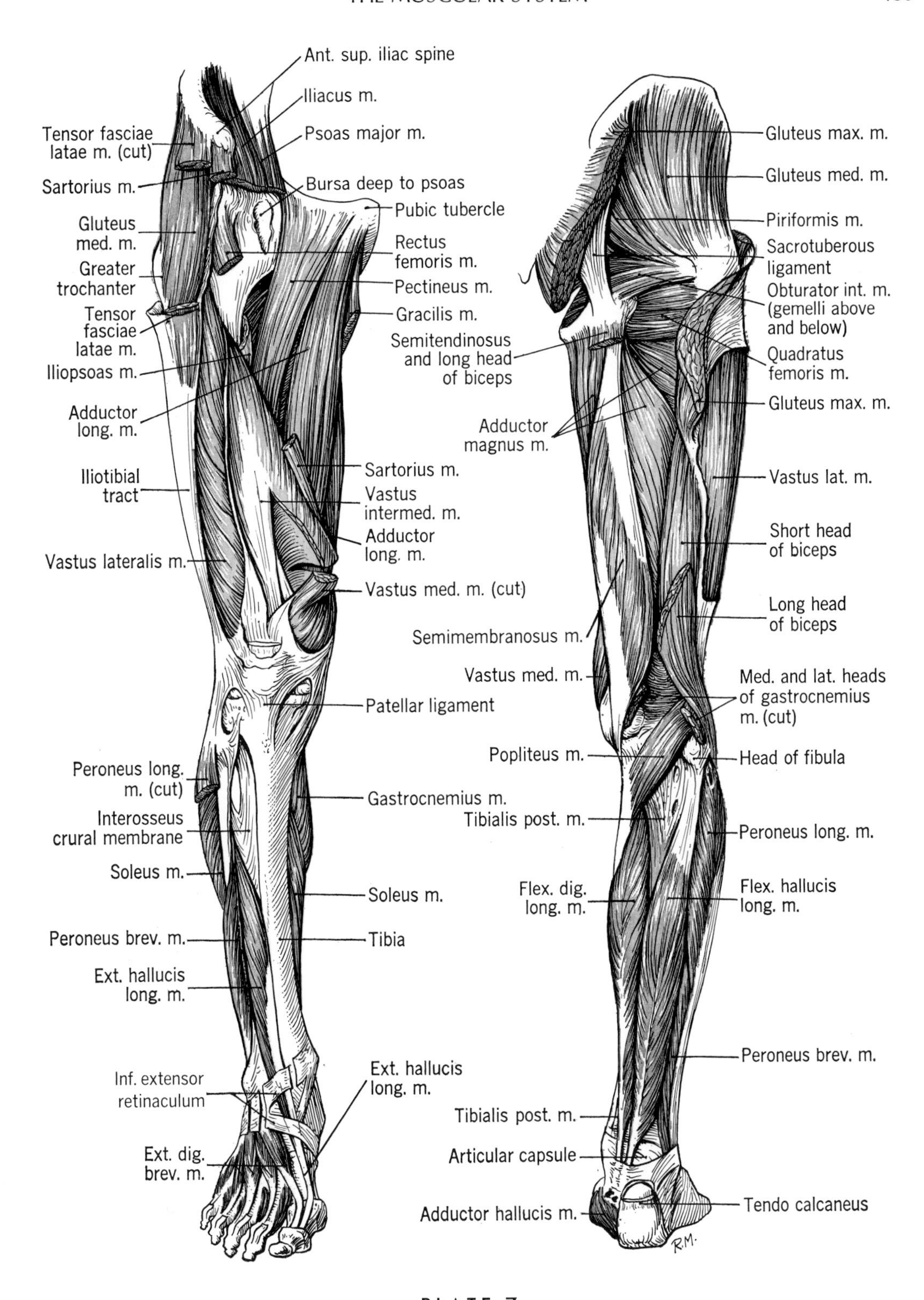

PLATE 7

Muscles of Right Lower Limb, Deep Dissection

Table 8-1. Summary of Skeletal Muscles

MUSCLE	ORIGIN	INSERTION	ACTION	INNERVATION
Abductor digiti minimi (of foot)	Calcaneus	Proximal phalanx of little toe	Abducts and flexes little toe	Lateral plantar
Abductor digiti minimi (of hand)	Pisiform	Proximal phalanx of little finger	Abducts little finger	Ulnar
Abductor hallucis	Calcaneus	Proximal phalanx of big toe	Abducts big toe	Medial plantar
Abductor pollicis brevis	Flexor retinaculum and trapezium	Proximal phalanx of thumb	Abducts thumb	Median
Abductor pollicis longus	Radius and ulna (posterior aspect)	Metacarpal 1	Abducts thumb	Radial
Adductor brevis	Pubis (body and inferior ramus)	Femur (upper linea aspera)	Adducts thigh	Obturator
Adductor hallucis	Tendon of peroneus longus and metatarsals 2–4	Proximal phalanx of big toe	Adducts big toe	Lateral plantar
Adductor longus	Pubis (body)	Femur (linea aspera on posterior aspect)	Adducts thigh	Obturator
Adductor magnus	Ischiopubic ramus and ischial tuberosity	Femur (linea aspera and adductor tubercle	Adducts and extends thigh	Obturator and sciatic (tibial portion)
Adductor pollicis	Metacarpal 3, metacarpal 2, capitate, and trapezoid	Proximal phalanx of thumb	Adducts thumb	Ulnar
Anconeus	Humerus (lateral epicondyle)	Olecranon	Assists in extending forearm	Radial
Biceps brachii	Scapula (coracoid process, supraglenoid tubercle)	Radial tuberosity	Flexes and supinates forearm	Musculocutaneous
Biceps femoris	Ischium (tuberosity) and femur (lateral aspect of linea aspera)	Fibula (head)	Extends thigh, flexes and laterally rotates leg	Sciatic (tibial and common peroneal)
Brachialis	Humerus (anterior aspect)	Ulna (coronoid process)	Flexes forearm	Musculocutaneous
Brachioradialis	Humerus (supracondylar ridge)	Radius (styloid process)	Flexes forearm	Radial
Buccinator	Maxilla, mandible, and pterygomandibular raphe	Angle of mouth	Compresses cheeks	Facial
Bulbospongiosus	Central tendon of perineum	Corpus spongiosum	Assists in maintaining erection, aids in expelling urine and semen	Pudendal
Coccygeus	Spine of ischium	Sacrum and coccyx	Assists in supporting pelvic viscera	Sacral 3, 4
Constrictor, inferior	Cricoid and thyroid cartilage	Median raphe	Constricts pharynx	Pharyngeal plexus
Constrictor, middle	Hyoid	Median raphe	Constricts pharynx	Pharyngeal plexus
Constrictor, superior	Sphenoid, mandible, and pterygomandibular raphe	Median raphe, occipital	Constricts pharynx	Pharyngeal plexus
Coracobrachialis	Scapula (coracoid process)	Humerus (medial aspect)	Flexes arm	Musculocutaneous
Cremaster	Inguinal ligament and internal oblique m.	Spermatic cord, testis	Raises testis	Genitofemoral
Deltoid	Clavicle, scapula (acromion and spine)	Humerus (lateral aspect)	Flexes, abducts and extends arm	Axillary
Depressor anguli oris	Mandible	Angle of mouth	Depresses angle of mouth	Facial
Depressor labii inferioris	Mandible	Lower lip	Depresses lower lip	Facial

MUSCLE	ORIGIN	INSERTION	ACTION	INNERVATION
Diaphragm	Sternum, costal cartilages, ribs, lumbar vertebrae	Central tendon	Respiration, increases size of thoracic cavity, decreases size of abdominal cavity	Phrenic
Digastric	Temporal (mastoid process)	Mandible	Raises hyoid, depresses mandible	Facial and mandibular division of trigeminal
Erector spinae	Lower vertebral column	Upper vertebral column, ribs, and skull	Extends and laterally bends vertebral column	Spinal nerves
Extensor carpi radialis brevis	Humerus (lateral epicondyle)	Metacarpals 2 and 3	Extends and abducts wrist	Radial
Extensor carpi radialis longus	Humerus (lateral epicondyle and supracondylar ridge)	Metacarpal 2	Extends and abducts wrist	Radial
Extensor carpi ulnaris	Humerus (lateral epicondyle)	Metacarpal 5	Extends and adducts wrist	Radial
Extensor digiti minimi	Humerus (lateral epicondyle)	Extensor expansion of digit 5	Extends digit 5	Radial
Extensor digitorum	Humerus (lateral epicondyle)	Extensor expansions of digits 2–5	Extends digits	Radial
Extensor digitorum brevis	Calcaneus (upper) and extensor retinaculum	Tendons of extensor digitorum longus	Extends toes	Deep peroneal
Extensor digitorum longus	Tibia (lateral condyle) and fibula (upper anterior aspect)	Extensor expansions toes 2–5	Extends toes 2–5 dorsiflexes foot	Deep peroneal
Extensor hallucis brevis	Calcaneus (upper) and extensor retinaculum	Proximal phalanx of big toe	Extends big toe	Deep peroneal
Extensor hallucis longus	Fibula (anterior middle aspect) and interosseous membrane	Distal phalanx of big toe	Extends big toe and aids dorsiflexion of foot	Deep peroneal
Extensor indicis	Ulna (posterior aspect)	Proximal phalanx of index finger	Extends index finger	Radial
Extensor pollicis brevis	Radius (posterior aspect)	Proximal phalanx of thumb	Extends proximal phalanx of thumb	Radial
Extensor pollicis longus	Ulna (posterior aspect)	Distal phalanx of thumb	Extends distal phalanx of thumb	Radial
Flexor carpi radialis	Humerus (medial epicondyle)	Metacarpals 2 and 3	Flexes and abducts wrist	Median
Flexor carpi ulnaris	Humerus (medial epicondyle), ulna	Pisiform and metacarpal 5	Flexes and adducts wrist	Ulnar
Flexor digiti minimi brevis (of foot)	Metatarsal 5 (base)	Proximal phalanx of little toe	Flexes little toe	Lateral plantar
Flexor digiti minimi brevis (of hand)	Hamate	Proximal phalanx of little finger	Flexes little finger	Ulnar
Flexor digitorum brevis	Calcaneus	Middle phalanges of toes 2–5	Flexes middle phalanges	Medial plantar
Flexor digitorum longus	Tibia (middle of posterior aspect)	Distal phalanges of toes 2–5	Flexes distal phalanges of toes 2–5	Tibial
Flexor digitorum profundus	Ulna (upper anterior aspect)	Distal phalanges of digits 2–5	Flexes distal phalanges	Ulnar and median
Flexor digitorum superficialis	Humerus (medial epicondyle), upper radius and ulna	Middle phalanges of digits 2–5	Flexes middle phalanges	Median
Flexor hallucis brevis	Cuboid, lateral cuneiform	Proximal phalanx of big toe	Flexes big toe	Medial plantar
Flexor hallucis longus	Fibula (posterior aspect)	Distal phalanx of big toe	Flexes distal phalanx of big toe	Tibial
Flexor pollicis brevis	Flexor retinaculum and trapezium	Proximal phalanx of thumb	Flexes thumb	Median and ulnar
Flexor pollicis longus	Radius (upper anterior aspect)	Distal phalanx of thumb	Flexes distal phalanx of thumb	Median

MUSCLE	ORIGIN	INSERTION	ACTION	INNERVATION
Frontalis	Epicranial aponeurosis	Skin of forehead	Raises eyebrows	Facial
Gastrocnemius	Femur (lateral and medial condyles)	Calcaneus	Plantar flexes foot, flexes knee	Tibial
Gemellus inferior	Ischium (lesser sciatic notch)	Tendon of obturator internus muscle	Laterally rotates thigh	Lumbar 5, sacral 1, 2
Gemellus superior	Ischium (spine and lesser sciatic notch)	Tendon of obturator internus muscle	Laterally rotates thigh	Lumbar 5, sacral 1, 2
Genioglossus	Mandible	Tongue	Protrudes and depresses tongue	Hypoglossal
Geniohyoid	Mandible	Hyoid	Elevates hyoid	Upper cervical
Gluteus maximus	Ilium, sacrum, coccyx	Femur (posterior aspect) and iliotibial tract	Extends thigh	Inferior gluteal
Gluteus medius	Ilium	Femur (greater trochanter, lateral surface)	Abducts and medially rotates thigh	Superior gluteal
Gluteus minimus	Ilium	Femur (greater trochanter, lateral surface)	Abducts and medially rotates thigh	Superior gluteal
Gracilis	Pubis (body and inferior ramus)	Tibia (upper medial aspect)	Adducts and flexes thigh, flexes and medially rotates leg	Obturator
Hyoglossus	Hyoid bone	Tongue	Depresses and retracts tongue	Hypoglossal
Iliacus	Ilium and sacrum	Femur (lesser trochanter)	Flexes thigh and trunk	Femoral
Iliopsoas (combined iliacus and psoas)	Ilium, sacrum, lumbar vertebrae	Femur (lesser trochanter)	Flexes thigh and trunk	Lumbar 1-3, and femoral
Infraspinatus	Scapula (infraspinous fossa)	Humerus (greater tubercle)	Laterally rotates arm	Suprascapular
Intercostals, external	Inferior border of rib	Superior border of rib below	Elevate ribs	Intercostals
Intercostals, innermost	Inferior border of rib	Superior border of rib below	Elevate ribs, draw ribs together	Intercostals
Intercostals, internal	Inferior border of rib	Superior border of rib below	Elevate ribs, draw ribs together	Intercostals
Interossei, dorsal (of foot)	Each from adjacent shafts of metatarsals	Proximal phalanges of toes 2-4	Abduct toes, flex proximal phalanges	Lateral plantar
Interossei, dorsal (of hand)	Each from adjacent shafts of metacarpals	Proximal phalanges of digits 2-4 and extensor expansions	Abduct fingers, flex proximal phalanges	Ulnar
Interossei, palmar	Metacarpals 2, 4, and 5	Extensor expansions	Adduct fingers, flex proximal phalanges	Ulnar
Interossei, plantar	Metatarsals 3-5	Proximal phalanges of toes 3-5	Adduct toes, flex proximal phalanges	Lateral plantar
Ischiocavernosus	Ischium (ramus)	Crus of penis or clitoris	Maintains erection	Pudendal
Latissimus dorsi	Lower thoracic vertebrae, thoracolumbar fascia, ilium, lower ribs	Humerus (intertubercular groove)	Extends, adducts and medially rotates arm	Thoracodorsal
Levator ani	Pubis, lateral wall of pelvis	Midline pelvic viscera, central tendon of perineum	Supports pelvic viscera, controls urination, defecation	Sacral 3, 4, pudendal
Levator labii superioris	Maxilla and zygomatic bone	Upper lip	Elevates upper lip and angle of mouth	Facial
Levator palpebrae superioris	Orbit	Upper eyelid	Raises upper eyelid	Oculomotor
Levator scapulae	Upper cervical vertebrae	Scapula (medial border)	Elevates scapula	Cervical 3, 4
Levator veli palatini	Temporal bone	Soft palate	Elevates soft palate	Pharyngeal plexus
Levatores costarum	Thoracic vertebrae	Adjacent ribs below	Elevate ribs	Intercostals
Lumbricals (of foot)	Tendons of flexor digitorum longus	Proximal phalanges, extensor expansions	Flex proximal phalanges, extend middle and distal phalanges	Medial plantar (for 1); lateral plantar (for 2-4)

MUSCLE	ORIGIN	INSERTION	ACTION	INNERVATION
Lumbricals (of hand)	Tendons of flexor digitorum profundus	Proximal phalanges, extensor expansions	Flex proximal phalanges, extend middle and distal phalanges	Median and ulnar
Masseter	Zygomatic arch	Mandible (lateral aspect)	Elevates mandible	Mandibular division of trigeminal
Mentalis	Mandible	Skin of chin	Protrudes lower lip	Facial
Musculus uvulae	Palatine bones and aponeurosis	Uvula	Elevates uvula	Pharyngeal plexus
Mylohyoid	Mandible	Median raphe and hyoid	Elevates hyoid, depresses mandible, raises floor of mouth	Mandibular division of trigeminal
Oblique, external	Ribs 5-12	Linea alba and iliac crest	Compresses abdomen, rotates and flexes vertebral column	Intercostals subcostal, and upper lumbar
Oblique, inferior	Orbit	Eyeball	Rotates eyeball	Oculomotor
Oblique, internal	Thoracolumbar fascia iliac crest, inguinal ligament	Lower ribs, linea alba, and pubis	Compresses abdomen, rotates and flexes vertebral column	Intercostals, subcostal and upper lumbar
Oblique, superior	Orbit	Eyeball	Rotates eyeball	Trochlear
Obturator externus	External surface of obturator foramen and hip bone	Femur (trochanteric fossa)	Laterally rotates thigh	Obturator
Obturator internus	Internal surface of obturator foramen and hip bone	Femur (greater trochanter, medial aspect)	Laterally rotates thigh	Lumbar 5, sacral 1, 2
Occipitalis	Occipital bone	Epicranial aponeurosis	Moves scalp backward	Facial
Omohyoid	Scapula	Hyoid	Depresses hyoid	Upper cervical
Opponens digiti minimi	Hamate	Metacarpal 5 (shaft)	Draws metacarpal 5 forward and deepens palm	Ulnar
Opponens pollicis	Flexor retinaculum and trapezium	Metacarpal 1 (shaft)	Opposes thumb to fingers	Median
Orbicularis oculi	Orbit	Upper and lower eyelids	Closes eyelids	Facial
Orbicularis oris	Upper and lower lips	Upper and lower lips	Closes and protrudes lips	Facial
Palatoglossus	Soft palate	Tongue	Elevates tongue	Pharyngeal plexus
Palatopharyngeus	Palate (soft and hard)	Pharynx and thyroid cartilage	Elevates pharynx	Pharyngeal plexus
Palmaris longus	Humerus (medial epicondyle)	Palmar aponeurosis	Tenses fascia and weakly flexes wrist	Median
Pectineus	Pubis (crest)	Femur (pectineal line)	Adducts thigh	Femoral and obturator
Pectoralis major	Sternum, clavicle, upper ribs	Humerus (intertubercular groove)	Adducts arm	Medial and lateral pectoral
Pectoralis minor	Ribs 3-5	Scapula (coracoid process)	Depresses shoulder and elevates ribs	Medial pectoral
Perinei, deep transverse	Ischium (ramus)	Median raphe	Helps constrict urethra	Pudendal
Perinei, superficial transverse	Ischium (ramus)	Central tendon of perineum	Fixes central tendon of perineum	Pudendal
Peroneus brevis	Fibula (lower lateral aspect)	Metatarsal 5	Everts foot	Superficial peroneal
Peroneus longus	Fibula (upper lateral aspect) and tibia (lateral condyle)	Medial cuneiform and metatarsal 1	Plantar flexes and everts foot	Superficial peroneal
Peroneus tertius	Fibula (lower aspect)	Metatarsal 5	Dorsiflexes foot	Deep peroneal (anterior tibial)
Piriformis	Sacrum, ilium	Femur (greater trochanter, upper border)	Laterally rotates thigh	Sacral nerves 1 and 2
Plantaris	Femur (lateral supracondylar ridge)	Tendo calcaneus or calcaneus	Assists gastrocnemius and soleus, plantar flexion	Tibial

MUSCLE	ORIGIN	INSERTION	ACTION	INNERVATION
Platysma	Upper fascia of thoracic region	Mandible and angle of mouth	Depresses angle of mouth and jaw	Facial
Popliteus	Femur (lateral condyle)	Tibia (upper posterior aspect)	Flexes and medially rotates leg	Tibial
Pronator quadratus	Lower ulna	Lower radius	Pronates forearm	Median
Pronator teres	Humerus (medial epicondyle)	Radius (lateral aspect)	Pronates and weakly flexes forearm	Median
Psoas major	Lumbar vertebrae	Femur (lesser trochanter)	Flexes thigh and trunk	Lumbar 1, 2, 3
Psoas minor	12th thoracic and 1st lumbar vertebrae	Pubic bone	Flexes trunk	Lumbar 1
Pterygoid, lateral	Sphenoid (pterygoid plate)	Mandible and capsule of temporomandibular joint	Protrudes and lowers mandible	Mandibular division of trigeminal
Pterygoid, medial	Sphenoid (pterygoid plate)	Mandible (medial aspect)	Elevates mandible	Mandibular division of trigeminal
Quadratus femoris	Ischium (tuberosity)	Femur (intertrochanteric crest)	Laterally rotates thigh	Lumbar 4, 5, sacral 1
Quadratus lumborum	Iliac crest and lumbar vertebrae	Rib 12	Flexes trunk laterally, fixes rib	Subcostal and upper lumbar
Quadratus plantae	Calcaneus	Tendons of flexor digitorum longus	Assists flexor digitorum longus	Lateral plantar
Rectus abdominis	Symphysis pubis and crest of pubis	Xiphoid process and costal cartilages 5–7	Flexes trunk	Lower intercostals and subcostal
Rectus femoris	Ilium (anterior inferior iliac spine)	Patella and tibial tuberosity	Extends leg and flexes thigh	Femoral
Rectus, inferior	Orbit	Eyeball	Depresses eyeball	Oculomotor
Rectus, lateral	Orbit	Eyeball	Abducts eyeball	Abducens
Rectus, medial	Orbit	Eyeball	Adducts eyeball	Oculomotor
Rectus, superior	Orbit	Eyeball	Elevates eyeball	Oculomotor
Rhomboid major	Upper thoracic vertebrae	Scapula (medial border)	Adducts scapula	Dorsal scapular
Rhomboid minor	7th cervical, 1st thoracic vertebrae	Scapula (medial border)	Adducts scapula	Dorsal scapular
Risorius	Parotid fascia	Angle of mouth	Retracts angle of mouth	Facial
Salpingopharyngeus	Auditory tube	Pharynx	Elevates pharynx	Pharyngeal plexus
Sartorius	Ilium (anterior superior iliac spine)	Tibia (upper medial aspect)	Flexes and laterally rotates thigh; flexes and medially rotates leg	Femoral
Scalenus anterior	Cervical vertebrae (3–6)	1st rib	Elevates 1st rib and rotates neck	Lower cervical
Scalenus medius	Lower cervical vertebrae	1st rib	Elevates 1st rib and rotates neck	Lower cervical
Scalenus posterior	Lower cervical vertebrae	2nd rib	Elevates 2nd rib and rotates neck	Lower cervical
Semimembranosus	Ischium (tuberosity)	Tibia (medial condyle)	Extends thigh, flexes and medially rotates leg	Sciatic (tibial portion)
Semitendinosus	Ischium (tuberosity)	Tibia (below medial condyle)	Extends thigh, flexes and medially rotates leg	Sciatic (tibial portion)
Serratus anterior	Ribs 1–8	Scapula (medial border)	Abducts scapula	Long thoracic
Serratus posterior inferior	Lower thoracic and upper lumbar vertebrae	Ribs 9–12	Depresses ribs	Thoracic 9–12
Serratus posterior superior	Ligamentum nuchae and upper thoracic vertebrae	Ribs 2–5	Elevates ribs	Thoracic 2–5
Soleus	Fibula (posterior aspect) and tibia	Calcaneus	Plantar flexes foot	Tibial
Sphincter urethrae	Pubis (ramus)	Median raphe, surrounds urethra (& vagina)	Constricts urethra	Pudendal
Splenius	Ligamentum nuchae, spines of upper thoracic and lower cervical vertebrae	Occipital and temporal bones, transverse processes of upper cervical vertebrae	Rotates head and neck	Dorsal rami of cervical

MUSCLE	ORIGIN	INSERTION	ACTION	INNERVATION
Sternohyoid	Sternum	Hyoid	Depresses hyoid and larynx	Upper cervical
Sternomastoid (sternocleido-mastoid)	Sternum, clavicle	Temporal (mastoid process)	Rotates and flexes head and neck	Accessory and cervical 2, 3
Sternothyroid	Sternum	Thyroid cartilage	Depresses thyroid	Upper cervical
Styloglossus	Temporal (styloid process)	Tongue	Retracts and elevates tongue	Hypoglossal
Stylohyoid	Temporal (styloid process)	Hyoid	Elevates hyoid	Facial
Stylopharyngeus	Temporal (styloid process)	Pharynx and thyroid cartilage	Elevates pharynx	Glossopharyngeal
Subclavius	1st rib	Clavicle	Depresses clavicle	Cervical 5
Subcostals	Angles of ribs	2–3 ribs below	Draw ribs together	Intercostals
Subscapularis	Scapula (subscapular fossa)	Humerus (lesser tubercle)	Medially rotates arm	Subscapular
Supinator	Humerus (lateral epicondyle and ulna)	Radius (anterior and lateral aspect)	Supinates forearm	Radial
Supraspinatus	Scapula (supraspinous fossa)	Humerus, greater tubercle	Laterally rotates arm	Suprascapular
Temporalis	Temporal	Mandible (coronoid process)	Elevates mandible	Mandibular division of trigeminal
Tensor fasciae latae	Ilium (crest, anterior superior iliac spine)	Iliotibial tract	Flexes and medially rotates thigh, tenses fascia lata	Superior gluteal
Tensor veli palatini	Sphenoid	Soft palate	Elevates soft palate	Mandibular division of trigeminal
Teres major	Scapula (lateral border)	Humerus (medial intertubercular groove)	Adducts and medially rotates arm	Lower subscapular
Teres minor	Scapula (lateral border)	Humerus (greater tubercle)	Laterally rotates arm	Axillary
Thyrohyoid	Thyroid cartilage	Hyoid	Depresses hyoid or elevates thyroid	Upper cervical
Tibialis anterior	Tibia (upper lateral aspect)	Medial cuneiform and metatarsal 1	Dorsiflexes and inverts foot	Deep peroneal
Tibialis posterior	Fibula (posterior aspect) and interosseous membrane	Navicular, cuneiforms, cuboid, and metatarsals 2–4	Inverts foot	Tibial
Transversospinal	Vertebral transverse processes	Vertebral spinous processes	Rotate trunk	Spinal nerves
Transversus abdominis	Thoracolumbar fascia, iliac crest, inguinal ligament	Lower ribs, linea alba, and pubis	Compresses abdomen	Intercostals, subcostal, and upper lumbar
Transversus thoracis	Sternum	Ribs 2–6 (costal cartilages)	Depresses ribs	Intercostals
Trapezius	Occipital, ligamentum nuchae, spines of thoracic vertebrae	Spine of scapula, acromion, clavicle	Elevates, adducts, rotates, and depresses scapula	Accessory and cervical 3, 4
Triceps brachii	Scapula (infraglenoid tubercle), humerus (posterior and lateral aspect)	Ulna (olecranon process)	Extends forearm	Radial
Vastus intermedius	Femur (anterior and lateral aspects)	Patella and tibial tuberosity	Extends leg	Femoral
Vastus lateralis	Femur (lateral aspect of linea aspera, greater trochanter)	Patella and tibial tuberosity	Extends leg	Femoral
Vastus medialis	Femur (medial aspect of linea aspera)	Patella and tibial tuberosity	Extends leg	Femoral
Zygomaticus	Zygomatic arch	Angle of mouth	Elevates angle of mouth	Facial

9

The Cardiovascular System

The cardiovascular system is designed to transport and distribute blood throughout the body. (Because of this function it is often grouped along with the lymphatic system as part of the circulatory system.)

The cardiovascular system consists of the heart which acts as a pump, and the blood vessels which carry blood to and from the tissues where an exchange of nutrients, gases, and waste products occurs. This system also provides a means for transporting hormones and for bringing defensive elements, such as white blood cells and antibodies, to areas susceptible to infection and invasion by foreign matter.

THE HEART

Gross Anatomy

The heart is located in the inferior region of the thorax. The thorax contains three closed sacs: two pleural sacs containing the lungs, and the pericardium (pericardial sac) containing the heart (Fig. 9-1A). Each pleural sac is situated laterally, and between the sacs is an interpleural space, the **mediastinum.** The mediastinum is subdivided into superior and inferior portions by a line drawn from the sternal angle (junction of manubrium and body of sternum) backward to the intervertebral disc between the fourth and fifth thoracic vertebrae (Fig. 9-1B). The inferior mediastinum is further subdivided into three portions: the anterior mediastinum, middle mediastinum, and posterior mediastinum. The pericardium occupies the middle mediastinum.

The **pericardium** encloses the heart and consists of an outer **parietal pericardium** composed of dense connective tissue lined by a serous membrane, and an inner **visceral pericardium** which is a continuation of the serous membrane onto the surface of the heart. Because of its close association with the heart tissue, the visceral pericardium is often called the **epicardium.** The pericardium can be visualized as a collapsed fluid-filled sac pressed against the heart. The outer layer of the sac is the parietal pericardium, the inner layer is the visceral pericardium, and the potential space between the two is the **pericardial cavity** which contains a thin lubricating film of serous fluid. Should the pericardial cavity suddenly become filled with an increased amount of fluid, the tough and fibrous parietal pericardium cannot yield to the increased pressure, and the heart becomes compressed (cardiac tamponade) and ceases to function. However, should there be a gradual increase in the volume of pericardial fluid, the pericardium can expand outward, thereby preventing compression of the heart.

In front, the parietal pericardium forms the posterior boundary of the anterior mediastinum; behind, it forms the anterior boundary of the posterior mediastinum. The parietal pericardium is attached to the diaphragm below.

The heart is a double pump consisting of a right half (represented by the right atrium and right ventricle), and a left half (represented by the left atrium and left ventricle) (Figs. 9-2 and 9-3). The **right atrium** receives deoxygenated blood from two large veins (superior vena cava and inferior vena cava) and from the coronary sinus of the heart (to be described later). The right atrium transmits the blood to the **right ventricle,** which pumps it out via the **pulmonary trunk** to the **pulmonary arteries** and then to the lungs, where the blood becomes oxygenated. The oxygenated blood passes by way of four **pulmonary veins** (two from each lung) to the **left atrium** and then to the **left ventricle** which pumps the blood out via the **aorta** for distribution to the other organs of the body. The circulation of blood to and from the lungs is often called the **pulmonary circuit,** while that to and from the rest of the body is the **systemic circuit.**

The heart is situated obliquely so that the two atria and their inflowing veins are located posterior to the two ventricles and their outflowing arteries. The **apex** or tip of the heart points anteriorly, inferiorly, and to the left (Fig. 9-3). Since the heart lies obliquely most of the anterior or sternocostal surface of the heart is made up of the right ventricle, while the posterior surface consists of the left atrium and a portion of the right atrium. The inferior or diaphragmatic surface is formed by the right and left ventricles.

A projection of the heart outline onto the surface of the thorax shows that much of the heart lies directly behind the sternum and extends more to the left than to the right (Fig. 9-4). Although the apex has been described as occurring at the left 4th or 5th intercostal space in the cadaver, it is subject to considerable variation in the living, depending on respiratory movements and the position of the body.

The right and left atria exhibit small earlike **auricular appendages (auricles)** which project anteriorly on the side of the aorta and pulmonary trunk (Fig. 9-3). (In the past, the term

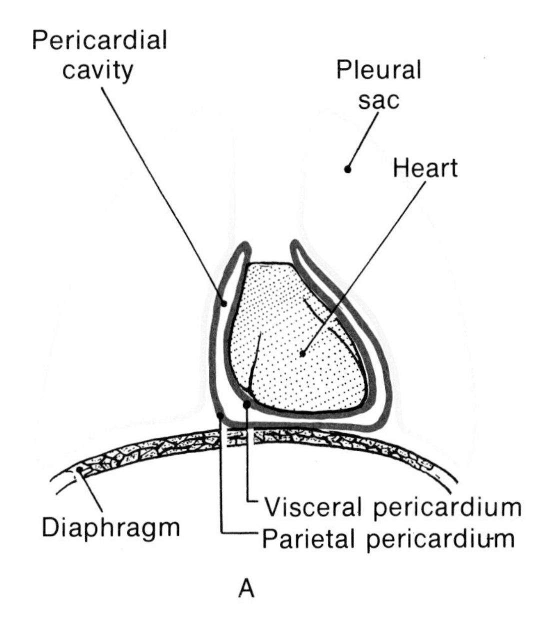

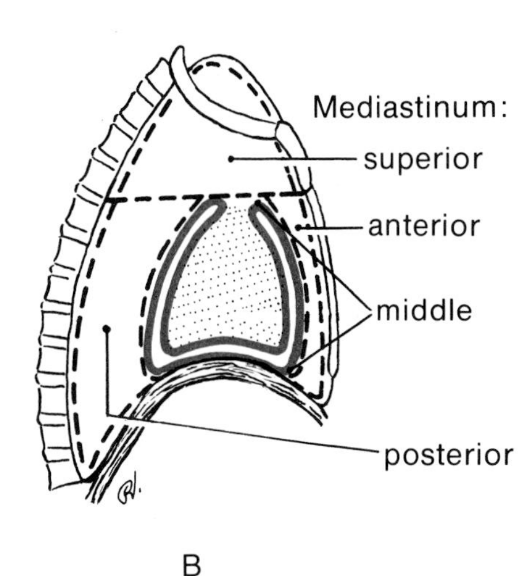

Fig. 9-1. Subdivisions of the thorax. (A) Anterior view. The mediastinum lies between two pleural sacs (outlined in yellow). The pericardium is in red. (B) Lateral view of the mediastinum. *Broken black line* demarcates subdivisions. The pericardium is in red.

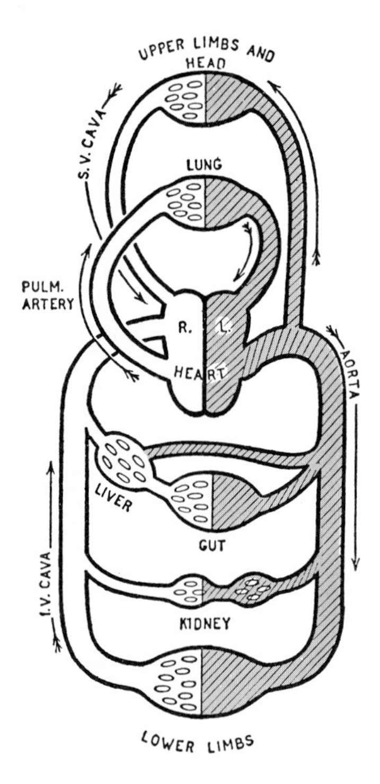

Fig. 9-2. Schematic diagram of the heart (as a double pump) and the venous and arterial circulations. S.V. Cava, superior vena cava; I.V. Cava, inferior vena cava. (From J. V. Basmajian, *Grant's Method of Anatomy,* Ed. 9, The Williams & Wilkins Co., Baltimore, 1975.)

"auricle" was used synonymously with atrium.) An **atrioventricular groove** separates each atrium from its ventricle, while **anterior** and **posterior interventricular** (longitudinal) **grooves** separate the two ventricles. These grooves contain coronary vessels and their branches and are often inlayed with fat in the epicardium (Fig. 9-5).

The arteries supplying the heart are termed **coronary arteries** because they encircle and embrace the heart like a crown (corona) (Fig. 9-6). The right and left coronary arteries originate from the base of the aorta and travel in the epicardium. Branches from the coronary arteries eventually penetrate and supply the heart muscle.

The **right coronary artery** passes along the right atrioventricular groove first on the anterior surface of the heart and then posteriorly onto its back surface (Figs. 9-5 and 9-6). The artery next gives off a **posterior interventricular (descending) branch** extending downward along the posterior interventricular groove. The right coronary artery continues in the atrioventricular groove and joins (forms an anastomosis) with the circumflex branch of the left coronary artery (see below). The right coronary artery supplies primarily the right atrium and right ventricle.

The **left coronary artery** originates from the aorta and almost immediately divides into two branches. One is the **anterior interventricular (descending) branch** which descends in the anterior interventricular groove. This branch then curves around the apex and ascends in the posterior interventricular groove to join the posterior interventricular branch of the right coronary artery. The other branch of the left coronary artery is termed the **circumflex branch** because it curves backward along the left atrioventricular groove to join the right coronary artery. The left coronary artery supplies most of the left ventricle and left atrium.

Anastomoses between the various branches of the coronary arteries are important in establishing a collateral circulation should one of the smaller vessels become occluded (Fig. 9-6). However, a sudden occlusion (as occurs when

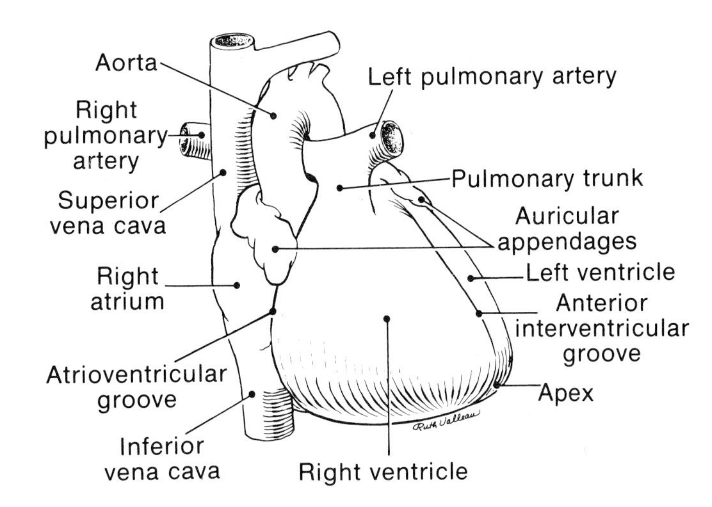

Fig. 9-3. Anterior view of the heart.

a blood clot blocks a vessel) is dangerous because the heart muscle may become damaged before an adequate adjustment can occur in the collateral circulation. Such damage to the heart muscle is called a **myocardial infarct.** Blood tests can now be used to determine the degree of destruction by measuring the amount of an enzyme released into the blood by damaged cardiac muscle cells.

Blood from the coronary arteries is returned to the heart via the **cardiac veins,** most of which accompany the coronary arteries (Figs. 9-5 and 9-7). Although a few cardiac veins empty directly into the right atrium, the majority empty indirectly by way of the coronary sinus. The **coronary sinus** is a short wide vessel lying posteriorly in the left atrioventricular groove. It receives blood from several cardiac veins, including the **great cardiac vein** which accompanies the anterior interventricular branch of the left coronary artery. The coronary sinus empties into the right atrium.

Internally the two atria are separated from one another by the **interatrial septum,** whose counterpart between the ventricles is the **interventricular septum.** The lining of the **right atrium** is smooth, except for its anterior portion and the auricular appendage where the lining is ridged with elevations termed **pectinate muscles** (Fig. 9-8). The sharp boundary between smooth and rough portions is the **crista**

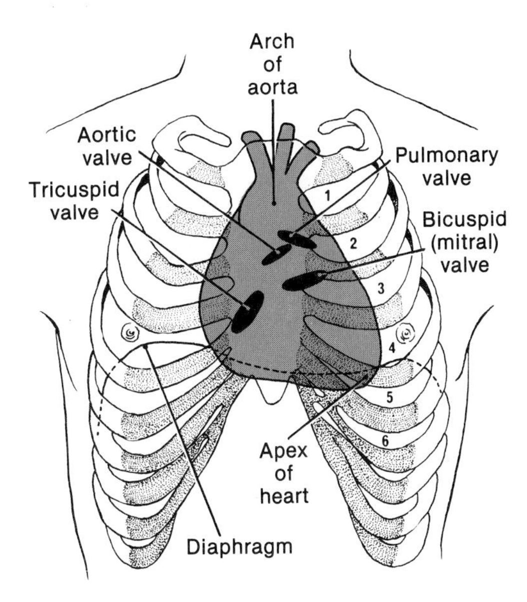

Fig. 9-4. Anterior view showing the heart and its valves in relation to the ribs and diaphragm. The first six intercostal spaces are indicated.

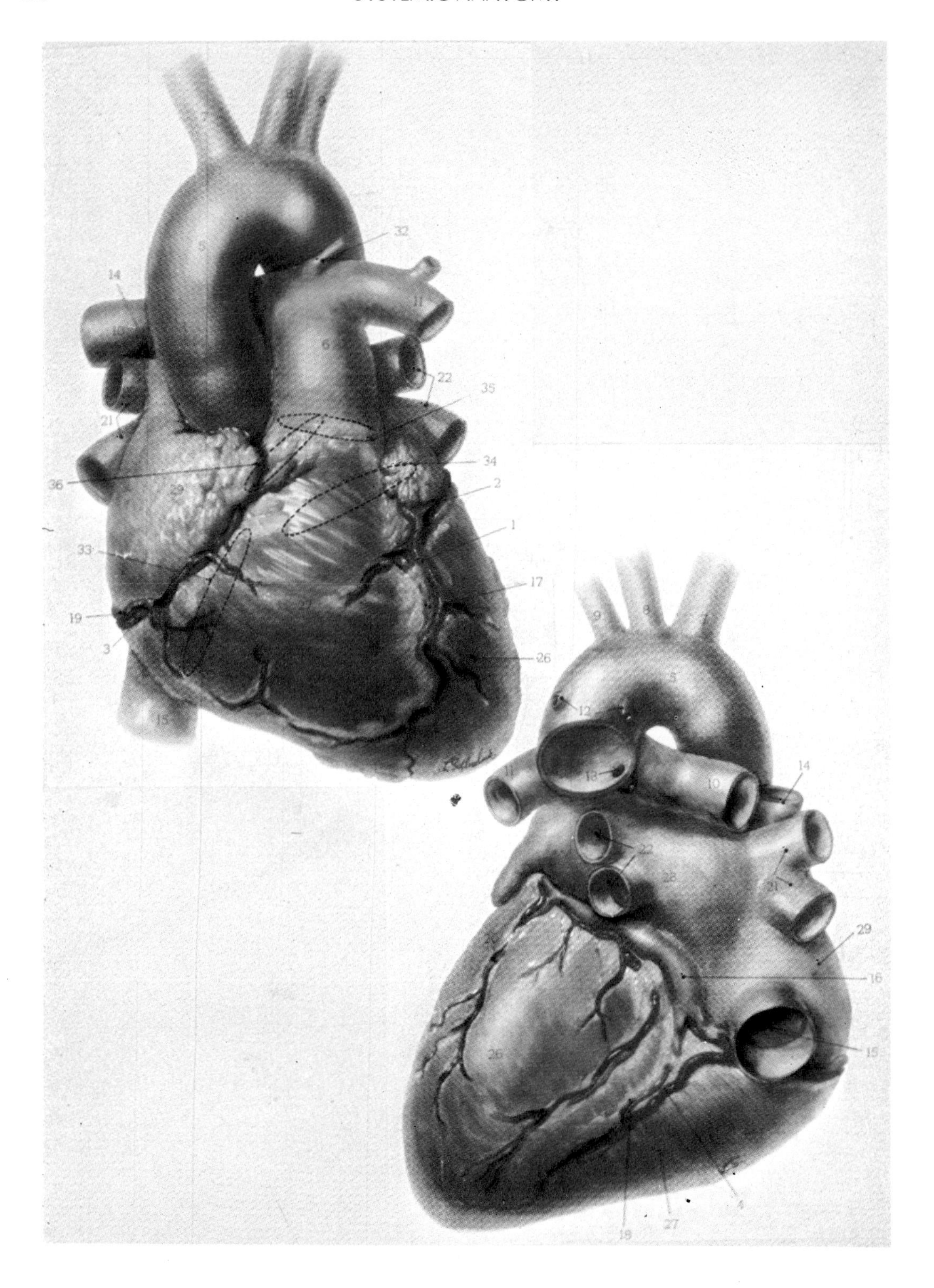

32
14
11
10
6
22
35
21
34
36
2
1
33
17
19
3
26
15
9
8
7
5
12
13
11
10
14
22
28
21
29
16
15
26
4
27
18

terminalis. The right atrium contains openings for three veins: the **superior vena cava** (SVC), **inferior vena cava** (IVC), and the **coronary sinus.** The latter collects blood from the heart itself, whereas the venae cavae bring blood from the upper and lower regions of the body. The right atrial aspect of the interatrial septum is marked by a depression, the **fossa ovalis,** which indicates the site where the two atria communicated with one another during prenatal life.

The right atrium communicates with the right ventricle by means of the atrioventricular opening (orifice) which is guarded by the **right atrioventricular valve.** This valve consists of three triangular flaps or cusps; hence it is also termed the **tricuspid valve.** The base of each cusp is attached to a ring of fibrous tissue around the periphery of the atrioventricular opening. The free apical portions of the cusps are connected to **tendinous cords (chordae tendineae)** from the right ventricle.

The **right ventricle** is characterized by thick walls and an irregular internal surface resulting from the upward projection of muscle bundles called **trabeculae carneae.** Some of these trabeculae are large and prominent and merit special attention. These are the **papillary muscles** (**anterior, posterior,** and **septal**). The chordae tendineae extend from these muscles to the cusps of the tricuspid valve. The ventricular aspect of this valve is similar to the canopy of a parachute, with the chordae tendineae acting to stabilize the tips of the cusps so as to prevent them from everting upward into the atrium. Near the apical region of the right ventricle a prominent trabecula known as the **septomarginal trabecula** (moderator band) passes from the interventricular septum to the base of the anterior papillary muscle. It transmits a part of the conducting system of the heart, to be described below. The outflow orifice from the right ventricle into the **pulmonary trunk** is guarded by the **pulmonary semilunar valve** consisting of three crescent shaped cusps.

The lining of the **left atrium** is smooth, except for the left auricular appendage which is ridged with pectinate muscles. Four openings for the right and left pairs of **pulmonary veins** occur on the walls of the left atrium (Fig. 9-9). The left atrioventricular orifice is guarded by the **left atrioventricular valve,** also called the **bicuspid valve** because of its two cusps. (The term **mitral valve** is sometimes used because of its resemblance to a bishop's hat or "miter"). As in the tricuspid valve, the bases of the bicuspid valve are attached to a fibrous ring around the left atrioventricular orifice, and the apices of the valve are stabilized from below by chordae tendineae.

The wall of the **left ventricle** is even thicker than that of the right ventricle so as to maintain higher pressure in the systemic circuit. Trabeculae carneae are present, as are an anterior and posterior papillary muscle to which the chordae tendineae pass from the cusps of the bicuspid valve. The outflow orifice to the aorta contains the **aortic semilunar valve** similar in appearance to the pulmonary semilunar valve.

It is important to keep in mind that the inflow and outflow orifices of each ventricle lie more or less in the same plane (Fig. 9-5). The tough fibrous rings of connective tissue sur-

Fig. 9-5. The heart, anterior view *(upper left)* and posterior view *(lower right).* The *broken lines* indicate the position of the heart valves. *1,* Anterior descending branch of left coronary artery; *2,* circumflex branch of left coronary artery; *3,* right coronary artery; *4,* posterior descending branch of right coronary artery; *5,* aorta; *6,* pulmonary trunk; *7,* brachiocephalic trunk (innominate artery); *8,* left common carotid artery; *9,* left subclavian artery; *10,* right pulmonary artery; *11,* left pulmonary artery; *12,* intercostal aa.; *13,* Bronchial a.: *14,* superior vena cava; *15,* inferior vena cava; *16,* coronary sinus; *17,* great cardiac v.; *18,* middle cardiac v.; *19,* small cardiac v.; *20,* L. posterior ventricular v.; *21,* R. pulmonary vv.; *22,* L. pulmonary vv.; *26,* L. ventricle; *27,* R. ventricle; *28,* L. atrium; *29,* R. atrium; *32,* ligamentum arteriosum; *33,* tricuspid valve; *34,* mitral valve (bicuspid); *35,* pulmonary valve (semilunar); *36,* aortic valve (semilunar). (Courtesy of the American Heart Association.)

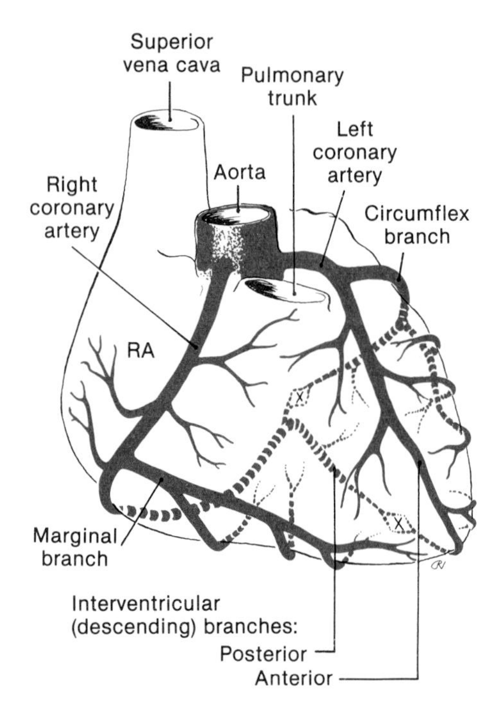

Fig. 9-6. Diagram of the right and left coronary arteries and their major branches, depicted as if the heart were transparent so that structures lying posteriorly *(broken lines)* can be seen from an anterior view. RA, right atrium. The X's indicate regions of anastomosis between major arteries. (Modified after Grant.)

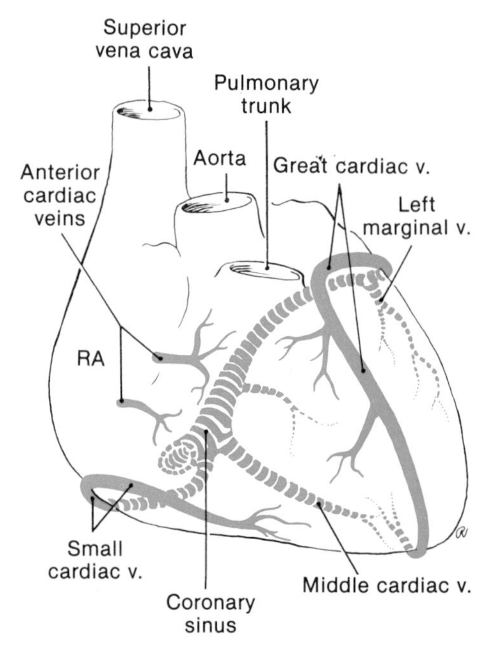

Fig. 9-7. Diagram of the major cardiac veins, depicted as if the heart were transparent so that structures lying posteriorly *(broken lines)* can be seen from an anterior view. RA, right atrium. (Modified after Grant.)

rounding these orifices are often termed the "**cardiac skeleton**" which prevents the orifices from stretching too much when blood is forced through them (Fig. 9-10). The cardiac skeleton also serves as a base of insertion for the cardiac muscle fibers.

Conducting System of Heart

In order for the various regions of the heart to beat synchronously, impulses are initiated in one region of the heart and then passed on to other regions. This is accomplished by a group of cardiac muscle fibers specialized for conduction. A small knot of these specialized fibers, known as the **sinu-atrial (S-A) node,** is located in the upper part of the right atrium near the entrance of the superior vena cava (Fig. 9-11). The impulse is initiated at the S-A node and then spreads over the two atria and reaches the **atrioventricular (A-V) node** in the right atrium just above the opening for the coronary sinus. From the A-V node the impulse passes along a bundle of conducting fibers, the **atrioventricular (A-V) bundle (of His)** in the upper part of the interventricular septum. The A-V bundle bifurcates into a right and a left branch which transmit the impulse to the right and left ventricles, respectively. These conducting fibers are termed **Purkinje fibers.**

Although the S-A node is responsible for initiating the impulses for contraction, the rate of contraction can be modified by extrinsic factors. For example, the vagus nerves of the parasympathetic nervous system slow the heart beat, whereas nerves from the sympathetic system speed it up. Hormones and chemicals can also affect the heart rate.

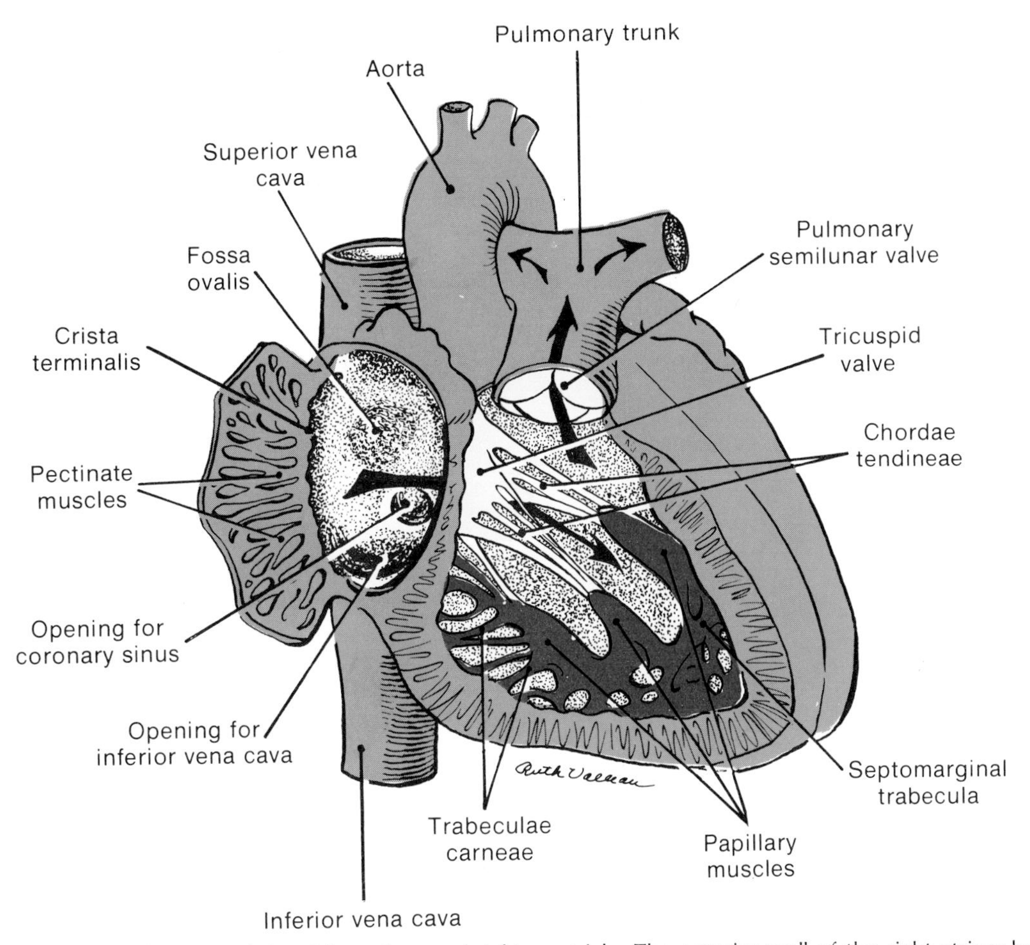

Fig. 9-8. Internal aspect of the right atrium and right ventricle. The anterior wall of the right atrium has been pulled back. The arrows show the direction of the blood flow through the atrioventricular opening surrounded by the tricuspid valve (yellow), and the pulmonary opening surrounded by the semilunar valve (yellow).

Great Vessels

The eight great vessels transmit blood into or out from the heart. They are: the **superior vena cava, inferior vena cava, pulmonary trunk, aorta,** and **four pulmonary veins.** Since the parietal pericardium is reflected onto the surface of these vessels, a portion of each lies within the pericardial cavity and a portion lies outside it. The great vessels will be described more fully in terms of their relationship with other vessels of the pulmonary and systemic circuits.

Microscopic Anatomy

The heart consists of three layers: epicardium (visceral pericardium), myocardium, and endocardium. The **epicardium** covers the heart surface and is composed of an outer layer of simple squamous epithelium (mesothelium) beneath which is a layer of loose fibrous connective tissue invested with varying amounts of fat. The epicardium serves as a bed for the coronary arteries and cardiac veins as they course on the surface of the heart (Fig. 9-12).

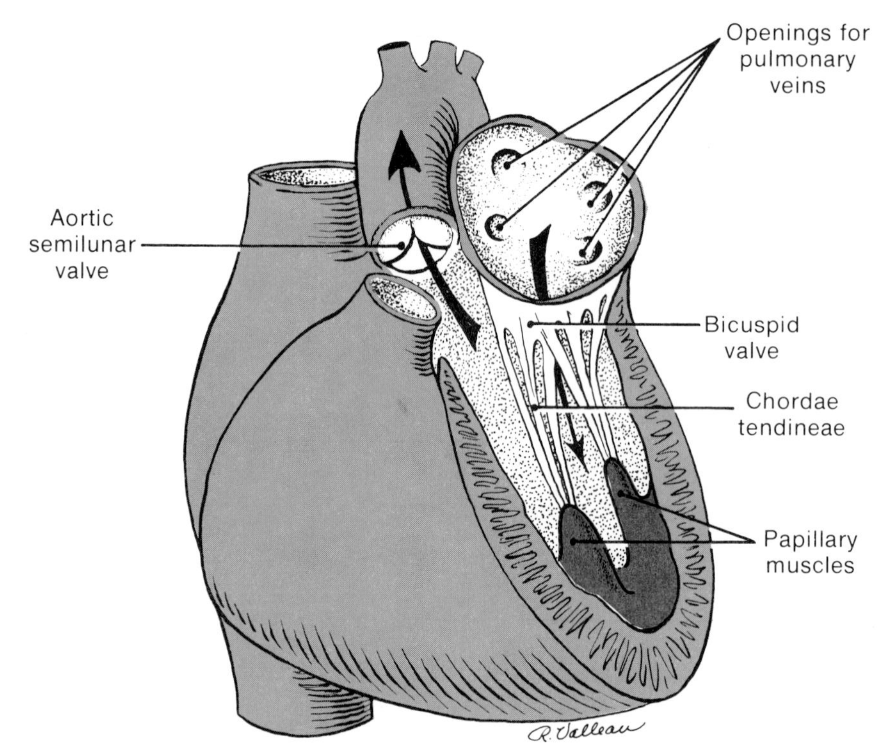

Fig. 9-9. Internal aspect of left atrium and left ventricle. The anterior walls of the left ventricle and atrium have been removed. The *arrows* show the direction of blood flow through the bicuspid and aortic semilunar valves (yellow).

The **myocardium** is composed of cardiac muscle (see Chapter 4). Cardiac muscle fibers are striated, contain centrally located nuclei, and are richly supplied with mitochondria. Intercalated discs seen with the light microscope represent tight junctions between individual muscle fibers. Since the two atria are basically reservoirs receiving blood, the myocardium in their walls is relatively thin, as compared with the thicker myocardium in the two ventricles which act as forceful pumps. These muscle fibers are arranged spirally so as to allow the blood to be propelled outward by a wringing action.

The **endocardium** lines the chambers of the heart and the valves and consists of a layer of simple squamous epithelium (endothelium) overlying loose fibrous connective tissue. Just beneath the endocardium are the Purkinje fibers of the impulse conducting system. These are large, pale, specialized cardiac muscle cells which have a vacuolated appearance. The S-A and A-V nodes as well as the A-V bundle are also composed of modified cardiac muscle fibers of the conducting system.

The pericardium, myocardium, and endocardium are subject to inflammation (pericarditis, myocarditis, endocarditis) which can impair proper functioning of the heart. In the case of pericarditis, the parietal pericardium and visceral pericardium (epicardium) may adhere to one another creating adhesions which restrict the heart contractions. This condition can be alleviated by surgically removing the pericardium. Endocarditis often produces faulty valves, since these structures are composed largely of endocardium.

BLOOD VESSELS

Blood vessels are the channels whereby blood is distributed throughout the body. Those vessels conducting blood away from the heart are arteries; those carrying blood to the heart are veins. The walls of large arteries and veins depend on a blood supply of their own and are thus served by smaller blood vessels termed **vasa vasorum** ("vessels of the vessels"). Most arteries carry oxygenated blood, while most veins carry deoxygenated blood. However, the situation is reversed in the pulmonary circuit where the pulmonary arteries conduct deoxygenated blood from the heart to the lungs and the pulmonary veins carry oxygenated blood from the lungs back to the heart.

Arteries become progressively smaller at greater distances from the heart, the smallest arteries being termed **arterioles.** Arteries and arterioles are composed of three basic coats (tunics). The outer coat is the **tunica adventitia** (or **externa**) consisting of loosely arranged fibrous connective tissue (Fig. 9-13). The middle coat, the **tunica media,** contains connective tissue and smooth muscle arranged circularly. The inner coat is the **tunica intima** (or **interna**) composed of a small amount of connective tissue and an endothelium (simple squamous epithelium) which lines the lumen.

The tunica media of **large arteries** contains substantial amounts of concentrically arranged elastic tissue in addition to muscle fibers, and this elasticity allows the arteries to expand passively with each contraction of the heart (systole) and then to return to normal size between contractions (diastole). Thus one can feel the "pulse" in arteries but not in veins. As the arteries get smaller, the relative amount of muscle in the tunica media gradually increases and the elastic tissue decreases. Such an artery (often called a **muscular artery**) still pulsates passively, but it can also control blood flow by actively changing the size of its lumen. In the **arterioles** the tunica media consists almost entirely of muscle; these vessels greatly decrease the blood pressure and regulate the flow of blood into the next portion of the vascular system, the capillaries.

Blood passes from arterioles into the smallest blood vessels, **capillaries** (Fig. 9-14), which form extensive anastomosing networks (capillary beds) where raw materials and waste prod-

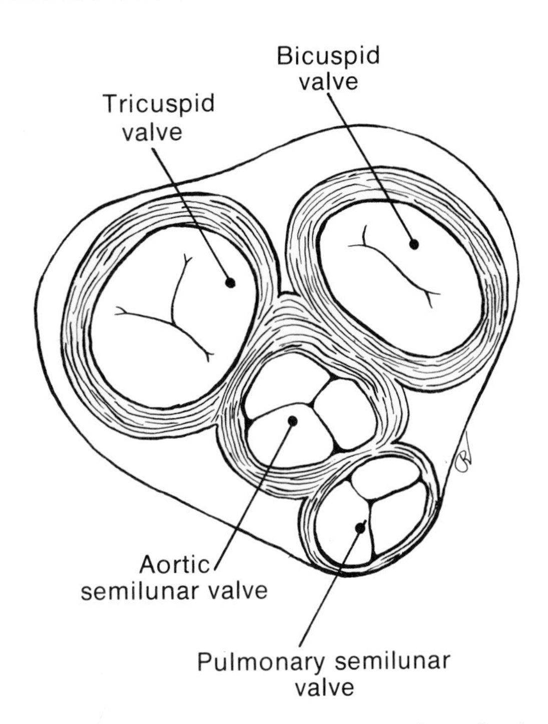

Fig. 9-10. The "cardiac skeleton" (in yellow) viewed from above and consisting of fibrous rings surrounding the heart valves.

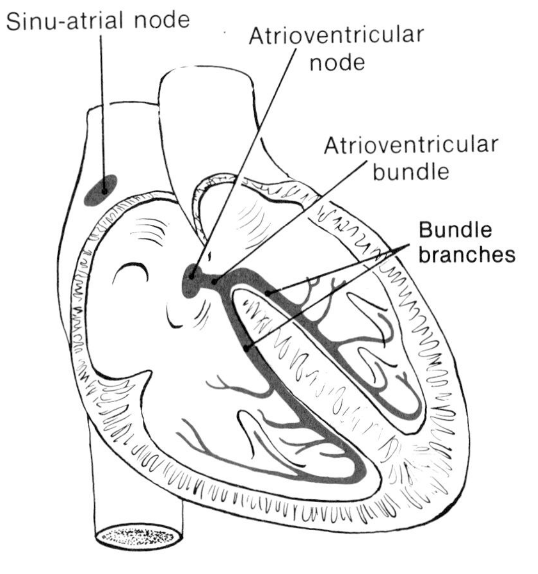

Fig. 9-11. The conducting system (in red) of the heart.

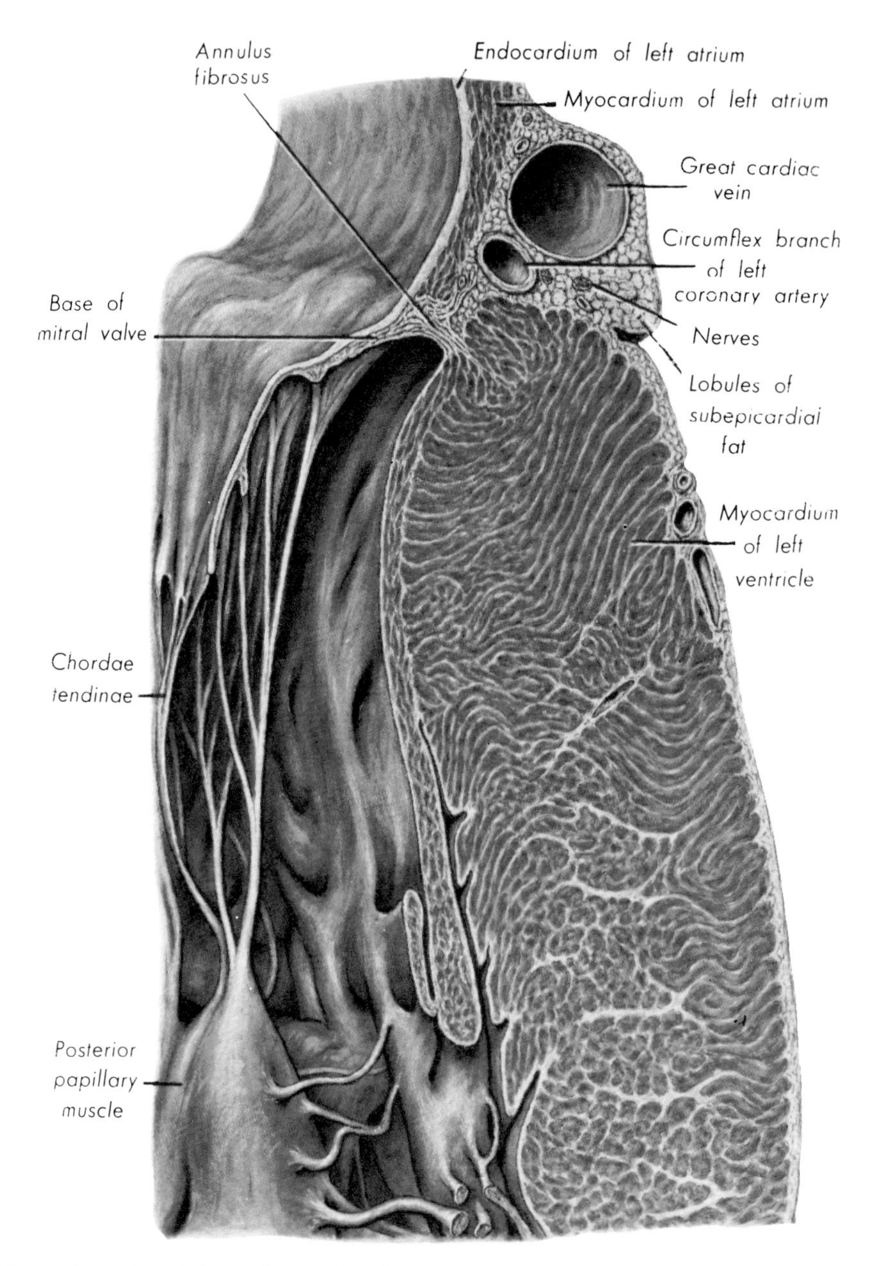

Fig. 9-12. Three dimensional view of a section through the left atrium and left ventricle in the region of the mitral valve. (From W. M. Copenhaver, R. P. Bunge, & M. B. Bunge, *Bailey's Textbook of Histology*, Ed. 16, The Williams & Wilkins Co., Baltimore, 1971.)

ucts are exchanged with the body tissues. In addition, the capillaries in some organs play a special role, such as those in the lungs where oxygen is taken in and carbon dioxide given off, or those in the intestine where nutritive substances are absorbed. The walls of capillaries consist only of a thin endothelium which facilitates the passage of materials between the blood in the lumen and the tissue fluid outside of the capillary.

The blood pressure in capillaries is very low, and the rate of flow is slower than in other blood vessels. Some capillaries may be closed or open, depending on the state of activity of the organs they supply. Although capillary beds are pervasive throughout the body, some structures such as the cornea are devoid of capillaries. Epithelia and cartilage also lack capillaries and depend on diffusion of substances via the tissue fluid.

From the capillary beds the blood passes back toward the heart first by means of tiny **venules** and then through **veins** of increasing size. The small venules contain some connective tissue in addition to endothelium, and as the venules get larger they gradually acquire additional coats. Although veins are composed of three basic coats, these generally are thinner than their counterparts in arteries (Fig. 9-13). In the largest veins, however, the tunica adventitia is quite thick and also contains large amounts of longitudinally arranged smooth muscle.

The lumen of a vein tends to be larger than that of its corresponding artery. Also, in contrast to arteries, many veins contain **valves** consisting of endothelial flaps pointing in the direction of blood flow (Fig. 9-15). Since the pressure in the veins is low, the propulsion of blood through the venous system often depends on the movement of nearby structures such as skeletal muscles which gently compress the walls of the veins and thereby move the blood forward for short distances. As the blood is pushed beyond a venous valve, the valves close to prevent a backflow. It is not surprising that there are numerous valves in the veins of the lower limbs so as to help counteract the force of gravity which tends to cause blood to pool when one stands or sits for long periods of time. Under such circumstances it is important to try to flex the limb muscles so as to facilitate the movement of blood through the veins. A lack of proper venous flow can eventually lead to the formation of potentially dangerous blood clots. These can become detached and transported to various regions of the cardiovascular system where they may lodge and occlude smaller blood vessels.

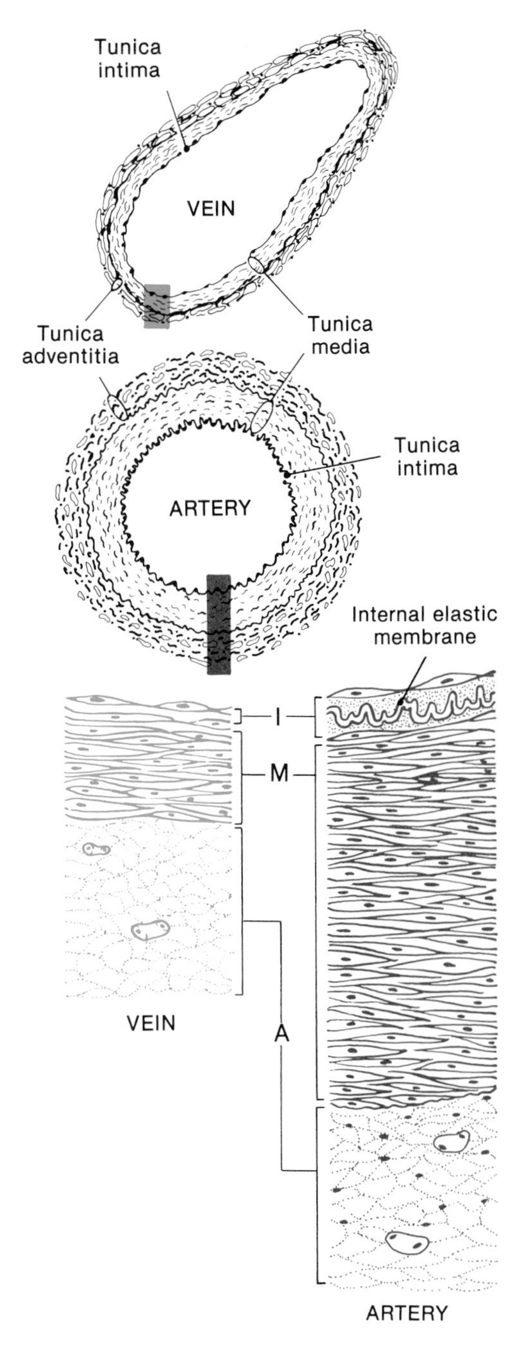

Fig. 9-13. Diagram of a cross section through a medium-sized vein and artery, showing the difference in thickness of their walls. The rectangles indicate a portion of the wall shown below at higher magnification. I, tunica intima, M, tunica media, A, tunica adventitia.

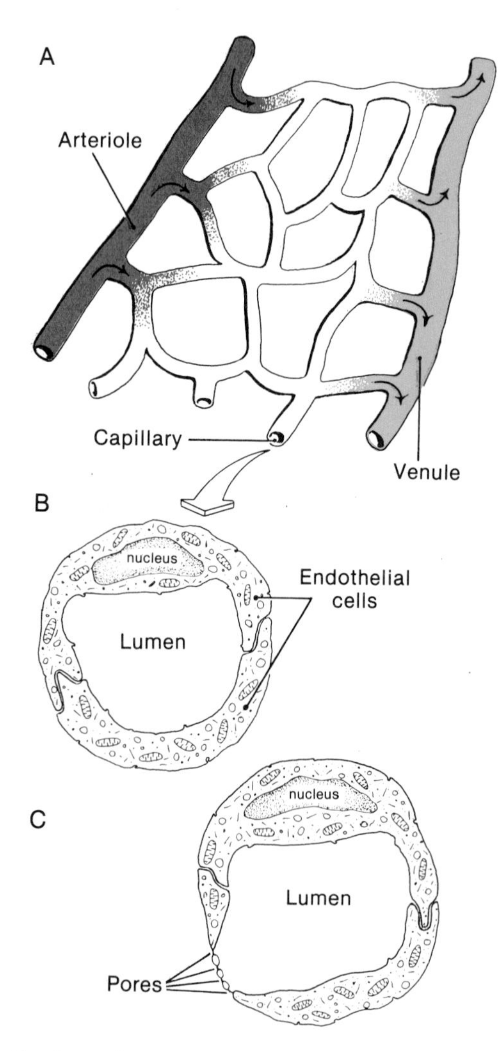

Fig. 9-14. (A) Diagram of a capillary bed located between an arteriole and a venule, (B) cross section through the wall of a capillary showing parts of two endothelial cells (one with a nucleus in the plane of section), (C) cross section through the wall of a capillary as in B, but with pores (fenestrations) in the wall.

Pulmonary Circuit

The pulmonary circuit begins with the single **pulmonary trunk** which emerges from the right ventricle and passes upward to bifurcate into the **right** and **left pulmonary arteries** to the right and left lungs, respectively (Fig. 9-3). Each pulmonary artery subdivides into smaller and smaller branches carrying deoxygenated blood to the pulmonary capillary beds, where carbon dioxide is released and oxygen is absorbed. The oxygenated blood then flows through pulmonary venules, small veins, and ultimately into the two **right** or two **left pulmonary veins** which empty into the left atrium. It should be noted that since the pulmonary arteries carry deoxygenated blood to the lungs, much of the lung tissue itself must receive oxygenated blood via a separate system of bronchial arteries from the systemic circuit (see below).

Systemic Circuit

Since the systemic circuit distributes blood throughout the body, it is more extensive and involves a greater number of named vessels than does the pulmonary circuit. Only the major arteries and veins will be cited briefly here, but some will be referred to again with reference to the organs and tissues which they supply. Also, since many of the arteries are accompanied by veins which are similarly named, it will be convenient to discuss both the arterial and venous circulation together with respect to various regions of the body.

Aorta

The aorta originates from the left ventricle, passes upward and slightly to the right as the **ascending aorta,** emerges from the pericardium, and becomes the **arch of the aorta** which curves posteriorly and to the left (Fig. 9-5).

Ascending Aorta. Because of its intrapericardial location, the ascending aorta is considered to be a constituent of the middle mediastinum. The right and left coronary arteries originate at the base of the ascending aorta from within the right and left aortic sinuses, respectively (Fig. 9-16). The **aortic sinuses** are the cup-shaped depressions formed by the cusps of the aortic semilunar valves. (The coronary arteries, as well as the cardiac veins, are discussed above with the heart.)

Arch of the Aorta. The arch of the aorta lies in the sagittal plane of the superior mediastinum. It gives off three large branches from which originate smaller arteries carrying blood to various parts of the head, neck, upper limbs, and thorax.

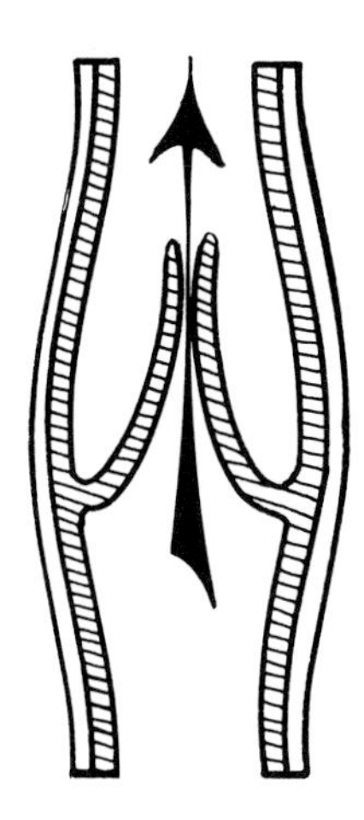

Fig. 9-15. Diagram of a venous valve, longitudinal section. *Arrow* indicates direction of flow.

Arteries of the Head, Neck, and Upper Limbs

The arch of the aorta gives rise to the brachiocephalic trunk, left common carotid, and left subclavian arteries (Fig. 9-5). Beyond the origin of the left subclavian artery the arch of the aorta is bound to the left pulmonary artery by the **ligamentum arteriosum (arterial ligament),** a fibrous remnant of an embryonic shunt between the pulmonary and systemic circuits. The **brachiocephalic trunk** (innominate artery) is short and soon divides into the right subclavian artery and right common carotid artery (Fig. 9-17). The **common carotid arteries** carry blood for the head and neck, whereas the **subclavian arteries** supply the upper limbs as well as some portions of the head, neck, and upper thorax.

Each **common carotid artery** extends upward through the neck. Near the angle of the mandible the common carotid bifurcates into an internal carotid and external carotid artery (Fig. 9-17). At the bifurcation is a small **carotid body** which detects changes in the oxygen content of the blood and can alert respiratory and cardiac centers in the brain to increase respiration and accelerate the heart rate.

The base of each **internal carotid artery** is dilated to form the **carotid sinus** which is sensitive to changes in blood pressure. The internal carotid artery continues upward without giving rise to any branches and soon enters the intracranial cavity via the carotid canal in the tem-

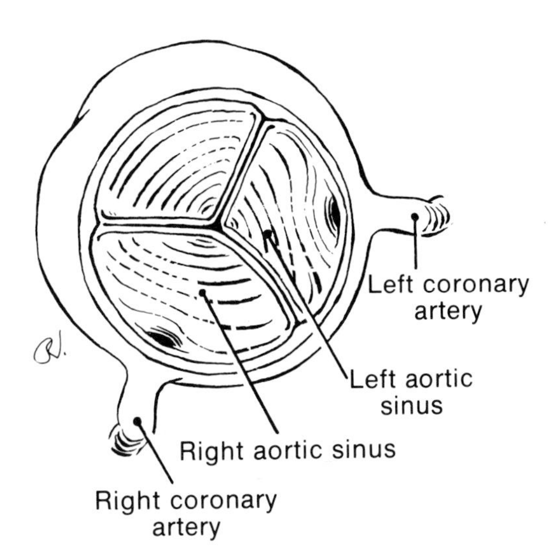

Fig. 9-16. The base of the aorta viewed from above. The right and left coronary arteries originate from the right and left aortic sinuses, respectively.

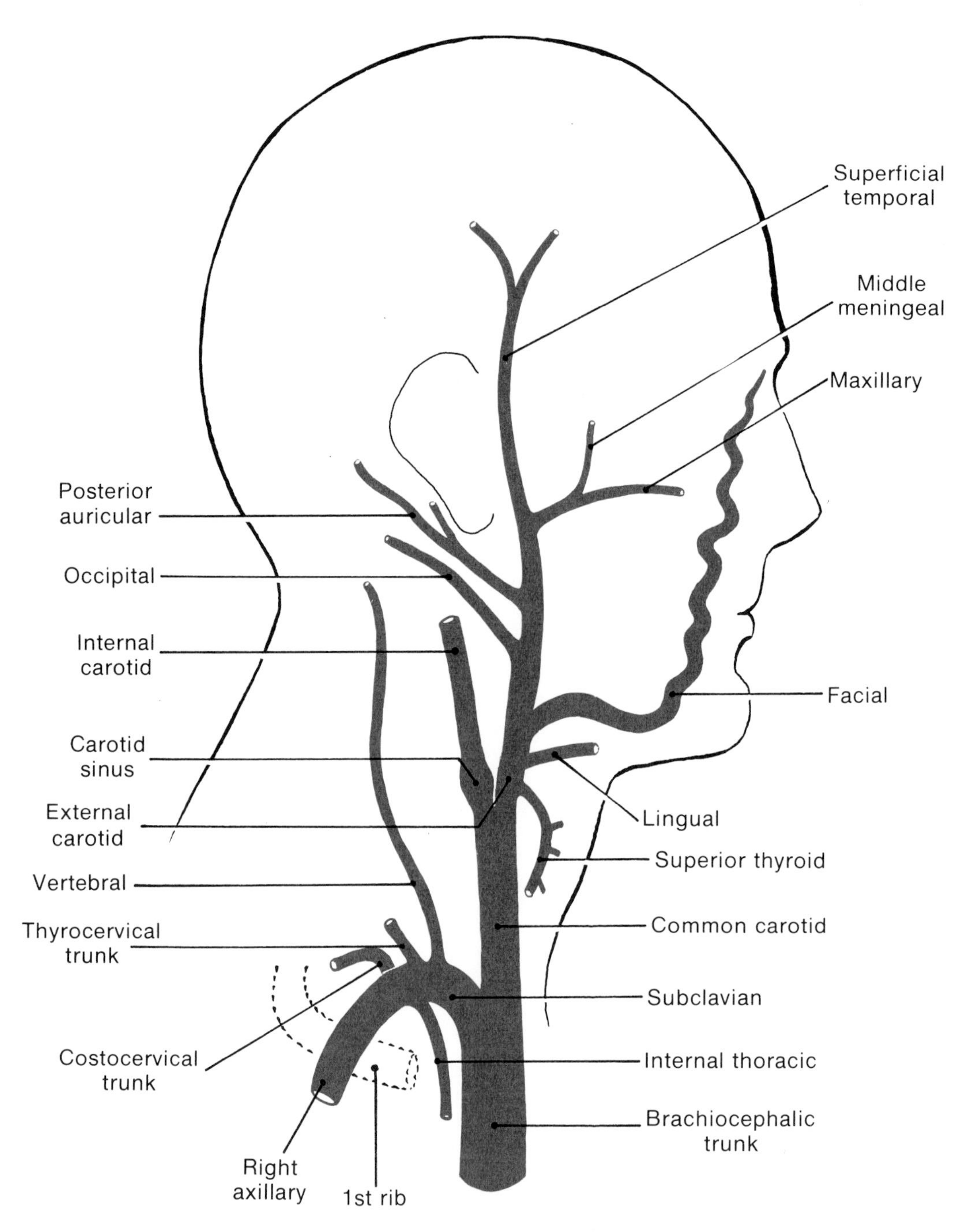

Fig. 9-17. Arteries of the head and neck, as viewed from the right side.

poral bone. The artery supplies the brain and orbit by means of a series of branches which are described in greater detail with reference to the central nervous system (Chapter 12).

Each **external carotid artery** is a major source of blood supply for the head and neck region, excluding the brain and orbit (Fig. 9-17). Branches of the external carotid are: (1) the **superior thyroid artery** to the thyroid gland; (2) a small **ascending pharyngeal artery;** (3) the **lingual artery** which passes beneath the tongue; (4) the **facial artery** running superficially and obliquely across the mandible to supply lower and upper lips, nose, palate, and muscles of facial expression; (5) the **occipital artery** to the back of the head; and (6) the **posterior auricular artery** supplying the region of the ear.

The external carotid artery ends by bifurcating into two additional branches: the **superficial temporal artery** which passes upward in front of the ear and supplies the temporal area of the head, and the **maxillary artery** which travels deep to the neck of the mandible and into the infraorbital region, supplying branches to the teeth, gums, and muscles of mastication. The connective tissue coverings of the brain (meninges) are supplied by an important branch of the maxillary artery, the **middle meningeal artery.** This vessel is often damaged by injuries to the head, and bleeding from the middle meningeal artery or from its branches can cause compression of intracranial structures. (The middle meningeal artery passes into the cranial cavity through the foramen spinosum of the skull.)

The right and left **subclavian arteries** have different origins, the right one arising from the brachiocephalic trunk and the left one directly from the arch of the aorta beyond the origin of the left common carotid artery. Since the course and distribution of each are the same, the following description applies to both vessels.

The subclavian artery arches upward behind the scalenus anterior muscle, passes deep to the clavicle (hence its name subclavian), and continues laterally until it reaches the lateral border of the first rib, at which point the subclavian artery becomes the **axillary artery** (Fig. 9-17). The branches of the subclavian artery which contribute to the supply of the head (including the brain), neck, and thorax are: (1) the **vertebral artery** which travels upward through the transverse foramina of the upper six vertebrae, enters the cranial cavity via the foramen magnum, and supplies branches to the brain and spinal cord; (2) the **internal thoracic (mammary) artery** running downward and behind the costal cartilages and contributing to the supply of the anterior thoracic wall, diaphragm, and abdominal wall (via the **superior epigastric artery**); (3) the **thyrocervical trunk** which in turn gives off an **inferior thyroid artery** to the thyroid gland and branches to the vertebrae, spinal cord, and scapular muscles; and (4) a **costocervical trunk** supplying the upper thorax and deep muscles of the neck.

The **axillary artery** is a continuation of the subclavian artery beyond the first rib (Fig. 9-17). It gives off a series of branches, the **thoracoacromial, subscapular,** and **anterior** and **posterior circumflex humeral arteries,** which form an extensive network for the shoulder muscles (Fig. 9-18). The axillary artery also gives rise to the **lateral thoracic artery** which supplies blood to the pectoral muscles and to the breast. When the axillary artery reaches the lateral border of the teres major muscle it is arbitrarily called the brachial artery, which courses through the arm.

The **brachial artery** passes along the medial aspect of the arm and is easily compressed against the humerus; hence it is commonly used to measure blood pressure. The artery gives off a **deep brachial artery** and also supplies additional branches to the arm muscles as well as to a rich network of vessels around the elbow. In the cubital region (the anterior aspect of the elbow) the brachial artery bifurcates into the radial artery and the ulnar artery.

The **radial artery** runs along the lateral aspect of the forearm beneath the brachioradialis muscle and becomes superficial near the wrist, where it is often used to measure the pulse. In the hand the radial artery forms an anastomosis

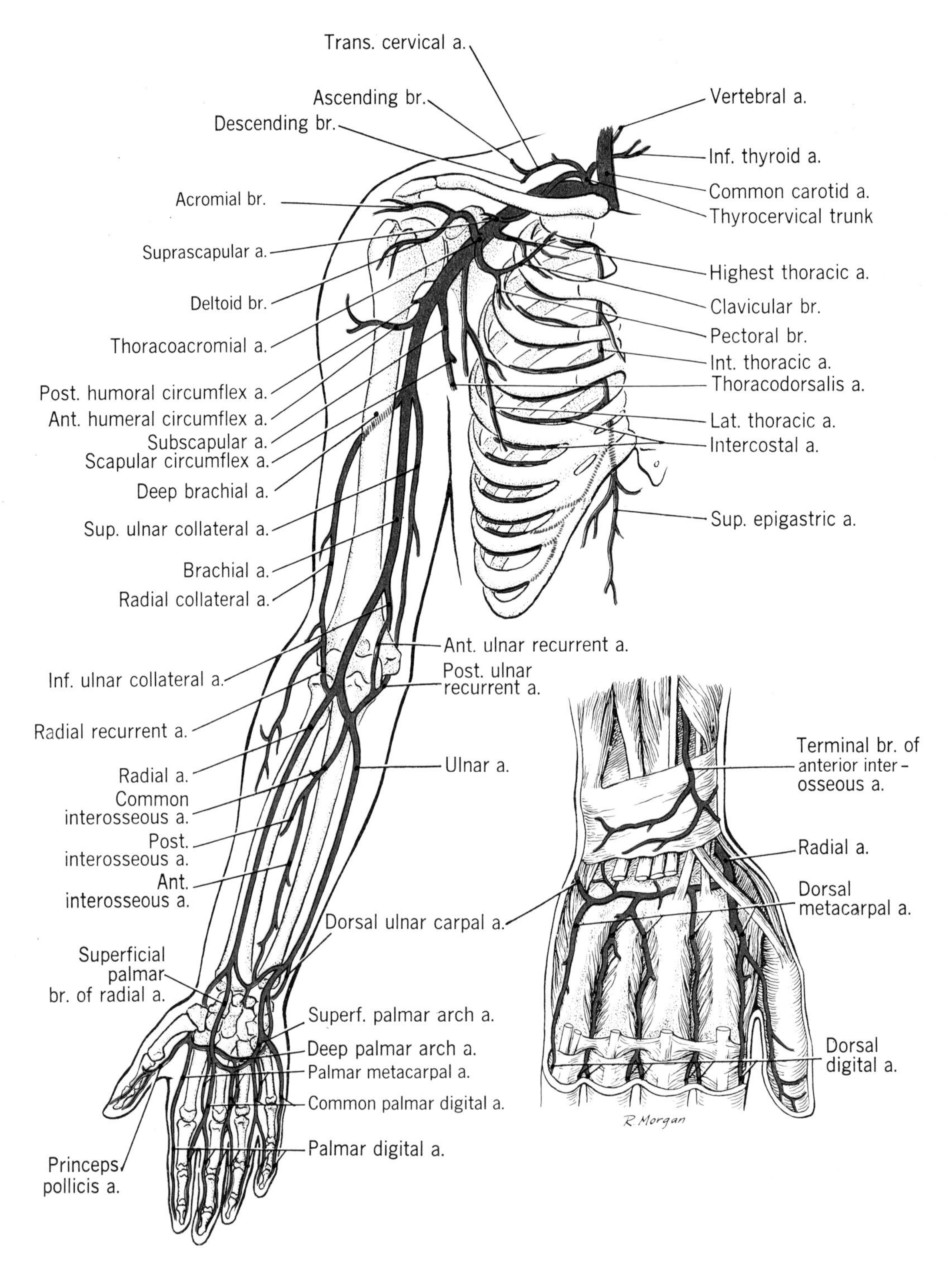

Fig. 9-18. Arteries of the shoulder region and upper limb. (From *Stedman's Medical Dictionary,* Ed. 23, The Williams & Wilkins Co., Baltimore, 1976.)

(communication) with the **deep palmar arch** and the **superficial palmar arch,** both of which curve medially across the palm. The deep and superficial palmar arches provide branches to the digits.

The **ulnar artery** travels along the medial aspect of the forearm under cover of several flexor muscles and likewise becomes superficial at the wrist. The ulnar artery also forms an anastomosis with the deep and superficial palmar arches.

Portions of several arteries in the head, neck, and upper limbs are located superficially and can be palpated. These vessels include the common carotid, facial, superficial temporal, brachial, radial, and ulnar arteries.

Veins of the Head, Neck, and Upper Limbs

In general, the veins which carry blood from the head, neck, and upper limbs often have the same names as the arteries they accompany. However, the veins tend to be more variable, and certain of the larger veins require special attention.

The counterparts of the carotid arteries are the jugular veins (Fig. 9-19). The right and left **internal jugular veins** receive tributaries from the brain, orbit, and face; the **external jugular veins** receive tributaries which accompany the branches of the external carotid arteries in the face and neck regions. Each external jugular vein runs obliquely and superficial to the sternocleidomastoid muscle and ends usually by joining the subclavian vein of the same side.

The **subclavian vein** receives branches from the upper limb. Many of these (such as the **brachial, radial,** and **ulnar veins**) are paired and tend to travel on each side of the companion artery. Such pairs of parallel veins are termed **venae comitantes** and are common in the upper and lower limbs. In addition to these veins, which are considered to be deep veins, there is a network of superficial veins which travel in the subcutaneous tissue and have no counterparts in the arterial system.

The **superficial veins** of the upper limb begin as a plexus on the dorsum of the hand, from which two prominent veins emerge. One of these is the **cephalic vein** which courses upward along the lateral aspect of the upper limb and eventually ends by turning deeply and joining the axillary vein near the clavicle (Fig. 9-20). The other prominent superficial vein is the **basilic vein** which travels upward along the medial aspect of the limb and passes deeply to join the brachial vein. An important plexus of superficial veins exists in the cubital region at the front of the elbow (Fig. 9-20). These are often used for intravenous injections, for withdrawing blood, or for introducing catheters for diagnostic purposes. Such catheters can be passed all the way into the heart via the superior vena cava.

The common vessel formed by the union of the subclavian vein with the external and internal jugular veins is called the **brachiocephalic (innominate) vein.** The right brachiocephalic vein is short and straight; the left brachiocephalic is longer and crosses obliquely toward the right side of the heart (Figs. 9-19 and 9-22). The right and left brachiocephalic veins join one another to become the **superior vena cava** which empties into the right atrium. Each brachiocephalic vein receives several tributaries, including vertebral, internal thoracic, and inferior thyroid veins.

Arteries of the Thorax and Abdomen

The **thoracic (descending) aorta** passes downward through the posterior mediastinum along the left side of the vertebral column (Fig. 9-21). It sends off consecutive pairs of **posterior intercostal arteries,** each of which travels along the lower border of a rib and supplies blood to muscles in the intercostal space. (In the anterior region of the thoracic wall, the posterior intercostal arteries anastomose with short **anterior intercostal arteries** originating from the internal thoracic arteries.) The thoracic aorta also gives rise to several small **superior phrenic arteries** which supply the upper surface of the diaphragm.

During its course through the thorax the

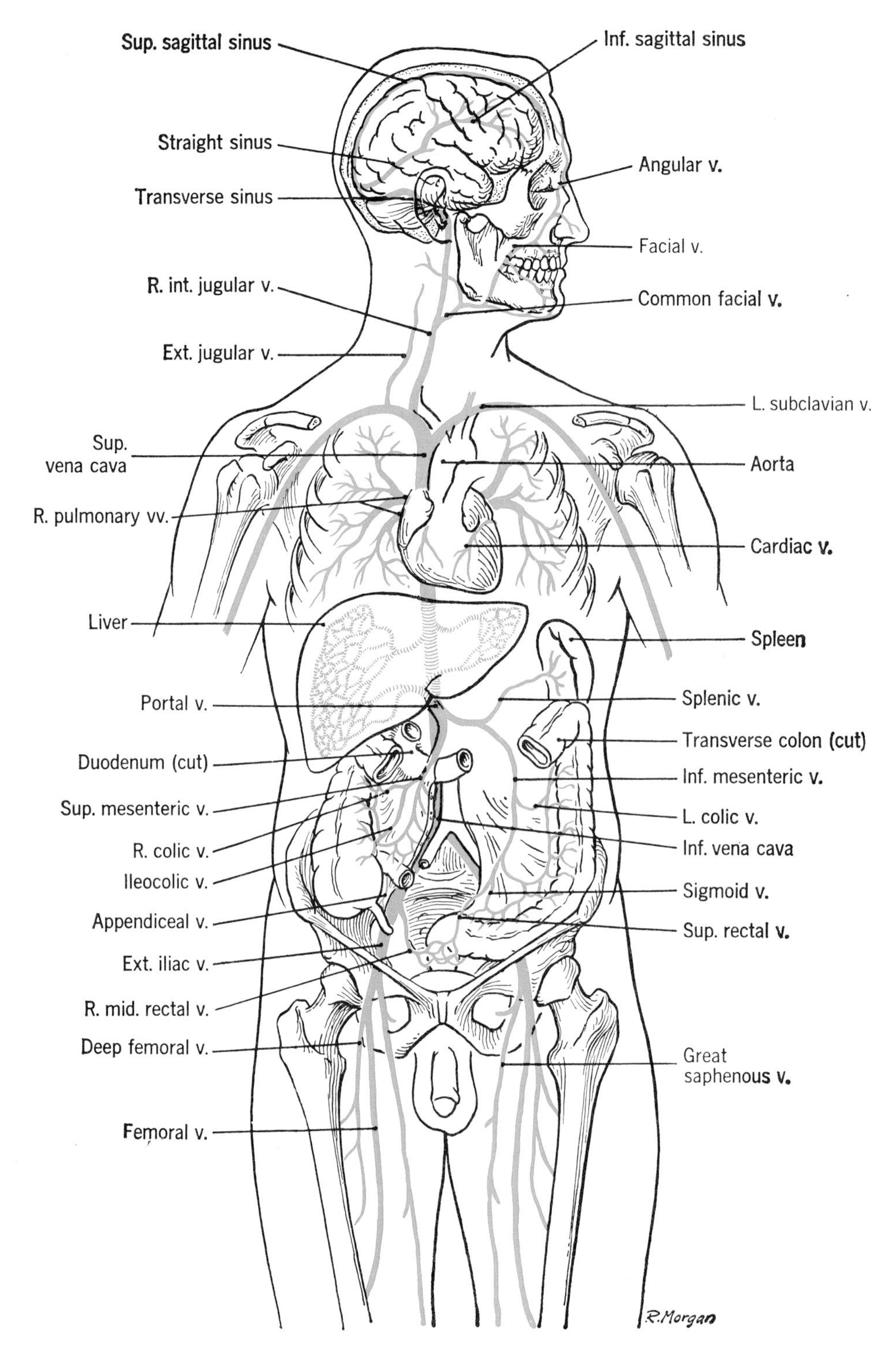

Fig. 9-19. Veins of the head, neck, thorax, and hepatic portal system. (From *Stedman's Medical Dictionary*, Ed. 23, The Williams & Wilkins Co., Baltimore, 1976.)

aorta gives off several **esophageal arteries** and **bronchial arteries** to the esophagus and much of the tissue of the lungs, respectively. The thoracic aorta passes through the aortic hiatus of the diaphragm and becomes the abdominal aorta.

The **abdominal aorta** extends along the anterior surfaces of the lumbar vertebral bodies. Upon entering the abdomen, the aorta almost immediately gives rise to the right and left **inferior phrenic arteries** which supply the inferior aspect of the diaphragm. A major visceral branch, the **celiac trunk,** is then given off and supplies a **left gastric artery** to the stomach, a large **splenic artery** to the spleen, and a **common hepatic artery** to the liver.

Just below the origin of the celiac trunk the aorta gives rise to the single **superior mesenteric artery** which supplies parts of the pancreas and small and large intestines. The aorta next sends off pairs of **middle suprarenal, renal,** and **gonadal arteries** to the suprarenal (adrenal) glands, kidneys, and gonads, respectively, and a single **inferior mesenteric artery** to the lower portion of the large intestine. These vessels are discussed more extensively with the various organs which they supply.

Four or five pairs of **lumbar arteries** pass from the aorta to the muscles of the posterior abdominal wall. The aorta then ends by bifurcating into a **right** and **left common iliac artery** at the level of the fourth lumbar vertebra. (Near the bifurcation, a very small sacral artery extends caudally a short distance in front of the sacrum and coccyx.)

Each common iliac artery runs laterally and soon divides into an internal and external iliac artery. The **internal iliac arteries** supply branches to the pelvic walls, the gluteal muscles, and the skin and muscles of the genital region. In addition, the internal iliac arteries also give off branches to various organs of the pelvis such as the urinary bladder, sex organs, and rectum.

The **external iliac arteries** carry blood for the lower limbs. They also give rise to the **inferior epigastric arteries** which turn upward and supply branches to muscles and skin of the

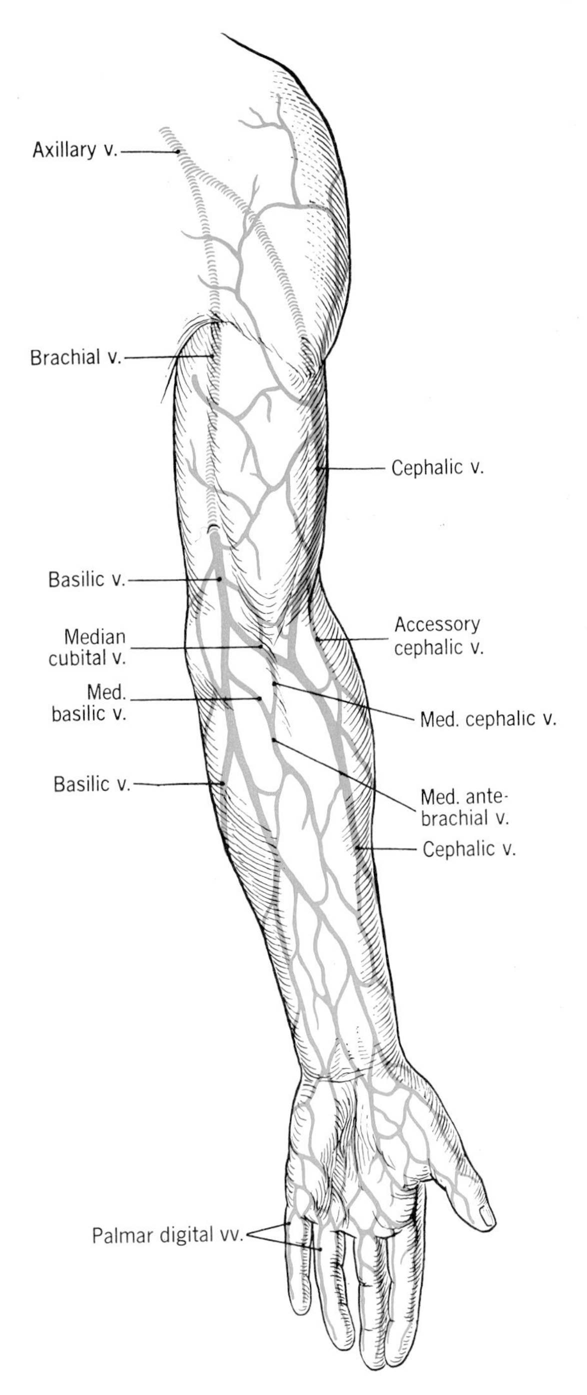

Fig. 9-20. Superficial veins of the left upper limb, anterior view. (From *Stedman's Medical Dictionary,* Ed. 23, The Williams & Wilkins Co., Baltimore, 1976.)

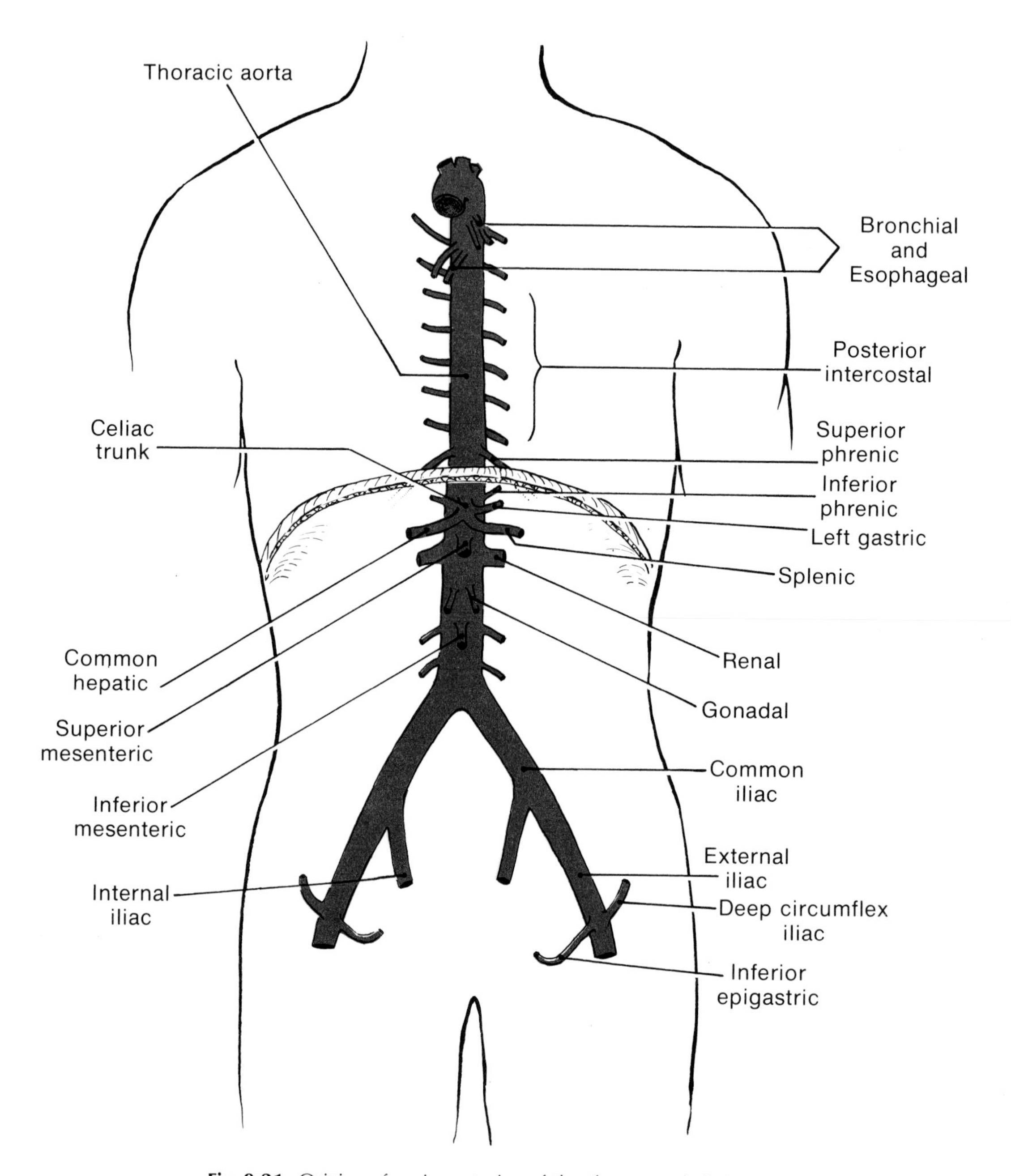

Fig. 9-21. Origins of major arteries of the thorax and abdomen.

anterior abdominal wall. In the upper region of the wall, the inferior epigastric arteries eventually anastomose with the superior epigastric arteries extending downward from the internal thoracic branches of the subclavian arteries.

Each external iliac artery also sends off a **deep circumflex iliac artery** to supply the lateral wall of the pelvis. The external iliac then passes behind the inguinal ligament and becomes the femoral artery.

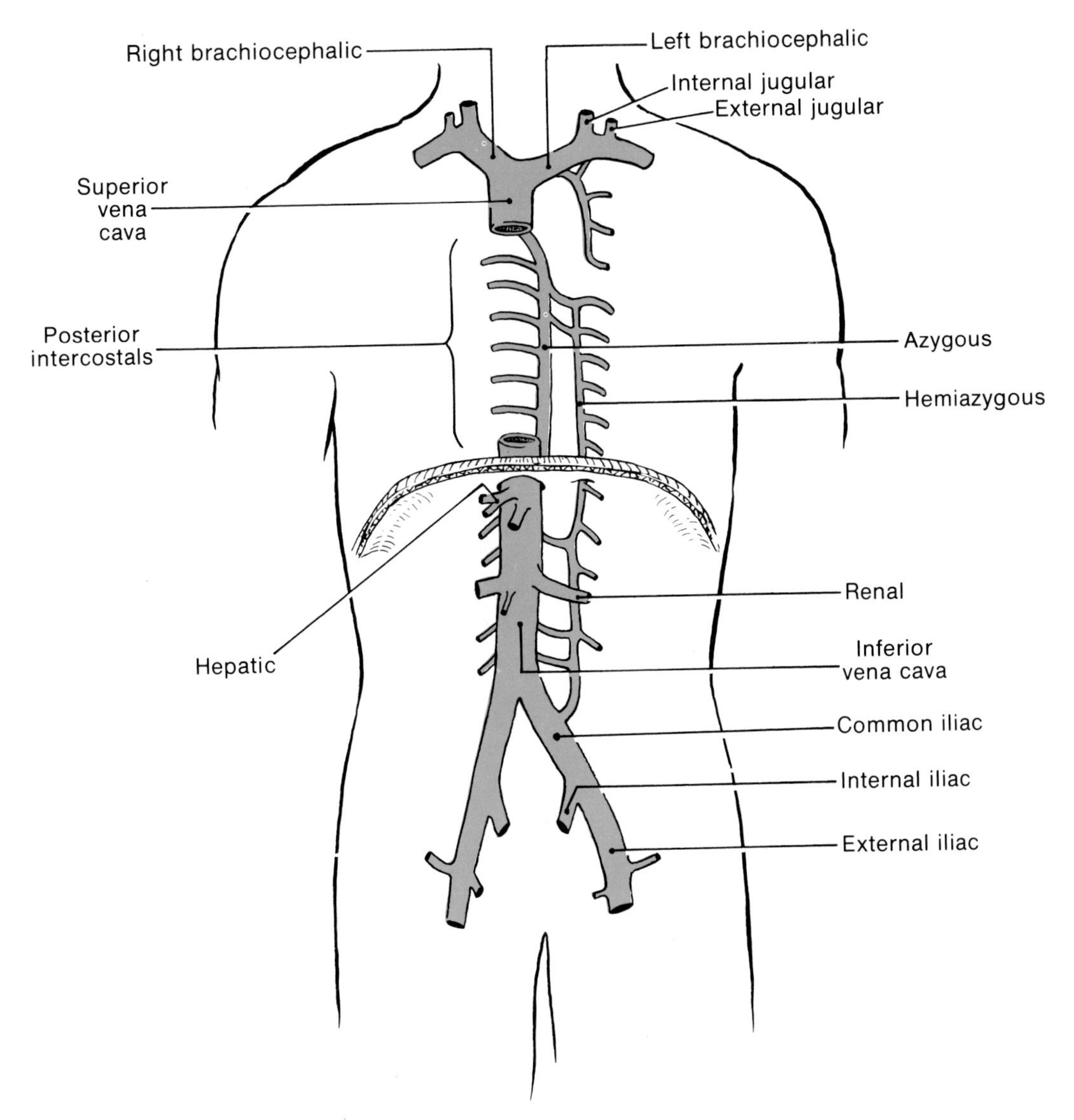

Fig. 9-22. Origins of major veins of the thorax and abdomen, not including the portal system.

Veins of the Thorax and Abdomen

The venous return from the thorax occurs primarily via a network of tributaries known as the azygous system (Fig. 9-22). Pairs of **posterior intercostal veins** travel along the ribs in company with the intercostal arteries. At the posterior thoracic wall, the intercostal veins from the right side of the thorax communicate with a longitudinal channel termed the **azygous vein** which runs along the vertebral column and empties into the superior vena cava. On the left side of the thorax the posterior intercostal veins drain into a variable **hemiazygous vein** joining the azygous vein by one or more cross connections. The azygous and hemiazygous veins also receive **bronchial** and **esophageal veins.**

Blood from the walls of the abdomen can drain into the azygous system by way of **ilio-**

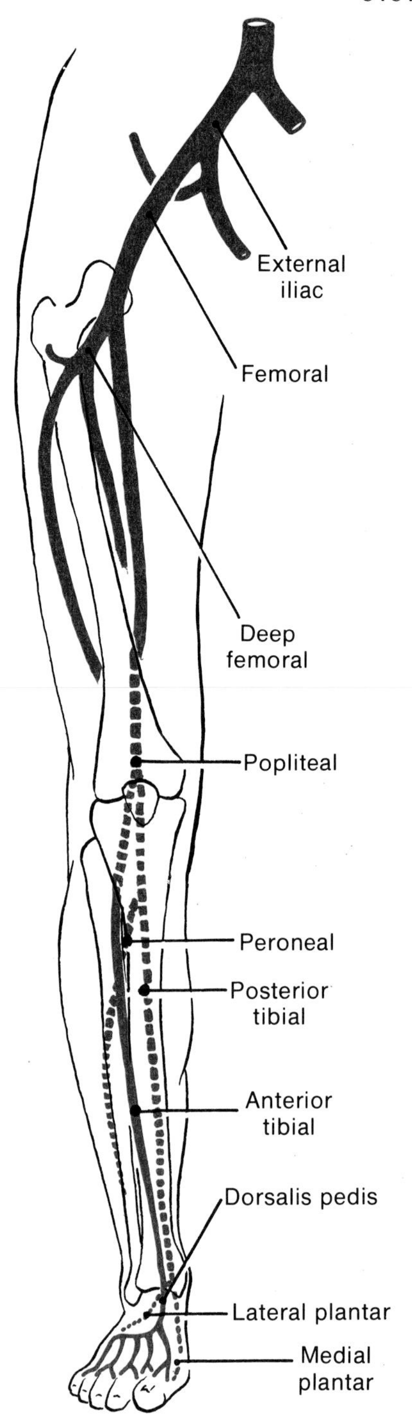

Fig. 9-23. Arteries of the lower limb, anterior view. *Dotted lines* represent arteries lying posteriorly.

lumbar, lumbar, and **ascending lumbar veins.** However, the major route of return is the **inferior vena cava,** a massive vein running upward along the right side of the lumbar vertebral column (Fig. 9-22). The inferior vena cava is formed by the union of the two **common iliac veins,** each of which in turn receives blood from an **internal** and **external iliac vein.** The internal iliac vein receives tributaries from the pelvic organs. The external iliac vein transmits blood from the lower limb and also receives the **inferior epigastric veins** which drain the anterior abdominal wall. The inferior vena cava also receives **lumbar, gonadal, renal, suprarenal, inferior phrenic,** and **hepatic veins.** The hepatic veins join the inferior vena cava just as it passes upward through the diaphragm to empty into the right atrium of the heart.

In addition to the abdominal portion of the azygous system and the inferior vena cava, the abdomen also utilizes a unique system of veins known as the **hepatic portal system.** Here the blood from the various digestive organs travels via **splenic, gastric, superior mesenteric,** and **inferior mesenteric veins** to a short wide vein termed simply the **portal vein** (Fig. 9-19; see also Fig. 14-28). This vein carries the venous blood from the digestive tract to the liver and breaks up into a second network of small vessels, the **liver sinusoids.** The blood then drains into **hepatic veins** which empty into the inferior vena cava. Since the portal system involves a network of small capillary-like vessels (the liver sinusoids) interposed between the capillary network in the digestive organs and the heart, it allows the liver to process substances which have been absorbed by the intestinal tract. However, the portal system poses a problem for the liver since metastases of cancer cells from malignancies in other digestive organs can readily be transmitted to the liver via the portal vein. Diseases of the liver can also create an obstruction in the portal system (portal hypertension) resulting in a backup of blood and enlargement of portal vessels and their tributaries.

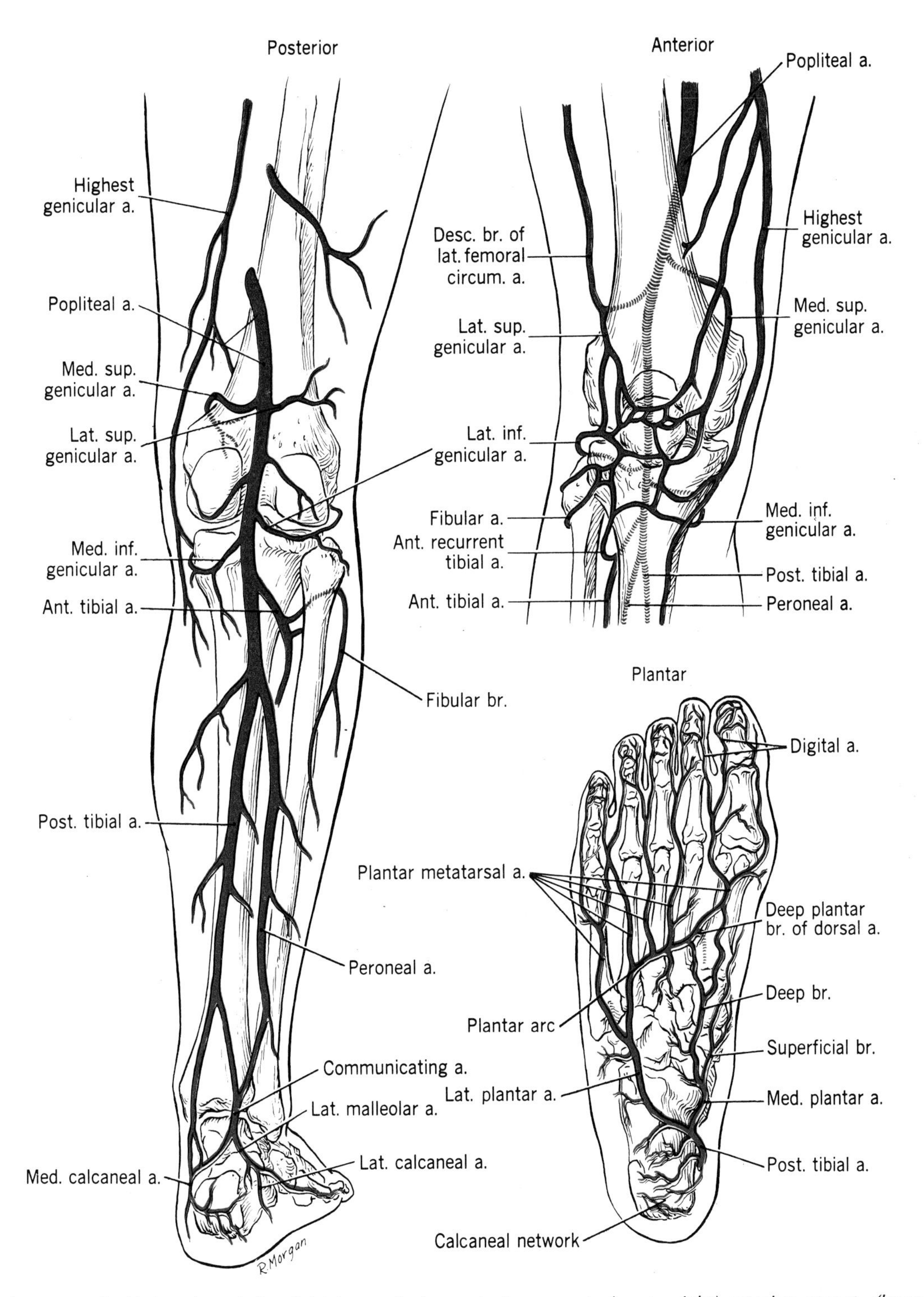

Fig. 9-24. *(Left)* Arteries of the right lower limb, posterior aspect, *(upper right)* anterior aspect. *(lower right)* arteries of the sole of the right foot. (From *Stedman's Medical Dictionary,* Ed. 23, The Williams & Wilkins Co., Baltimore, 1976.)

Arteries of the Lower Limbs

The external iliac arteries pass behind the inguinal ligaments and become the **femoral arteries,** which supply the lower limbs (Figs. 9-23 and 9-24). Each femoral artery travels along the medial aspect of the thigh under cover of the sartorius muscle and gives off a **deep femoral artery** and other branches to the thigh muscles. The femoral artery then passes to the popliteal fossa at the back of the knee where it becomes known as the **popliteal artery,** which gives off branches to the knee joint and divides into the anterior and posterior **tibial arteries.**

The **anterior tibial artery** passes along the anterior face of the interosseous membrane between the tibia and fibula and supplies adjacent muscles on the anterior surface of the leg. It becomes superficial as the **dorsalis pedis artery** near the inner aspect of the ankle and forms branches which supply the dorsum of the foot and which anastomose with branches from the posterior tibial artery. The large **posterior tibial artery** travels beneath the soleus and gastrocnemius muscles, gives off a **peroneal artery** to the lateral side of the leg and eventually divides into **medial** and **lateral plantar arteries** for the sole of the foot (Figs. 9-23 and 9-24). The lateral plantar artery forms the **plantar arch** which supplies metatarsal and digital arteries to the toes.

Veins of the Lower Limbs

The **deep veins** of the lower limbs consist of venae comitantes which are similar in name and distribution to the arteries of the limb. However, as in the upper limbs, there are also **superficial veins** beginning as a plexus in the foot, from which emerge a small saphenous vein laterally and a great saphenous vein medially. The **small saphenous vein** runs up the back of the leg and penetrates deep into the popliteal fossa to join the popliteal vein. The **great saphenous vein** continues upward along the medial aspect of the leg and thigh and eventually communicates with the femoral vein (Fig. 9-25). The length and easy accessibility of the great saphenous vein allow it to be used surgically as vessel grafts for other parts of the body.

Superficial veins communicate with the deep veins of the lower limb by means of perforating veins. The blood flows from the superficial to the deep system of veins, and both systems are well supplied with valves. If the valves become incompetent, then the superficial veins enlarge as **varicose veins** which bulge out from the surface of the limb. Standing or sitting for long periods of time may be stressful to the valves in the legs, as is the back pressure resulting from obstructions to the outflow of blood from this region. Hence, varicose veins sometimes occur during and after pregnancies or in the presence of large abdominal or pelvic masses.

DEVELOPMENTAL AND CLINICAL ANATOMY OF THE CARDIOVASCULAR SYSTEM

A brief discussion of the embryonic cardiovascular system can aid in understanding the adult anatomy and also can help to explain some of the more common anomalies which occur in this system. In the embryo, the heart and major blood vessels develop from splanchnic mesoderm (Chapter 5). The **heart** begins as a pair of hollow tubes underlying the foregut. These tubes soon fuse to form a single endothelial tube whose cranial portion becomes the **truncus arteriosus,** caudal to which are four bulges named the **bulbus cordis, ventricle, atrium,** and **sinus venosus** (Fig. 9-26). The walls of the tube gradually thicken, forming a thin myocardial layer around the endothelial (endocardial) lining.

Meanwhile, a system of solid strands of mesodermal cells forms throughout the embryonic body, and these strands soon become hollow, thereby producing a network of thin-walled blood vessels in the form of a capillary bed. These vessels communicate with similar ones in the yolk sac, where blood cells and

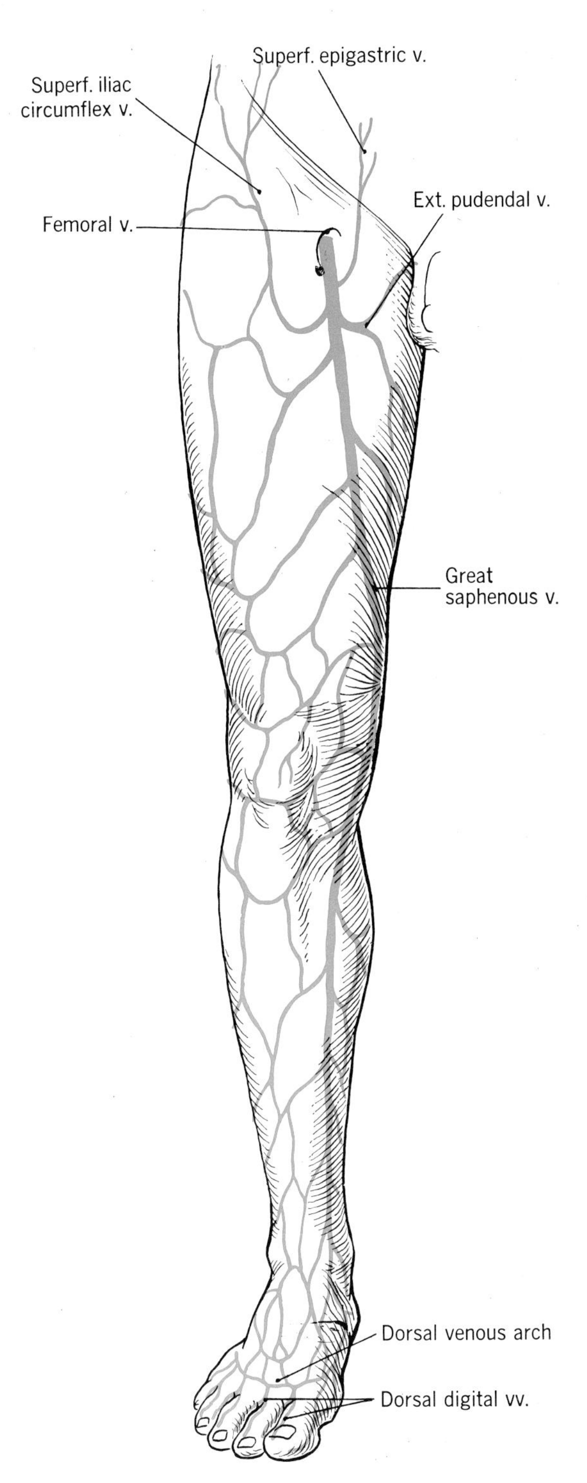

Fig. 9-25. Superficial veins of the lower limb, anterior view. (From *Stedman's Medical Dictionary,* Ed. 23, The Williams & Wilkins Co., Baltimore, 1976.)

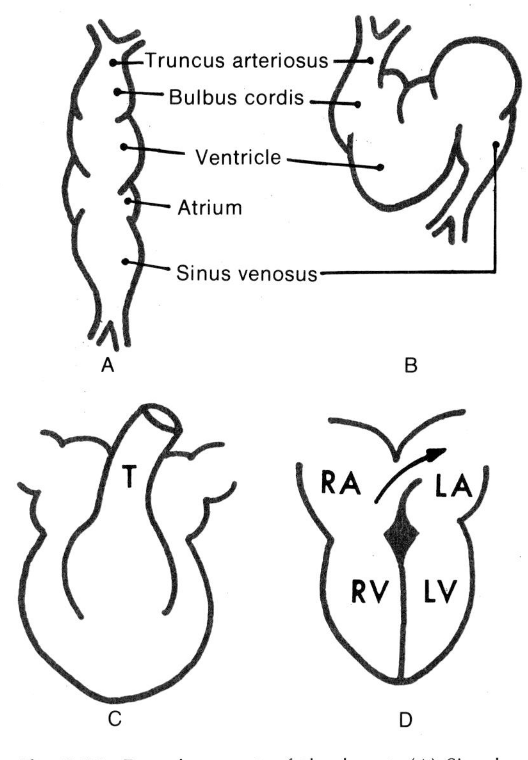

Fig. 9-26. Development of the heart. (A) Simple heart tube, (B) cardiac loop forms, (C) truncus (T) and bulbus move anterior to the ventricle and atrium, (D) section through the heart showing partitioning into two atria and two ventricles. *Arrow* indicates shunt of blood from right to left atrium via foramen ovale.

plasma are being produced, and blood begins to circulate freely throughout the vessels of the yolk sac and into the capillary network of the embryo (see Chapter 5, Fig. 5-10). The embryonic heart shows erratic, uncoordinated contractions which provide some propulsive force for the circulation, even as early as the fourth week of gestation.

Blood enters the heart caudally by way of the sinus venosus and exits cranially through the bulbus and truncus arteriosus. The heart then forms a cardiac loop, and a complex series of changes takes place so that the sinus venosus, atrium, and ventricle come to lie posterior to the bulbus and truncus. The sinus venosus also gradually becomes associated with the right side of the atrium.

Next, the heart becomes subdivided into right and left halves by the formation of an interatrial and interventricular septum. The **interatrial septum** does not completely separate the two atria, since an aperture called the **foramen ovale** remains in the septum and allows some blood to flow from the right atrium directly into the left atrium throughout embryonic and fetal life.

In contrast, the **interventricular septum** completely separates right and left ventricles. The interventricular septum also unites with a partition which subdivides the interior of the bulbus and truncus into a right half (the pulmonary trunk) and a left half (the aorta). In this manner, the right ventricle communicates with the pulmonary trunk as its outflow tract while the left ventricle communicates with the aorta.

The pulmonary trunk sends out a right and left pulmonary artery, but since the placenta performs the respiratory function for the embryo, there is no advantage in having much blood pass through the pulmonary circuit to the embryonic lungs. Thus, some of the blood in the right atrium is shunted directly into the left atrium via the foramen ovale. The remainder of the blood does pass into the right ventricle and pulmonary trunk, but most of the remainder is shunted directly into the systemic circuit by means of a duct which occurs between the pulmonary artery and the aorta (Fig. 9-27). This second shunt is termed the **ductus arteriosus** and, like the foramen ovale, functions throughout embryonic and fetal life.

While changes are taking place in the heart region, the directional flow of blood through the capillary networks of the body results in the selection and enlargement of certain channels which become the major blood vessels of the arterial and venous systems. The embryonic vascular system is also connected to the placental circulation where the metabolic waste products from the embryonic tissues are exchanged for nutrients and oxygen. For this purpose, two **umbilical arteries** originate from the internal iliac artery and carry deoxygenated blood out to the placenta, whereas a single **umbilical vein** brings oxygenated blood from the placenta back to the embryo (Fig. 9-27).

The umbilical vein passes through the liver and empties the oxygenated blood into the ductus venosus which in turn empties into the inferior vena cava which is carrying deoxygenated blood from the lower portions of the body. The inferior vena cava enters the right atrium, and most of its oxygenated blood is immediately shunted via the foramen ovale to the left atrium and then to the left ventricle. Meanwhile the deoxygenated blood in the right atrium passes to the right ventricle and out the pulmonary trunk. Most of this blood eventually passes into the systemic aorta via the ductus arteriosus beyond the origins of the carotid and subclavian arteries. The heart, head, neck, and upper limbs thus receive a relatively higher concentration of oxygenated blood (from the left ventricle) than do other parts of the body (Fig. 9-27). The pressure in the right atrium is higher than in the left atrium, since the right atrium not only receives the blood from the embryonic venous system but also the blood from the umbilical vein. In contrast, the pulmonary veins bring little blood back to the heart from the nonfunctioning lungs. Hence the right to left shunt is maintained.

In the few weeks before birth, increasing amounts of blood pass to the embryonic lungs, although they still do not function as respira-

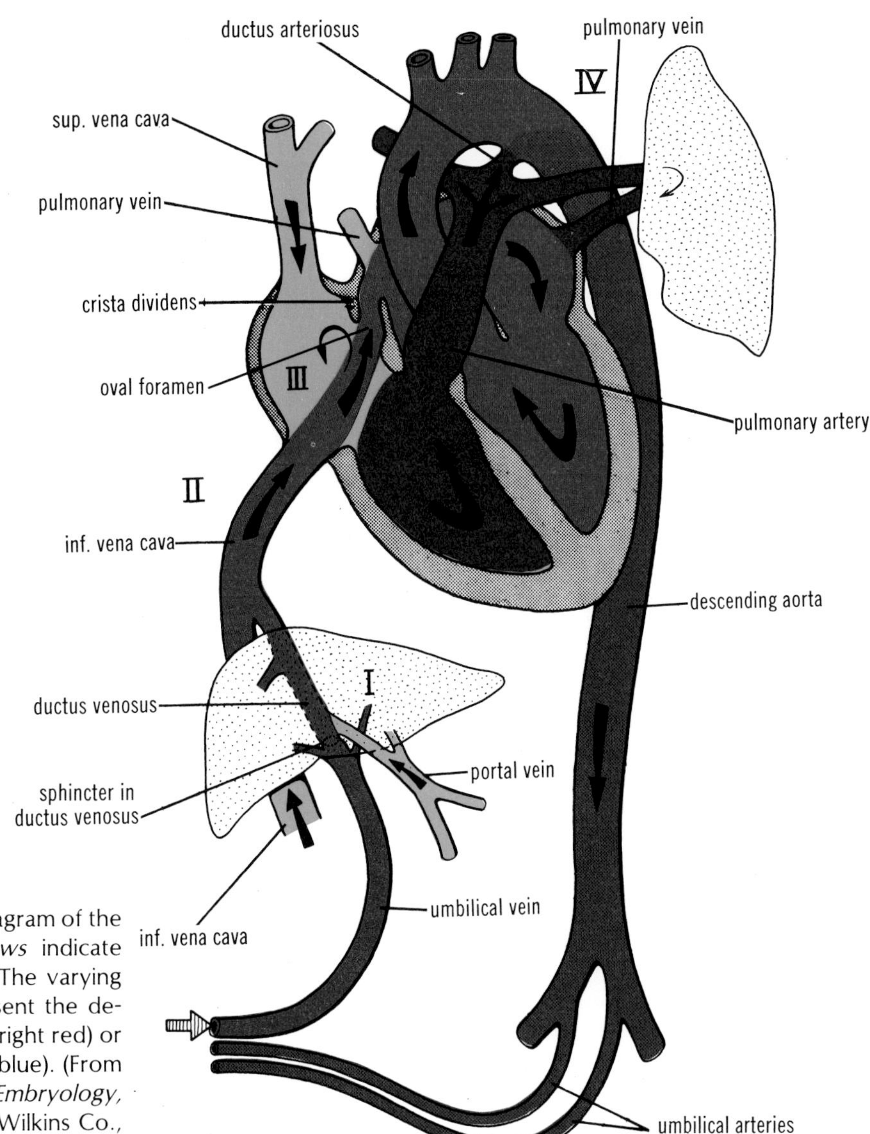

Fig. 9-27. Schematic diagram of the fetal circulation. *Arrows* indicate the direction of flow. The varying shades of color represent the degree of oxygenation (bright red) or deoxygenation (bright blue). (From J. Langman, *Medical Embryology,* Ed. 3, The Williams & Wilkins Co., Baltimore, 1975.)

tory organs, and the ductus arteriosus becomes narrower. At the time of birth the lungs expand with the first breath, and the blood in the pulmonary trunk bypasses the ductus arteriosus and is drawn to the lungs. The ductus arteriosus then closes down and becomes converted into the fibrous **ligamentum arteriosum** (arterial ligament) of the adult (Fig. 9-28). Large amounts of blood now pass via the pulmonary veins from the lungs to the left atrium. When the umbilical cord is cut, there is no longer an input of blood from the umbilical vein to the right atrium, and thus the pressures in the two atria equalize and the foramen ovale closes. The **fossa ovalis** of the adult interatrial septum marks the site of the embryonic foramen ovale.

Some of the most common congenital anomalies affect the heart and great vessels.

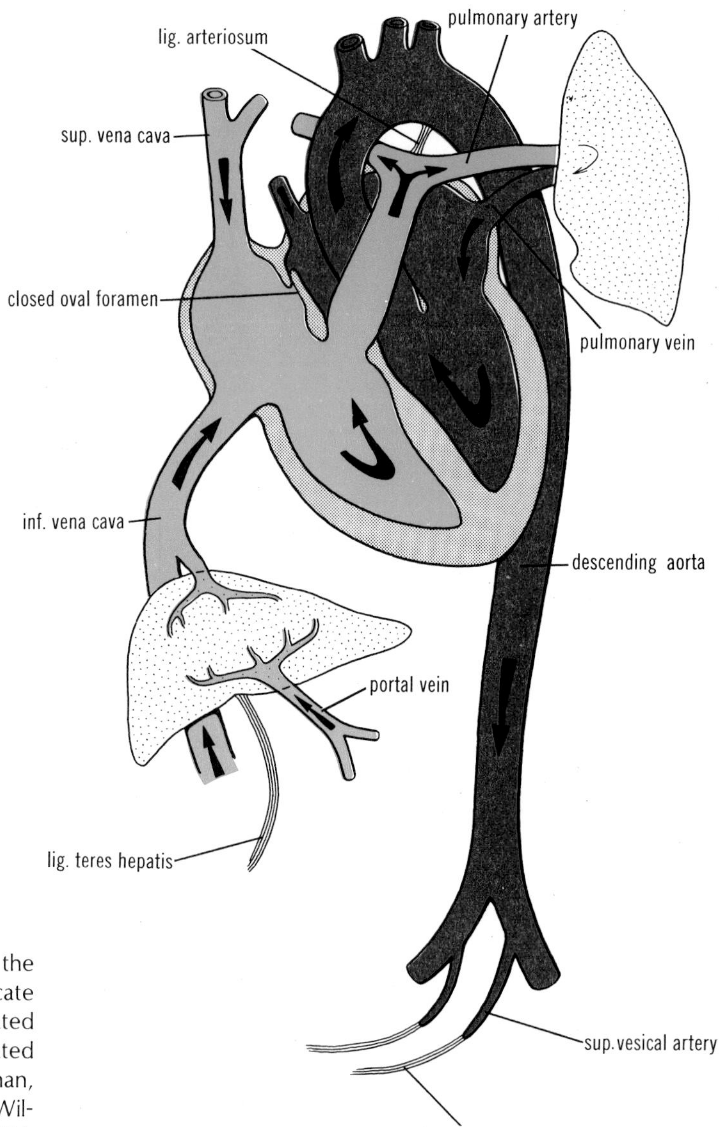

Fig. 9-28. Schematic diagram of the circulation after birth. *Arrows* indicate the direction of flow of oxygenated blood (bright red) and deoxygenated blood (bright blue). (From J. Langman, *Medical Embryology,* Ed. 3, The Williams & Wilkins Co., Baltimore, 1975.)

These include atrial septal defects, ventricular septal defects and persistent truncus arteriosus and/or persistent foramen ovale. Such abnormalities may result in a mixing of venous with arterial blood after birth, so that the child develops **cyanosis** (commonly called a "blue baby"). One rather complex condition is the **tetralogy (of Fallot)** which consists of four defects resulting from an unequal partitioning of the truncus and bulbus. These defects are: pulmonary stenosis (narrowing), right ventricular hypertrophy (enlargement), interventricular septal defect, and overriding aorta. Since the aorta receives blood from both the right and left ventricles, cyanosis occurs. Although cyanosis can be compatible with life, the inefficient oxygen supply to the viscera and muscles creates severe disability. Fortunately, with the advent of open heart surgery many congenital heart defects can now be corrected.

Numerous structural defects may also occur in the heart after birth. The valves may become rigid or stenotic (narrowed) due to inflammation (bacterial endocarditis), and the resulting valvular stenosis often prevents sufficient amounts of blood from passing through the narrowed opening. Valves can also become stretched or defective in closing, so that blood is allowed to pass backward (valvular insufficiency).

The efficiency of valves can be determined by listening to the heart sounds through a stethoscope. There are two sounds with each heartbeat. The first occurs with the closure of the atrioventricular valves and sounds like "lubb." The second occurs with the closure of the aortic and pulmonary semilunar valves and sounds like "dup." If the valves are insufficient, then the regurgitation of the blood may be heard as a heart "murmur."

Cardiac function can also be impaired by an inadequate blood supply from the coronary arteries. These arteries can become constricted by a thickening in their walls. The latter condition is referred to as **arteriosclerosis** and can likewise occur in other blood vessels of the body. When arteriosclerosis is due to fatty deposits in the inner wall of the vessel, this is termed **atherosclerosis.** These conditions generally deprive the heart of a sufficient blood supply, resulting in pain **(angina pectoris)**. If a coronary blood vessel becomes completely occluded, as from a blood clot, the heart muscle can die from a lack of blood. This results in a "heart attack" or "coronary" which can be fatal if the damage is extensive.

The conducting system of the heart sometimes becomes defective, so that the heart contracts erratically. Cardiac muscle itself has an intrinsic capacity for contraction, and localized uncoordinated activity can occur so as to produce a rapid, fluttering beat known as **fibrillation.**

A variety of diseases can affect the blood vessels of the body, including arteriosclerosis as mentioned above with reference to the coronary arteries. An artery or vein can also develop an **aneurysm** which is due to a weakness in its wall. A sac thus balloons out and, in the case of arteries, the sac may pulsate with each heartbeat. Aneurysms can rupture and cause serious or fatal hemorrhages. Veins are subject to the condition known as **thrombophlebitis** which involves an inflammation with subsequent clot formation. Such clots pose a hazard because of their tendency to become dislodged and carried as **emboli** to distant parts of the body. The veins of the lower limbs are most vulnerable to this type of clot formation, and emboli from this site then travel upward to the right atrium by way of the inferior vena cava. Should they be carried via the pulmonary arteries to the lungs, the emboli can clog the pulmonary vessels and seriously impair pulmonary function.

10

The Lymphatic System

The lymphatic (lymphoreticular) system encompasses a group of organs and tissues which are widely scattered throughout the body. This system includes lymphatic vessels, lymphatic tissue, and lymphatic (lymphoid) organs.

LYMPHATIC VESSELS

Lymphatic vessels collect and transport excess fluid, much of which has escaped from the blood vessels into the intercellular spaces. This fluid is eventually returned to the blood stream (Fig. 10-1). The smallest lymphatic vessels are the **lymphatic capillaries** which are thin-walled tubes in the connective tissue of most regions of the body. In the villi of the small intestine, the lymphatic capillaries are called **lacteals** because they collect a white milky fluid **(chyle),** consisting of modified fats absorbed from the cavity (lumen) of the intestine (Fig. 10-2). The lacteals have a small amount of smooth muscle to help propel the chyle into larger vessels of the lymphatic system.

The lymphatic capillaries form an interconnecting network which leads into larger lymphatics termed **collecting lymphatic vessels**. The collecting vessels eventually drain into one of two main lymphatic trunks: the **thoracic duct** and the **right lymphatic duct** (Fig. 10-1). The thoracic duct lies adjacent to the vertebral column and begins inferiorly in the abdomen as an irregular dilated sac called the **cisterna chyli**. Collecting lymphatic vessels from the lower limbs and abdomen (including those carrying chyle from the intestinal lacteals) empty into the cisterna chyli and the lower end of the thoracic duct. The thoracic duct extends upward through the thorax, receives tributaries from the left side of the thorax, and arches upward into the lower region of the neck, where it receives tributaries from the left side of the neck and head and from the left upper limb. The thoracic duct then empties into the left subclavian vein or the left internal jugular vein. The right lymphatic duct is smaller and often consists of an irregular plexus of lymphatic channels draining lymph from the right side of the thorax, neck, and head, and from the right upper limb. The right lymphatic duct usually empties into the right subclavian vein or the right internal jugular vein.

Although the thoracic duct ordinarily serves a greater area of the body than does the right lymphatic duct, the situation can be reversed should the thoracic duct become constricted or surgically ligated. In such cases the numerous anastomoses among the lymphatics in the thorax and neck region enable a collateral circulation to be established, and the right lymphatic duct takes over the territory of the thoracic duct. In general, most lymphatic vessels travel alongside blood vessels. The flow of lymph through the lymphatic vessels is aided

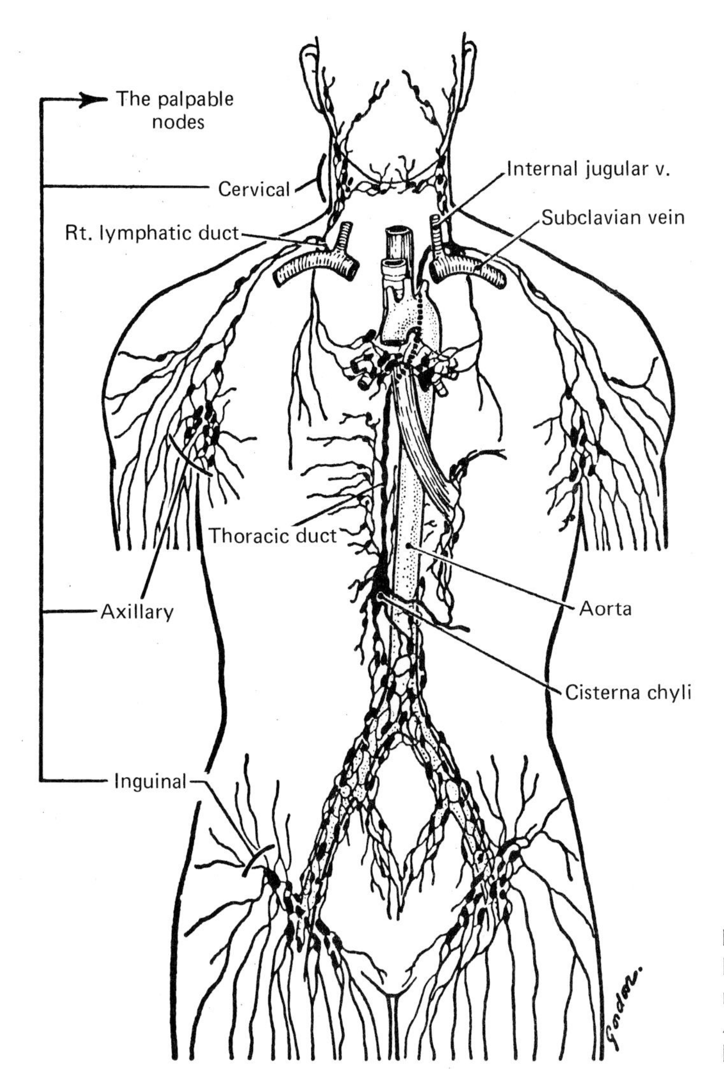

Fig. 10-1. The thoracic duct, major lymphatic vessels, and palpable lymph nodes. (From J. V. Basmajian, *Primary Anatomy,* Ed. 7, The Williams & Wilkins Co., Baltimore 1976).

by compression from nearby muscles and by respiratory and cardiac movements in the thorax. The main lymphatic ducts also contain valves which point in the direction of flow and thereby prevent backflow.

Blockage of lymphatic vessels results in an accumulation of lymph **(lymphedema)** in the region normally drained by the lymphatics. The accumulated fluid can create a swelling of considerable magnitude. This occurs when the lymphatic vessels become obstructed by certain roundworm parasites (in the disease commonly called "elephantiasis") or when they are obstructed by encroaching tumors or even from some surgical procedures. Since cells can pass fairly easily into the lymphatic capillaries, this system can also serve as a pathway for the dissemination of malignancies.

Microscopic Anatomy

The walls of the **lymphatic capillaries** consist only of an extremely thin layer of endothelium lying on a basement membrane. **Collecting lymphatic vessels** contain three layers: (1) an inner **tunica intima** consisting of an endothe-

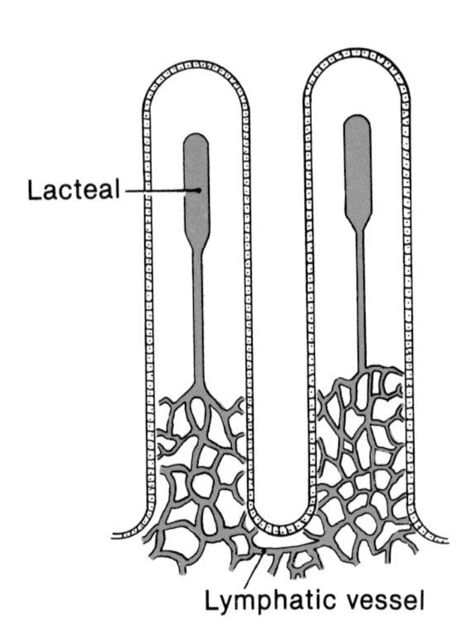

Fig. 10-2. Diagram of a vertical section through two intestinal villi, showing a lacteal in each villus.

lium, basement membrane, and sparse elastic tissue; (2) a **tunica media** with circular and longitudinal smooth muscle tissue; and (3) a **tunica adventitia** composed of loose connective tissue with some longitudinal smooth muscle. The walls of the thoracic duct and right lymphatic duct are structurally similar to those of veins of comparable size.

LYMPHATIC TISSUE

Lymphatic (lymphoid) tissue consists of **reticular connective tissue** (reticular cells and reticular fibers) and lymphocytes. The reticular cells (also known as fixed macrophages) are capable of engulfing harmful material. The lymphocytes play an important role in immunity.

There are two kinds of lymphocytes, both of which are initially produced by the bone marrow and released into the blood stream. One type of lymphocyte travels to the thymus, which provides the environment necessary for these cells to differentiate into **T-cells** (thymus-dependent cells). The T-cells then migrate via the blood stream to the spleen and lymph nodes, where they occupy specific zones (T-cell zones). T-cells are capable of attacking and destroying foreign cells, and they travel freely via the blood and lymphatic circulation to sites where they are needed.

The other type of lymphocyte is the **B-cell**. In birds, a pouch of the intestine called the bursa of Fabricius provides the appropriate environment for the differentiation of B-cells; in mammals the B-cells apparently depend on the bone marrow itself for differentiation, although it has been suggested that various accumulations of lymphoid tissue in the mammalian intestine may act in a manner similar to that of the bursa of Fabricius in birds. Like the T-cells, B-cells eventually pass via the blood stream to the spleen and lymph nodes where they occupy their own territory in B-cell zones. However, unlike T-cells, B-cells give rise to **plasma cells** which produce and release circulating antibodies into the blood. Despite their functional differences, T-cells and B-cells have not as yet been morphologically distinguishable from one another.

Lymphatic tissue may be diffusely distributed or localized in discrete structures such as solitary lymph nodules, aggregate lymph nodules, and tonsils. Lymphoid organs are those in which the lymphatic tissue predominates; these include the lymph nodes, spleen, and thymus.

Diffuse Lymphatic Tissue

Diffuse lymphatic tissue commonly occurs in the connective tissue layer (lamina propria) of mucous membranes in the digestive and respiratory tracts. The meshwork of reticular cells, fibers, and lymphocytes blends imperceptibly into the surrounding connective tissue. It gives the appearance of loose connective tissue except for the larger numbers of lymphocytes.

Lymphatic Nodules

Lymphatic nodules are rounded accumulations of lymphatic tissue and are often embedded in the diffuse lymphatic tissue of the digestive and respiratory tracts. The lymphatic nodule also serves as a building block found in more elaborate structures of the lymphatic system. It may occur singly as a **solitary nodule** or may be grouped with others in **aggregate nodules**. Aggregate nodules are especially well developed in the lamina propria of the ileum of the small intestine where they are called **Peyer's patches** (Fig. 10-3).

Each nodule is approximately 2 mm in diameter and is composed of densely packed darkly staining lymphocytes. In the center of each nodule there may be a paler staining area called a **germinal center**. Here the lymphocytes are immature and contain more cytoplasm. As they mature, the lymphocytes become smaller and move into the periphery of the nodule.

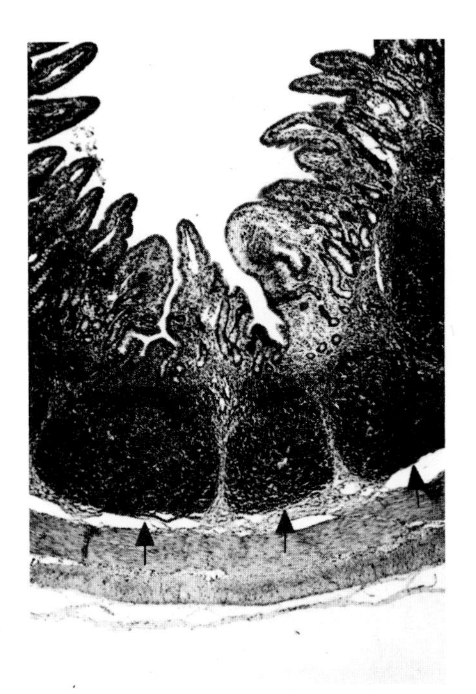

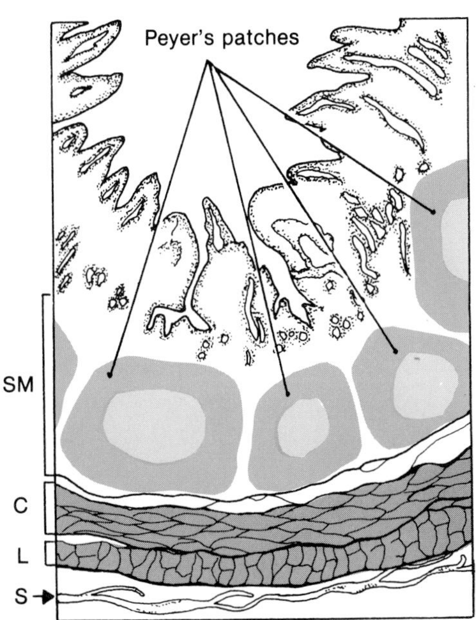

Fig. 10-3. *(Above)* Microscopic section of ileum showing Peyer's patches (three dark masses indicated by arrows). (From W. J. Banks, *Histology and Comparative Organology,* The Williams & Wilkins Co., Baltimore, 1974.) (Below) Diagram of microscopic section. SM, submucosa, C, circular layer of muscle, L, longitudinal layer of muscle, S, serosa.

TONSILS

The tonsils are modified aggregate nodules partially encapsulated with connective tissue. There are two **palatine tonsils**, one **pharyngeal tonsil**, and a **lingual tonsil**, all of which form an irregular, discontinuous ring of lymphatic tissue at the entrance to the pharynx ("throat"). These structures produce lympho-

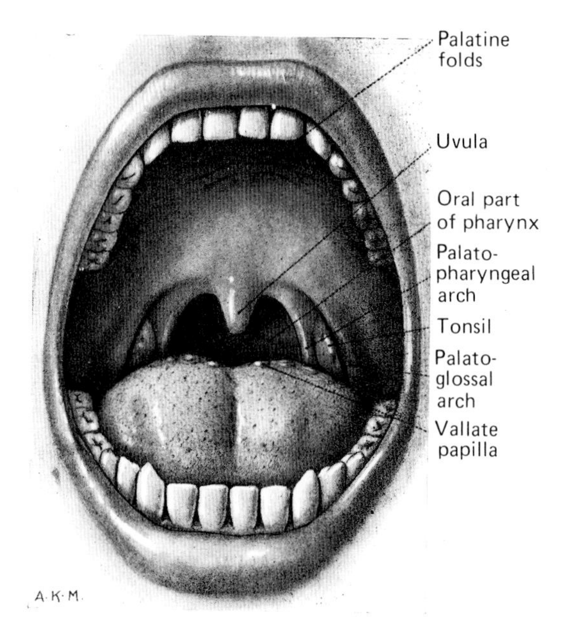

Fig. 10-4. Anterior view into the oral cavity, showing the palatine tonsils situated laterally between the palatoglossal and palatopharyngeal arches. (From W. J. Hamilton, G. Simon, and S. G. I. Hamilton, *Surface and Radiological Anatomy*, Ed. 5, The Macmillan Press, London, 1971.)

cytes and plasma cells and thus serve as a line of defense against harmful foreign matter entering the body through the nose and mouth.

Each palatine tonsil is located laterally at the back of the mouth between two arches of soft tissue (the palatoglossal and palatopharyngeal arches) (Fig. 10-4). The pharyngeal tonsil lies above the soft palate and in the upper part of the nasopharynx, the passageway which connects the nasal cavities with the back of the mouth. An enlargement of a pharyngeal tonsil is known as **adenoids** and can interfere with nasal breathing. The lingual tonsil is located at the base of the tongue.

The tonsils consist of clusters of lymphatic nodules (containing germinal centers) separated from deeper structures by a layer of fibrous connective tissue (Fig. 10-5). The free surface of each tonsil is covered with an epithelium characteristic of the region in which it resides. Thus, the palatine and lingual tonsils are covered by stratified squamous epithelium, while the pharyngeal tonsil is covered by pseudostratified ciliated epithelium. The surfaces of the palatine and lingual tonsils also show deep invaginations termed **crypts**.

Tonsils are usually highly developed in children but then gradually involute in adults and become mostly replaced by fibrous connective tissue. The crypts trap and accumulate foreign matter and bacteria; therefore, they can also become focal sites of infection.

LYMPH NODES

Lymph nodes are encapsulated, oval bodies of lymphatic tissue situated in the pathways of lymphatic vessels. The nodes tend to be grouped in certain areas of the body, such as in the cervical, axillary, and inguinal regions (Figs. 10-1 and 10-6). The thoracic and abdominal cavities also contain clusters of nodes, especially in the regions of the lungs, in the mesentery of the intestine, and along the aorta.

Like tonsils, the lymph nodes are sites of lymphocyte and plasma cell production. However, unlike other lymphoid organs, the lymph nodes are the only ones located in the pathways

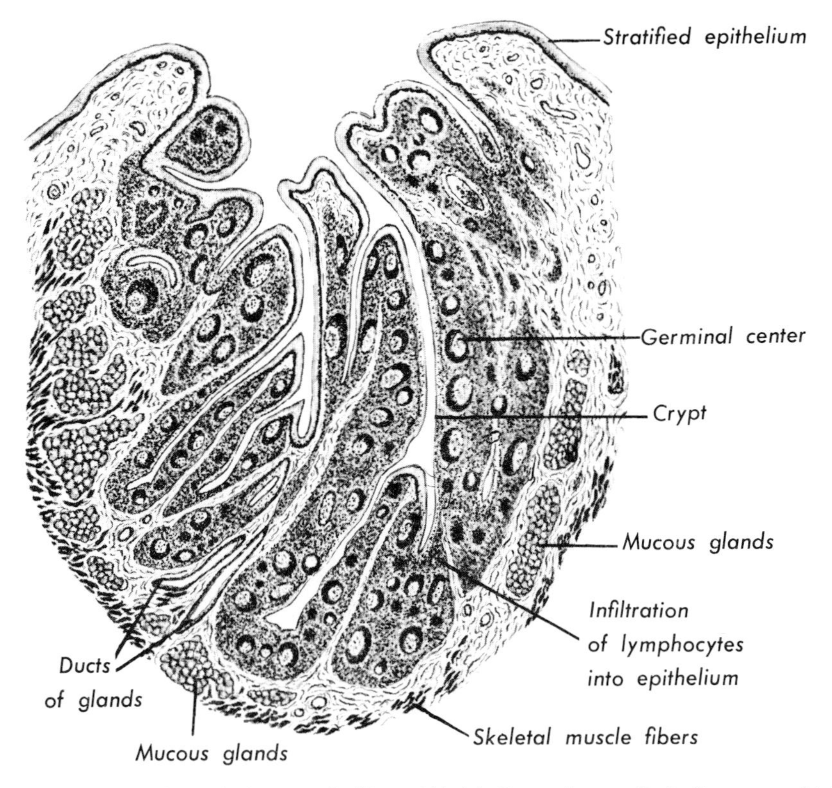

Fig. 10-5. Section through the palatine tonsil. (From W. M. Copenhaver, R. P. Bunge, and M. B. Bunge, *Bailey's Textbook of Histology,* Ed. 16, The Williams & Wilkins Co., Baltimore, 1971.)

of lymphatic vessels. Thus, they remove foreign matter, including bacteria and degenerating cells, from the lymph brought to the nodes via **afferent lymphatic vessels**. The lymph filters through each node and leaves by way of **efferent vessels**. In regions of the body exposed to large amounts of particulate matter, such as in the lungs, the phagocytic cells in the lymph nodes may become blackened by accumulations of carbon.

Cancer cells may accumulate in lymph nodes situated in the pathway of lymph vessels draining a malignancy. For example, the axillary nodes are common sites where malignant cells from a breast cancer may be found (Fig. 10-6). Consequently, these nodes may be surgically removed along with the malignant tissue with the hope of preventing further dissemination of cancer cells via the lymphatic system.

Each lymph node is surrounded by a connective tissue capsule from which septa pass inward to subdivide it into compartments (Figs. 10-7 and 10-8). Numerous afferent lymphatic vessels enter the node along its convex surface; fewer efferent lymphatic vessels leave the node at the **hilus**, a concave indentation on the opposite side of the node. The hilus also serves as an entrance and exit for blood vessels. The outer portion of the node is the **cortex** which contains typical lymphatic nodules. The central region is the **medulla** in which the lymphatic tissue is arranged as **medullary cords**. Both the cortex and medulla exhibit fluid-filled passageways, the **lymphatic sinuses**, which transmit the lymph through the node.

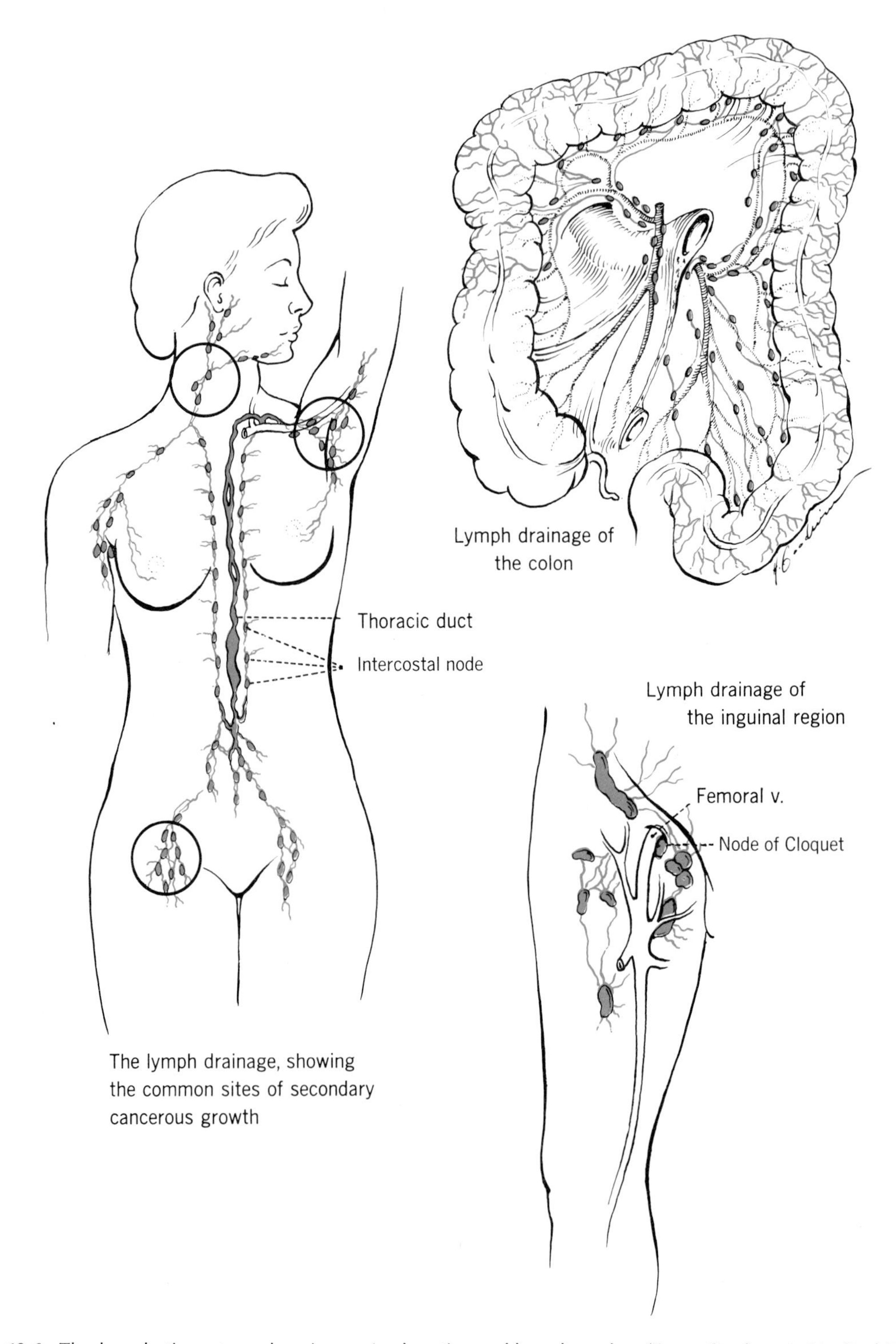

Fig. 10-6. The lymphatic system showing major locations of lymph nodes. (From *Stedman's Medical Dictionary*, Ed. 23, The Williams & Wilkins Co., Baltimore, 1976.)

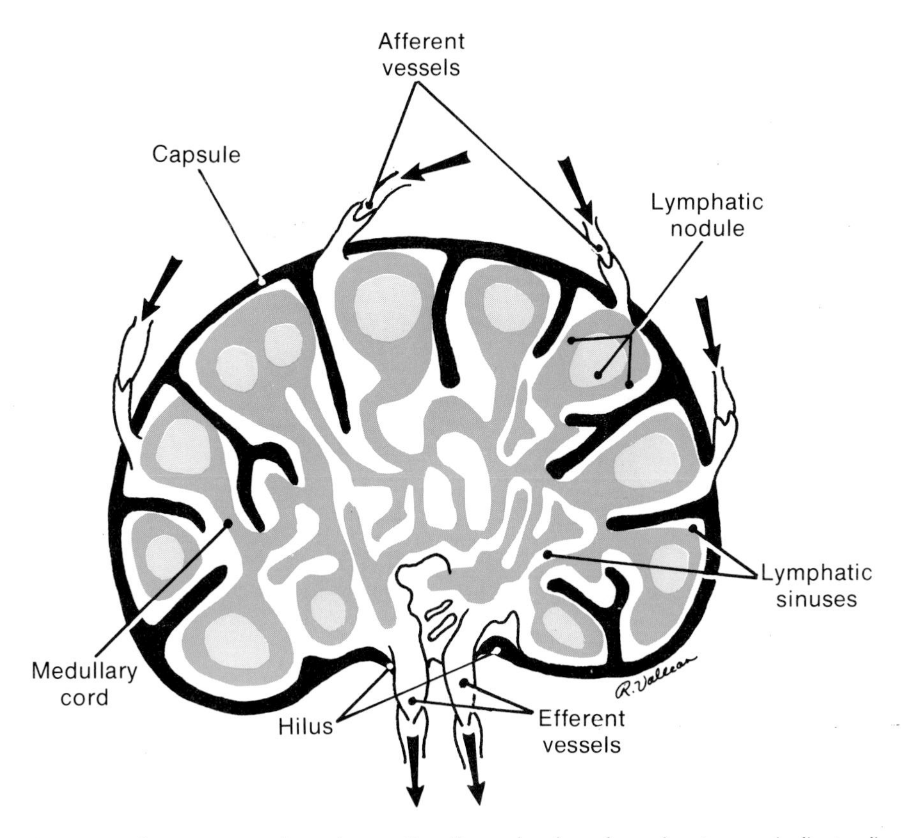

Fig. 10-7. Diagrammatic representation of a section through a lymph node. *Arrows* indicate direction of flow.

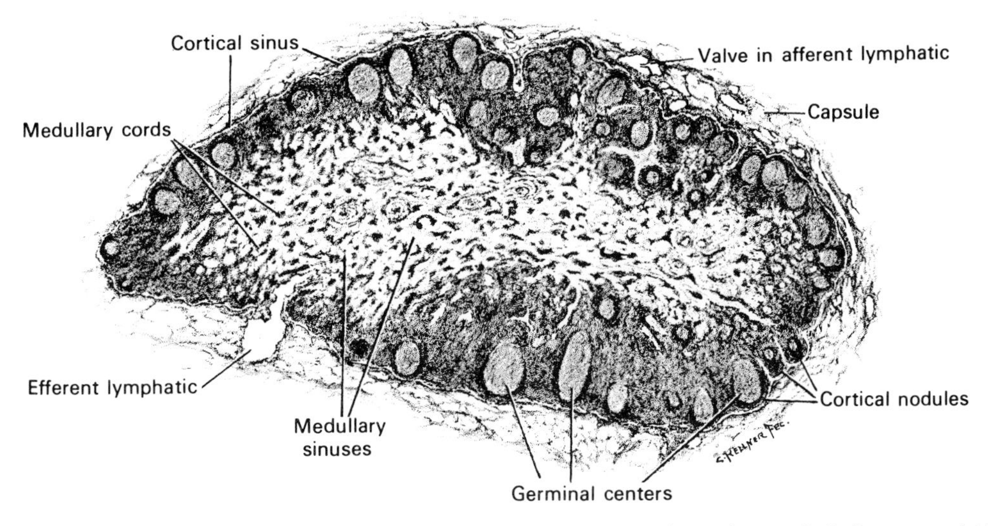

Fig. 10-8. Microscopic section through a lymph node. (From W. M. Copenhaver, R. P. Bunge, and M. B. Bunge, *Bailey's Textbook of Histology,* Ed. 16, The Williams & Wilkins Co., Baltimore, 1971.)

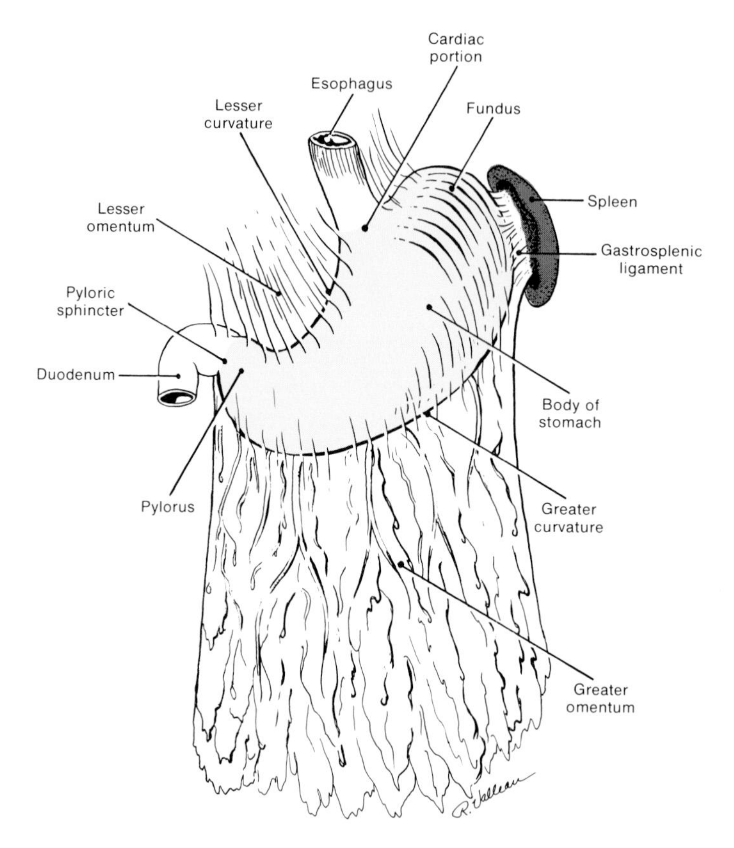

Fig. 10-9. The spleen (in red) suspended by a mesentery (the gastrosplenic "ligament") from the stomach.

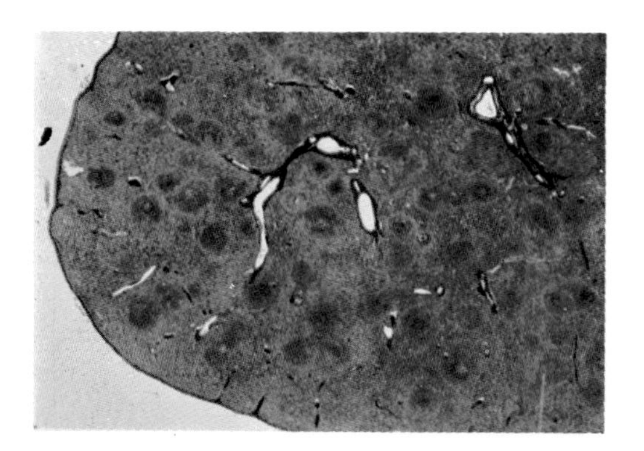

Fig. 10-10. Low magnification of a microscopic section through the spleen, showing nodules of white pulp (stained purple) and red pulp (stained light pink). The capsule, trabeculae, and walls of the blood vessels are stained blue. (Courtesy of Dr. Walter A. Stultz, University of California, San Diego.)

The lymphocytes which leave the node via the efferent lymphatic vessels eventually reach the blood stream via the thoracic duct and right lymphatic duct, which empty into the venous system. The lymphocytes ultimately are carried back to the lymph nodes via blood vessels which supply the nodes, and the cells then pass through the walls of the blood vessels and into the lymphatic sinuses, thereby reentering the lymphatic circulation.

SPLEEN

The spleen is the largest lymphatic organ and is suspended by a mesentery (the gastrosplenic "ligament") from the posterior aspect of the stomach (Fig. 10-9). In addition to its lymphoid functions the spleen also serves as a reservoir and filter for blood and as a site where aged

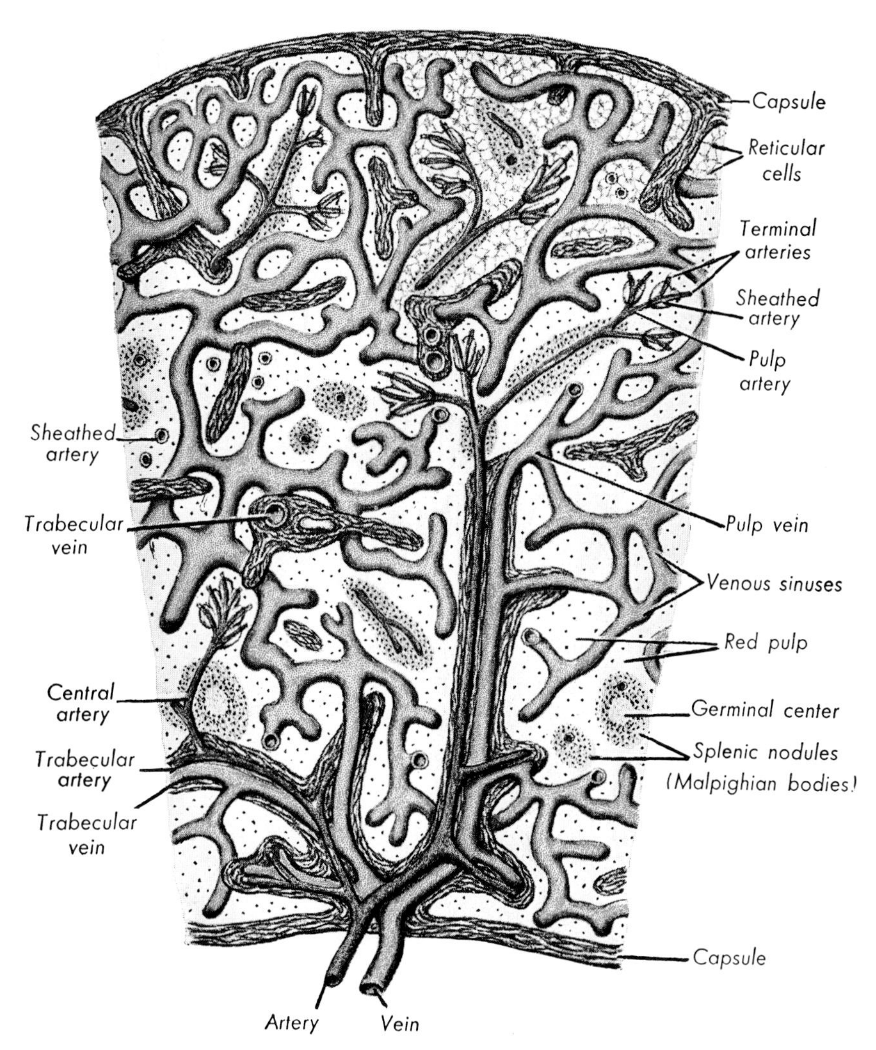

Fig. 10-11. Schematic diagram of a portion of the spleen. The white pulp is indicated in yellow. (From W. M. Copenhaver, R. P. Bunge, and M. B. Bunge, *Bailey's Textbook of Histology,* Ed. 16, The Williams & Wilkins Co., Baltimore, 1971.)

blood cells are destroyed. The spleen is situated in the pathway of blood vessels, the splenic arteries and veins, which enter and leave at a deep indentation (hilus) on one side. (In contrast, the lymph nodes are situated in the pathway of lymphatic vessels.)

Microscopic Anatomy

The spleen is surrounded by a fibromuscular **capsule** from which partitions **(trabeculae)** radiate inward to form compartments (Figs. 10-10 and 10-11). The spongelike tissue of the spleen is known as **splenic pulp**, of which there are two types: white pulp and red pulp. The **white pulp** (Fig. 10-10) exists in the form of patches containing typical lymphatic nodules (splenic nodules) and loose strands of lymphatic tissue.

The **red pulp** consists of cords of reticular tissue with an abundance of **reticular cells** (fixed macrophages) lining venous sinuses filled

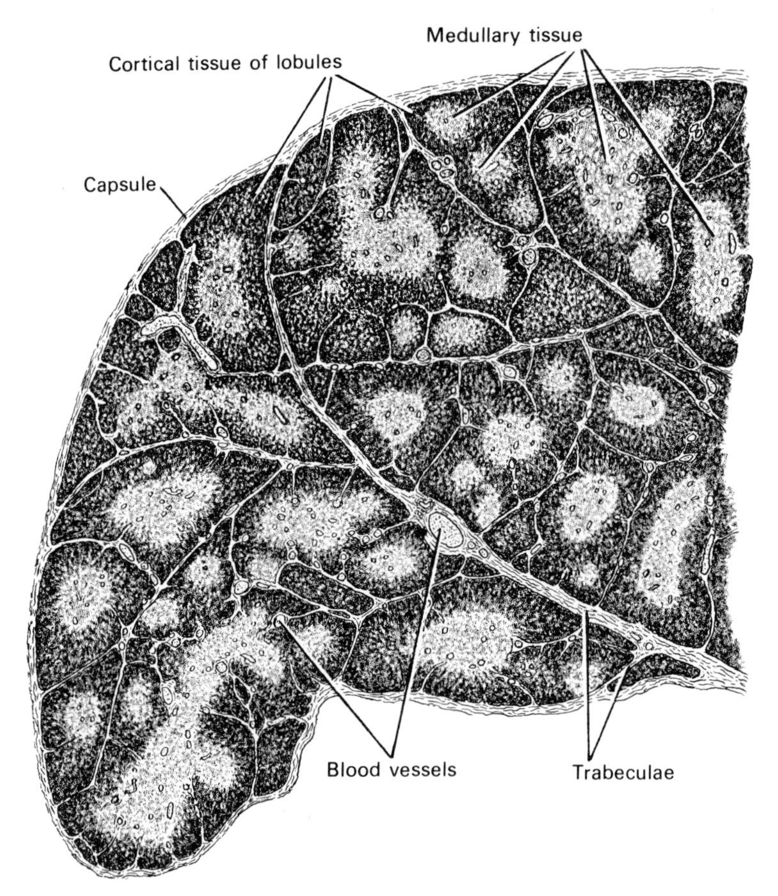

Fig. 10-12. Microscopic section of the thymus gland, low magnification. (From W. M. Copenhaver, R. P. Bunge, and M. B. Bunge, *Bailey's Textbook of Histology,* Ed. 16, The Williams & Wilkins Co., Baltimore, 1971.)

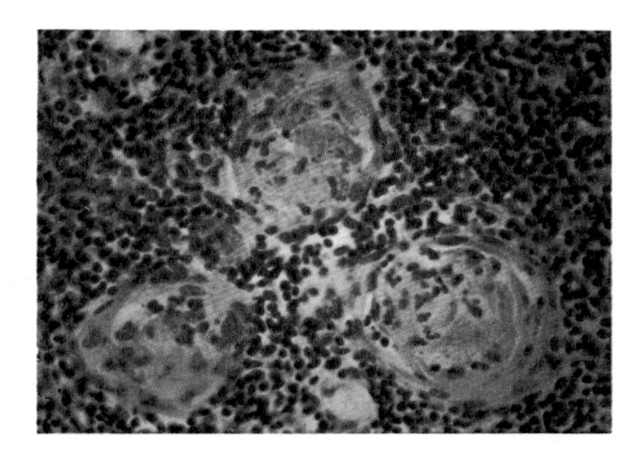

Fig. 10-13. Microscopic section of the medulla of the thymus gland, showing thymic corpuscles, high magnification. (From the teaching collection, Department of Anatomy, College of Physicians and Surgeons, Columbia University.)

with blood. These cells are important in attacking and removing microorganisms from the blood as it passes through the spleen. The reticular cells also destroy old red blood cells, thereby releasing their hemoglobin into the blood stream for use ultimately in producing new red blood cells. The pulp and sinuses of the spleen are also sites where considerable amounts of blood are stored. Under certain circumstances, this blood can be released quickly from the spleen, as in response to hemorrhage.

Although the spleen performs a variety of functions, it is not essential for life. If it is removed, some of its lymphoid functions are compensated for by other lymphatic organs. Its role as a blood reservoir is also not necessary to maintain life.

THYMUS

The thymus is a large well-developed organ in the infant and child but begins to involute during adolescence and becomes largely replaced by fibrous connective tissue and fat in the adult. It consists of two lobes and is located behind the sternum. As indicated previously, the thymus provides an environment necessary for the proper differentiation of lymphocytes known as T-cells. It also is believed to stimulate lymphocyte production in other lymphatic tissues by producing a hormonelike substance (thymosin) which is carried to them in the blood stream. The thymus thus plays a vital role in the development of the body's immune capability. Congenital absence of the thymus or a thymic malfunction in infants and children results in an immunologic deficiency which leaves the body defenseless against infection and disease.

Microscopic Anatomy

Each lobe of the thymus is subdivided by connective tissue into numerous lobules, each of which contains a cortex and medulla (Fig. 10-12). The **cortex** consists of dense clusters of rapidly proliferating T-cells (lymphocytes), which are often called "thymocytes." The **medulla** contains loosely arranged T-cells (thymocytes) as well as peculiar, concentrically arranged cells in the form of **thymic (Hassall's) corpuscles** (Fig. 10-13). Their function is debatable, although they become larger and more prominent with age. Throughout both the cortex and medulla there is also a modified type of reticular cell, which however is not phagocytic. It is possible that these special cells produce the thymic hormonelike substance mentioned above.

11

The Respiratory System

The respiratory system transports air into and out of the body and provides the means for gases such as oxygen and carbon dioxide to be exchanged between the air and the blood. The respiratory system also is important in maintaining the proper acid-base balance of body tissues, in excreting water in limited amounts, and in producing vocal sounds (phonation).

The respiratory organs include the nasal cavities, pharynx, larynx, trachea, bronchi, and lungs (Fig. 11-1). All of these serve as conducting passageways which warm, moisten, and filter the air, whereas the actual site of gaseous exchange takes place only in specialized saclike structures (alveoli) in the lungs. In addition, such structures as the diaphragm, thoracic cage, and intercostal muscles play an important role in inspiration (inhaling) and expiration (exhaling).

Much of the respiratory system is lined by a mucous membrane (mucosa) which, in the larger passages, consists of **pseudostratified ciliated columnar epithelium (respiratory epithelium)** overlying a connective tissue layer (lamina propria) (Fig. 11-2). In some regions the lamina propria is highly vascular and thus warms the air as it passes by. The respiratory epithelium is studded with mucus-producing goblet cells. The mucus provides moisture to the air and also filters it by trapping particulate matter. Moisture is also provided by numerous **seromucous glands** which extend downward from the epithelium into the lamina propria and submucosa and produce a serous, watery secretion as well as mucus. The secretions are constantly being moved by ciliary action toward the pharynx where they can be swallowed and disposed of via the digestive tract.

NOSE, PARANASAL SINUSES, AND PHARYNX

Gross Anatomy

Nose

The nose consists of an external portion projecting outward from the face and an internal portion containing two nasal cavities (Figs. 11-1 and 11-4). The external nose is covered with skin. Beneath the skin are nasal cartilages, except in the uppermost region of the nose ("bridge") where the two **nasal bones** are situated. Inferiorly the flared portion of the external nose consists of the **alae** (singular: ala) which flank the nostrils (Fig. 11-3).

The two nasal cavities are passageways which lead from the nostrils anteriorly to the nasopharynx posteriorly. The nasal cavities are separated from one another by the nasal septum consisting of the **septal cartilage**, the **vomer bone**, and the perpendicular plate of the **ethmoid bone**. The anteriormost portion of each nasal cavity contains a small cup-shaped area, the **vestibule** (Fig. 11-5), which is bounded laterally by the alae. The nasal chambers are separated from the oral cavity below

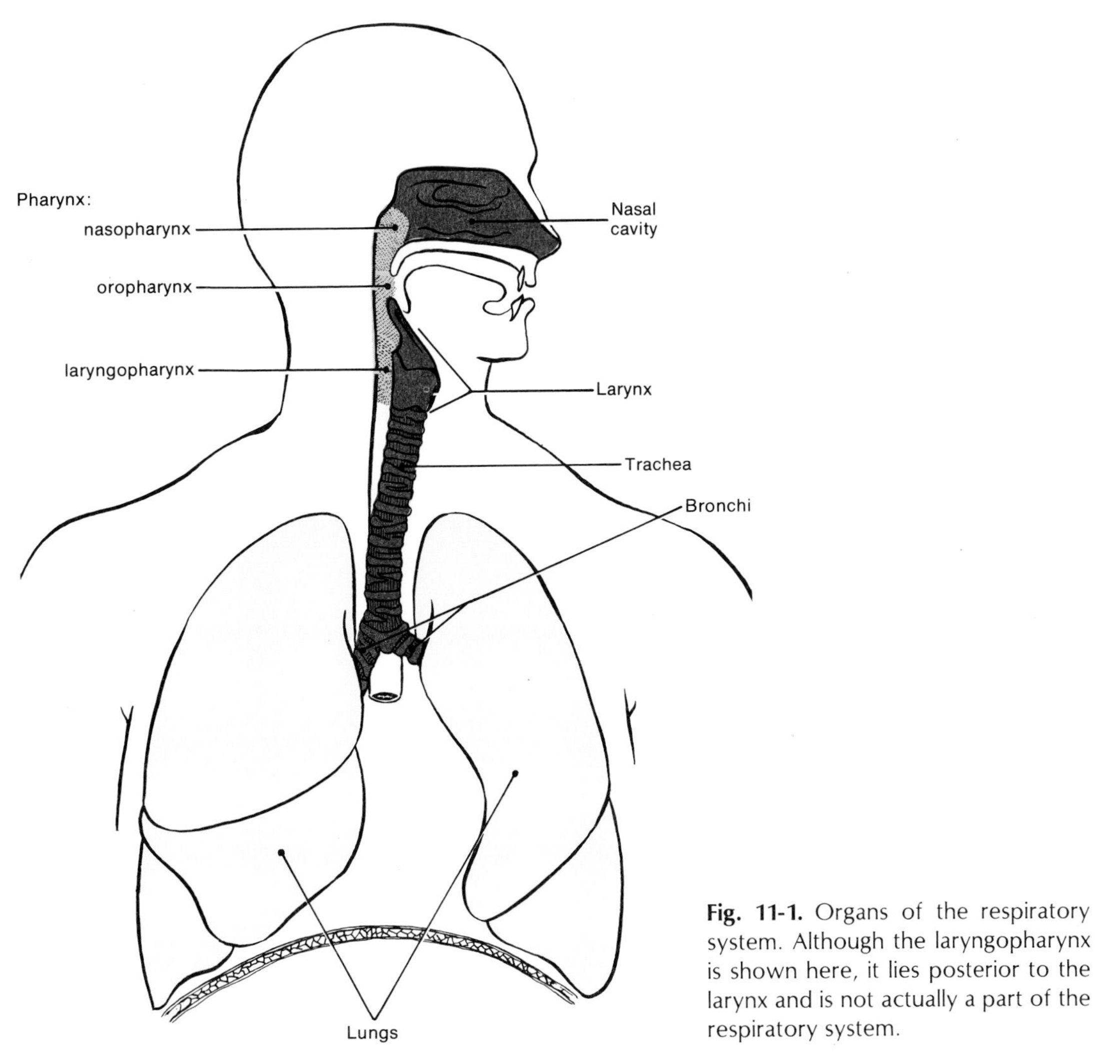

Fig. 11-1. Organs of the respiratory system. Although the laryngopharynx is shown here, it lies posterior to the larynx and is not actually a part of the respiratory system.

by the **hard palate**. Three bony projections, the **conchae**, occur along the lateral wall of each nasal cavity. The **superior** and **middle conchae** are parts of the ethmoid bone, whereas the **inferior concha** is a separate bone (see Chapter 7, Fig. 7-13). These curved structures increase the surface area and are highly vascularized; they thus are important in warming the air on its way to the lungs.

Paranasal Sinuses

Associated with the nasal cavities are four pairs of paranasal sinuses, each bearing the name of the bone in which it resides: **maxillary**, **frontal**, **ethmoidal**, and **sphenoidal** (Fig. 11-4). Each sinus communicates with the nasal cavity via a duct and tiny opening, thereby allowing serous fluid and mucus to drain downward, particularly from the frontal, ethmoidal, and sphenoidal sinuses. Drainage from the maxillary sinus is more difficult because its opening is located high on its medial wall. Each nasal cavity also receives the termination of the **nasolacrimal duct** which carries tears away from the eyes (see Chapter 12, Fig. 12-37).

Pharynx

The nasal cavities communicate posteriorly with the **nasopharynx**, which also contains an opening from each **pharyngotympanic (audi-**

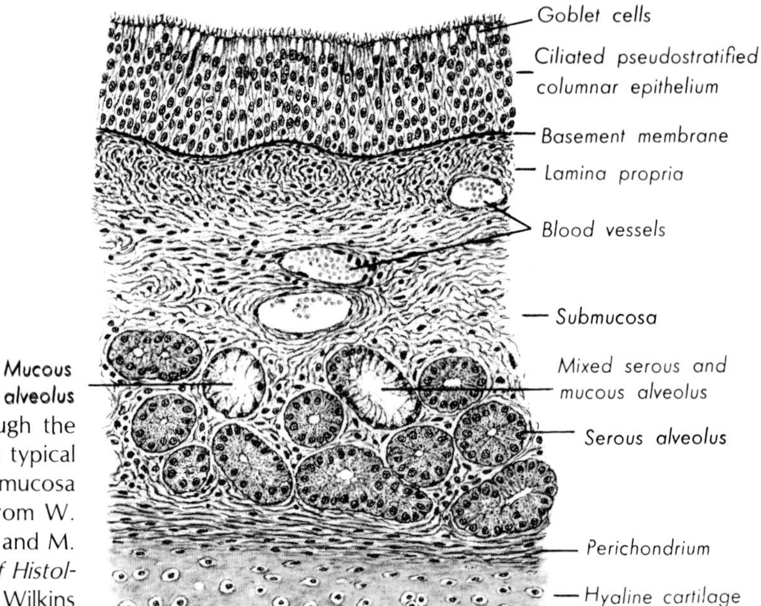

Fig. 11-2. Cross section through the wall of the trachea showing a typical respiratory mucosa and submucosa overlying hyaline cartilage. (From W. M. Copenhaver, R. P. Bunge, and M. B. Bunge, *Bailey's Textbook of Histology,* Ed. 16, The Williams & Wilkins Co., Baltimore, 1971.)

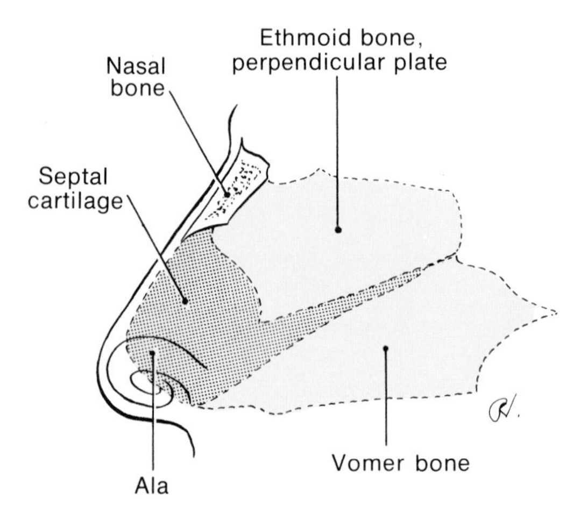

Fig. 11-3. Lateral view of the nasal septum indicated in yellow, of which the cartilaginous portion is stippled. The left ala is superimposed laterally.

tory, Eustachian) tube coming from the middle ear (Fig. 11-5). This provides a means for equalizing air pressure on the tympanic membrane (eardrum). The nasopharynx also contains masses of lymphoid tissue, the **pharyngeal tonsil**. Enlargement of this tissue **(adenoids)** can obstruct the nasopharynx and interfere with nasal breathing, thus forcing one to breathe through the mouth.

The **oropharynx** lies below the nasopharynx and is separated from it by the soft palate. It is a common chamber for both the respiratory and digestive systems. The **soft palate** is a fleshy plate of tissue which projects backward and slightly downward from the hard palate and permits air to pass from the nasopharynx to the oropharynx and larynx. When food or liquids are swallowed, the soft palate swings upward to prevent them from entering the nasopharynx.

A third portion of the pharynx is the **laryngopharynx** which lies behind the larynx (Fig. 11-1) and which communicates below with the esophagus of the digestive tract. The laryngopharynx is thus not considered a part of the respiratory system.

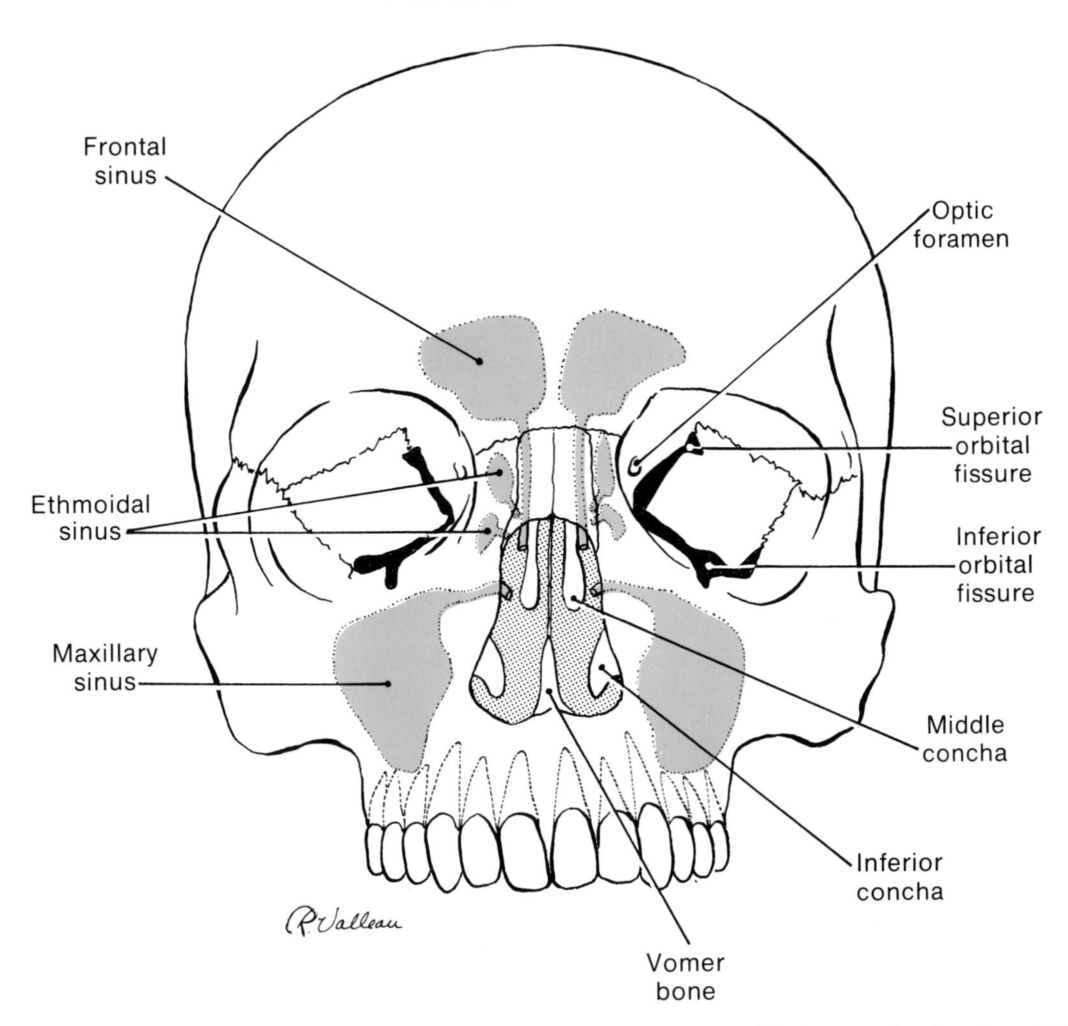

Fig. 11-4. Anterior view of the nasal cavities, orbits, and paranasal sinuses (blue) except for the sphenoidal sinus which is not indicated.

Microscopic Anatomy

The various regions of the nose are lined by epithelium, beneath which are variable amounts of connective tissue binding it to cartilage or bone. The vestibule of the nose is lined with a stratified squamous epithelium similar to the epidermis of the skin. It also contains numerous short thick hairs which are important as a first line of defense in trapping large particles of dirt. Most of each nasal cavity, including the conchae, is lined with typical respiratory epithelium (pseudostratified ciliated columnar epithelium with goblet cells and seromucous glands). A rich network of blood vessels occurs in the connective tissue beneath the epithelium, and these vessels help to warm the air as it passes along the walls of the passageways. Unfortunately, the vessels often become dilated in response to a virus infection, thereby creating nasal congestion. Moreover, this rich vascular network, as well as the larger vessels which supply it, may occasionally rupture, resulting in a nosebleed.

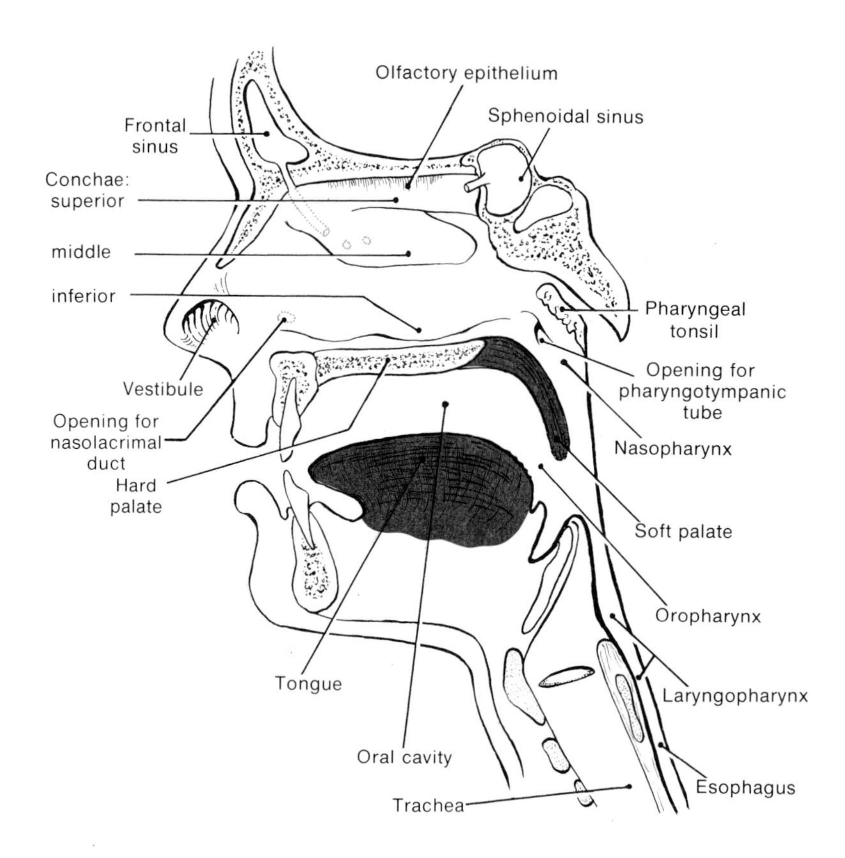

Fig. 11-5. Sagittal section of the head, with the nasal septum removed, showing the right lateral wall of the nasal cavity. *Dotted blue lines* indicate locations of openings for drainage from the paranasal sinuses and nasolacrimal duct.

In the uppermost region of the nasal cavities the epithelium is a specialized **olfactory epithelium** containing pseudostratified columnar **supporting cells** and spindle-shaped **nerve cells**. The nerve cells receive olfactory stimuli and transmit them to the brain via the olfactory nerve. When the nasal cavities are congested, air cannot reach the olfactory epithelium and one's sense of smell (olfaction) is dulled. The sensation of taste also depends on olfaction; therefore food may seem to be "tasteless" when the nasal cavities are swollen.

The paranasal sinuses and nasopharynx are lined with typical respiratory epithelium similar to that in the nasal cavities. However, in the nasopharynx there may be stratified squamous epithelium in localized regions where surfaces constantly come in contact (as in the region where the posterior border of the soft palate pushes against the wall of the nasopharynx). The oropharynx is lined with stratified squamous epithelium similar to that which lines the mouth. Both the nasopharynx and oropharynx are surrounded by connective tissue and by skeletal muscle fibers of the pharyngeal constrictor muscles.

LARYNX, TRACHEA, AND MAIN BRONCHI

Gross Anatomy

Larynx

The larynx transmits air to and from the oropharynx and trachea and is situated in the neck in front of the laryngopharynx and just inferior to the hyoid bone (Fig. 11-1). The larynx is composed primarily of cartilaginous plates and skeletal muscle arranged in the form of a triangular box, with the tapered end pointing downward. The three largest cartilages are unpaired: the thyroid, epiglottis, and cricoid. In addition, there are three pairs of smaller cartilages: arytenoid, corniculate, and cuneiform.

The **thyroid cartilage** is easily palpated since it occupies most of the anterior aspect of the larynx and contains a **median (thyroid) notch** on its upper border (Fig. 11-6). Inferior to the notch is a ridge, the **laryngeal prominence** (popularly called the "Adam's apple" and more prominent in males). The upper and lower borders of the thyroid cartilage bear horns (cornua) at each end. Each **superior horn** projects upward at right angles to the body of the hyoid bone, while each **inferior horn** forms a hingelike joint below with the cricoid cartilage, thereby allowing the thyroid cartilage to be tilted forward and backward.

The **epiglottis** is a leaf-shaped cartilage attached by means of a narrow stalk to the posterior surface of the thyroid cartilage (Fig. 11-6). The expanded portion of the epiglottis passes upward behind the hyoid bone toward the root of the tongue.

The **cricoid cartilage** marks the boundary between the larynx above and the trachea below. It also demarcates the level at which the laryngopharynx joins the esophagus. The cricoid cartilage is ring-shaped with a posterior expansion, on which sit the two **arytenoid cartilages**. These are triangular in shape, and each bears a small **corniculate cartilage** at its apex. The corniculate cartilages are embedded at the base of a fold of mucous membrane, the **aryepiglottic fold**, which extends upward from the apex of each arytenoid cartilage to the apex of the epiglottis. Also embedded in the aryepiglottic folds is a pair of **cuneiform** cartilages.

The larynx contains a pair of musculofibrous bands, the **vocal folds** ("true" vocal cords) which stretch in an anteroposterior direction between the bases of the arytenoid cartilages and the back of the thyroid cartilage (Fig. 11-6). A pair of larger **vestibular (ventricular) folds** ("false" vocal cords) is located just above the vocal folds. The vocal folds are vital in the production of sound (phonation) and surround an aperture of varying size (the **rima glottidis**). When one speaks, this aperture is reduced to a narrow slit as the vocal folds are brought together to vibrate in close approximation (Fig. 11-7). The vestibular folds are largely protective in function. They also help to close the larynx so as to produce an increase in intrathoracic and abdominal pressure, as occurs during straining or just prior to coughing and sneezing. Between the vestibular folds and vocal folds is a canoe-shaped cavity, the **ventricle**, from which a small **saccule** projects anteriorly. The saccule contains glands which help to lubricate the vocal folds and is sometimes called the "oil can" of the vocal folds.

The **laryngeal muscles** are skeletal muscles and can be divided into two groups: **extrinsic muscles** responsible for elevating or depressing the larynx (see Chapter 8), and a complex set of **intrinsic muscles** which produce changes in the length, position, and tension of the vocal folds.

Trachea

The trachea begins just inferior to the larynx and extends downward to the level of about the 5th thoracic vertebra where it divides into two main bronchi (Fig. 11-1). In the neck, the upper part of the trachea can be easily palpated. The trachea lies anterior to the esophagus and contains a series of 16–20 C-shaped cartilaginous rings which are incomplete pos-

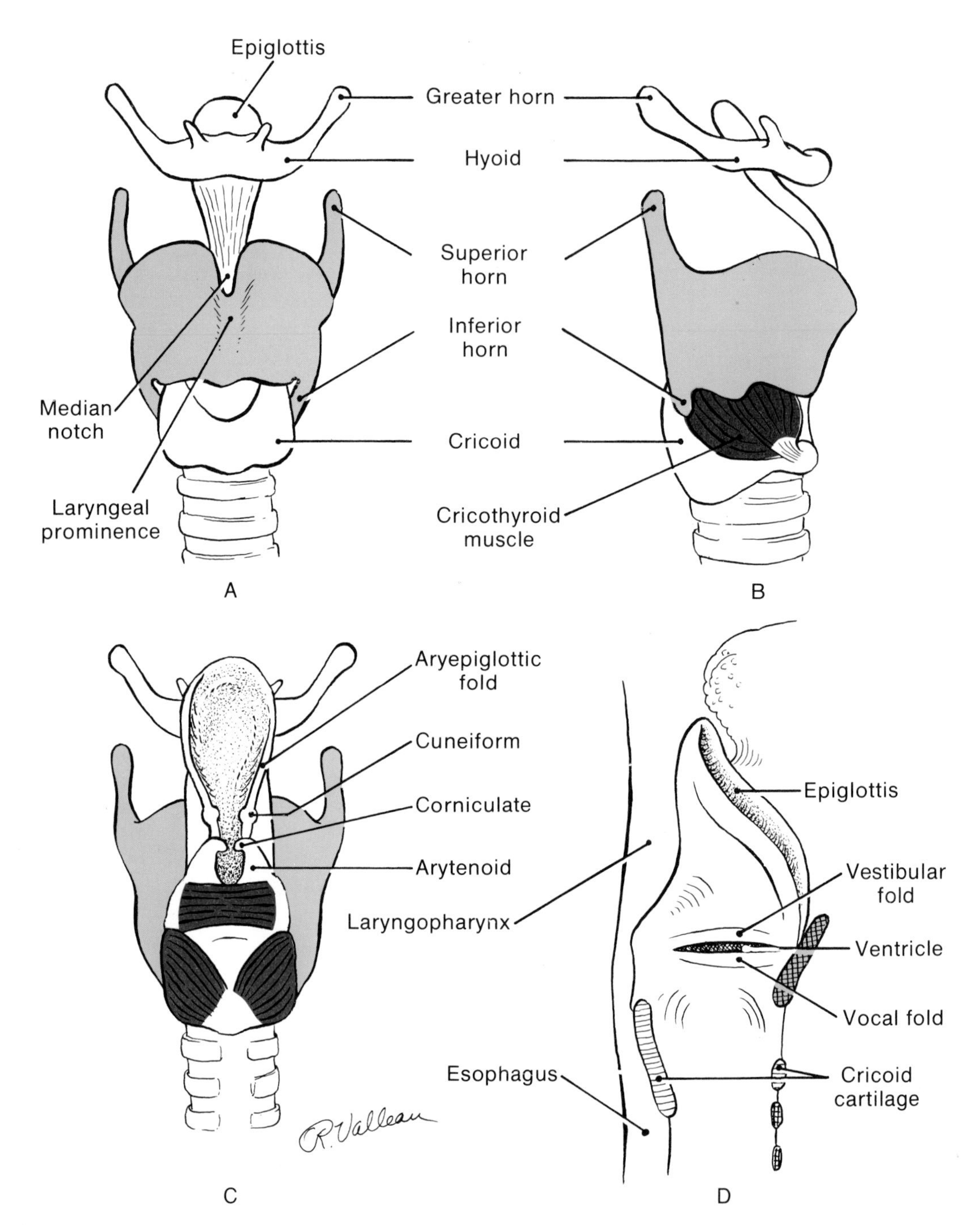

Fig. 11-6. Larynx. The thyroid cartilage is indicated in blue. (A) Anterior view, (B) lateral view, (C) posterior view, (D) sagittal section. Various intrinsic laryngeal muscles are indicated in B and C.

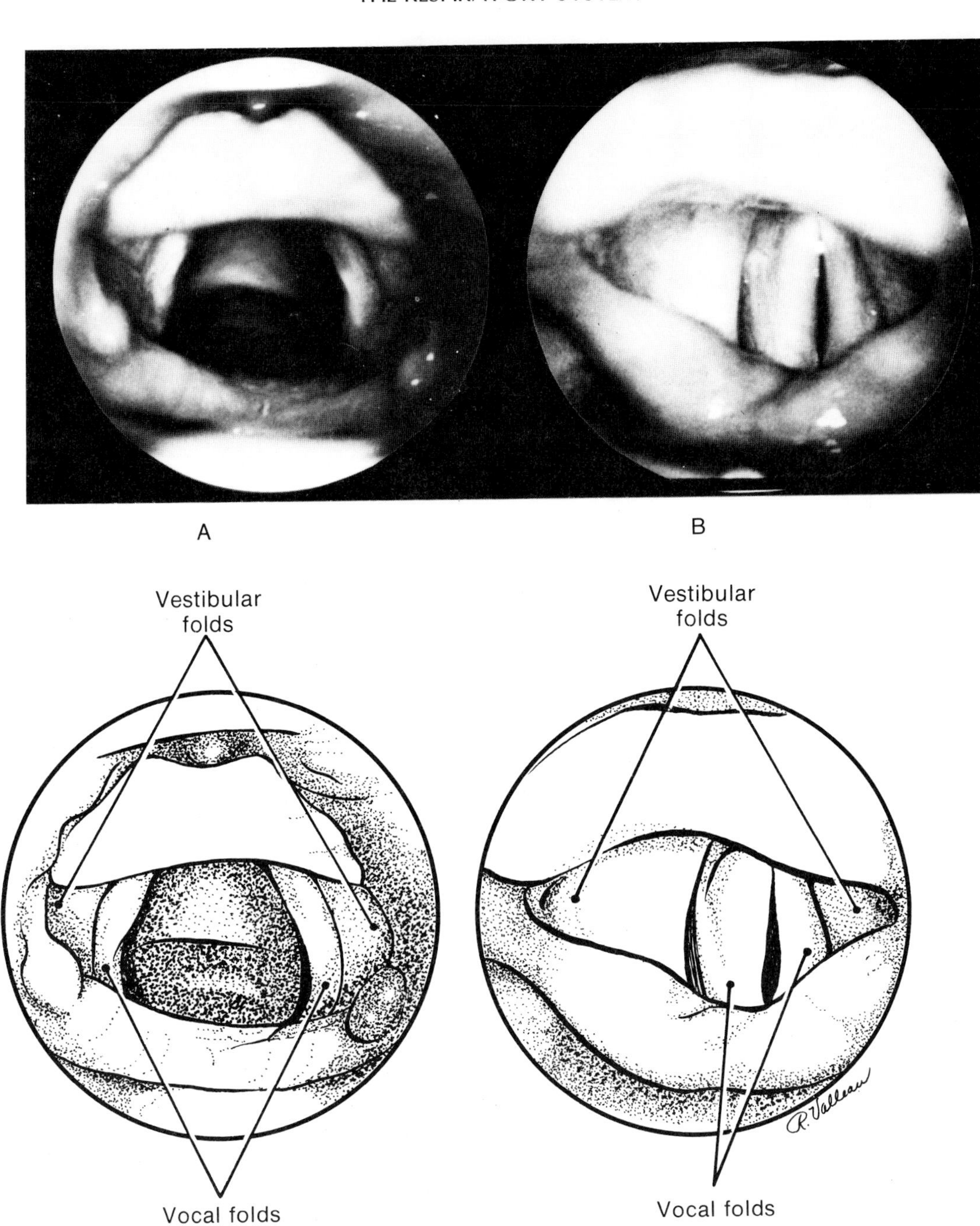

Fig. 11-7. Surface view of the glottis. (A, B) Viewed indirectly by means of a mirror placed against the posterior pharyngeal wall. In A, the vocal folds are open during respiration. In B, the folds are in approximation, as during speaking. (From E. D. Gardner, D. J. Gray, and R. O'Rahilly, Ed. 4, *Anatomy,* W. B. Saunders Co., Philadelphia, 1975.) (C, D) Diagrammatic sketches of views A and B.

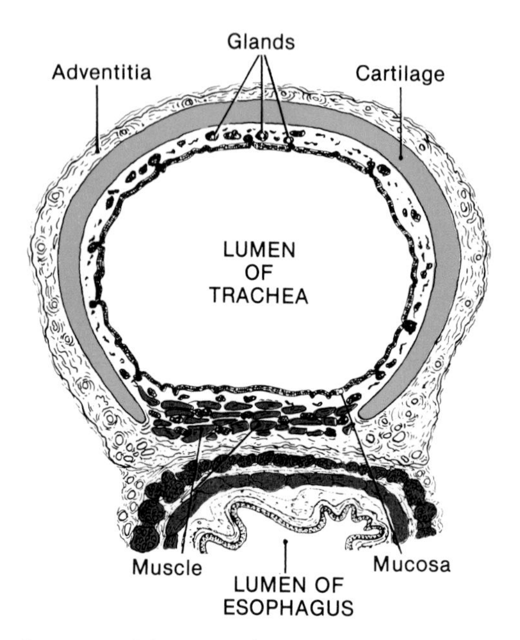

Fig. 11-8. Diagram of a transverse section through the trachea and anterior portion of the esophagus. (Modified after Copenhaver.)

teriorly. The gap between the open ends of the cartilages is bridged by connective tissue and a mass of smooth muscle (the trachealis muscle). The cartilage provides support and maintains an open airway, whereas the fibromuscular tissue permits the posterior wall of the trachea to accommodate to bulges produced by food passing downward in the esophagus lying immediately posterior to the trachea (Fig. 11-8).

Main Bronchi

Each main bronchus passes from the trachea to the lung. The right main bronchus is shorter and wider than the left one (Fig. 11-1). Also, the right main bronchus extends downward from the trachea in a more vertical plane; thus foreign objects are more likely to drop from the trachea into the right main bronchus. Both bronchi are structurally similar to the trachea but contain fewer cartilaginous rings.

Microscopic Anatomy

The larynx, trachea, and main bronchi are lined by respiratory mucosa consisting mainly of pseudostratified ciliated columnar epithelium with goblet cells overlying a lamina propria of connective tissue. Seromucous glands are common, and in the trachea they extend downward as tracheal glands into the submucosa (Figs. 11-2 and 11-8). In some parts of the larynx the epithelium is stratified squamous, particularly where surfaces continually come in contact with one another.

Much of the cartilage in the larynx is of the hyaline type, although the epiglottis, corniculate, and cuneiform cartilages are elastic. The tracheal and bronchial rings are composed of hyaline cartilage. The outer layer of the trachea and bronchi is called **adventitia** (fibrosa) and consists of loose connective tissue.

LUNGS

Gross Anatomy

The two lungs are situated in the thoracic cavity just above the diaphragm. Each lung is

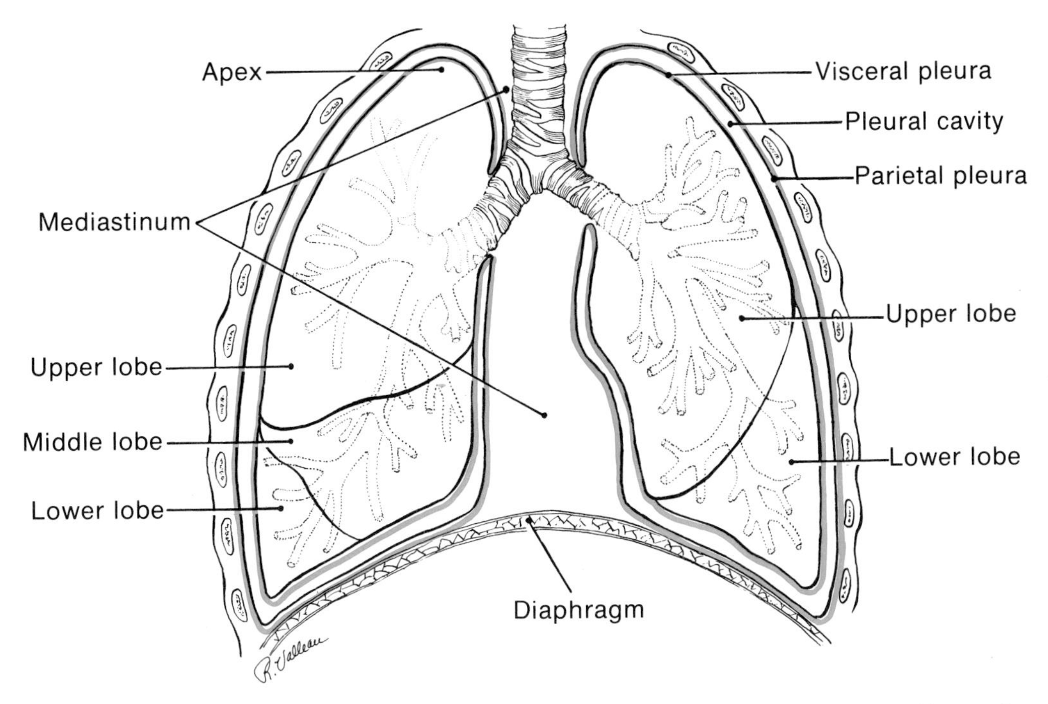

Fig. 11-9. The lungs within the thorax. The pleural cavities are exaggerated in size. *Dotted lines* indicate branching of bronchi.

housed within a **pleural sac** composed of a serous membrane. One portion of the sac is in close contact with the lung tissue and represents the **visceral pleura**; the other portion is in contact with the walls of the thoracic cage and upper surface of the diaphragm and is termed the **parietal pleura** (Fig. 11-9). The visceral and parietal pleura are closely associated with one another and are separated only by a thin film of fluid in a potential space, the **pleural cavity**. In the midline between the right and left pleural sacs is a wide area called the **mediastinum**, which contains a variety of structures, including the trachea, main bronchi, and pulmonary vessels.

The right lung consists of three **lobes** (upper, middle and lower) and the left lung consists of two (upper and lower). In both lungs much of the lower lobe lies posteriorly and thus cannot be easily seen from an anterior view. The **apex** of each lung projects upward into the neck. The **base** of each lung contains a concave diaphragmatic surface which follows the contour of the diaphragm. The costal surface of the lung lies against the thoracic cage, whereas the mediastinal surface faces the mediastinum.

Each lung is suspended by a main bronchus and pulmonary vessels leaving and entering the medial aspect of the lung at a region called the **hilus**. The right main bronchus divides into three **lobar bronchi**, one for each of the three lobes of the right lung; the left main bronchus divides into two lobar bronchi. Each lobar bronchus in turn divides into smaller branches called **segmental bronchi** which in turn undergo numerous subdivisions into smaller and smaller tubes to form the "bronchial tree." The linings of the trachea, main bronchi, lobar bronchi, and segmental bronchi can be viewed by means of **bronchoscopy** which involves passing a flexible tube (bronchoscope) along them.

A segmental bronchus supplies a discrete area of the lung termed a **bronchopulmonary segment** (Fig. 11-10). These segments are important clinically since a diseased segment can be removed surgically without interfering with the functioning of other portions of the lung.

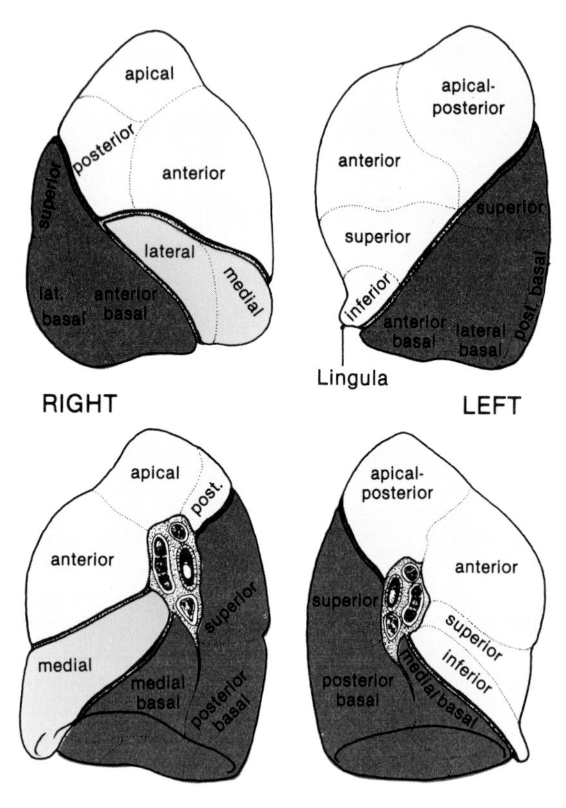

Fig. 11-10. Bronchopulmonary segments of the right and left lungs viewed laterally (*top*) and medially (*bottom*). Yellow, upper lobe; red, lower lobe; blue, middle lobe. (Modified after Grant.)

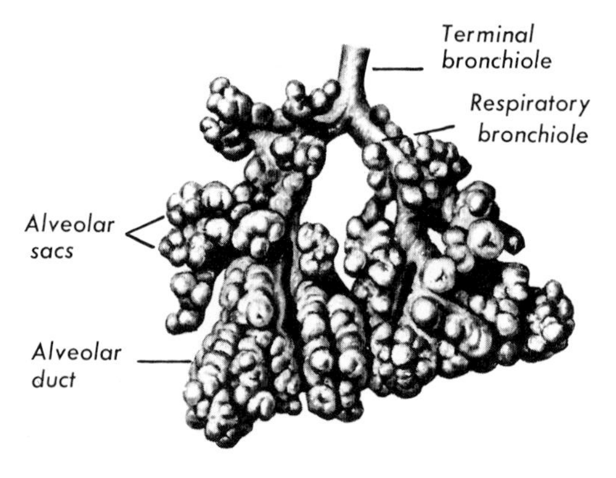

Fig. 11-11. Cast of a terminal bronchiole, respiratory bronchioles, alveolar ducts, and alveolar sacs. (Braus, after Loeschcke, from W. M. Copenhaver, R. P. Bunge, and M. B. Bunge, *Bailey's Textbook of Histology,* Ed. 16, The Williams & Wilkins Co., Baltimore, 1971.)

Microscopic Anatomy

The lobar and segmental bronchi are structurally similar to the main bronchi except that the cartilage is in the form of irregular, discontinuous plates rather than rings. The amount of cartilage gradually decreases in the more distal subdivisions of the bronchi while the amount of smooth muscle increases. During normal respiration, this smooth muscle contracts with expiration and relaxes with inspiration and thereby aids the flow of air. If the smooth muscle contracts abnormally, as in response to an irritant, bronchospasm may result.

When the cartilage disappears completely, the passageways are about 1 mm in diameter and are termed **bronchioles**. Further subdivisions of the bronchioles produce still smaller tubes called **terminal bronchioles**. At this point the epithelium is simple columnar or cuboidal, cilia are still present, but goblet cells and seromucous glands are lacking.

The terminal bronchioles lead into **respiratory bronchioles**, which have a few thin sacs (alveoli) bulging from their walls (Figs. 11-11 and 11-12). The respiratory bronchioles undergo further subdivisions, lose their cilia, and eventually lead into **alveolar ducts** whose walls consist entirely of alveoli.

Each **alveolus** is a sac composed mainly of simple squamous epithelium (type I cells) surrounded by a delicate network of elastic tissue and a capillary plexus. The extremely thin walls of the alveolar epithelium and capillary endothelium serve as a blood-air diffusion barrier, across which gases are exchanged between the air in the alveolus and the blood in the capillaries (Fig. 11-13). The alveolar epithelium has some cuboidal cells called great alveolar cells (type II cells) which produce surfactant, a substance which reduces surface tension. Surfactant production begins prenatally at about six months of gestation, and an absence or reduced amount of surfactant can lead to **hyaline membrane disease**, a major cause of death in premature infants. The alveolar epithelium also contains a phagocytic type of cell ("dust cell") serving as a scavenger to engulf particulate matter which may have slipped

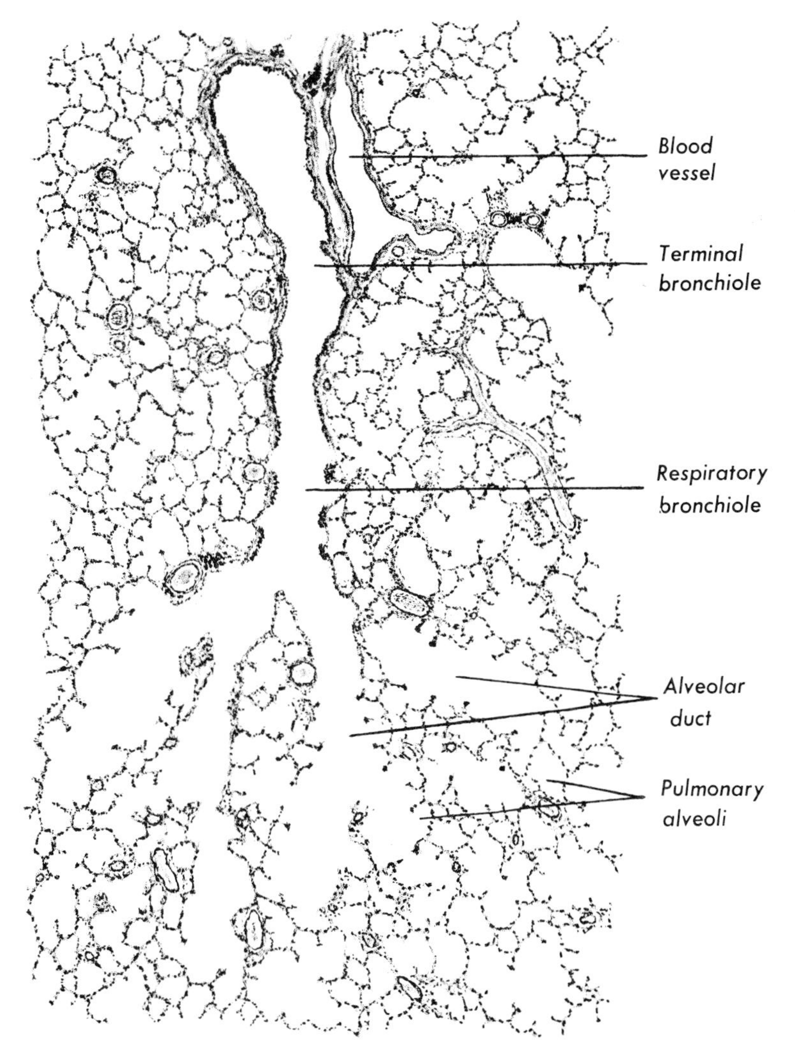

Fig. 11-12. Microscopic section through portion of a lung, including a terminal bronchiole, respiratory bronchiole, alveolar ducts, and alveoli. (From W. M. Copenhaver, R. P. Bunge, and M. B. Bunge, *Bailey's Textbook of Histology,* Ed. 16, The Williams & Wilkins Co., Baltimore, 1971.)

past the defenses of the upper respiratory passageways.

Blood Supply to the Lungs

Blood is brought to the lungs by two routes: the pulmonary arteries and the bronchial arteries. Each **pulmonary artery** divides into a number of branches which follow closely the bronchial tree (Fig. 11-14). The branches eventually form a capillary plexus around the alveoli, and the blood then drains back to the heart via **pulmonary veins**. Since the pulmonary arteries carry only deoxygenated blood, the walls of the bronchial tree depend on a separate system of **bronchial arteries** carrying oxygenated blood from the aorta.

BREATHING AND PHONATION

Normal breathing depends on a number of factors, including an efficient diaphragm and tho-

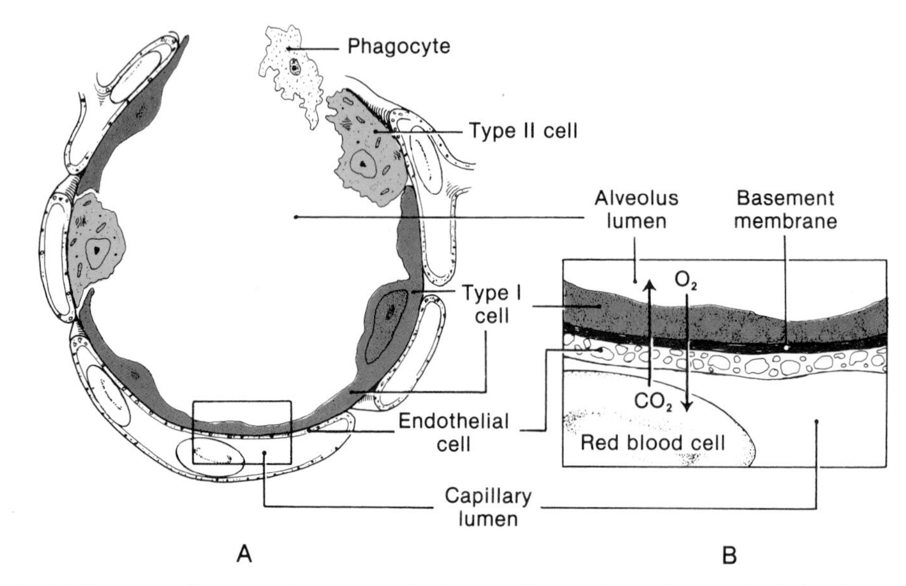

Fig. 11-13. (A) Diagram of an alveolus surrounded by capillaries. A portion of the "blood-air" barrier is enclosed by the rectangle and is shown at higher magnification in B.

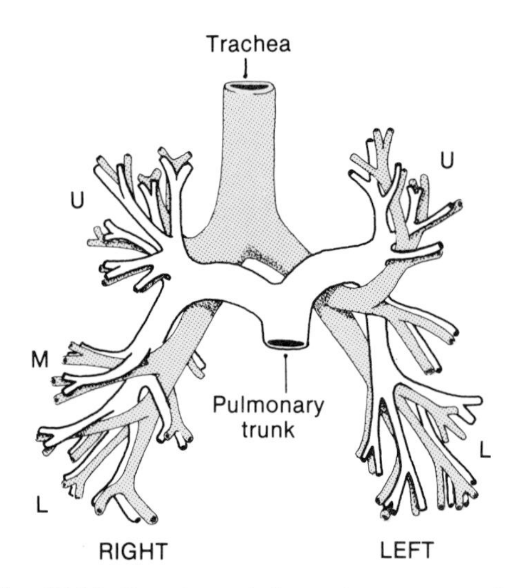

Fig. 11-14. Branches of the pulmonary arteries and their relationships to the bronchi, anterior view. U, M, L, branches to upper, middle, and lower lobes. (Modified after Grant.)

racic cage, a negative intrathoracic pressure, and elasticity of the lungs. Upon inspiration, the diaphragm contracts and moves downward and the ribs move upward, thereby increasing the volume of the thoracic cavity and lowering the intrathoracic pressure. As a result, additional air is passively drawn into the respiratory passageways, further expanding the elastic tissue of the lungs (Fig. 11-15). During expiration the diaphragm relaxes and moves upward and the ribs move downward, resulting in a decrease in the size of the thoracic cavity. Much of the air is thereby forced out of the lungs, and the elastic tissue recoils. However, a certain amount of air is always retained in the lungs as residual air.

Phonation (vocalization) involves the production of sound, as in speaking or singing. During expiration the air passes upward through the trachea and larynx, causing the vocal folds to vibrate. The tension and position of the vocal folds is controlled by the laryngeal muscles. (The vocal folds in males are somewhat longer than in females and thus produce a lower pitch.) The pharyngeal, oral, and nasal cavities as well as the paranasal sinuses serve as

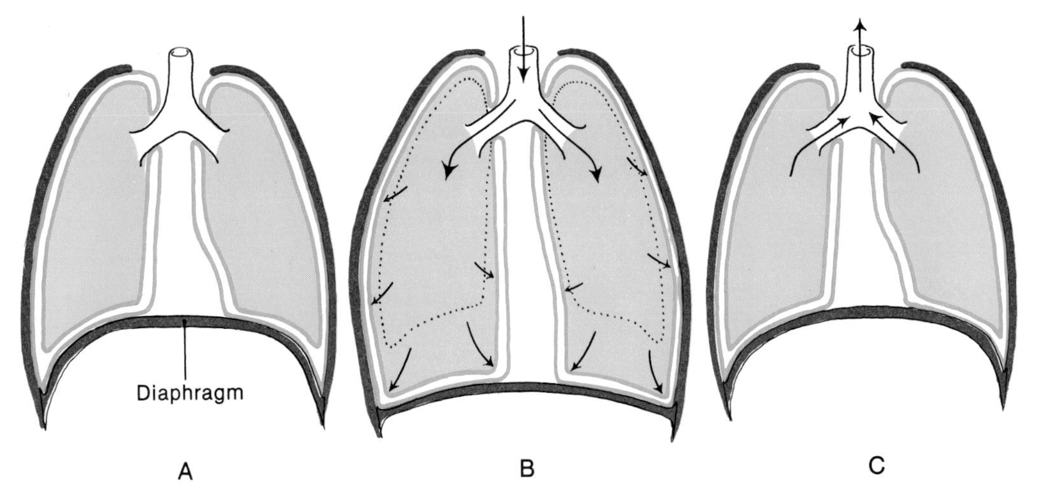

Fig. 11-15. The mechanics of breathing. (A) "Resting" position. (B) Inspiration: the diaphragm contracts and descends, and the ribs elevate, thereby increasing the size of the thoracic cavity, and air is drawn into the lungs. The *dotted lines* represent the initial size of the lungs, and the *arrows* show the direction and degree of expansion. (C) Expiration: the diaphragm relaxes and ascends, and the ribs return to their "resting" position, thereby decreasing the size of the thoracic cavity, and air rushes out of the lungs.

resonating chambers. The importance of these cavities becomes obvious when they become congested, producing the dull sounds typical of someone with a common cold. The tongue, soft palate, and lips are responsible for producing the wide range of vowels and consonants characteristic of human speech.

DEVELOPMENTAL AND CLINICAL ANATOMY

The major portion of the respiratory system develops initially as an endodermally lined tube from the ventral aspect of the foregut (Fig. 11-16). The upper portion of this tube becomes the larynx and retains its connection with the foregut, whereas the remainder of the tube separates from the foregut and develops into the trachea which bifurcates distally into two **lung buds**. The lung buds continue to subdivide and ultimately form the bronchial tree.

Occasionally the trachea does not separate completely from the portion of the foregut which becomes the esophagus. A communication or fistula thus occurs between the trachea and esophagus, allowing digestive contents to get into the respiratory system and possibly leading to pneumonia in the newborn infant. However, with early diagnosis such congenital defects can be surgically corrected before the condition becomes fatal.

The lining of the pharynx and posterior portion of the oral cavity are endodermally derived from the upper foregut; the lining of the anterior portion of the oral cavity is ectodermally derived from an invagination known as the **stomodeum** (see Chapter 14). The nasal cavities are also ectodermal derivatives which develop from indentations **(olfactory pits)** of the epidermis above the stomodeum.

A number of difficulties can occur postnatally in the respiratory system. Breathing can be impaired if the diaphragm or thoracic muscles are injured or become paralyzed. Also, if the pleural cavity is punctured, the atmospheric air rushes inward and creates a condition known as **pneumothorax** whereby the pressure in the cavity increases, and the lung becomes compressed and collapses. Since each lung is surrounded by its own pleural cavity, a

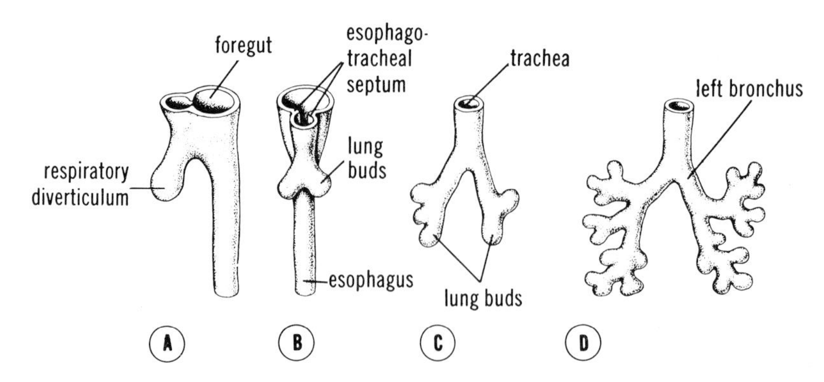

Fig. 11-16. Development of the trachea and lungs. (A) Lateral view showing the respiratory diverticulum from the foregut, (B, C, D) anterior views at successive stages of development. The trachea bifurcates into lung buds which then subdivide to form the bronchial tree. (From J. Langman, *Medical Embryology*, Ed. 3, The Williams & Wilkins Co., Baltimore, 1975.)

pneumothorax on one side will not affect the function of the opposite lung.

Occasionally the pleurae may become irritated and inflamed, resulting in **pleurisy**. If large amounts of fluid are secreted into the pleural cavity **(pleural effusion)**, the lung can become compressed. **Emphysema** involves an abnormal expansion of the alveoli (usually in response to chronic irritation, as in smoking) so that the alveolar membrane becomes damaged, whereas **pneumonia** results from an infection in which the alveoli become filled with fluid. In both instances the exchange of gases is impaired. **Bronchitis** is an inflammation of the bronchial passageways; **laryngitis** specifically affects the larynx.

12

The Nervous System

The nervous system is the most complex and least understood organ system in the body. Indeed, an entire subdivision of the field of anatomy, **neuroanatomy**, is devoted to the study of the nervous system. Nervous tissue is characterized by its capacity to conduct impulses. It serves an important function in keeping the body in touch with its external environment while at the same time regulating the activities of other organ systems so that vital bodily functions are coordinated with one another. In addition, the nervous system provides each of us with a sense of awareness or "consciousness" and enables us to think, reason, remember, and to perceive and experience emotions.

Nervous tissue consists of two basic cell types: **neurons** (nerve cells) which conduct impulses, and **supporting cells** which are nonconducting cells assisting the neurons. Each neuron consists of a **nerve cell body** (which contains the nucleus and surrounding cytoplasm) and cytoplasmic extensions (processes) of various lengths (Fig. 12-1). One of these processes, the **axon**, tends to be longer than the others and usually conducts impulses away from the nerve cell body. Other processes called **dendrites** are shorter, more numerous than axons, and carry impulses to the cell body.

Neurons communicate with one another via specialized areas called **synapses** (Fig. 12-2). Chemicals known as neurotransmitter substances are released from tiny vesicles at the end of an axon of one neuron, flow across the synaptic area, and initiate an impulse in the dendrite or the cell body of a second neuron. Some nerve cell processes are ensheathed by elaborate layers of plasma membranes from supporting cells and are thus said to be **myelinated** nerve fibers. Processes which lack this elaborate covering of membranes are **unmyelinated** fibers.

Both myelinated and unmyelinated fibers may be bundled together outside of the brain and spinal cord in structures called **nerves**. Concentrations of nerve cell bodies outside of the brain and spinal cord are termed **ganglia** (Fig. 12-3). Within the brain and spinal cord, bundles of nerve fibers are termed **tracts**, whereas clusters of nerve cell bodies are called **nuclei**. Details on the microscopic anatomy of nervous tissue are presented in Chapter 4.

The nervous system is organized into two basic subdivisions: (1) the **central nervous system (CNS)** consisting of the brain and spinal cord, and (2) the **peripheral nervous system (PNS)** consisting of the cranial and spinal nerves plus other nerve cell processes and cell bodies lying outside the central nervous system. One should keep in mind that the CNS and PNS are interconnected and that portions of an individual neuron may be found in both systems (Fig. 12-3). The nervous system can also be subdivided functionally into the **somatic** nervous system which controls primarily vol-

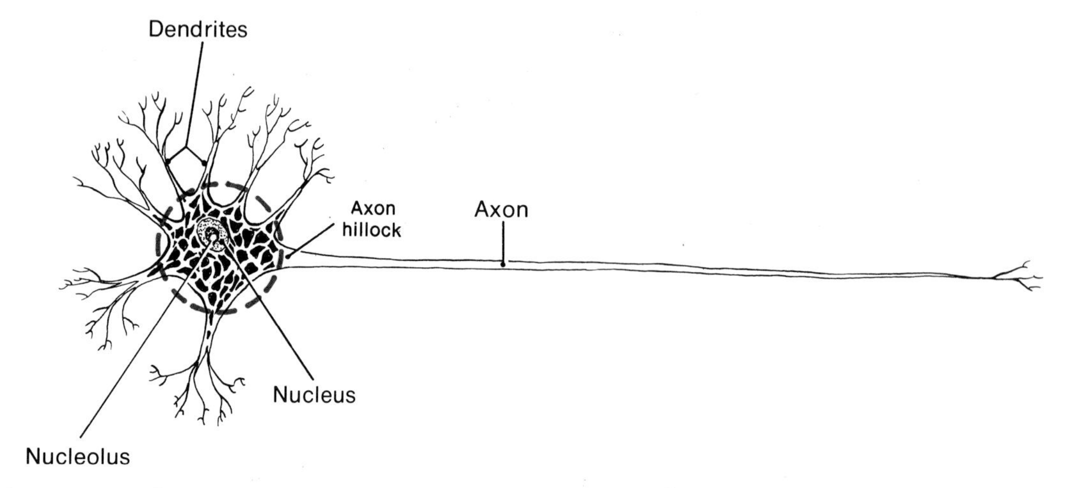

Fig. 12-1. Diagram of a typical neuron. The red *broken line* delimits the nerve cell body. The axon is usually considerably longer than depicted here.

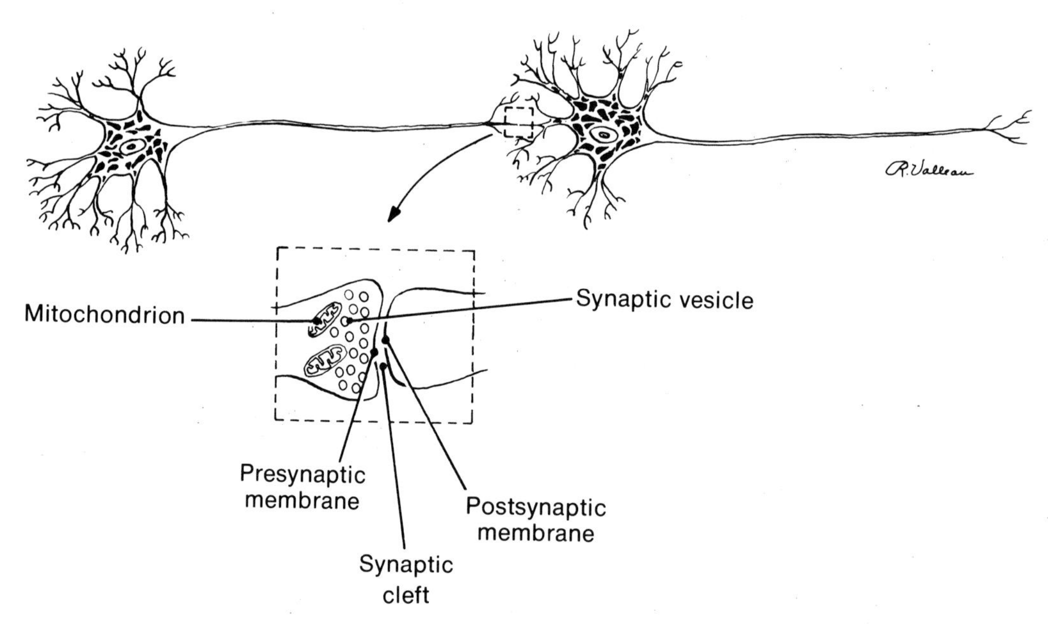

Fig. 12-2. Two neurons, with synaptic area enclosed in rectangle. *Arrow* points to higher magnification of the synaptic area. (Axon is on left; dendrite on right.)

untary activities and the **autonomic** nervous system which controls primarily involuntary activities. The autonomic nervous system is further subdivided into **sympathetic** and **parasympathetic** portions, both of which will be described in detail later.

The nervous system consists of a network of neurons interacting with each other via synapses and neurotransmitters. This interaction is illustrated by a **simple reflex arc** where sensory and motor neurons form a functional pathway. Impulses originating in the PNS are carried by **sensory (afferent)** neurons to the CNS. **Internuncial** neurons, located entirely within the CNS, receive the impulses from sensory neurons and transmit them to motor neurons or to other neurons in the CNS. **Motor (efferent)** neurons carry impulses away from the CNS via the PNS to effector organs (muscles and glands).

An example of a simple reflex arc which involves three neurons in sequence occurs in response to a painful stimulus. If you place your finger on a hot burner, the sensory impulses are carried along sensory nerve fibers into the spinal cord where they are transferred to internuncial neurons which transmit the impulses to motor neurons. The motor neurons carry motor impulses out to the periphery and cause skeletal muscle fibers to contract and to reflexively pull your finger away from the source of pain. (Meanwhile sensory impulses also travel up the spinal cord to higher centers located in the brain and you become aware of heat and pain.)

An even simpler reflex involves only two consecutive neurons and occurs as the well-known **patellar reflex (knee jerk)** when the knee is in the flexed position and the tendon below the patella (kneecap) is lightly tapped (Fig. 12-4). This causes stretch receptors (called muscle spindles) in the associated muscles to send an impulse along sensory nerve fibers to the spinal cord. In the spinal cord the impulse is transferred directly to a motor neuron to be carried out to the limb muscles which contract and cause the flexed leg to kick forward. If this reflex is reduced or absent, then it is likely that there is damage somewhere in the reflex arc.

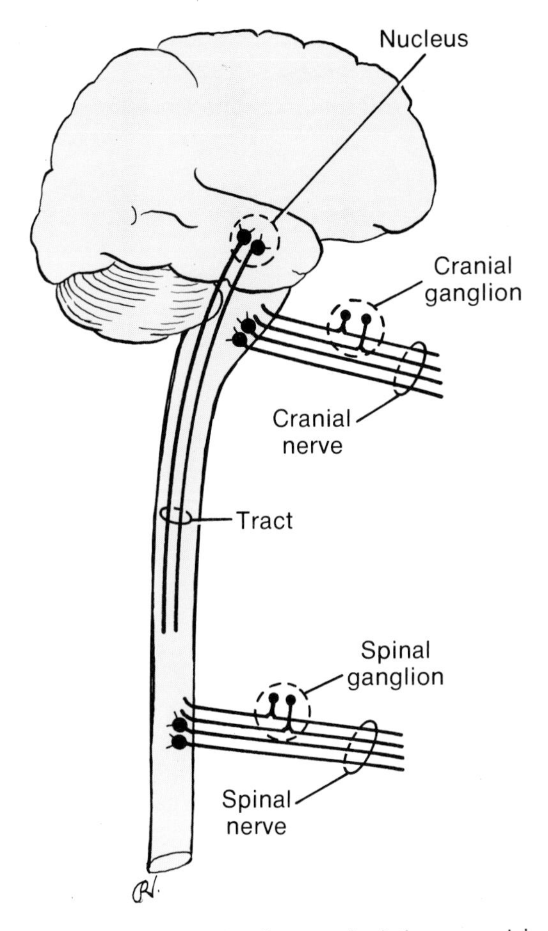

Fig. 12-3. Schematic diagram depicting a cranial ganglion, cranial nerve, spinal ganglion, spinal nerve, nucleus, and tract. These structures are shown greatly enlarged relative to the size of the brain and spinal cord (in blue).

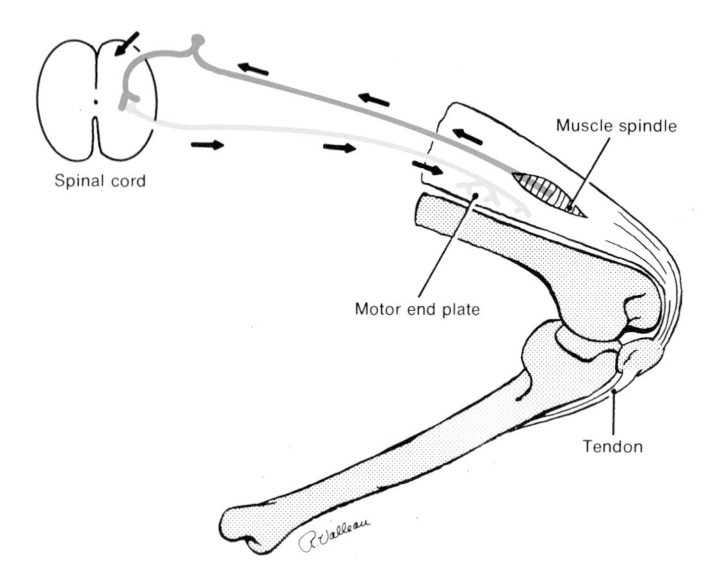

Fig. 12-4. Pathway of the reflex arc for the patellar reflex (knee jerk). *Arrows* indicate the direction of flow along one sensory (afferent) neuron (blue) and one motor (efferent) neuron (yellow).

Although this reflex does not depend on the brain, the force of the contraction is modulated by mild inhibitory impulses coming from the brain. If there is some damage to the pathway carrying this modulation, then the reflex is exaggerated. For this reason, the patellar reflex is routinely tested not only to indicate whether the reflex arc is intact, but also to determine whether higher centers of modulation are functioning properly.

Some pathways in the nervous system carry sensory impulses from the periphery into the spinal cord and from there upward into the brain where they are perceived. Such **sensory pathways** are often characterized by three consecutive neurons: a first order neuron (most of which lies in the PNS), a second order neuron in the spinal cord, and a third order neuron in the brain. Other pathways carry motor impulses from the brain down the spinal cord and out to peripheral effector organs. These **motor pathways** are also frequently represented by three neurons: a first order neuron which initiates the impulse in the brain, a second order neuron in the brain or spinal cord, and a third order neuron whose nerve cell body is in the spinal cord but whose axon passes out from the CNS as part of a peripheral nerve in the PNS.

CENTRAL NERVOUS SYSTEM (CNS)

The brain and spinal cord are housed within and protected by the skull and vertebral column, respectively. In addition, there are three layers of connective tissue membranes called **meninges** which immediately surround and protect the brain and spinal cord. The outermost layer of the meninges is the **dura mater**, a tough fibrous membrane which adheres closely to the inner aspect of the skull and vertebral column (Fig. 12-5). In the skull the dura mater shows inner and outer layers, and in some regions the inner layer of the dura mater dips inward to form a septum partially separating portions of the brain. One example is the **falx cerebri** which passes downward between the two cerebral hemispheres.

The two layers of the dura mater are ordinarily in close contact, except in regions where they enclose venous sinuses (such as the superior sagittal sinus). The sinuses carry venous blood from the brain and meninges back to the heart via veins in the neck (internal jugular veins).

In the region of the vertebral column the dura mater is separated from the bony wall of the vertebral canal by an **epidural space** con-

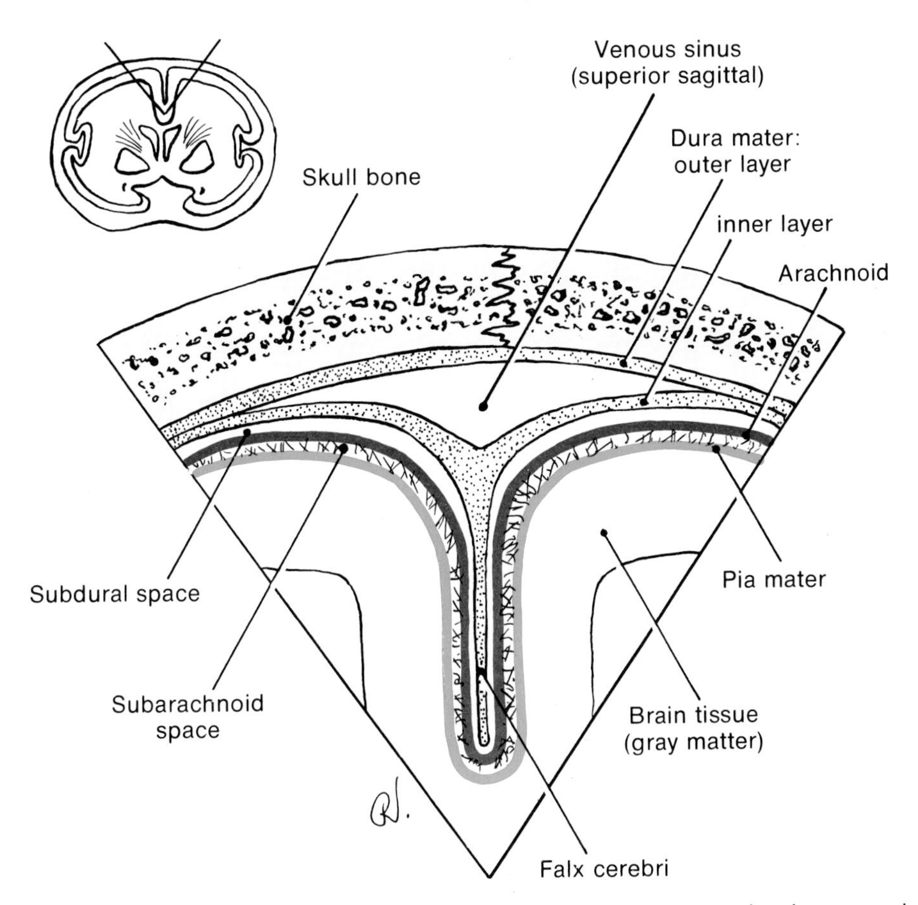

Fig. 12-5. Meninges of the brain in the region indicated by V-shaped wedge on sketch at upper left. (The subdural space is exaggerated.)

taining vertebral venous sinuses. In the skull there normally is no epidural space unless bleeding occurs from damaged meningeal blood vessels, in which case the blood artificially creates an epidural space as it seeps between the dura mater and skull bones. Such an epidural hemorrhage poses a serious threat as it develops into a clot (epidural hematoma) which eventually can compress the brain.

The middle layer of meninges is the **arachnoid**, a weblike filmy membrane which is separated from the dura mater by a potential space, the **subdural** space. (A subdural hematoma can form here if blood seeps into the space from injured meningeal vessels.) Beneath the arachnoid is a substantial cavity, the **subarachnoid space** containing **cerebrospinal fluid** as well as some delicate connective tissue fibers. The innermost layer of the meninges is the **pia mater** which adheres closely to the surface of the brain and spinal cord.

Spinal Cord

The spinal cord extends caudally from the foramen magnum, the opening at the base of the skull, to approximately the level of the first or second lumbar vertebra. Beyond this point the pia mater continues caudally a short distance as a connective tissue projection, the **filum terminale** (Fig. 12-6). The subarachnoid space, arachnoid, and dura mater extend downward

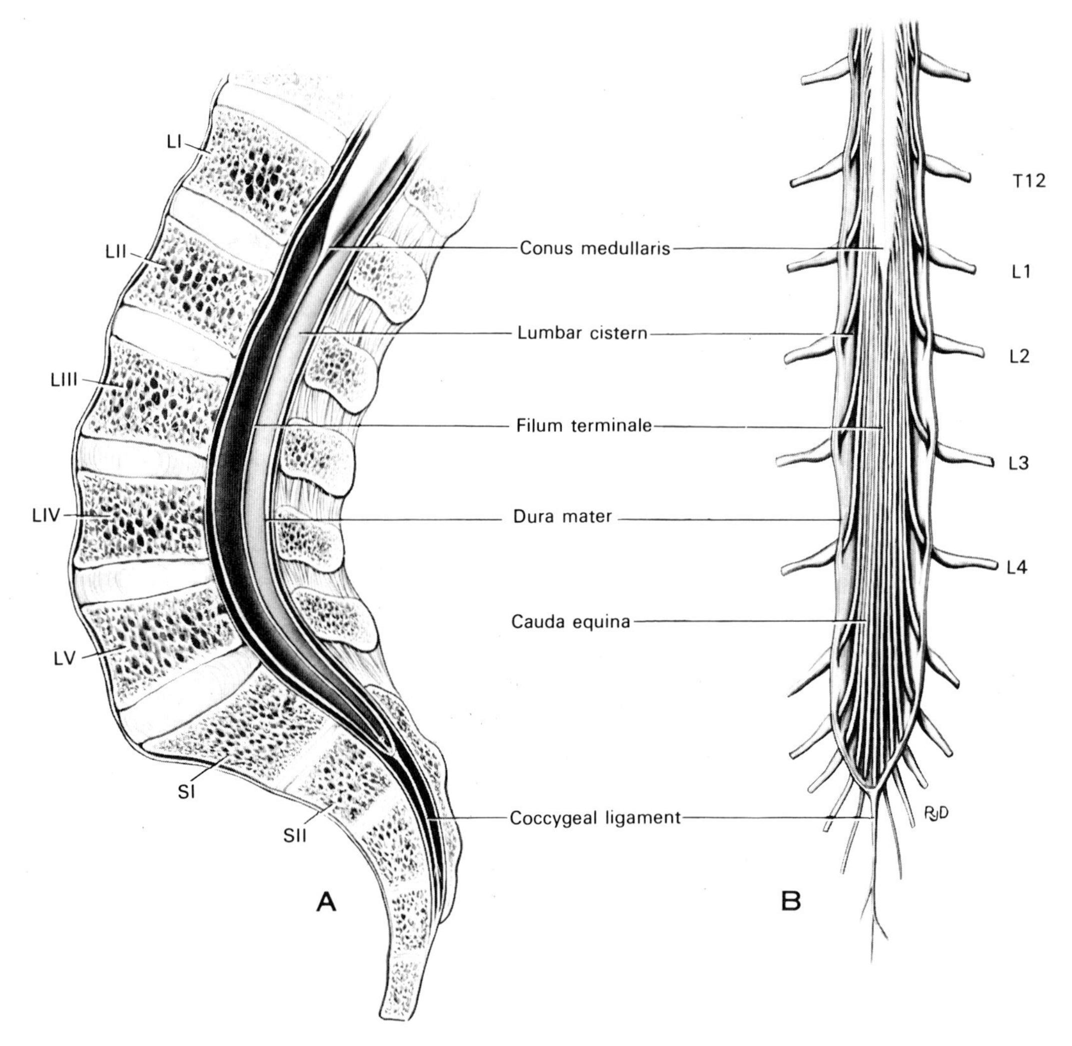

Fig. 12-6. (A) Sagittal section of lower portion of spinal cord and vertebral column, (B) posterior view of lower portion of spinal cord. (From M. B. Carpenter, *Human Neuroanatomy,* Ed. 7, The Williams & Wilkins Co., Baltimore, 1976.)

well beyond the ending of the spinal cord. For this reason, cerebrospinal fluid can be withdrawn from the subarachnoid space in the lower lumbar region by means of a diagnostic procedure known as a lumbar puncture ("spinal tap") without risk of damage to the spinal cord.

The spinal cord exhibits a prominent enlargement in the cervical region and in the lumbar region (Fig. 12-7). These reflect the large numbers of nerve cell bodies which give rise to the pairs of spinal nerves supplying the upper and lower limbs. At the lowermost levels of the cord the spinal nerves take a downward course before emerging from the vertebral canal. This vertical mass of spinal nerves is called the **cauda equina** because of its resemblance to a horse's tail (Figs. 12-6 and 12-7).

A cross section of the spinal cord shows an H-shaped mass of **gray matter** surrounded by a rim of **white matter** (Fig. 12-8). The gray matter consists mainly of nerve cell bodies; the white matter contains axons, most of which are myelinated. In the middle of the crossbar of the H is a tiny **central canal** which may be partially or completely obliterated. The anterior aspect of the spinal cord is characterized by a wide indentation, the **anterior median fissure**, whereas the posterior aspect contains merely a narrow slit, the **posterior median sulcus**.

The gray matter is organized into two posterior (dorsal) horns and two anterior (ventral) horns. The **posterior horns** contain nerve cell bodies of neurons which receive sensory impulses passing into the spinal cord. The neurons in the posterior horns then transmit the impulses to other regions of the central nervous system and are designated as **internuncial neurons**. The nerve cell bodies in the **anterior horns** transmit motor impulses out from the spinal cord. In the thoracic and upper lumbar regions there is also a **lateral horn** composed of neurons belonging to the autonomic system.

The white matter is organized into anterior, lateral, and posterior columns called **funiculi**. Each funiculus contains bundles of axons known as **tracts**. Those tracts which ascend from lower regions of the spinal cord to higher regions or to the brain tend to be sensory; those which descend downward from the brain and upper regions of the cord are usually motor.

Each tract carries impulses of like nature. This is clinically important since the site of damage to the spinal cord can be determined on the basis of which sensations or motor functions are disturbed. Tracts are often named on the basis of the direction in which the impulses pass; thus, the spinothalamic tract sends impulses from the spinal cord upward to the thalamic region of the brain, whereas the corticospinal tract transmits impulses from the cortex of the brain to the spinal cord.

Ascending tracts

The following are some of the more important ascending tracts which carry sensory impulses from lower regions upward to the brain. The **fasciculus gracilis** and **fasciculus cuneatus** are situated in the posterior funiculus (dorsal column) (Fig. 12-8). These two tracts carry impulses concerned with touch, pressure, and a

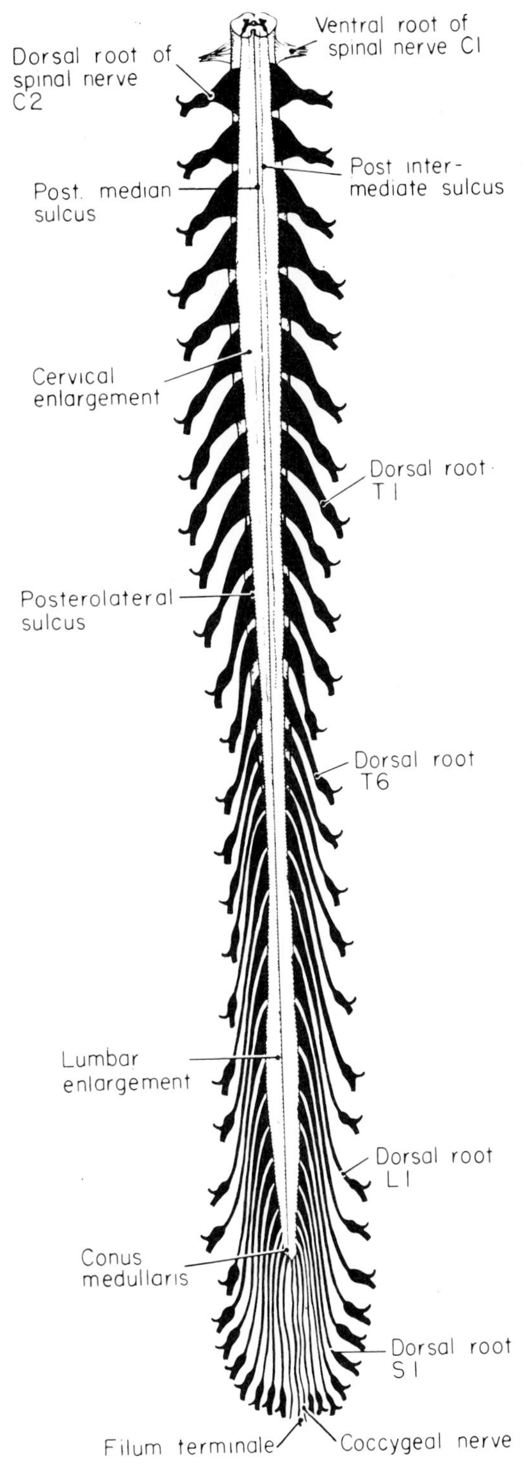

Fig. 12-7. Spinal cord and nerve roots, posterior view. (From M. B. Carpenter, *Human Neuroanatomy,* Ed. 7, The Williams & Wilkins Co., Baltimore, 1976.)

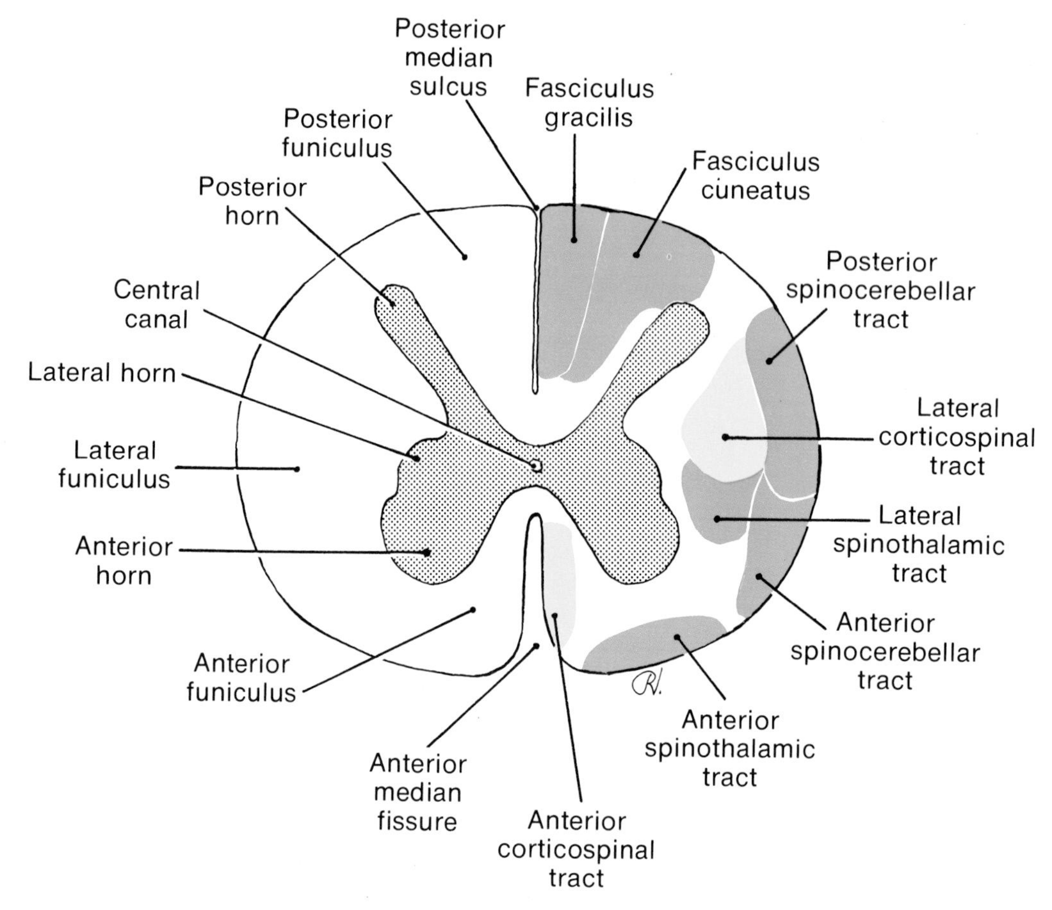

Fig. 12-8. Schematic cross section of spinal cord showing arrangement of gray matter (stippled gray) and white matter. Major ascending (sensory) tracts of the white matter are indicated in blue; major descending (motor) tracts are in yellow.

sense of position and movement (kinesthesis). These sensations are ultimately perceived in upper regions of the brain.

Ascending tracts in the lateral funiculus include the **anterior** and **posterior spinocerebellar tracts** which transmit impulses concerning the position of various portions of the body. Although this information is not consciously perceived, it enables the cerebellar region of the brain to coordinate complex movements. The lateral funiculus also carries the **lateral spinothalamic tract** which is very important in that it conveys impulses for pain and heat. An **anterior spinothalamic tract** runs in the anterior funiculus and is concerned with light touch.

Descending Tracts

Various descending tracts carry motor impulses from the brain or upper regions of the spinal cord to lower regions of the body. The most important descending tracts are the **lateral corticospinal tract** and **anterior corticospinal tract**, which are located in the lateral and anterior funiculi, respectively. These tracts convey voluntary motor impulses from the brain. (In the cervical and upper thoracic levels of the spinal cord there are also motor tracts

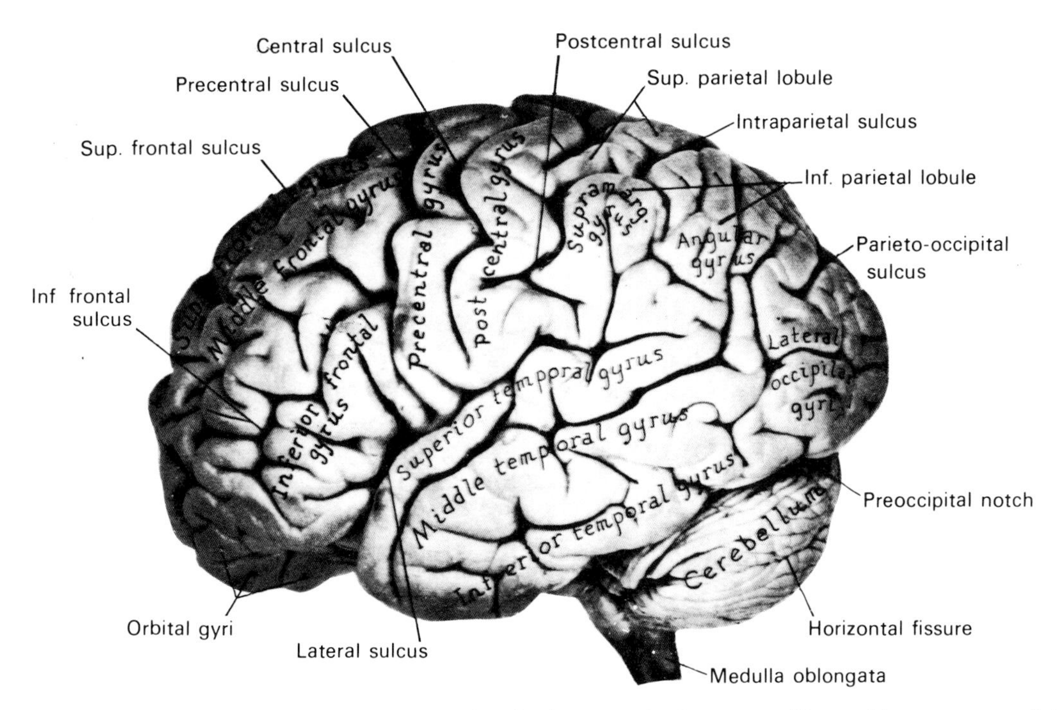

Fig. 12-9. Lateral view of the brain from the left side. (From M. B. Carpenter, *Human Neuroanatomy,* Ed. 7, The Williams & Wilkins Co., Baltimore, 1976.)

concerned with the regulation of muscle tone and with adjustments in posture.)

Brain

General Features

The brain receives and processes sensory information, controls voluntary and involuntary movements, and is the site of various ill-defined attributes such as consciousness, emotions, memory, and thought. The brain consists of three basic regions: the cerebral hemispheres, brain stem, and cerebellum. The **cerebral hemispheres** and **cerebellum** show similarities to one another in that the gray matter is located in the periphery and the white matter lies centrally, in contrast to the situation in other regions of the brain and in the spinal cord where the gray matter occupies a central position with the white matter located peripherally. The cerebral hemispheres and cerebellum also show a series of ridges on their external surfaces (Fig. 12-9). The **brain stem** is the median portion of the brain which connects the cerebral hemispheres and cerebellum to the spinal cord (Fig. 12-10).

Cerebral Hemispheres

The two cerebral hemispheres together are termed the **cerebrum**, the largest portion of the human brain. The hemispheres are separated from each other in the median plane by the **longitudinal fissure**, except for a transverse band of fibers, the **corpus callosum**, which connects the two hemispheres ventrally (Fig. 12-11). The longitudinal fissure contains the **falx cerebri**, a sheet of dura mater extending downward between the cerebral hemispheres (Fig. 12-5).

The external surfaces of the cerebral hemispheres are characterized by ridges called **gyri** (singular: gyrus) which are partially separated from one another by shallow fissures termed **sulci** (sulcus). The gyri and sulci are responsi-

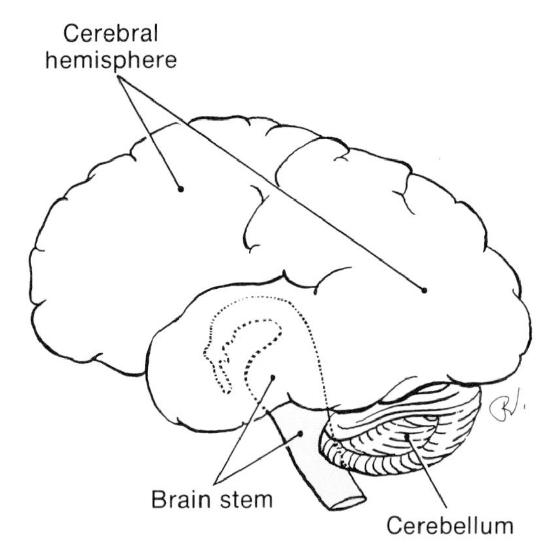

Fig. 12-10. Lateral view of the left side of the brain showing the left cerebral hemisphere, cerebellum, and brain stem (in yellow).

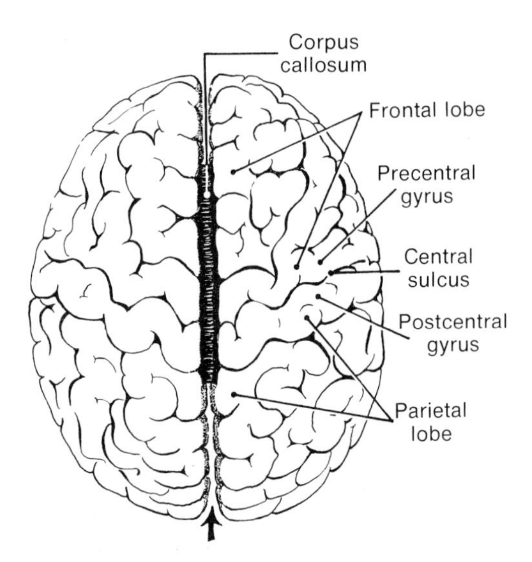

Fig. 12-11. Superior view of the brain. *Arrow* indicates the longitudinal fissure. The two hemispheres have been spread apart slightly along the longitudinal fissure to reveal the corpus callosum.

ble for the relatively large amount of surface area on the cerebral hemispheres, and many of them have been given special names (Fig. 12-9).

Several sulci are particularly deep and serve as convenient landmarks for distinguishing subdivisions or lobes of the cerebrum. The **central sulcus** lies on the dorsal and dorsolateral surface of each hemisphere, perpendicular to the longitudinal fissure (Figs. 12-9, 12-10, and 12-11). The central sulcus separates the **frontal lobe** cranially from the **parietal lobe** caudally. The prominent **precentral gyrus** occurs on the frontal lobe just in front of the central sulcus, and the **postcentral gyrus** occurs on the parietal lobe just behind the sulcus.

On the lateral surface of each hemisphere the **lateral sulcus** separates the **temporal lobe** below from the frontal and parietal lobes above (Fig. 12-9). The **occipital lobe** occupies the most caudal pole of the cerebrum, but it is not well delineated from the parietal lobe.

Another subdivision of each hemisphere is the **insula** ("island"), a lobe which is buried deeply within the lateral sulcus and thus hidden from a lateral view of the brain (Fig. 12-12). A poorly defined area of the cerebrum is the **limbic lobe** formed by medial portions of the frontal, parietal and temporal lobes and believed to be involved in emotional behavior and possibly in recent memory and learning.

The cerebral hemispheres consist of a cortex of gray matter and a subcortical layer of white matter (Fig. 12-13). The **cortical gray matter** contains nerve cell bodies, dendrites, and short axons arranged in horizontal layers. In most regions of the cerebrum there are six cortical layers consisting of three basic neuron types named according to their shapes: pyramidal, stellate, and spindle cells.

The **white matter** of the cerebrum consists mainly of large myelinated axons connecting the cortex with other regions of the CNS. The afferent (incoming) axons bring in sensory impulses, whereas efferent (outgoing) axons carry out motor impulses. Afferent and efferent fibers are grouped together and radiate upward toward the cortex as a fan-shaped structure

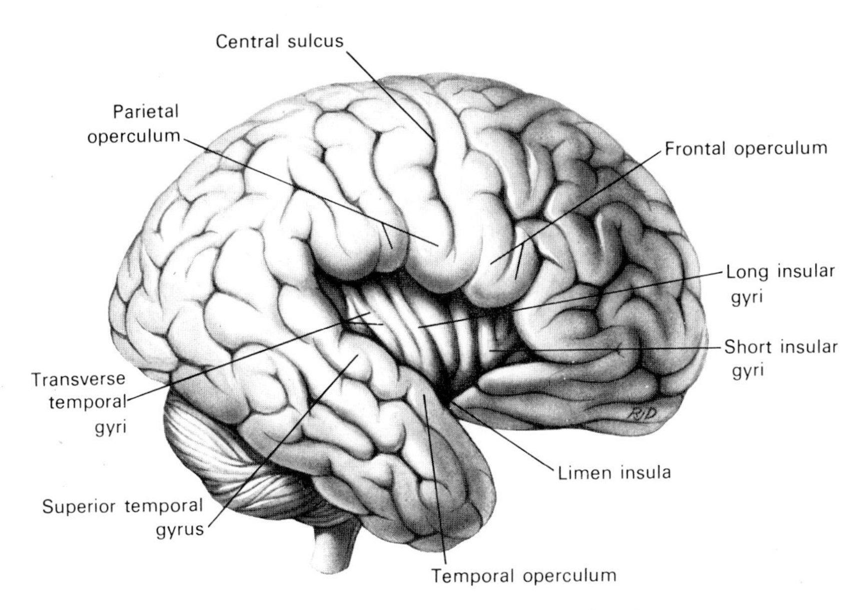

Fig. 12-12. Right side of the brain, lateral view. The lateral sulcus has been spread apart to reveal the insula and its gyri (long and short) lying deep to the temporal and frontal lobes. (From M. B. Carpenter, *Human Neuroanatomy*, Ed. 7, The Williams & Wilkins Co., Baltimore, 1976.)

called the **corona radiata** (Fig. 12-13). The lower region of this fan forms a compact mass of fibers, the **internal capsule**. Shorter axons connect and integrate various regions within the cerebral hemispheres. There are also commissural fibers which connect corresponding regions of the two hemispheres.

Masses of gray matter termed the **basal nuclei** (sometimes called basal ganglia) occur in the white matter of the cerebral hemispheres (Fig. 12-13). (The more important basal nuclei are the **caudate nucleus**, **lentiform nucleus**, and **amygdala**.) The basal nuclei regulate motor functions and muscle tone. Diseases which affect these nuclei result in **dyskinesia**, characterized by tremors and abnormal involuntary movements. **Parkinson's disease** is an example of such a disturbance.

Although the specific functions of much of the cerebrum are still unknown, certain functions have been attributed to distinct regions of the cerebral cortex. Among these are **primary sensory areas** where sensory impulses are initially received by the cortex. **Secondary sensory areas** are usually located immediately adjacent to the primary areas and are responsible for further perception and integration. Lesions in the secondary areas produce relatively mild disturbances in comparison to the more severe deficits produced by damage to primary sensory areas. **Primary motor areas** initiate and control movements of skeletal muscles and are aided by nearby **secondary** and **supplementary motor areas. Association areas** are those believed to be concerned with complex behavioral attributes such as intelligence and language expression.

Sensory Areas. The **primary visual area** is located in the occipital lobe, whereas the **primary auditory area** occurs in a portion of the temporal lobe buried deeply in the lateral sulcus (Fig. 12-14). The postcentral gyrus of the parietal lobe contains the **primary general sensory area** which receives a variety of incoming stimuli such as pain, touch, position of body parts, and temperature. Within the postcentral gyrus there are also secondary sensory areas which are believed to enable one to

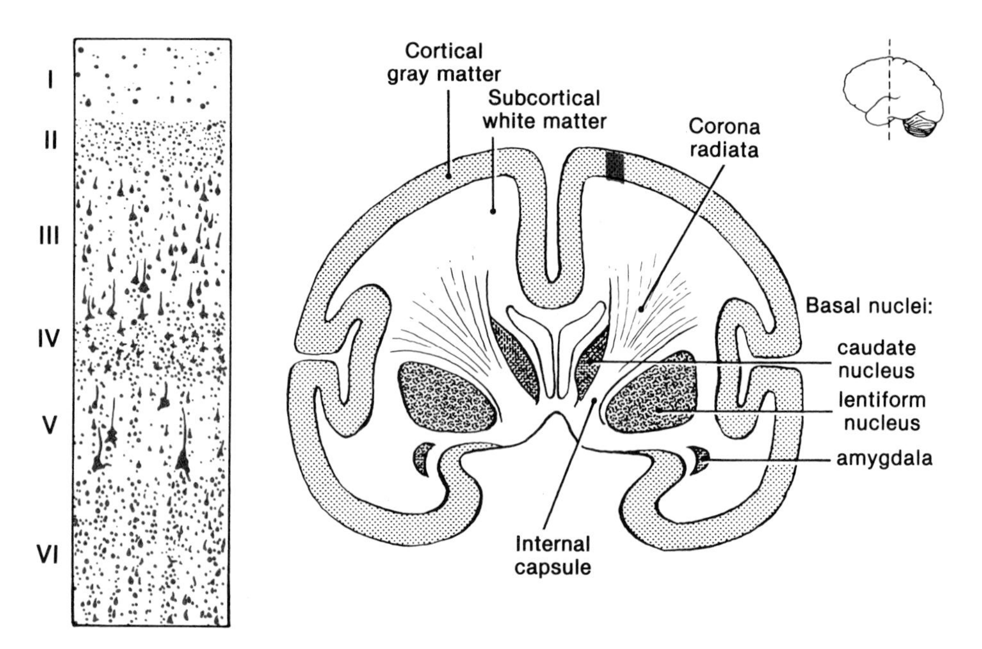

Fig. 12-13. Arrangement of gray matter and white matter in the cerebral hemispheres (coronal section). Small sketch *(upper right)* indicates the plane of section. Diagram *(left)* shows arrangement of the six basic layers of an area of the cerebral cortex represented by the red rectangle.

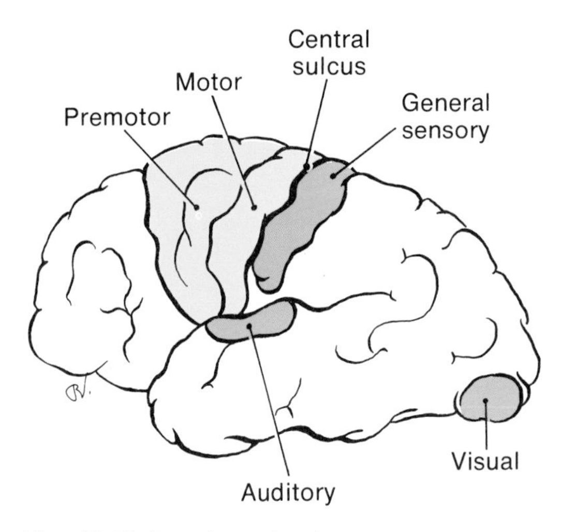

Fig. 12-14. Location of primary sensory areas (blue) and motor areas (yellow) in the cerebral cortex.

discriminate the intensity and location of these stimuli.

The inferior regions of the parietal lobe and nearby areas of the temporal lobe integrate a variety of stimuli which enable one to comprehend language and are thus considered as **sensory speech centers.** Much of the remainder of the parietal lobe is involved in **stereognosis**, enabling one to determine the nature of an object by touch alone without visual stimuli. This ability is particularly well developed in sightless individuals.

Motor Areas. Although most regions of the cerebral cortex send motor impulses to other regions of the CNS, an important motor area is situated in the precentral gyrus of the frontal lobe (Fig. 12-14). Here very large **pyramidal neurons** send out motor impulses along their axons (the corticospinal fibers) to the brain stem via the internal capsule. Since most of these fibers eventually cross over the midline to the opposite side, the motor cortex of each side is said to control contralateral movements. The regions controlled by the motor areas show a

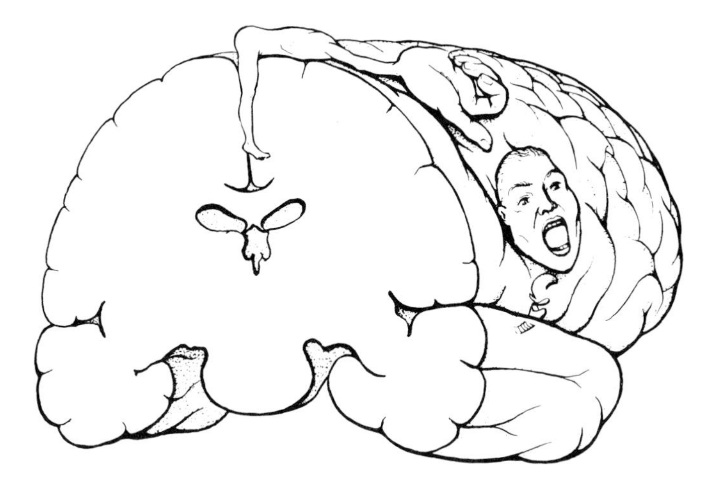

Fig. 12-15. Schematic diagram showing parts of the body drawn in proportion to the extent to which they are represented in the motor area of the cortex. Note the large area represented by the hand (particularly the thumb) and the face. (After Penfield and Rasmussen. '50, from M. B. Carpenter, *Human Neuroanatomy,* Ed. 7, The Williams & Wilkins Co., Philadelphia, 1976.)

preponderance of face and hand structures, as is the case with the sensory representation of these regions (Fig. 12-15).

A **premotor area** lies just in front of the precentral gyrus and is concerned mainly with movements affecting posture. Another specific area of the frontal lobe controls voluntary movements of the eyes. Still another important region is the **motor speech area** lying in front of and inferior to the premotor cortex and controlling movements of the larynx and mouth.

In most individuals the capacity for speech tends to reside in the left cerebral hemisphere regardless of whether one is right or left handed. This is known as cerebral dominance, and in such cases disturbances in the speech area in the right hemisphere have no effect on language ability. The loss of ability to communicate is termed **aphasia.** This can involve an inability to express oneself in speech or writing. Aphasia also can involve an inability to understand speech or written words.

Neocortex. Certain areas of the frontal, parietal, and occipital lobes are considered to have developed relatively recently in terms of the evolutionary history of the brain. These areas are collectively called the neocortex, in contrast to the older areas (paleocortex and archicortex). Much of the neocortex contains ill-defined association areas representing intelligence and learning ability. A portion of the cortex of the frontal lobe, in particular, is highly developed in man and is believed to be responsible for an individual's emotional makeup, persistence, and drive. Thus, should lesions occur in this region or should its outgoing fibers be surgically severed (a frontal lobotomy), an individual may become emotionally passive and unresponsive.

Brain Stem

The brain stem provides the pathways for ascending fibers to pass upward into the cerebrum and for descending fibers from the cerebrum to pass downward to the spinal cord. The brain stem also contains clusters of nerve cell bodies whose axons pass out of the brain as motor fibers of the cranial nerves. The major subdivisions of the brain stem are the diencephalon, midbrain, pons, and medulla oblongata.

Diencephalon. The most cranial portion of the brain stem is the diencephalon, although most of it is hidden from view by the overlying cerebral hemispheres. The lateral walls of the diencephalon constitute the thalamus, the roof is the epithalamus, and the floor the hypothalamus (Fig. 12-16). In general, the **thalamus** consists of a cluster of nerve cell bodies which act as relay stations by receiving sensory impulses from ascending tracts and sending the impulses to the appropriate sensory areas of the

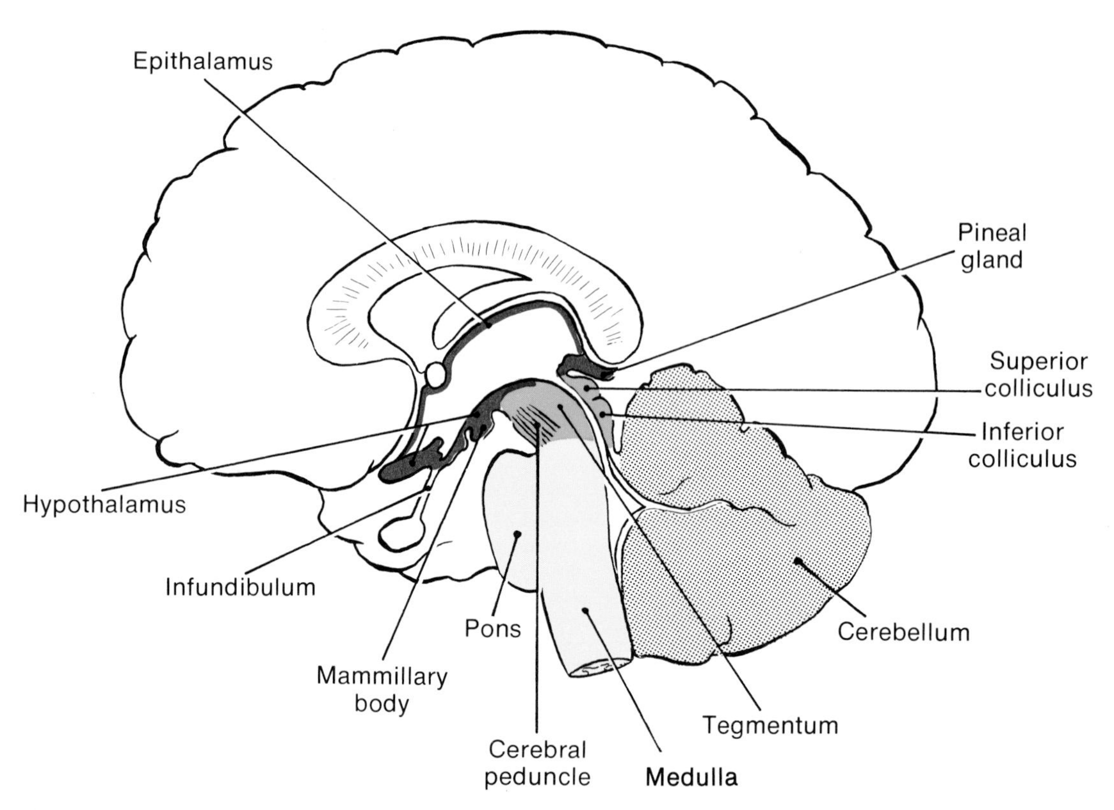

Fig. 12-16. Sagittal section of the brain. Various portions of the diencephalon are indicated in red; the midbrain is in blue, the pons and medulla in yellow, and the cerebellum in gray. (Modified after Carpenter).

cerebral cortex. The thalamus also receives various descending fibers from the cerebral cortex.

The **epithalamus** contains a small projection, the **pineal gland** (epiphysis). Although the functions of the pineal gland are not completely known, it is usually classified with the endocrine system and seems to exert some effects on the reproductive organs.

The **hypothalamus** lies just behind the optic chiasma and contains a downward projection (the infundibulum) and a pair of rounded **mammillary bodies** (Fig. 12-17). The **infundibulum** suspends the pituitary gland and also serves as a pathway for axons which originate from the hypothalamus. Some of these axons produce substances which regulate the secretory activities of the anterior lobe of the pituitary gland. Other axons secrete substances which ultimately affect smooth muscle cells in distant target organs such as the uterus. In addition to its effects on the pituitary gland, the hypothalamus controls many other involuntary activities of the body, including temperature regulation, water balance, appetite, and feeding behavior. It also influences the functions of the autonomic nervous system and seems to be involved with various emotions, particularly rage and fear.

Midbrain. The midbrain passes caudally from the diencephalon to the pons and gives origin to two pairs of cranial nerves (nerves III and IV). The dorsal aspect of the midbrain is the **tectum** and is characterized by two pairs of swellings, the **superior** and **inferior colliculi.** The superior colliculi, and the area immediately in front of them, mediate reflexes involving the visual system, such as constriction of the pupils in response to bright light. The inferior

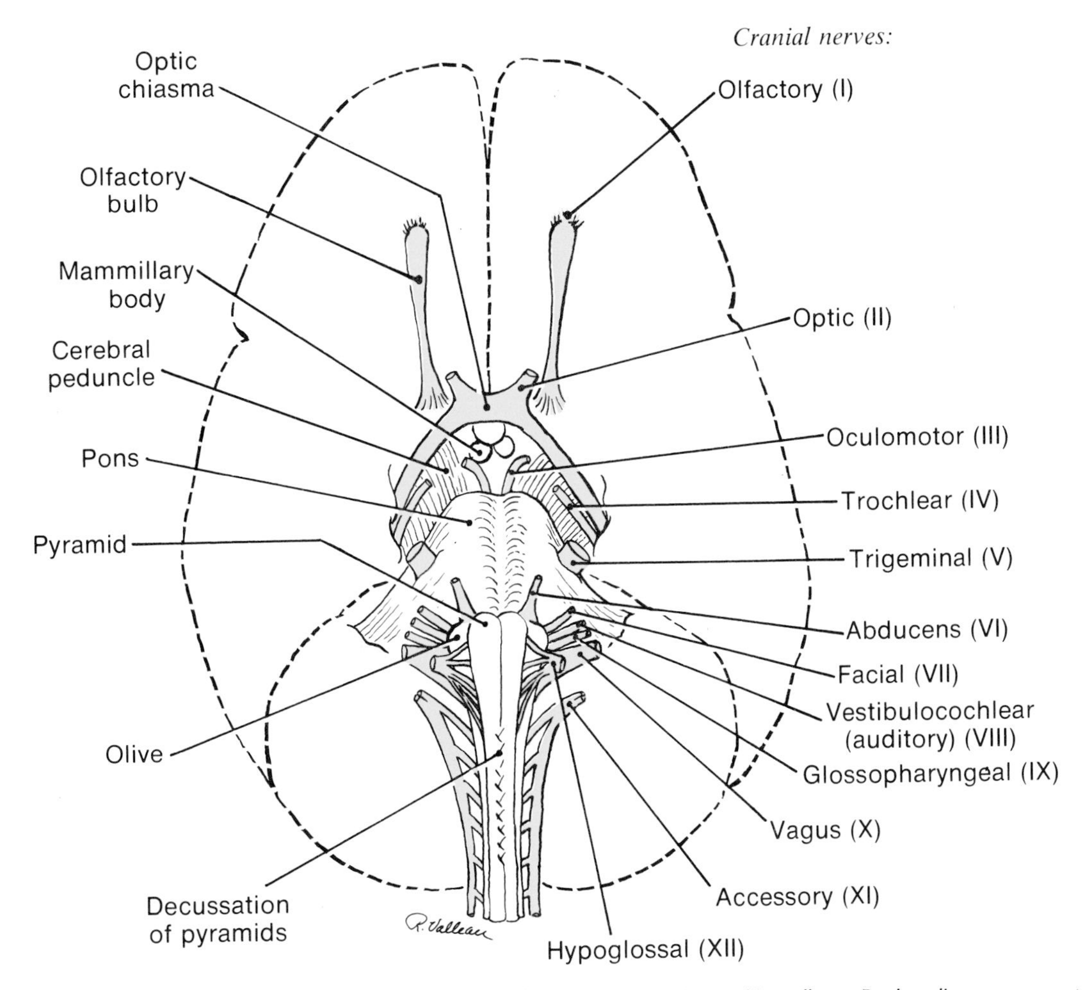

Fig. 12-17. Ventral aspect of brain stem with the cranial nerves indicated in yellow. *Broken lines* represent position of cerebral hemispheres and cerebellum. (Modified after Carpenter.)

colliculi are involved in auditory reflexes, for example those which might occur in reaction to a loud noise.

The ventral aspect of the midbrain exhibits two large bundles of fibers, the **cerebral peduncles** (crura cerebri) (Figs. 12-16 and 12-17), which pass downward from the cerebral hemispheres to the brain stem and spinal cord. The ventral portion of the midbrain is the **tegmentum** and contains groups of neurons which are part of the **reticular formation,** an ill-defined area extending throughout the brain stem and regulating many autonomic functions.

Pons. The pons is the short thick portion of the brain stem extending caudally from the midbrain to the medulla (Figs. 12-16 and 12-17). The pons ("bridge") is so named because it contains bundles of transverse fibers which help to bridge the gap between the cranial portions of the two cerebellar hemispheres which lie dorsal to it. The dorsal region of the pons contains masses of neurons which belong to the reticular formation. The ventral region of the pons serves as the site of origin for several cranial nerves (V, VI, VII and VIII) and also transmits corticospinal fibers as they descend from the cerebral cortex to the spinal cord.

Medulla Oblongata. The medulla extends

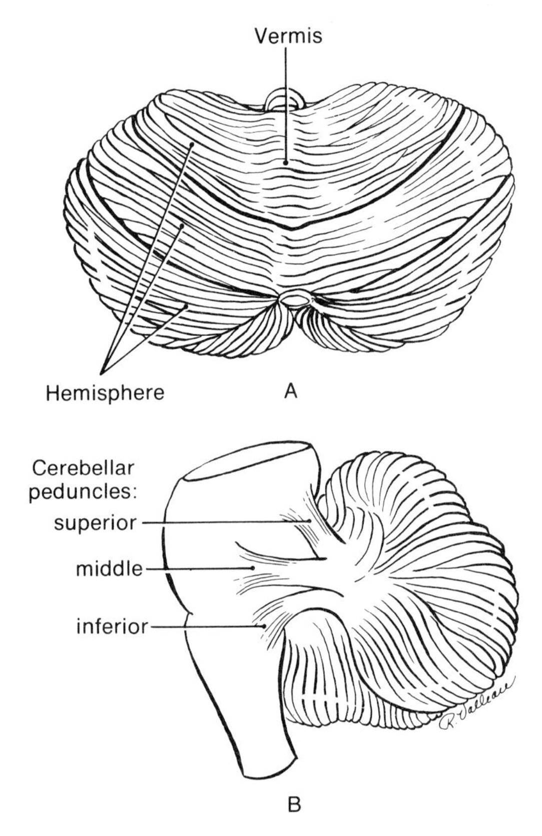

Fig. 12-18. The cerebellum. (A) Superior view, (B) lateral view.

from the caudal boundary of the pons to the beginning of the spinal cord at the foramen magnum. The dorsal region of the medulla consists of a thin membrane, dorsal to which are the caudal portions of the cerebellum (Fig. 12-16). The ventral aspect of the medulla shows a pair of lateral swellings (the **olives**), medial to which are two elongate masses called the **pyramids** which lie on either side of the midline (Fig. 12-17).

Much of the medulla is occupied by the reticular formation which extends cranially from the medulla into the pons and midbrain, and which controls such vital functions as respiration and heart rate. The medulla also gives rise to cranial nerves IX, X, a portion of XI, and XII. The pyramids contain descending corticospinal fibers, the majority of which cross over the ventral midline to the opposite side. This area is therefore known as the **decussation of the pyramids.** Neurons located in the olives give rise to axons which also cross the midline but ascend upward into the cerebellum.

Cerebellum

The cerebellum is situated dorsal to the pons and medulla and consists of two lateral lobes (the **cerebellar hemispheres**) and a median portion called the **vermis** (Fig. 12-18). The cerebellum is attached to the midbrain, pons, and medulla by means of three pairs of fiber bundles: the **superior, middle,** and **inferior cerebellar peduncles,** respectively. The external surfaces of the cerebellar hemispheres and vermis are marked by deep fissures subdividing them into lobes and lobules, which in turn are organized into narrow leaflike ridges (folia).

The cerebellar cortex consists of gray matter, beneath which is a core of white matter. The cortex contains three prominent layers: an outer **molecular layer** with sparsely scattered neurons, a **Purkinje cell layer** with one or two rows of large neurons (Purkinje cells), and a **granular layer** densely packed with very small neurons (granule cells) (Fig. 12-19). Much of the molecular layer consists of elaborately branched dendrites from the Purkinje cells.

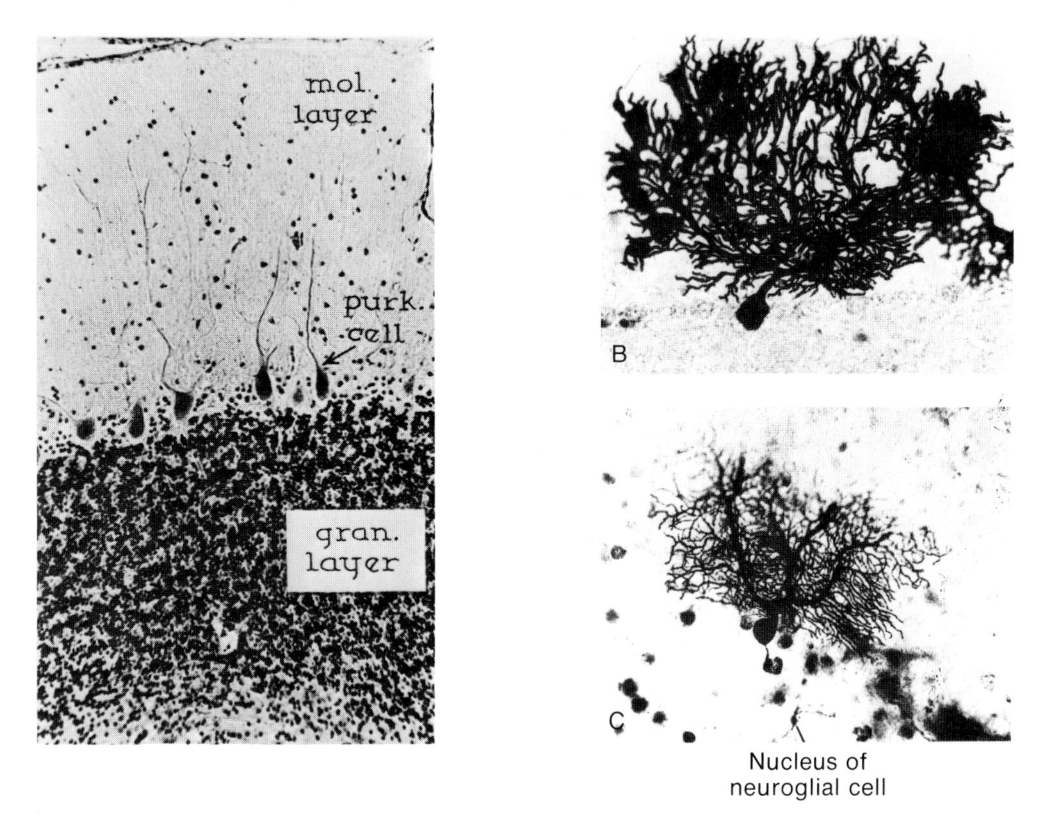

Fig. 12-19. Microscopic anatomy of the cerebellum. (A) Low magnification, showing molecular *(mol.)* layer, Purkinje *(purk.)* cell layer, and granular *(gran.)* layer. (From A. W. Ham and D. H. Cormack, *Histology,* Ed. 8, J. B. Lippincott Co., Philadelphia, 1979.) (B, C) Purkinje cells specially stained to show dendritic arborizations. (From E. D. Gardner, *Fundamentals of Neurology,* Ed. 6, W. B. Saunders Co., Philadelphia, 1975.)

The axons from the Purkinje cells contribute to the white matter, which also contains clusters of nerve cell bodies known as the **deep cerebellar nuclei.**

The cerebellum coordinates voluntary muscular activity and also is involved with equilibrium and muscle tone. Disturbances in cerebellar function are likely to produce ataxia consisting of distorted and uncoordinated movements, particularly in walking. Cerebellar lesions are also likely to produce decreased muscle tone (flaccidity) and tremors.

Ventricles

In the embryo, the central nervous system develops as a long hollow tube. Remnants of the cavity within this tube can be found in most of the adult CNS, and these are lined by a thin layer of epithelial cells, the **ependyma.** In some regions the cavity attains considerable size and is termed a ventricle.

In the adult, each cerebral hemisphere contains a **lateral ventricle** (often designated as ventricle 1 or 2), which communicates via an

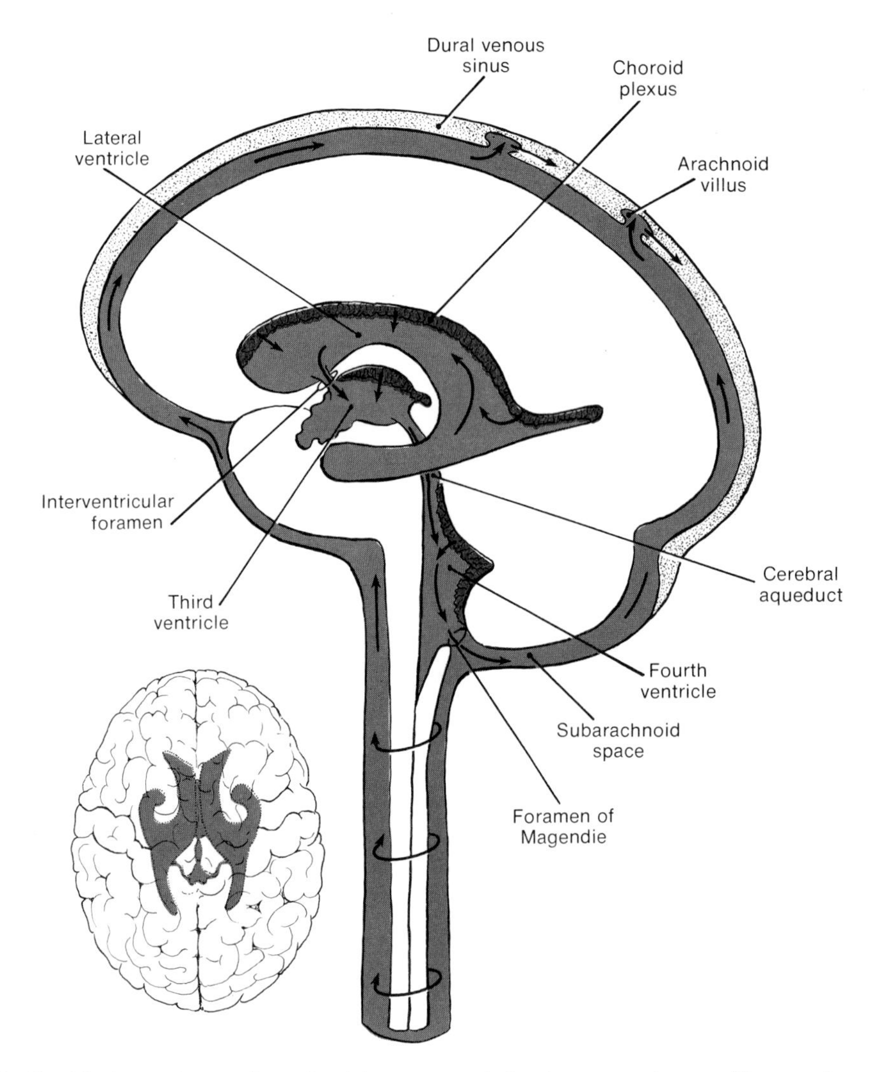

Fig. 12-20. Ventricular system, subarachnoid space, and dural venous sinuses. The cerebrospinal fluid flows in the direction indicated by the *arrows.* Dark red areas represent choroid plexuses. The diagram *(lower left)* shows a superior view of the ventricular system superimposed on a sketch of the brain.

interventricular foramen (of Monro) with the **third ventricle** within the diencephalon (Fig. 12-20). The third ventricle joins the narrow **cerebral aqueduct (of Sylvius)** within the midbrain; the aqueduct in turn joins the **fourth ventricle** (in the pons and medulla). Just dorsal to the fourth ventricle is the cerebellum. The fourth ventricle continues into the minute **central canal** of the spinal cord.

The ventricular system of the central nervous system is filled with **cerebrospinal fluid** (**CSF**) which is a clear, colorless liquid somewhat similar to blood plasma. CSF is secreted into the ventricles by the **choroid plexuses** consisting of specialized ependymal cells and blood vessels in the walls of the lateral, third, and fourth ventricles. The CSF circulates through the ventricular system of the central nervous system and leaves it via a cluster of tiny openings (which include the foramina of

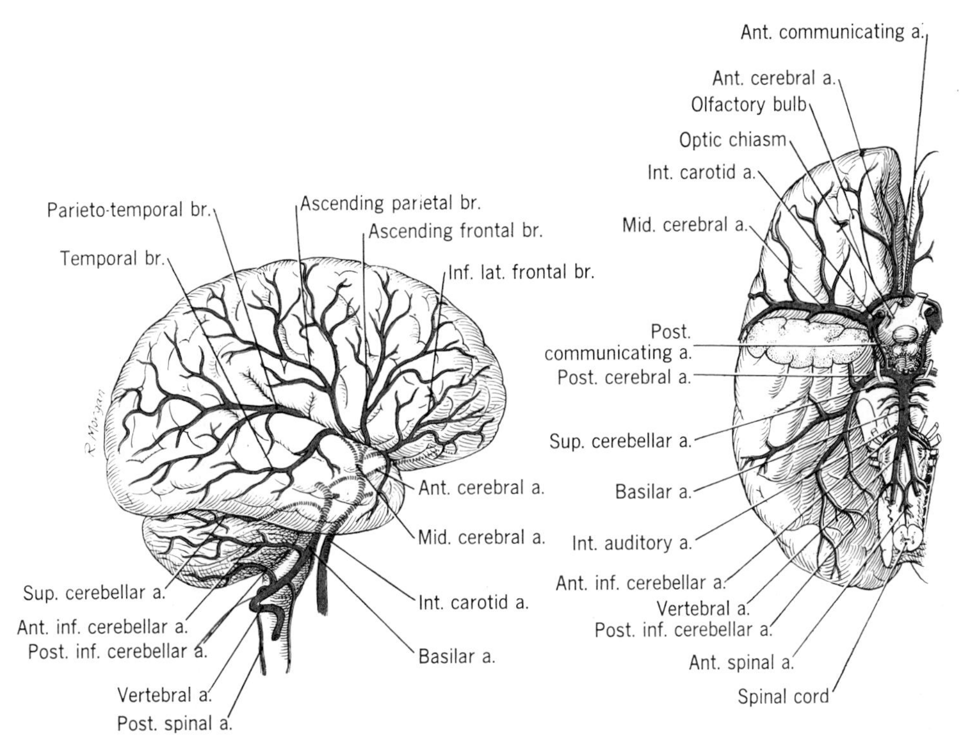

Fig. 12-21. Arterial supply of the brain. *(Left)* Lateral view, *(right)* inferior view. (From *Stedman's Medical Dictionary,* Ed. 23, The Williams & Wilkins Co., Baltimore, 1976.)

Magendie and Luschka) in the roof of the fourth ventricle, thereby passing into the subarachnoid space around the brain and spinal cord. Fingerlike extensions (villi) of the arachnoid project upward into the venous sinuses of the dura mater, and the CSF passes through these villi into the sinuses and is thereby returned to the vascular system. The brain and spinal cord are protected by the CSF acting as a cushion in the event of blows or sudden changes in position. The CSF may also be of metabolic significance to the central nervous system.

A sample of cerebrospinal fluid may be withdrawn from the subarachnoid space by a lumbar puncture so as to test the fluid for the presence of blood cells, bacteria, or changes in composition. A lumbar puncture can also be used to measure the pressure of the fluid, in which case an elevation in pressure may indicate the presence of a tumor or obstruction in the pathway of the CSF circulation. Gases may also be introduced (pneumoencephalography) so as to visualize the subarachnoid cavity by X-rays and thereby detect abnormalities. Anesthetics and radiopaque dyes can also be introduced via a lumbar puncture.

Blood Supply of the Brain

The blood supply of the brain is of great importance since nervous tissue is particularly sensitive to a decrease in oxygen. Even a temporary loss of blood flow to the brain can cause severe damage. For this reason the body has a defense mechanism in the form of fainting, since the flow of blood to the brain is facilitated in the recumbent position.

The brain receives its blood supply from the **internal carotid arteries** which enter the skull via the carotid canal and from the **vertebral arteries** via the foramen magnum (Fig. 12-21). The major branches of each internal carotid artery are the **anterior cerebral artery** and **middle cerebral artery** which supply blood to much of the cerebral hemispheres. The anterior cerebral arteries are also connected to each other by an **anterior communicating artery.**

The vertebral arteries supply branches to the medulla and to portions of the cerebellum. In the caudal region of the brain the two vertebral arteries fuse in the midline to form the **basilar artery** which distributes branches along the ventral surface of the pons and cerebellum. The cranial end of the basilar artery bifurcates into a pair of **posterior cerebral arteries.** Each posterior cerebral artery supplies caudal regions of the cerebral hemispheres and also joins a **posterior communicating artery** which may connect it with either the middle cerebral artery or the stem of the internal carotid artery.

The various anastomosing arteries in the ventral region of the diencephalon and midbrain are arranged in a somewhat circular configuration and thus are called the **cerebral arterial circle** (of Willis). The circle serves as a connection between the internal carotid arteries and the vertebral arteries. Under normal conditions the cerebrum is supplied by the internal carotids and vertebral arteries whereas the brain stem and cerebellum are supplied mainly by the vertebral arteries. However, should one of the vertebral or carotid pathways become occluded, it is possible for blood to be shunted to the affected area via alternate routes provided by the cerebral arterial circle.

The cerebral arteries divide into smaller and smaller vessels which eventually penetrate the brain tissue and become capillaries. These cerebral capillaries are unusual in that some substances which ordinarily pass easily into most tissues are prevented from entering brain tissue. This phenomenon is known as the **blood-brain barrier.**

The venous drainage of the brain consists of **cerebral veins** which accompany the cerebral arteries. The cerebral veins empty into several large venous sinuses in the dura mater. These include the **superior sagittal sinus** in the upper margin of the falx cerebri between the two cerebral hemispheres, the **inferior sagittal sinus** in the lower margin of the falx cerebri, and the **straight (rectus) sinus** extending backward from the inferior sagittal sinus (Fig. 12-22). These sinuses flow together into a common sinus (termed the **confluence**) at a central point on the internal surface of the occipital bone. Extending laterally from this point are two **transverse sinuses,** each of which passes along a groove on the inner surface of the occipital bone. The transverse sinuses become S-shaped **sigmoid sinuses** which also receive other venous tributaries and then communicate with the internal jugular veins. Many of the dural venous sinuses also connect with **emissary veins** which pass outward through tiny foramina in the skull to empty into the extracranial venous system.

The spinal cord receives its blood supply from the **anterior spinal artery** passing along the anterior median fissure (Fig. 12-23). In the uppermost region of the spinal cord the anterior spinal artery is fed by branches from each vertebral artery; the lower regions of the anterior spinal artery receive **segmental spinal arteries** entering the vertebral canal via the intervertebral foramina. These branches arise from various sources, including the vertebral, posterior intercostal, and lumbar arteries. The posterior aspect of the spinal cord contains an irregular pair of **posterior spinal arteries** which are likewise fed by segmental spinal branches.

The blood is returned from the spinal cord to the heart via a system of veins which takes a course similar to that of the spinal arteries. The segmental veins ultimately unite with thoracic and abdominal veins.

PERIPHERAL NERVOUS SYSTEM (PNS)

The peripheral nervous system consists of cranial and spinal nerves, their associated ganglia, and portions of the autonomic nervous system. Long cytoplasmic processes of neurons and their coverings are often termed nerve **fibers,** and bundles of these fibers which lie outside of

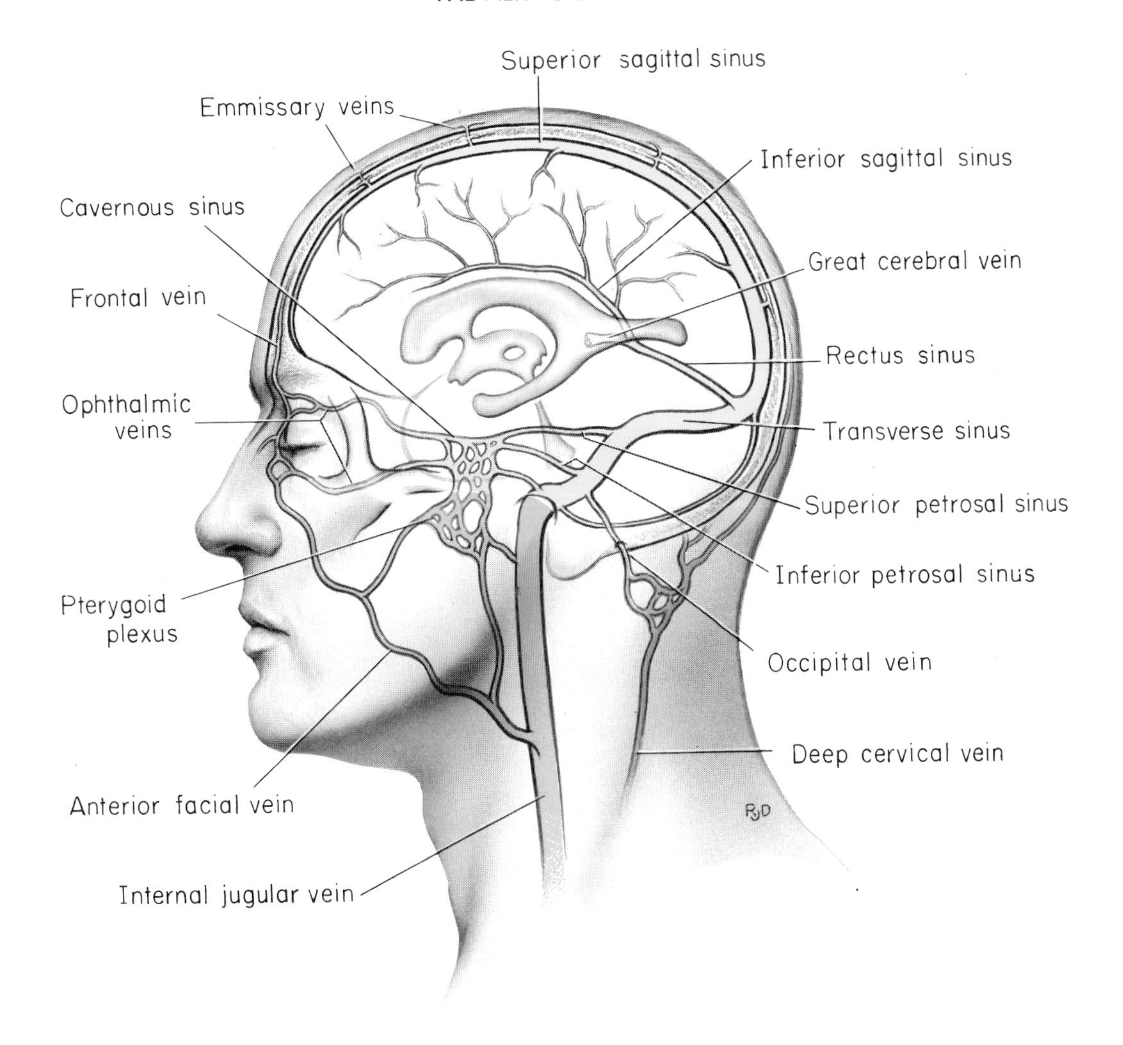

Fig. 12-22. The dural sinuses and major veins of the cranium. (From M. B. Carpenter, *Human Neuroanatomy,* Ed. 7, The Williams & Wilkins Co., Baltimore, 1976.)

the CNS are called **nerves.** (Bundles of fibers contained wholly within the CNS are **tracts.**) Within a peripheral nerve, each fiber consists of a nerve cell process (axon) and a covering called a **neurilemma** composed of **Schwann cells.** The neurilemma cells rotate around the processes to form many layers of plasma membranes which constitute **myelin,** thus resulting in a myelinated fiber. If the neurilemma fails to rotate around the process, then the fiber is nonmyelinated. Individual nerves may contain both myelinated and nonmyelinated fibers.

Surrounding the neurilemma of each fiber is a thin layer of connective tissue called an **endoneurium** (Fig. 12-24). Several fibers are bundled together by a connective tissue investment called a **perineurium.** A similar covering around the periphery of the nerve is called the **epineurium.** These connective tissue layers communicate with each other and carry blood vessels for the fibers and their coverings.

Although some nerves may consist entirely of sensory or entirely of motor fibers, most nerves contain fibers of both types and are thus

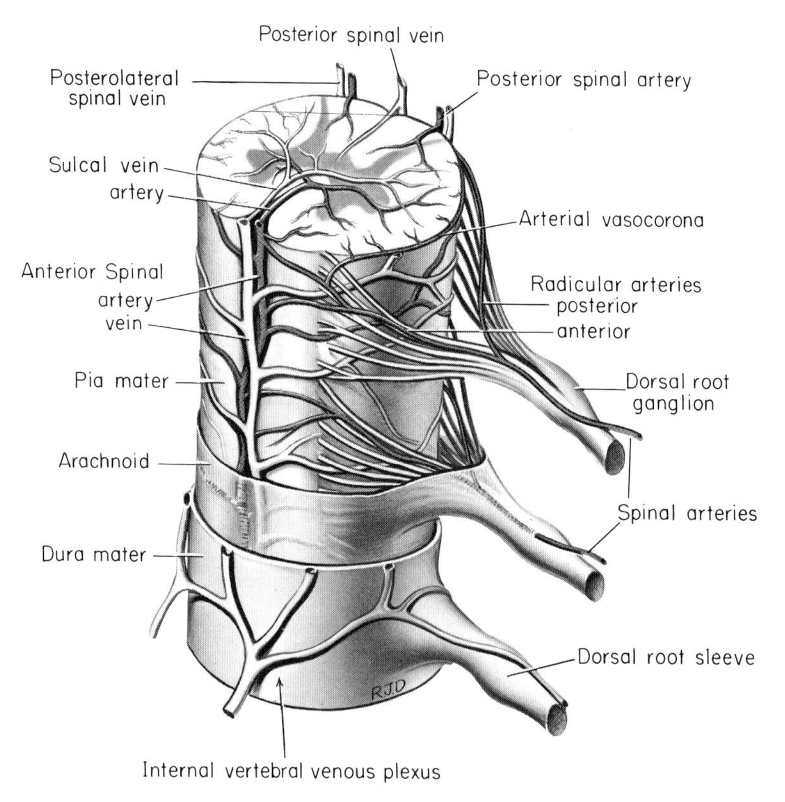

Fig. 12-23. Arterial supply and venous drainage of the spinal cord, oblique view. (From M. B. Carpenter, *Human Neuroanatomy,* Ed. 7, The Williams & Wilkins Co., Baltimore, 1976.)

considered to be **mixed.** Also, nerves may be classified as **somatic** if they are associated with voluntary activities or **autonomic** (visceral) if they involve involuntary activities. Some nerves are termed **special** (as opposed to **general**), if they are concerned with special senses such as sight, hearing, olfaction (smell), and taste.

Cranial Nerves

There are 12 pairs of cranial nerves numbered from I to XII in a cranial to caudal sequence (Fig. 12-17). The cell bodies of the sensory components of these nerves are located primarily in ganglia outside of the CNS; the cell bodies of the motor components occur within the brain.

I. The **olfactory nerve** is sensory and carries olfactory impulses which originate from the olfactory epithelium in the upper region of the nasal cavity. The olfactory epithelium contains neurons whose axons constitute the olfactory nerve. These axons pass upward through minute openings in the cribriform plate of the ethmoid bone in the anterior part of the skull and end in the olfactory bulb on the inferior surface of the frontal lobe (Fig. 12-17).

II. The **optic nerve** has its origin in the retina of the eye where sensory neurons receive visual impulses and transmit them to the brain along axons representing the optic nerve. Some of the axons from each optic nerve cross over to the opposite side of the brain, thereby forming the **optic chiasma** in front of the infundibulum of the diencephalon (Fig. 12-17).

III. The **oculomotor nerve** is a motor nerve which originates from the floor of the midbrain

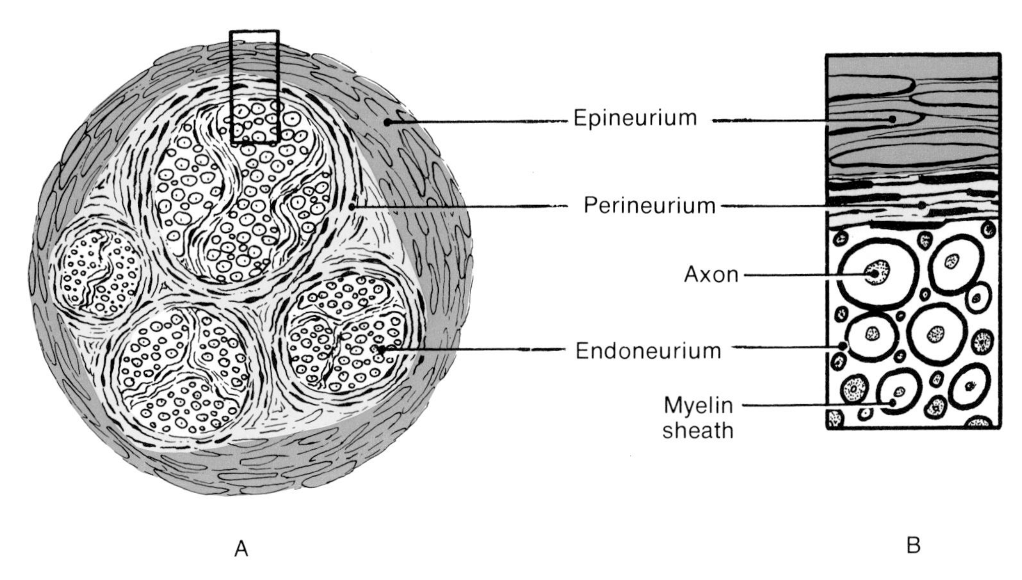

Fig. 12-24. (A) Diagram of a cross section of a nerve showing connective tissue investments and partitions; (B) higher magnification of area enclosed by the rectangle in A.

(Fig. 12-17). This nerve innervates most of the skeletal muscles responsible for moving the eyeball (inferior oblique, superior rectus, medial rectus, inferior rectus), as well as the levator palpebrae muscle in the upper eyelid. It also innervates smooth muscles involved in adjusting the shape of the lens and the size of the pupil.

IV. The **trochlear nerve** is a slender motor nerve which emerges from the dorsal region of the midbrain (Fig. 12-17). It supplies a single skeletal muscle (the superior oblique) which moves the eyeball.

V. The **trigeminal nerve** is a massive mixed nerve associated with the pons (Fig. 12-17). It contains three portions: the ophthalmic, maxillary, and mandibular divisions. The **ophthalmic division** carries general sensory impulses (pain, touch, pressure, temperature) from the orbit and much of the face and scalp, and the **maxillary division** carries general sensory impulses from a portion of the face, upper mouth region (including the upper lips, and teeth), and the nasal cavities (Fig. 12-25). The nerve cell bodies for these two divisions of the trigeminal nerve are situated in the **trigeminal** (Gasserian) **ganglion** just lateral to the pons. The **mandibular division** contains a motor component supplying the muscles associated with chewing (mastication) and a sensory component conveying general sensation from the lower lip, teeth, gums, mouth, and face.

VI. The **abducent nerve** is motor and originates from the ventral aspect of the pons and supplies a single skeletal muscle (the lateral rectus) which moves the eyeball (Fig. 12-17).

VII. The **facial nerve** arises near the junction of the pons and medulla (Fig. 12-17). It is a mixed nerve supplying motor fibers which innervate the muscles of facial expression, the sublingual and submandibular salivary glands, and the lacrimal gland. The sensory component of the facial nerve carries taste (gustatory) impulses from the anterior two-thirds of the tongue (Fig. 12-25). The **geniculate ganglion** contains the nerve cell bodies for the sensory fibers of this nerve.

VIII. The **vestibulocochlear (auditory, acoustic) nerve** carries only sensory components and originates close to the origin of the facial nerve near the junction of the pons and medulla (Fig. 12-17). The vestibular portion

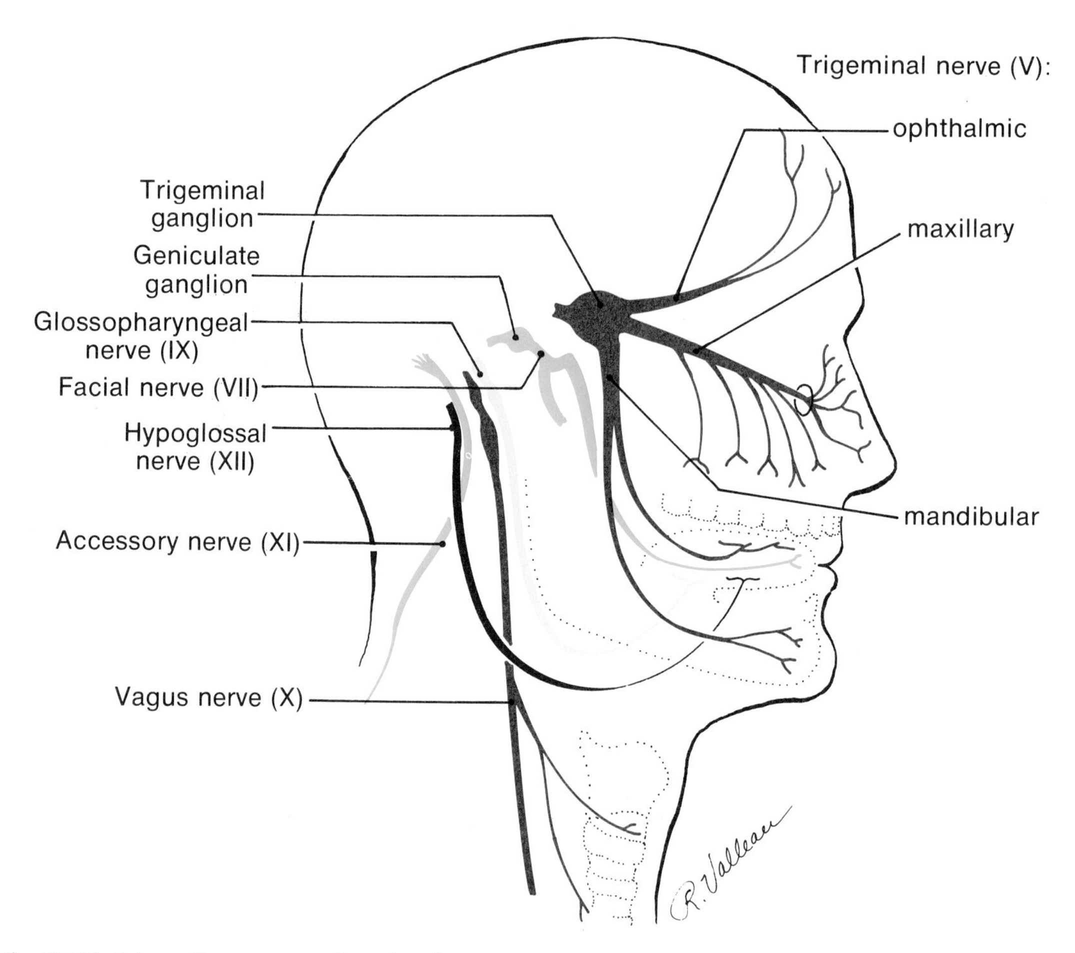

Fig. 12-25. Schematic representation of pathways of cranial nerves V, VII, IX, X, XI, and XII. (Modified from Hamilton, Boyd, and Mossman.)

conveys the sense of equilibrium; the cochlear portion carries auditory impulses. The cell bodies of these two components reside in ganglia associated with the inner ear.

IX. The **glossopharyngeal nerve** is a mixed nerve emerging from the medulla (Figs. 12-17 and 12-25). The sensory fibers carry taste impulses from the posterior one-third of the tongue and general sensory impulses from the pharyngeal region. The motor fibers supply one of the salivary glands (the parotid, although this gland may also receive a few fibers from cranial nerve VII) and a small muscle in the pharynx.

X. The **vagus** is a mixed nerve originating from the medulla and showing an extensive motor and sensory distribution to thoracic and abdominal viscera (Figs. 12-17, 12-25, and 12-31). It also carries motor and sensory fibers to structures in the pharynx and larynx.

XI. The **accessory nerve** is motor and originates as a series of rootlets along the medulla and upper cervical portion of the spinal cord (Fig. 12-17). These fibers join to form a single nerve trunk which then subdivides again into two divisions. One division travels with the vagus nerve to supply motor fibers to pharyngeal and laryngeal muscles. The other division supplies two muscles in the neck region: the sternocleidomastoid and trapezius muscles.

XII. The **hypoglossal nerve** is a purely motor nerve which originates from the medulla and innervates the muscles of the tongue (Figs. 12-17 and 12-25).

Spinal Nerves

The spinal nerves are arranged in 31 pairs which originate at regular intervals throughout the length of the spinal cord (Fig. 12-7). These pairs of nerves supply sensory and motor fibers to structures in the neck, trunk, and limbs. The nerves can be grouped regionally into 8 cervical, 12 thoracic, 5 lumbar, 5 sacral, and 1 coccygeal.

At its origin from the spinal cord, each spinal nerve consists of 2 parts: a **dorsal (posterior) root** carrying sensory (afferent) axons and a **ventral (anterior) root** carrying motor (efferent) axons (Fig. 12-26). Associated with each dorsal root is a **spinal ganglion** containing the cell bodies of the sensory neurons. The cell bodies of the motor neurons are located in the anterior horn of the spinal cord. The dorsal root and ventral root join with each other to form the spinal nerve which emerges from the intervertebral foramen. Each spinal nerve then divides into a small **dorsal ramus** (plural: rami) and a large **ventral ramus**.

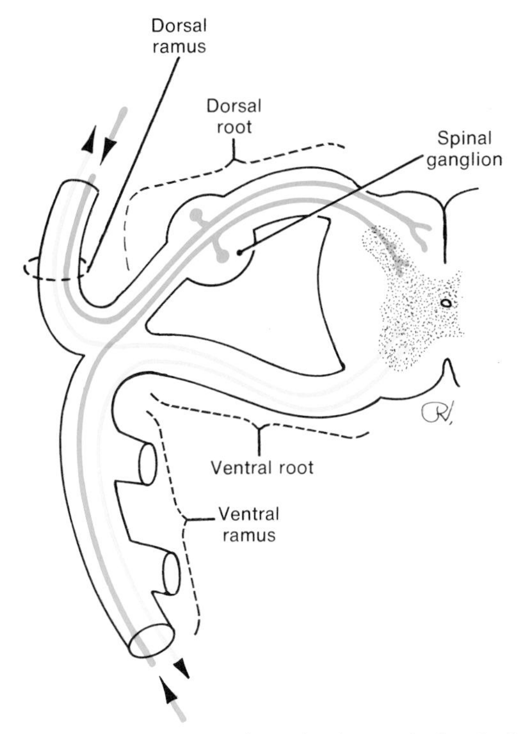

Fig. 12-26. Roots and rami of a typical spinal nerve. The sensory neurons are indicated in blue; motor neurons are in yellow. (Modified after *Grant's Method.*)

The **dorsal rami** of the spinal nerves supply sensory and motor fibers to the muscles and skin along the dorsal region of the neck and trunk. The **ventral rami** carry motor and sensory fibers to the remainder of the body, except the head. Some of the ventral rami form a system of communicating branches known as a **plexus** from which emerge a number of nerves which are named. The major plexuses are the cervical plexus, brachial plexus, and the lumbosacral plexus.

The **cervical plexus** is formed by the upper four cervical nerves and gives off fibers supplying muscles and skin of the neck region (Fig. 12-27). Cervical nerves 3–5 also give rise to the **phrenic nerve** which passes downward through the neck and thoracic region to innervate the diaphragm.

The **brachial plexus** is formed by cervical nerves 5–8 and thoracic nerve 1 (Fig. 12-27).

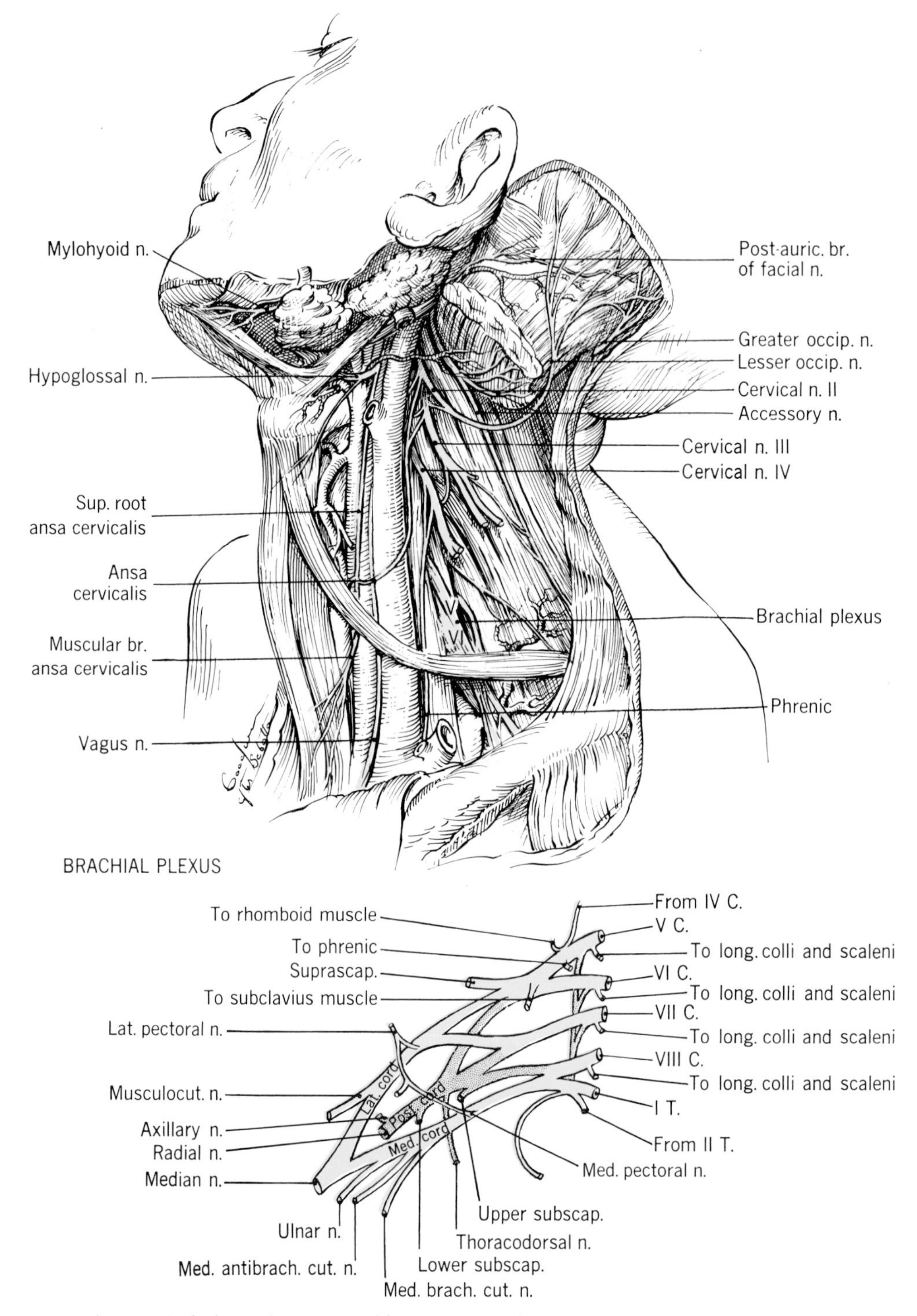

Fig. 12-27. The cervical plexus (greater and lesser occipital nerves and cervical nerves II, III, and IV) and the brachial plexus (cervical nerves V, VI, VII, VIII, and thoracic nerve I). (From *Stedman's Medical Dictionary,* Ed. 23, The Williams & Wilkins Co., Baltimore, 1976.)

(Tiny branches from cervical nerve 4 and thoracic nerve 2 may also participate in the plexus.) This plexus gives off branches to the scapular and pectoral regions, as well as the following important nerves for the upper limbs: the **radial nerve** (supplying extensor muscles), the **musculocutaneous nerve** (to the flexors of the forearm), the **axillary nerve** (to shoulder muscles), and the **median** and **ulnar nerves** to the flexors of the wrist and fingers (Fig. 12-28).

The **lumbosacral plexus** is formed by the lumbar nerves and sacral nerves (Fig. 12-29). This plexus innervates the hip and pelvic regions, and includes the **pudendal nerve** which supplies sensory and motor fibers to the external genitalia. The lumbosacral plexus also gives rise to the following major nerves for the lower limbs: the **femoral nerve** (Figs. 12-29 and 12-30) supplying anterior thigh muscles, the **obturator nerve** (Fig.12-29) to the adductor muscles on the medial aspect of the thigh, and the **sciatic nerve** (Figs. 12-30 and 19-9), which supplies the back of the thigh and then divides into the **tibial** and **common peroneal nerves** for the leg and foot. The sciatic nerve is the largest nerve in the body and passes downward beneath the gluteus maximus muscle before entering the thigh. Its course through the gluteal region is of clinical importance, since intramuscular injections in the buttocks can damage the sciatic nerve if they are improperly administered. The sciatic nerve is also vulnerable as it passes close to the hip joint and can be damaged when the hip is dislocated or fractured. It is also subject to inflammation resulting in the condition of **sciatica** characterized by pain radiating down the back of the leg.

Some of the ventral rami of spinal nerves do not participate in plexuses but instead pass directly out to their end organs. Among these are the second through twelfth **thoracic (intercostal) nerves** which innervate muscles and skin in the thoracic and abdominal walls.

AUTONOMIC NERVOUS SYSTEM

The autonomic nervous system controls the functions of visceral organs. An important center of autonomic control appears to reside in the **limbic system** of the brain and includes the basal nuclei, thalamus, hypothalamus, and poorly understood areas in the frontal and temporal lobes of the cerebrum. Also, the **reticular formation** in the brain stem contains autonomic centers which regulate respiration and activities of the circulatory system such as the heart rate. Motor impulses initiated by these higher centers are sent to lower levels of organization consisting of nerve cell bodies which give rise to fibers in some of the cranial nerves and in the spinal nerves. These lower pathways of autonomic outflow are classified into two subdivisions, the sympathetic and parasympathetic divisions, which differ from the voluntary or somatic peripheral nervous system in that two neurons occur in sequence between the central nervous system and the end organ (Fig. 12-31).

Sympathetic System

The nerve cell bodies of the sympathetic system occur in two regions: the spinal cord and the sympathetic ganglia. The sympathetic cell bodies in the spinal cord are located in the lateral horns of the thoracic and upper lumbar regions; the sympathetic system is thus often termed the **thoracolumbar system.** Axons of these neurons are known as **preganglionic fibers** and exit from the spinal cord via the spinal nerves. These fibers then almost immediately leave the spinal nerve and pass by means of a **white ramus communicans** to a sympathetic ganglion (Fig. 12-32).

The **sympathetic ganglia** are arranged at regular intervals along the lateral aspect of the vertebral column and are interconnected to form the **sympathetic trunk** (Fig. 12-31). Each ganglion contains sympathetic nerve cell bodies whose axons are termed **postganglionic fibers.** Some of these postganglionic fibers pass outward from the ganglia to innervate abdominal and pelvic visceral organs. (In the cervical region, the uppermost portion of the sympathetic trunk contains a particularly large ganglion, the **superior cervical ganglion,** which

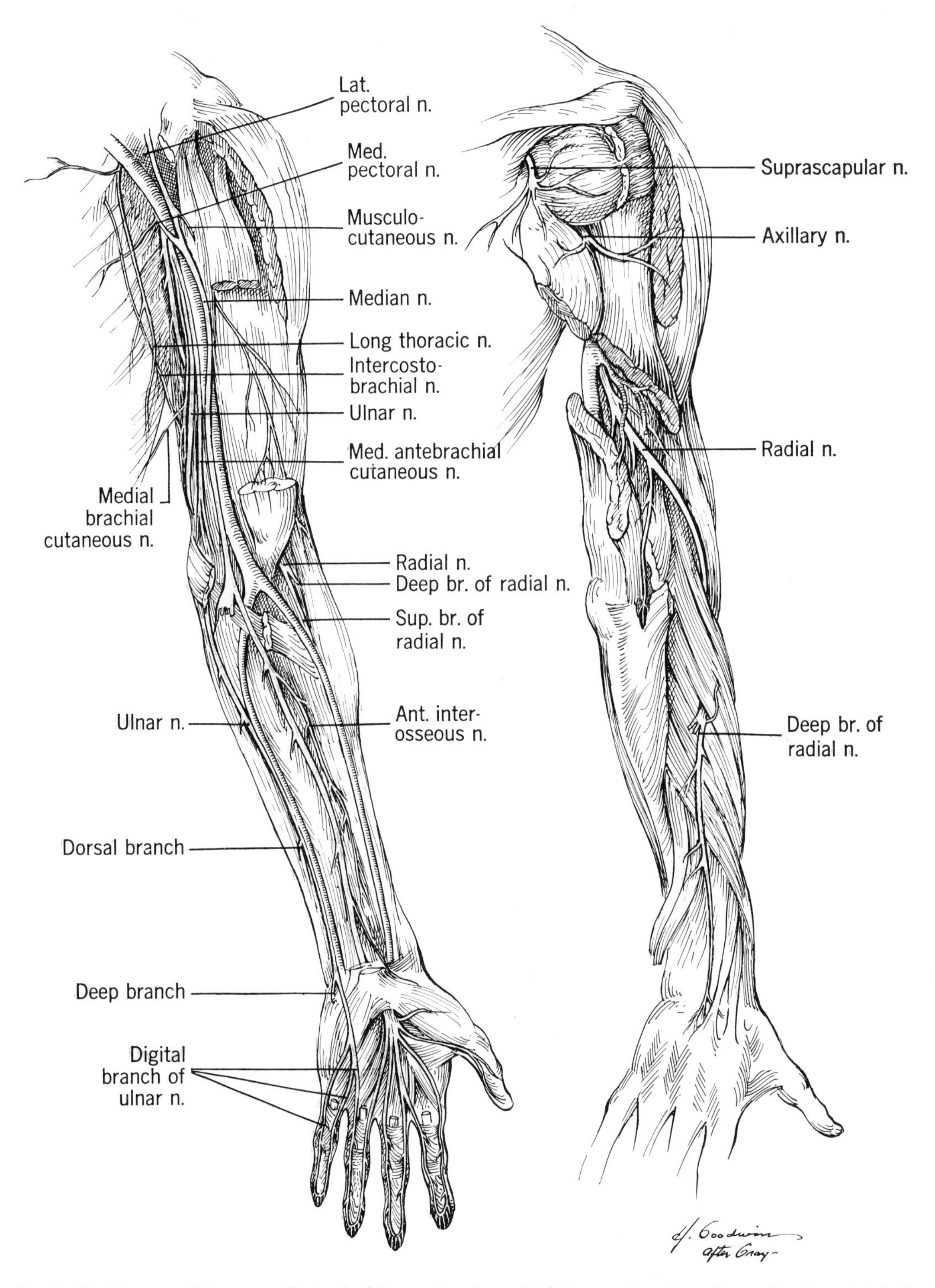

Fig. 12-28. Nerves of the upper limb. *(Left)* Anterior view, *(right)* posterior view. (From *Stedman's Medical Dictionary,* Ed. 23, The Williams & Wilkins Co., Baltimore, 1976.)

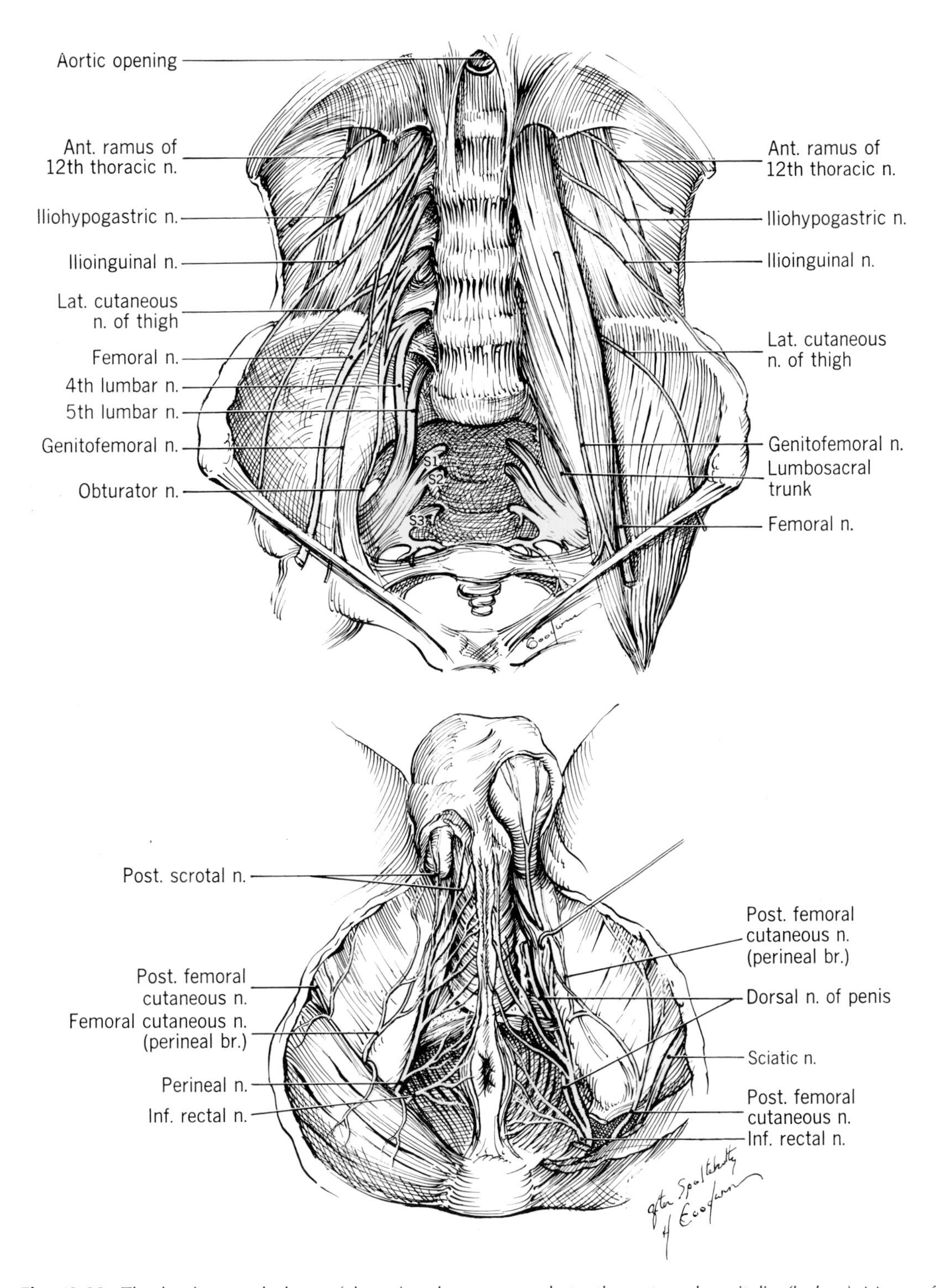

Fig. 12-29. The lumbosacral plexus *(above)* and nerve supply to the external genitalia *(below)*. Many of the nerves to the external genitalia are branches of the pudendal nerve. (From *Stedman's Medical Dictionary*, Ed. 23, The Williams & Wilkins Co., Baltimore, 1976.)

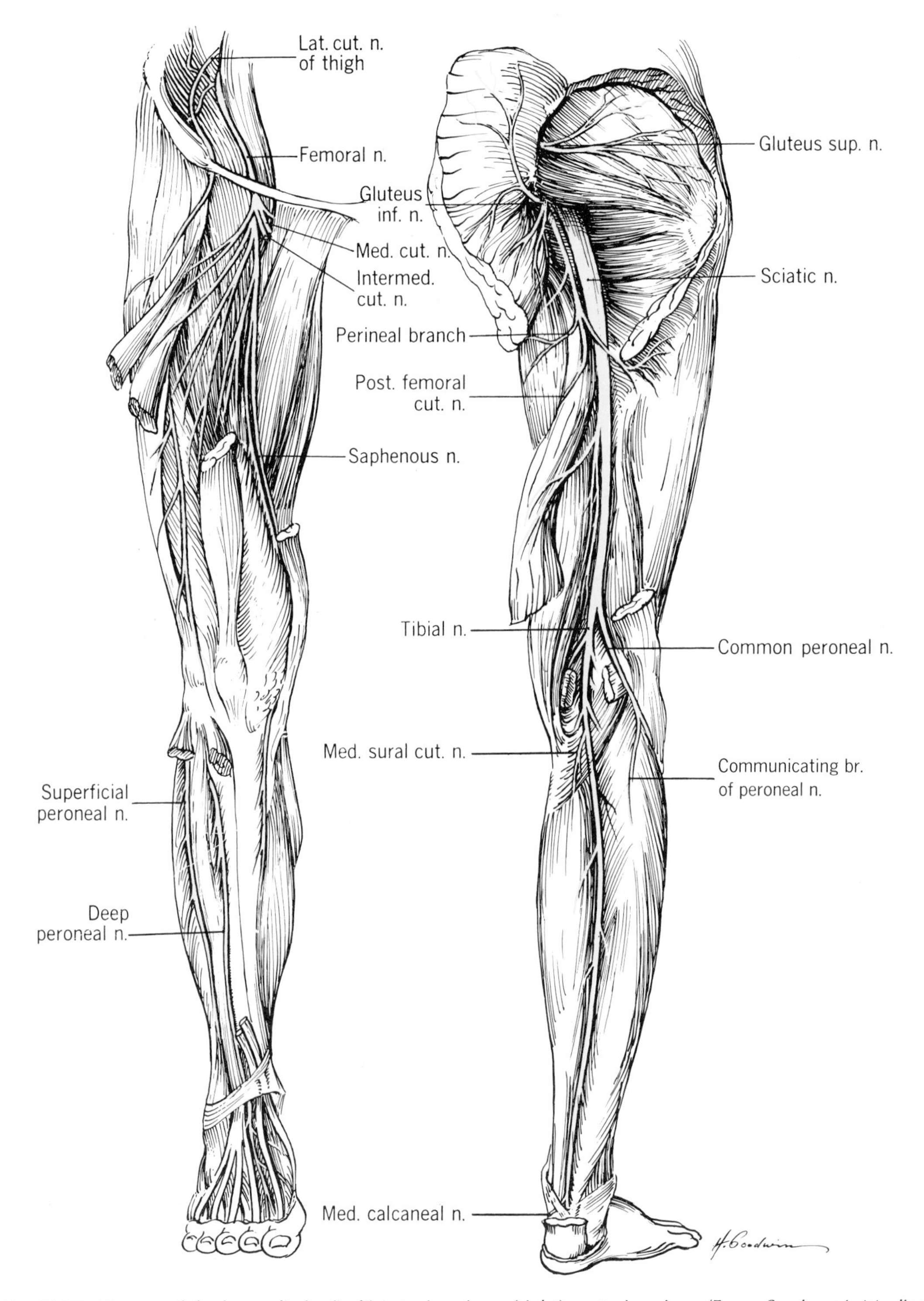

Fig. 12-30. Nerves of the lower limb. *(Left)* Anterior view, *(right)* posterior view. (From *Stedman's Medical Dictionary,* Ed. 23, The Williams & Wilkins Co., Baltimore, 1976.)

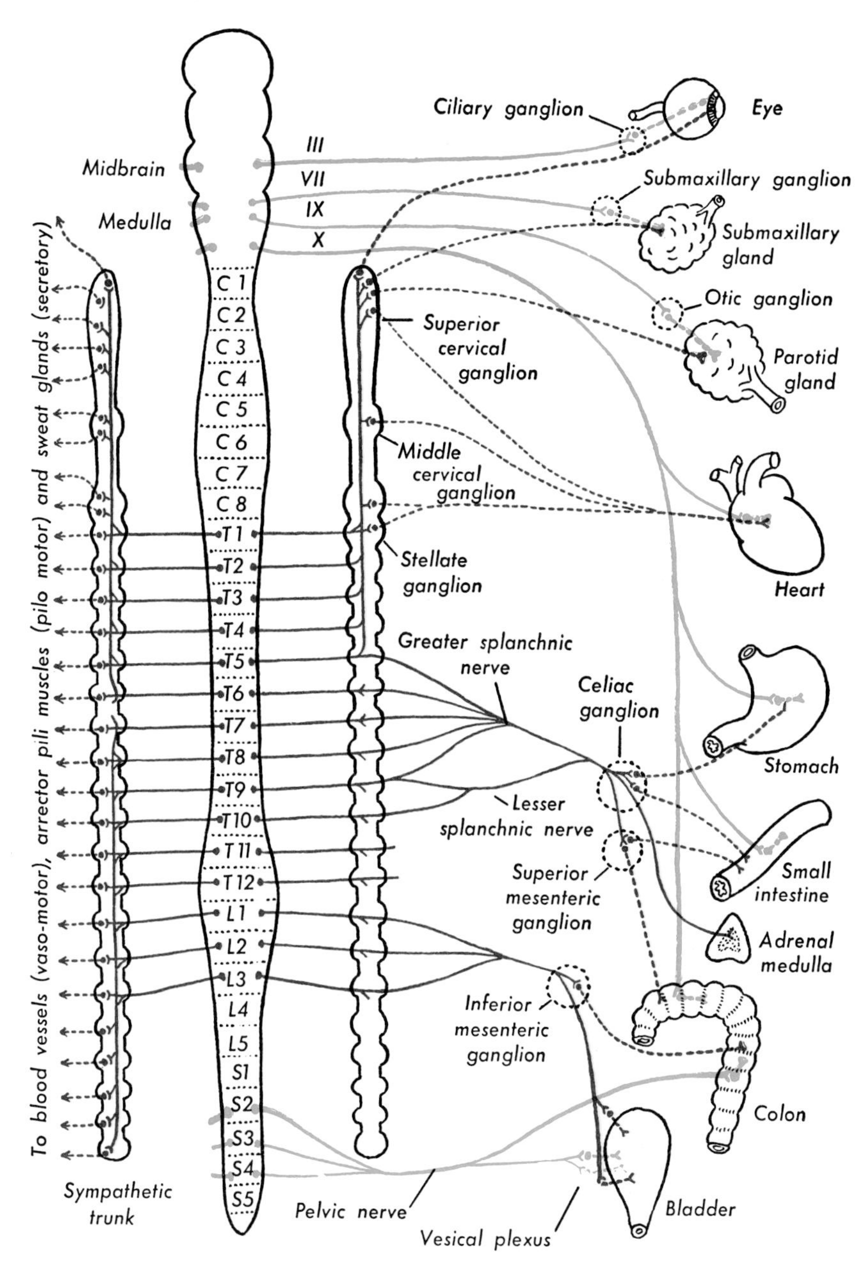

Fig. 12-31. The autonomic nervous system. Sympathetic components are in red; parasympathetic components are in blue. *Solid lines* represent preganglionic fibers; *broken lines* represent postganglionic fibers. For purposes of simplification the *left* side of the diagram shows the sympathetic trunk sending sympathetic fibers to the blood vessels, smooth muscle, and glands in peripheral regions of the body. On the *right* side of the diagram the sympathetic trunk shows fibers passing to the viscera. Also, the pathways of the parasympathetic elements are depicted only on the *right* side of the diagram. (From W. M. Copenhaver, R. P. Bunge, and M. B. Bunge, *Bailey's Textbook of Histology,* Ed. 16, The Williams & Wilkins Co., Baltimore, 1971.)

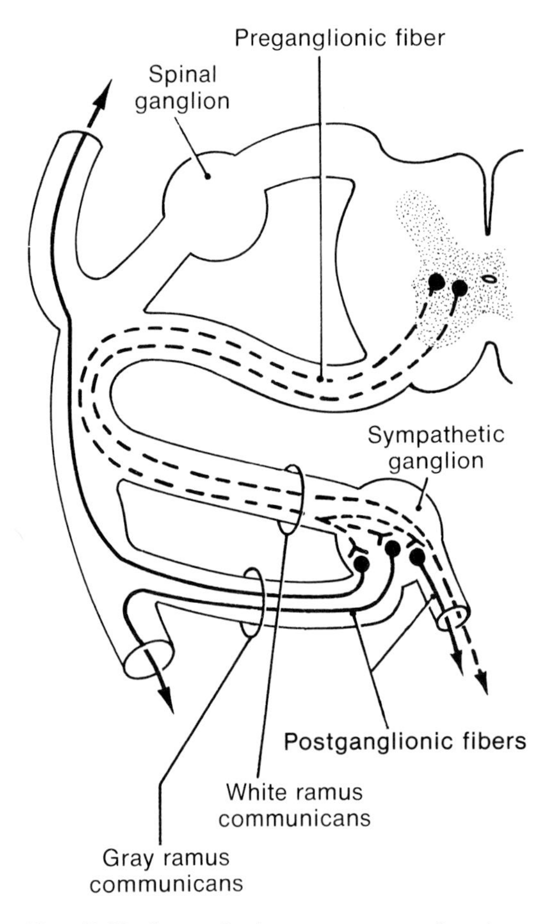

Fig. 12-32. Sympathetic components of a thoracic or lumbar nerve. (Modified after *Grant's Method*.)

sends out postganglionic sympathetic fibers to much of the head and neck regions.) From each sympathetic ganglion there are some postganglionic fibers which pass back to the spinal nerve via a **gray ramus communicans** and thereby travel outward with the spinal nerves to innervate blood vessels, sweat glands, or smooth muscle fibers in peripheral regions of the body (Fig. 12-32).

Some preganglionic sympathetic fibers pass either upward or downward via the sympathetic trunk and synapse in nearby sympathetic ganglia. Other fibers do not synapse in the sympathetic ganglia but instead pass to more distant groups of cell bodies such as the **celiac ganglia** located behind the stomach (Fig. 12-31). These ganglia give off fibers which form the **celiac (solar) plexus** and innervate various abdominal viscera.

Parasympathetic System

The nerve cell bodies of this system occur in the brain and sacral spinal cord and in parasympathetic ganglia situated at some distance from the CNS. Since the parasympathetic nerve cell bodies in the CNS send out preganglionic fibers via some of the cranial and sacral spinal nerves this system is often termed the **craniosacral system.** The preganglionic fibers enter parasympathetic ganglia situated very close to or within the viscera. Neurons in the **parasympathetic ganglia** then transmit the impulses via very short postganglionic fibers in the walls of the organs (Fig. 12-31).

Of the cranial nerves which carry parasympathetic fibers, the most extensive is the **vagus** (Fig. 12-31). This nerve conveys impulses to the heart, lungs, and most of the abdominal viscera, including the gastrointestinal tract to the distal part of the transverse colon. The remainder of the abdominal organs, as well as the pelvic viscera, receive parasympathetic innervation from the second, third, and fourth sacral nerves.

Both the sympathetic and parasympathetic systems innervate most organs, although there are no parasympathetic fibers to peripheral glands and to the smooth muscle of the skin and of its blood vessels. The effects of the sympathetic and parasympathetic system tend to be antagonistic. Thus, the sympathetic system dilates the pupils of the eyes, speeds the heart rate, and inhibits activities of the digestive tract. The parasympathetic system constricts the pupils, slows the heart, and promotes digestive processes. In general, sympathetic activities are associated with emergency "flight or fight" situations, while parasympathetic activities generally are concerned with vegetative and metabolic functions of the body.

The chemical neurotransmitter **acetylcholine** is released at the preganglionic endings of both the sympathetic and parasympathetic systems, as well as at the postganglionic endings of the parasympathetic system; however, the postganglionic endings of the sympathetic system release **norepinephrine.** The sympathetic system and the medulla of the **adrenal (suprarenal) gland** enhance one another functionally. Thus sympathetic stimulation causes the adrenal medulla to secrete epinephrine and norepinephrine which exert the same effect on organs as do impulses transmitted by sympathetic axons. (They also both show a similar embryonic origin.)

NERVE ENDINGS

Motor Nerve Endings

Axons which innervate effector structures in the periphery show various types of endings. Some terminate freely in or on such structures as glands, smooth muscle, and cardiac muscle. Those which innervate skeletal muscle show a more elaborate ending known as a **motor end plate (myoneural** or **neuromuscular junction)** (Fig. 12-33).

In the vicinity of the motor end plate, each axon branches repeatedly and each branch in turn subdivides into tiny filaments whose terminal swellings are filled with synaptic vesicles containing neurotransmitter substances (see Chapter 4). The swellings indent the postsynaptic membrane (sarcolemma) of the muscle cell and transmit the impulse from nerve to

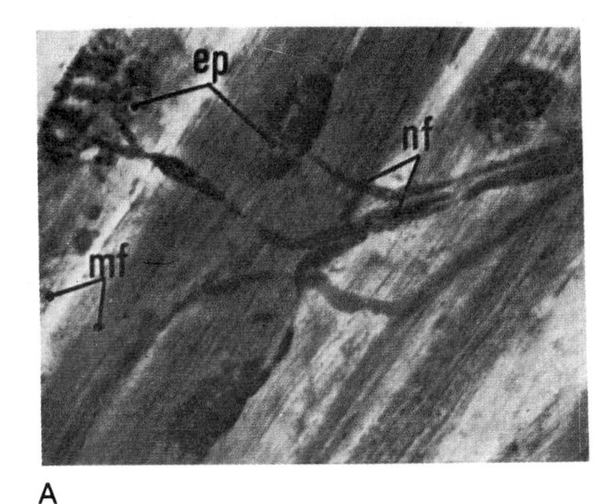

A

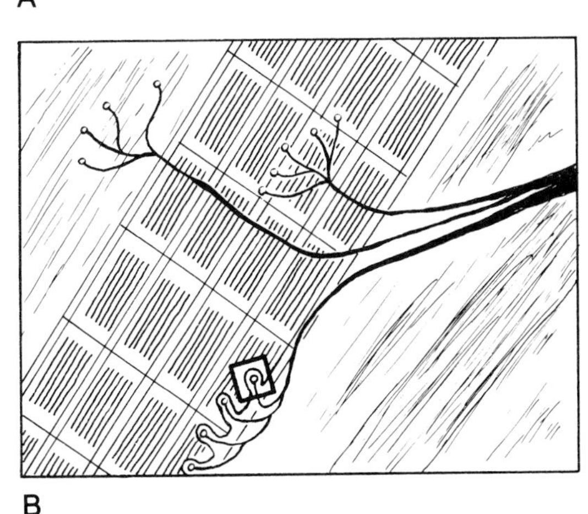

B

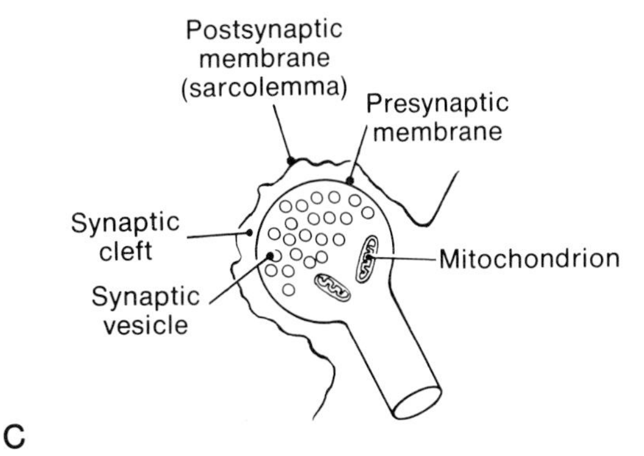

C

Fig. 12-33. (A) Micrograph of motor end plates (neuromuscular junctions): *nf*, nerve fibers; *ep*, end plates; *mf*, muscle fibers. (From M. B. Carpenter, *Human Neuroanatomy,* Ed. 7, The Williams & Wilkins Co., Baltimore, 1976.) (B) Diagram of some of the motor end plates shown in A. An axon divides into several branches, which subdivide into filaments with terminal swellings. (C) Higher magnification showing the synaptic area of the terminal swelling enclosed by the rectangle in B. (Modified after Gardner.)

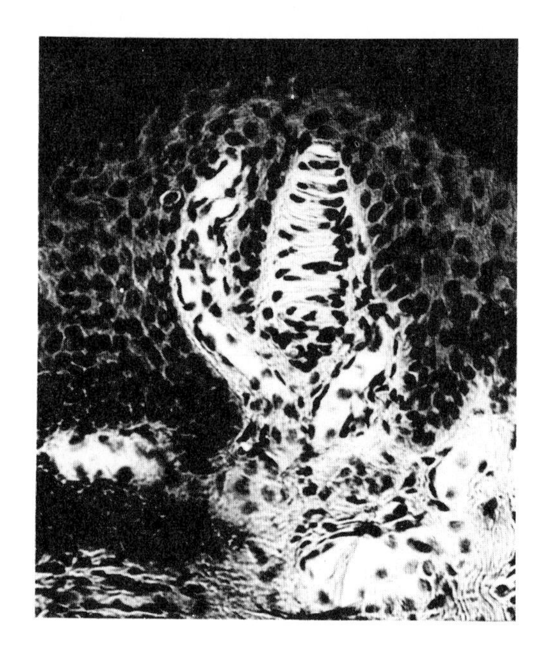

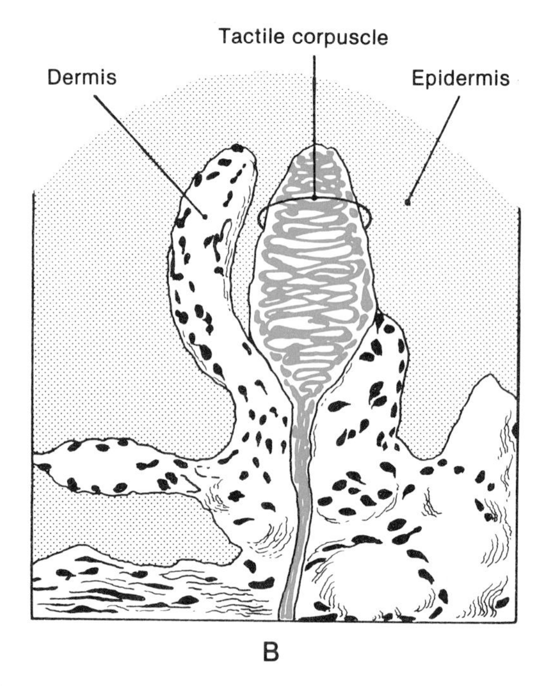

Fig. 12-34. (A) Microscopic section through the skin showing a tactile corpuscle (of Meissner). (From M. B. Carpenter, *Human Neuroanatomy,* Ed. 7, The Williams & Wilkins Co., Baltimore, 1976.) (B) Sketch of section shown in A.

muscle. In some skeletal muscles which control delicate movements (such as eye movements) many nerve fibers supply a relatively small number of muscle fibers. In other muscles such as those concerned with posture, there are fewer nerve fibers supplying relatively large numbers of muscle fibers.

Sensory Receptors

Sensory receptors receive stimuli and initiate impulses which are sent along nerve fibers to the central nervous system. Many receptors are actually specialized endings of nerve fibers which end freely in the skin (Fig. 6-3). These include receptors for **pain** and some for **temperature.** Other receptors may consist of nerve endings which are encapsulated with various amounts of connective tissue; examples are deep touch and vibration receptors **(Pacinian corpuscles)** and **tactile corpuscles (of Meissner)** for light touch (Fig. 12-34). Still others are unusually complex and represent proprioceptive receptors sensitive to the state of muscle contraction **(muscle spindles)** or the position of joints (Fig. 12-35). Highly specialized receptors also are located in the organs of special sense and are discussed below.

ORGANS OF SPECIAL SENSE

The organs of special sense include the eyes (vision), ears (hearing and equilibrium), olfactory epithelium (smell), and taste buds (taste). These structures receive sensory stimuli and transmit sensory impulses via cranial nerves to appropriate regions of the brain where they can be perceived and acted upon.

Eye

The eye contains an elaborate system for collecting and focusing light rays on a highly sensitive group of sensory cells located in the **ret-**

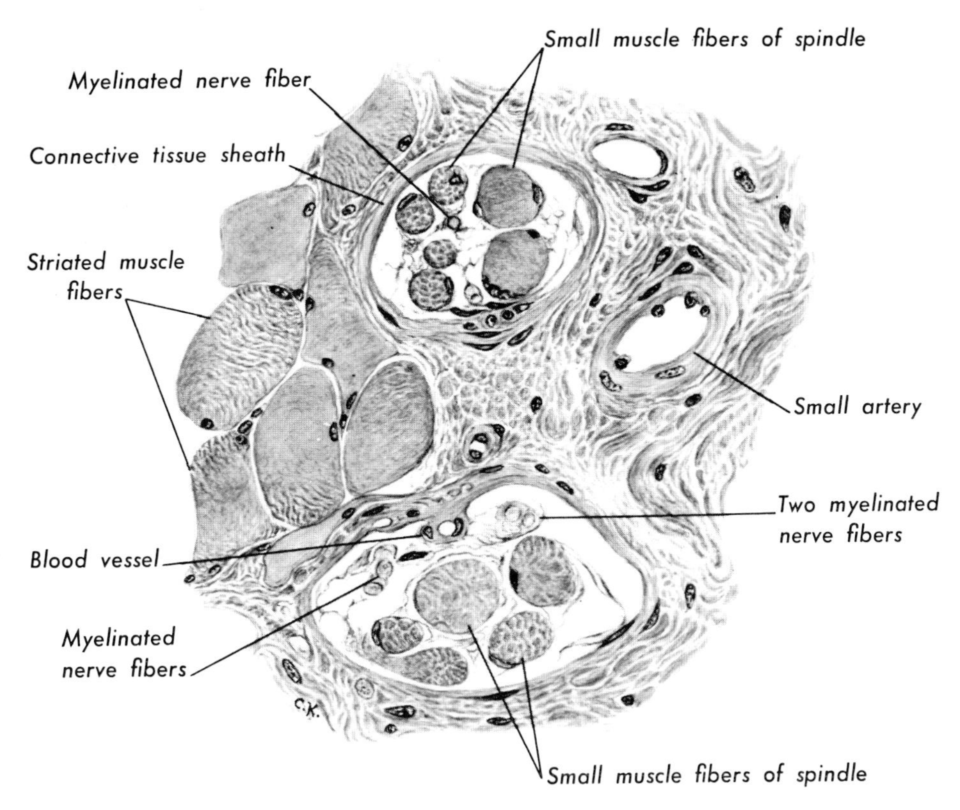

Fig. 12-35. Cross section showing two muscle spindles within skeletal muscle. The spindles consist of modified small muscle fibers and myelinated nerve fibers surrounded by a connective tissue sheath. (From W. M. Copenhaver, R. P. Bunge, and M. B. Bunge, *Bailey's Textbook of Histology,* Ed. 16, The Williams & Wilkins Co., Baltimore, 1971.)

ina. As in a camera, the eyeball is a dark light-tight box with an aperture, the **pupil,** surrounded by a diaphragm, the **iris.** The light rays pass through the pupil and are focused by the lens onto the retina acting as the photographic film. The retina represents the nervous component of the eye; the other portions are considered to be non-nervous.

Each eyeball is situated in its own bony orbit and is moved by six **extrinsic (extraocular)** skeletal muscles (Fig. 12-36). These muscles originate from the walls of the orbit and insert into the outermost coat of the eyeball. There are four **rectus** muscles: **superior, inferior, medial,** and **lateral,** which raise, lower, adduct, and abduct the eye, respectively. The **superior oblique** and **inferior oblique** muscles rotate each eye clockwise or counterclockwise.

The upper and lower **eyelids** (palpebrae) contain connective tissue and the **orbicularis oculi** muscle which constricts the slit between the eyelids. The upper lid also contains the **levator palpebrae superioris** muscle which raises the lid and thereby opens the slit. Damage to this muscle or to its innervation from the oculomotor nerve may result in an inability to keep the eye open. The margins of the upper and lower lids contain stout hairs (eyelashes), and a series of modified sebaceous and sweat glands called **ciliary glands.** Infection and inflammation of these produce a sty. Modified sebaceous and sweat glands are also found in a red fleshy body termed the **lacrimal caruncle,**

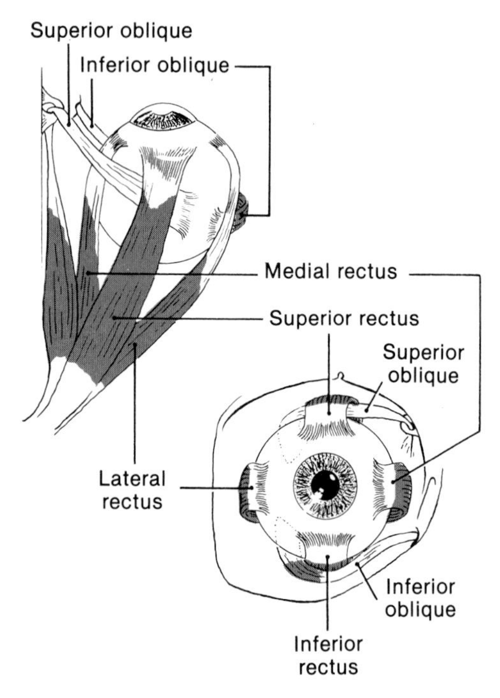

Fig. 12-36. The extrinsic eye muscles. *(Upper left)* Superior view of right eyeball, *(lower right)* anterior view of right eyeball. (Modified after Basmajian.)

which lies near the medial ends of the upper and lower lids (Fig. 12-37).

Lacrimal Apparatus

The **lacrimal gland** is hidden from view in the upper lateral region of the orbit between the frontal bone and the nearby extrinsic eye muscles (Fig. 12-37). A small portion of the gland projects into the lateral part of the upper eyelid. Lacrimal secretions provide moisture for the eye by passing over the anterior surface of the eyeball and draining into a tiny hole, the **punctum,** at the medial edge of each eyelid. Each punctum leads into a **lacrimal canaliculus,** which unite with one another to form the **lacrimal sac** at the medial aspect of the orbit. The sac in turn communicates with the **nasolacrimal duct** which carries the secretions downward to empty into the inferior region (meatus) of the nasal cavity. When one cries, the overabundance of lacrimal fluid spills over the lower eyelid in the form of tears. Much of the fluid, however, passes to the nasal cavity via the nasolacrimal duct.

Conjunctiva

The inner surfaces of the eyelids and much of the anterior surface of the eyeball are covered with a thin mucous membrane, the **conjunctiva** (Fig. 12-38). The conjunctiva is transparent and allows the whitish color of the outer coat of the eyeball to show through. If the conjunctiva becomes inflamed **(conjunctivitis)** the white area of the eye appears reddish because of the dilated blood vessels in the conjunctiva. At the medial angle of the eye the conjunctiva forms the **semilunar fold** which helps to trap foreign particles (Fig. 12-37). The particles are then passed on to the lacrimal caruncle, whose sticky secretions immobilize the material so that it can be wiped away from the eye.

Pupil and Iris

In the center of the anterior surface of the eyeball is a black, rounded aperture, the **pupil** (Fig. 12-37). Just peripheral to the pupil is the colored portion of the eye, the **iris.** The color of the iris depends on the amount of pigment

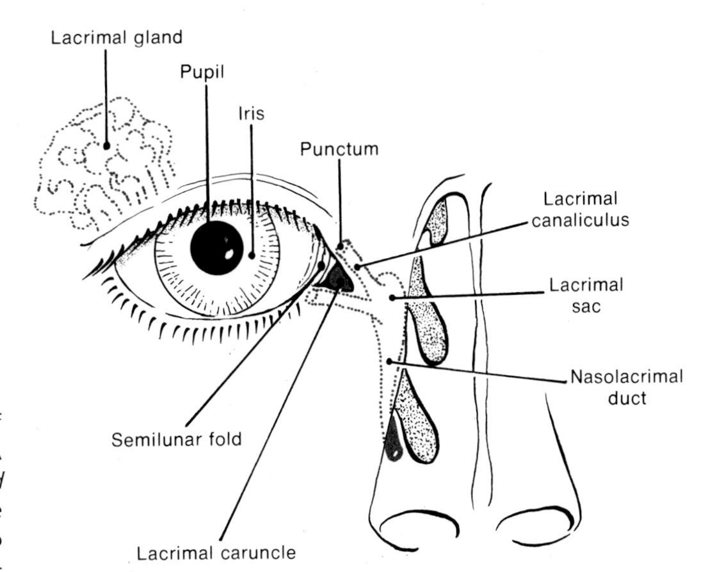

Fig. 12-37. Schematic anterior view of the eye showing lacrimal apparatus. A portion of the lacrimal gland *(dotted lines)* lies within the upper eyelid. The lacrimal canaliculi are located deep to the skin; the lacrimal sac and nasolacrimal duct are lodged in bone.

present, e.g., blue or gray eyes contain little pigment, brown eyes contain much. When pigment is completely lacking, as in albinos, the blood vessels in the iris give it a pink color. The iris also contains two groups of smooth **intrinsic muscles.** One is the **dilator pupillae** which increases the size of the pupil and is under sympathetic control. The other is the **sphincter pupillae** which constricts the pupil in response to bright light and is under parasympathetic control from the oculomotor nerve. Prior to an eye examination eyedrops containing atropine are often used to overcome the reflex sphincter action so as to allow the interior of the eyeball to be inspected with a bright light.

Cornea

The iris and pupil are covered anteriorly by the cornea, which is actually a transparent continuation of the outer coat of the eyeball. However, the conjunctiva stops at the periphery of the cornea (Fig. 12-38). The cornea lacks blood vessels and depends upon diffusion for its nutrients. It is readily transplantable and can be stored after death to be used in place of diseased corneas in the living.

Lens

Behind the pupil and iris is the lens, an oval, crystalline structure responsible for focusing light onto the sensory portion of the eye (Fig. 12-38). The lens is suspended by fibers called the **ciliary zonule.** These pass from the periphery of the lens to a muscular **ciliary body.** The contraction of smooth muscle fibers within the ciliary body enables the lens to change shape so as to accommodate one's sight to near or distant objects. As an individual gets older the lens hardens, and accommodation to near objects becomes more difficult. This is termed **presbyopia.** Should the lens become opaque, it is known as a **cataract.**

The wall of the eyeball is composed of three tunics (Fig. 12-38). The outermost is a layer of dense connective tissue known as the **sclera.** This constitutes the "white of the eye." The middle tunic is the **choroid,** a highly vascular and pigmented layer. The innermost tunic is the **retina** where the sensory cells are located.

Between the cornea and the iris is the **anterior chamber;** immediately behind the iris is

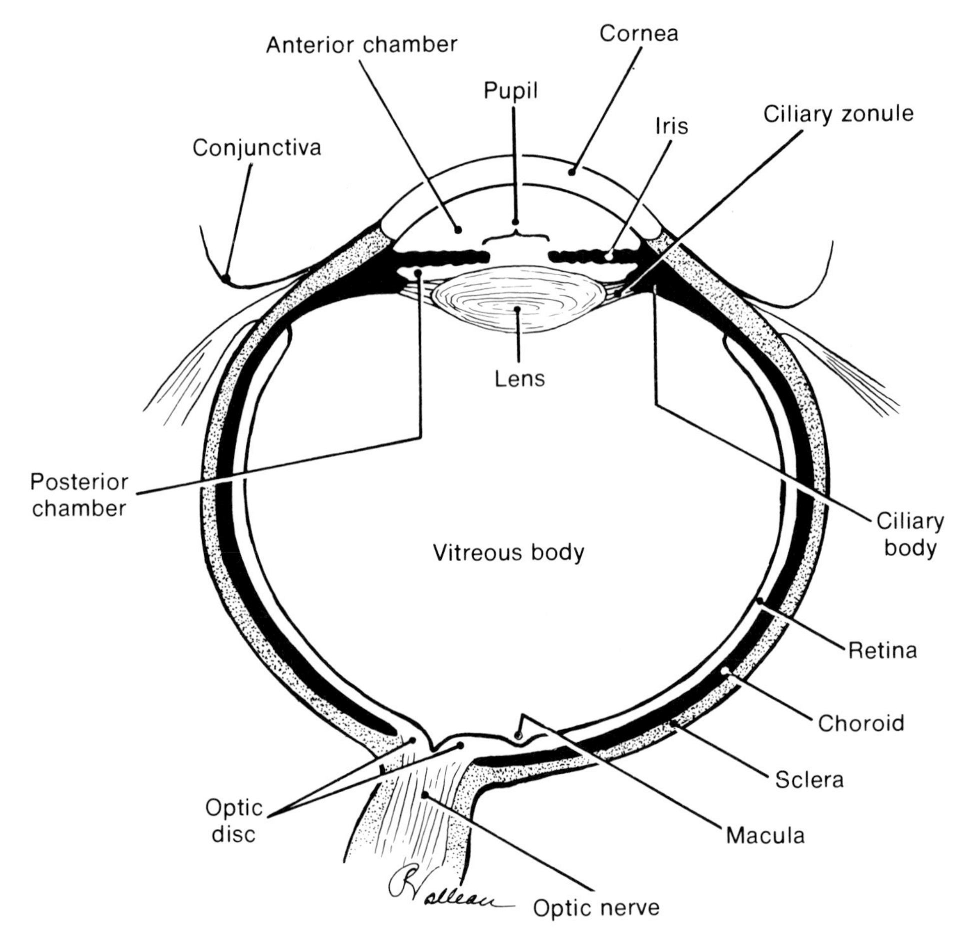

Fig. 12-38. Horizontal section through the right eyeball.

the **posterior chamber,** which lies between the iris and the lens. A watery fluid called **aqueous humor** is formed in the posterior chamber and passes to the anterior chamber. This fluid is constantly absorbed at the angle between the cornea and iris. Should a blockage occur, the abnormal accumulation of aqueous humor results in **glaucoma** which can lead to blindness because of eventual damage to the retina. The large space between the lens and the retina contains the **vitreous body** composed of a viscous material which provides shape and support to the walls of the eyeball.

Retina

The retina is the innermost coat of the eyeball and represents the sensory portion of the eye. With an instrument known as an ophthalmoscope one can shine light through the pupil and observe the condition of the surface of the retina (Fig. 12-39). This surface is often termed the **fundus.** In the center of the fundus is a yellowish spot, the **macula lutea,** which contains a slight depression, the **fovea.** It is here that the sharpest sense of vision occurs. Thus when one reads or watches a moving object the eyes are moved along so as to focus the image on this most sensitive portion of the retina.

Medial to the macula lutea is a whitish area, the **optic disc.** This represents the point at which the retinal arteries enter the eyeball and the optic nerve and retinal veins leave the eyeball. The retinal blood vessels radiate outward from the disc and are easily viewed with the

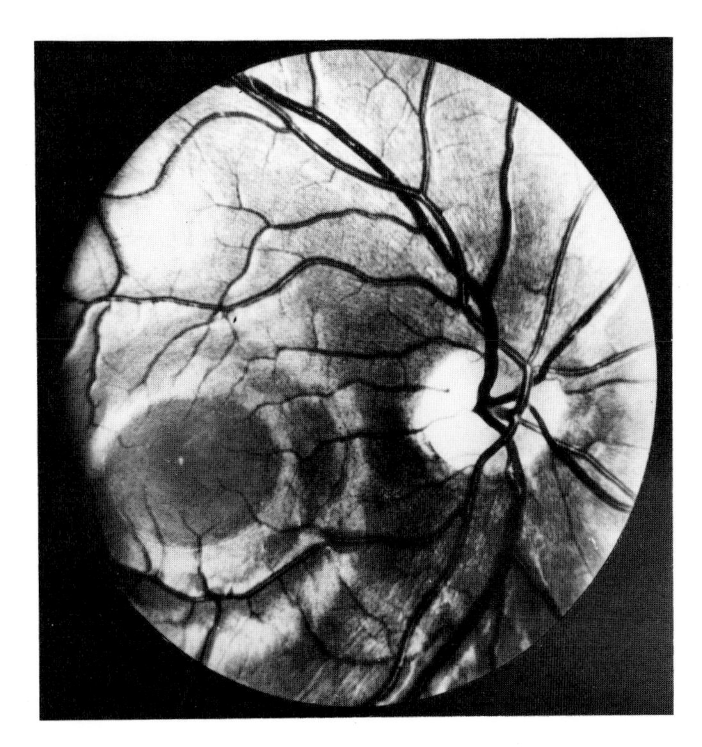

Fig. 12-39. A portion of the fundus of the right eye, as viewed with an ophthalmoscope. The dark circle on the left side of the photograph is the macula. The white circle on the right side of the photograph is the optic disc with retinal vessels radiating outward from it. (Courtesy of Dr. Hans Littmann and Carl Zeiss, Inc. From E. D. Gardner, D. J. Gray, and R. O'Rahilly, *Anatomy,* Ed. 4, W. B. Saunders Co., Philadelphia, 1975.)

ophthalmoscope. Since early pathological changes such as those associated with diabetes may be detected in the retinal blood vessels, an ophthalmoscopic examination provides important information not only on the condition of the fundus but also on the overall state of the vascular system.

Although the retina shows a complex arrangement of cells, these can be grouped into several layers (Fig. 12-40). The outermost layer is the **pigment layer of the retina** which is in contact with the choroid tunic (also containing pigment). These two pigmented layers trap the light rays and prevent them from passing beyond the retina.

Just internal to the pigment layer of the retina are layers of highly modified neurons known as cones and rods. These two types of cells are the sensory receptors of the retina. **Cones** contain the pigment iodopsin and are adapted for sharp vision (acuity) in light and for color vision. The cones are most highly concentrated in the fovea. **Rods** contain the pigment rhodopsin and are specialized for vision in dim light. Vitamin A is important for the formation of rhodopsin; therefore a deficiency of this vitamin often results in night blindness. The rods are most numerous in the periphery of the retina but are relatively sparse in the macula lutea. For this reason objects can be seen more easily in dim light if one does not look directly at them. Also, exposure to bright light impedes rod function, and if one goes from bright light to a darkened room it may take several minutes to adapt to the dim light.

The sensory impulses from the rods and cones are transmitted to the next layer of the retina consisting of **bipolar neurons.** These in turn pass the impulse to the innermost layer of neurons termed **ganglion cells.** The axons from the ganglion cells converge toward the optic disc and from there they exit from the eyeball as the optic nerve (cranial nerve II). Since rods and cones are absent from the optic disc, this area is often called the "blind spot."

The layered arrangement of retinal neurons is peculiar in that light rays must pass through the more superficial layers of the retina in order to reach the receptor cells (rods and cones) located in the deepest layer of neu-

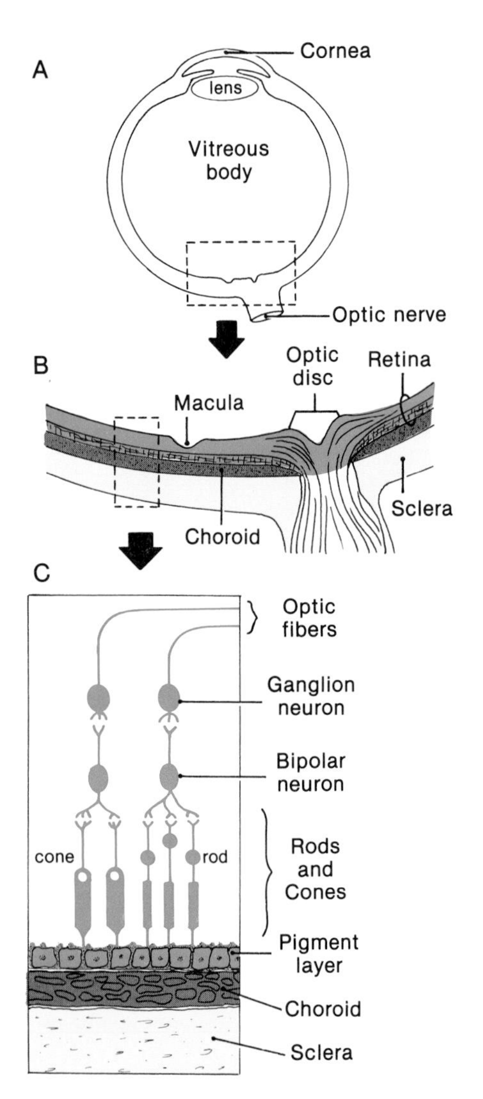

Fig. 12-40. (A) Horizontal section of the eye. The area enclosed by the rectangle is shown in B. (B) Higher magnification of the posterior portion of the eye. The rectangle encloses the area shown in C. (C) Higher magnification of the retina, choroid, and sclera.

rons. The impulses are then passed back to the most superficial layer containing the optic nerve axons. These axons ultimately pass through the wall of the eyeball on their way to the brain via the optic nerve.

Ear

Each ear contains two types of sensory receptors: those concerned with hearing and those concerned with the sense of equilibrium. In addition, the ear consists of numerous non-nervous structures which are supportive for the sensory portions and which also serve to collect, modify, and amplify incoming sound waves. The ear is conveniently subdivided into three regions: the external, middle, and internal (inner) ear (Fig. 12-41).

External Ear

The external ear consists of an outer flaplike structure (the **auricle** or **pinna**) and the **external acoustic (auditory) canal (meatus),** an oblique channel passing downward and inward to the **tympanic membrane** (eardrum). The auricle varies in shape and size and is composed of elastic cartilage covered by skin. The lower fleshy portion lacks cartilage and is termed the **lobule** ("earlobe"). The auricle helps to collect sound waves which pass down the external acoustic canal. The lateral portion of this channel is broad and cartilaginous; the medial portion is narrower and bony. Both regions are lined by skin containing hair and **ceruminous glands** which secrete the waxy substance **cerumen.** The hair and cerumen are important in trapping foreign particles so as to prevent them from reaching the tympanic membrane.

The **tympanic membrane** forms the boundary between the external and middle ear. The outer aspect of the membrane is covered with skin, the core of the membrane consists of fibrous connective tissue, and its inner aspect is lined with mucous membrane. The tympanic membrane vibrates according to the force of sound waves against it and transmits them to structures in the middle ear.

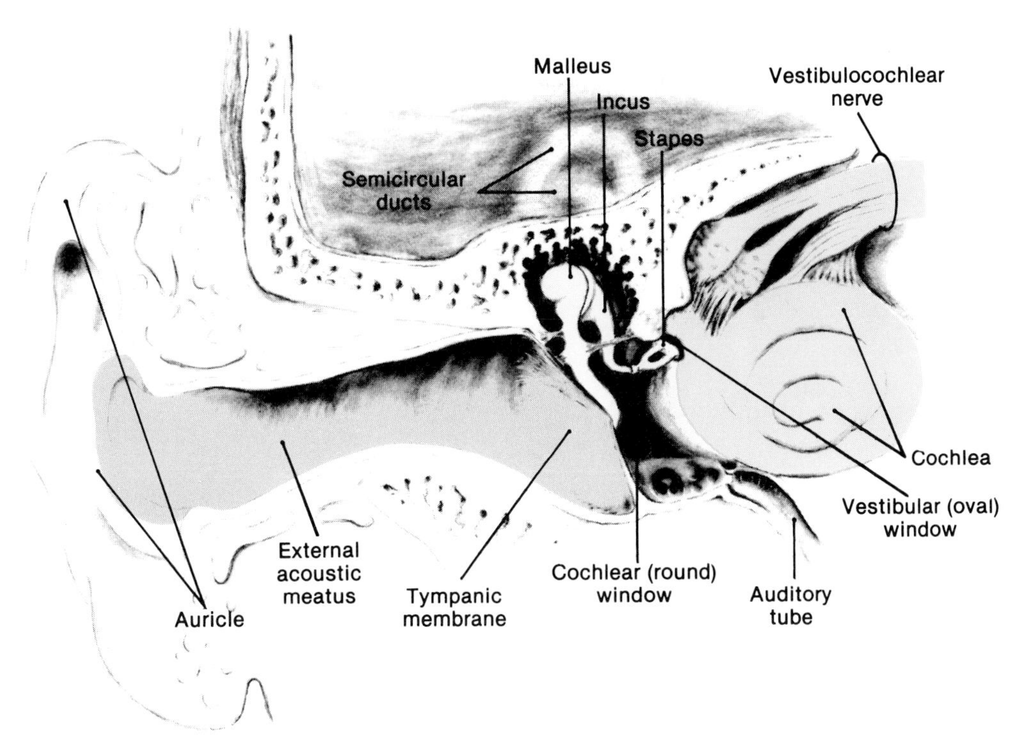

Fig. 12-41. The ear: external (red), middle (yellow), and internal (blue) portions.

Middle Ear

The middle ear includes a mucous membrane-lined chamber called the **tympanic cavity** containing three tiny bones **(ossicles).** These bones are arranged in end to end sequence and are responsible for transmitting and amplifying the sound waves to the internal ear. The first bone **(malleus)** is attached at one end to the tympanic membrane and at the other end to the second bone (the **incus**). The incus connects with the third bone (the **stapes**), which abuts against an aperture (**vestibular** or **oval window**) leading to the internal ear.

In order to prevent damage to the tympanic membrane, the air pressure against the outer surface of the membrane must be equalized by air pressure in the middle ear. This is accomplished by the **pharyngotympanic** (**Eustachian** or **auditory**) **tube** connecting the tympanic cavity with the pharynx. The tympanic cavity also communicates with a system of air-filled spaces in the mastoid portion of the temporal bone. Middle ear infections may spread into these spaces, producing an inflammation termed mastoiditis.

Internal (Inner) Ear

The internal ear is composed of an elaborate system of fluid-filled ducts termed the **membranous labyrinth** housed in a bony system of canals termed the **osseous labyrinth.** The upper portion of the membranous labyrinth contains three **semicircular ducts** which communicate with a saclike **utricle** below (Fig. 12-42). The utricle in turn joins the **saccule,** whose distal end communicates with a coiled tube, the **cochlear duct (cochlea).**

The membranous labyrinth contains a fluid, the **endolymph.** Clusters of special sensory cells occur at one end of each semicircular duct and in various regions of the utricle and saccule. These cells contain tiny hairs which are stimulated by the movement of endolymph

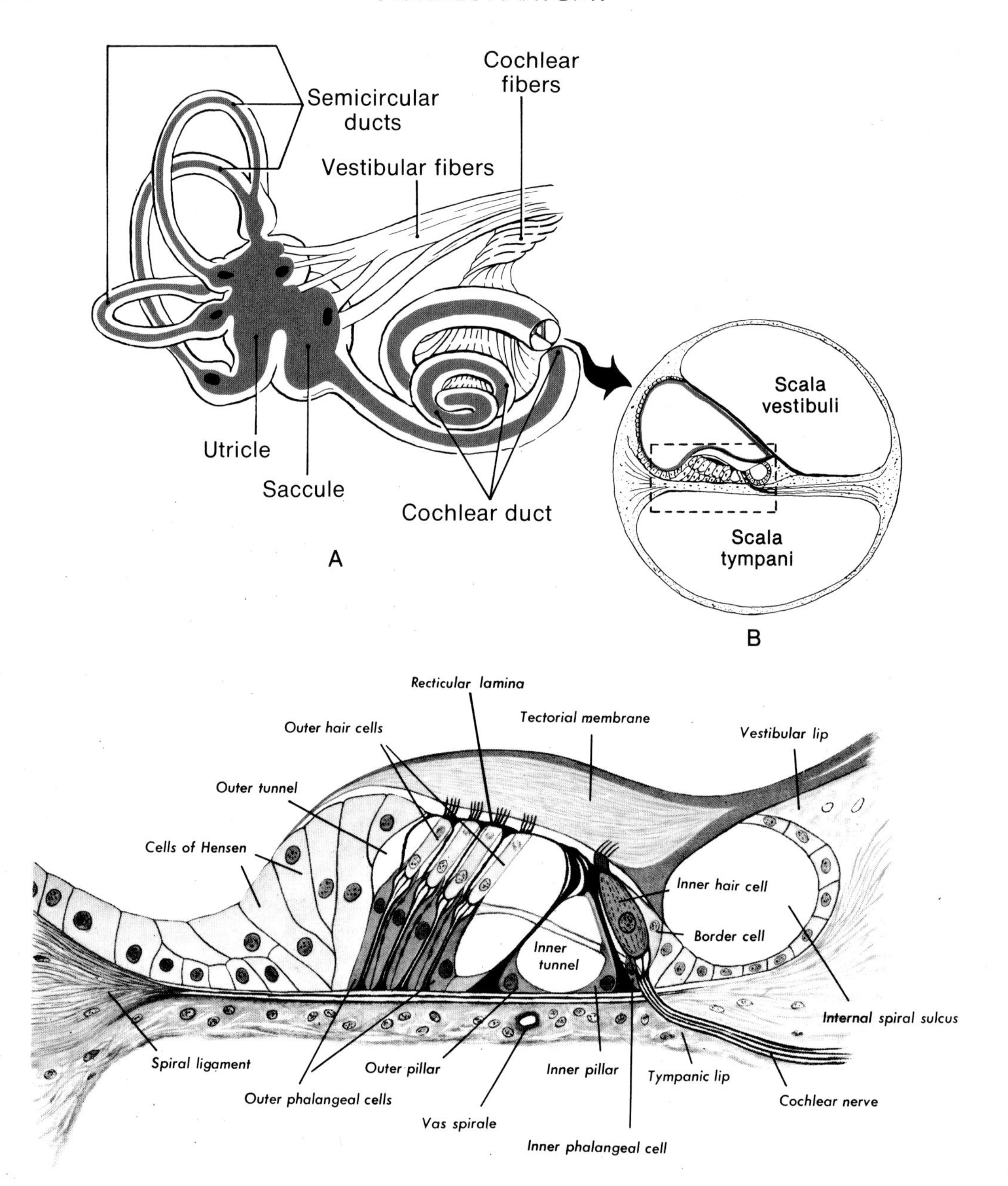

Fig. 12-42. The inner ear. (A) The membranous labyrinth (in red) lies within the osseous labyrinth. The dense black areas within the membranous labyrinth represent the locations of sensory cells. A portion of the cochlea is cut to reveal its internal structure depicted in cross section in B. (B) The broken line rectangle encloses the organ of Corti. (C) Microscopic section of the organ of Corti. (From W. M. Copenhaver, R. P. Bunge, and M. B. Bunge, *Bailey's Textbook of Histology,* Ed. 16, The Williams & Wilkins Co., Baltimore, 1971.)

when the head moves in different directions. Impulses concerned with equilibrium are then transmitted from these sensory cells to the **vestibular fibers** of the **vestibulocochlear nerve** (cranial nerve VIII).

The cochlear duct contains an elaborate and extremely complex sensory structure termed the **spiral organ of Corti** (Fig. 12-42). This consists of sensory cells with hairs projecting upward into a gelatinous shelflike structure (the **tectorial membrane**). These hairs are stimulated by movement of endolymph within the cochlea, and auditory impulses are then transmitted along the **cochlear fibers** of the vestibulocochlear nerve.

The membranous labyrinth is contained within and protected by the osseous labyrinth, a system of bony canals and sacs which follow the contours of the membranous labyrinth. The osseous labyrinth is filled with the fluid **perilymph,** acting as a cushion for the more delicate membranous labyrinth. The osseous labyrinth of the internal ear communicates with the middle ear by means of two membrane-covered apertures: the **vestibular (oval) window,** and the **cochlear (round) window** (Fig. 12-41).

Hearing occurs when sound waves are collected by the external ear and cause the tympanic membrane and ossicles of the middle ear to vibrate. The stapes pushes against the vestibular window, and the perilymph in the osseous labyrinth is thereby set in motion, transmitting pressure waves to the endolymph. Movement of the endolymph stimulates the hairs on the sensory cells in the spiral organ of Corti. The cochlear (round) window serves to equalize the endolymphatic pressure.

Diseases of the internal ear may affect either the vestibular or the cochlear portion or both. Difficulties with equilibrium may be attributable to damage of vestibular mechanisms, so that one experiences a dizzy swirling sensation **(vertigo).** Hearing deficits may result from a variety of causes, including damage to or malfunction of the spiral organ, vestibulocochlear nerve, ossicles of the middle ear, or tympanic membrane.

Olfactory Epithelium

The olfactory epithelium is located in the roof of the nasal cavities. It consists of non-nervous supporting cells and sensory receptor cells, the latter having minute hairlike processes. The axons of these sensory cells constitute cranial nerve I and pass upward into the cranial cavity via tiny holes in the cribriform plate of the ethmoid bone.

Taste Buds

The taste buds are small specialized structures which occur on the tongue, pharynx, larynx, and palate. The buds consist of specialized epithelial cells surrounding nerve endings which transmit the impulses to the brain. Further details on the distribution and function of these structures are provided in Chapter 14.

FUNCTIONAL CONSIDERATIONS OF THE NERVOUS SYSTEM

The nervous system serves as a means for communication among various portions of the body as well as with the external environment. For this reason it is difficult to understand how the nervous system functions unless one attempts to tie together and correlate the various regions and structures which have been presented individually. The following is a brief synopsis of some major functional pathways of the nervous system.

Sensory Pathways

Touch

The sense of touch is received at specialized endings of peripheral sensory nerve fibers. These are fibers of first order neurons which transmit the impulses into the spinal cord via the dorsal spinal roots of spinal nerves. From there they may take several pathways on their way to the brain (Fig. 12-43). Some impulses continue upward in the **fasciculus cuneatus** and **fasciculus gracilis** of the spinal cord to synapse with second order neurons in the me-

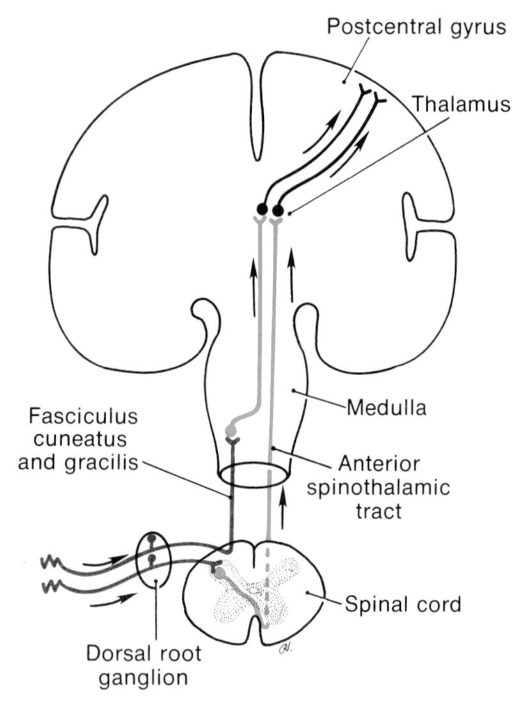

Fig. 12-43. Schematic diagram of pathways carrying touch impulses from the periphery to cerebral cortex. First order neurons are in red, second order in blue, third order in black.

dulla. The fibers of these second order neurons cross the midline and ascend to the thalamus to synapse with third order neurons whose fibers send the impulses to the postcentral gyrus of the cerebrum. Some impulses take a different pathway in the spinal cord by synapsing with neurons whose fibers cross immediately to the opposite side of the cord and ascend to the thalamus via **anterior spinothalamic tracts.** Regardless of the pathway taken the sensation of touch is ultimately perceived in the postcentral gyrus.

Pressure

The sense of pressure is transmitted by peripheral fibers which are different from those which carry the sense of touch. However, the central pathways taken by these two types of fibers are similar.

Temperature and Pain

The sensations of temperature and pain are carried along separate fibers which travel along similar central pathways. Temperature and pain receptors transmit impulses via sensory neurons whose fibers pass into the spinal cord by means of the dorsal roots. Many of these synapse with dorsal horn cells (second order neurons) whose axons cross the midline and ascend to the thalamus in the **lateral spinothalamic tracts** (Fig. 12-44). Impulses are then carried via third order neurons from the thalamus to the postcentral gyrus.

The pain and temperature pathways are crossed; thus if the lateral spinothalamic tract is cut, pain and temperature sensation will be lost on the opposite (contralateral) side of the body at levels below the transection. This procedure is sometimes used in cases where severe and constant pain cannot be alleviated by other methods.

Kinesthesis

The kinesthetic sense enables one to know the position of one's body and its various parts in space. Receptors for this are located primarily in joints and ligaments. These receptors send impulses via peripheral nerves and their dorsal roots into the spinal cord and from there upward along the **fasciculus cuneatus** and **fasciculus gracilis** to the medulla. Second order neurons then carry the impulses to the thalamus on the opposite side. Third order neurons in the thalamus transmit the impulses to the postcentral gyrus. The pathway for kinesthesis thus appears to be similar to one of the pathways for touch and pressure. The **spinocerebellar** tracts (anterior and posterior) are also involved in kinesthesis. However, since these pathways end in the cerebellum, the sensory impulses are not consciously perceived. Instead, the impulses provide the cerebellum with the spatial information necessary for coordinated limb movements to occur.

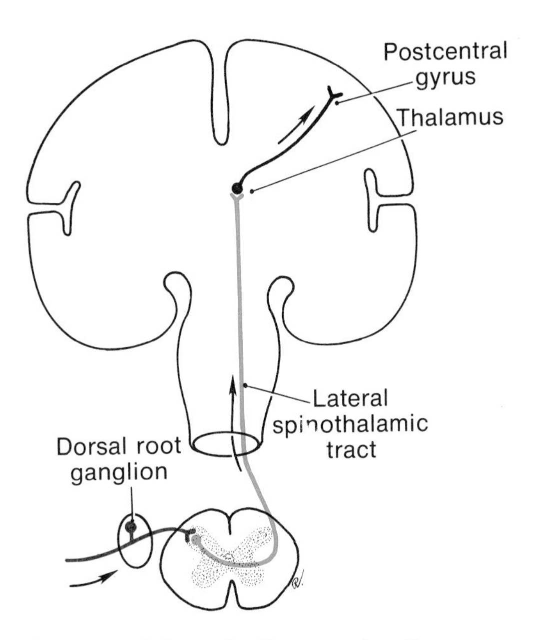

Fig. 12-44. Schematic diagram of pathway carrying pain and temperature impulses from periphery to cerebral cortex. First order neuron is in red, second order in blue, third order in black.

Pathways for the Special Senses

The **visual pathway** begins in the retina, where the sensory receptors (rods and cones) are stimulated by light and transmit the impulses first to the bipolar cells and then to the ganglion cells, whose axons leave the retina and travel back toward the brain as the optic nerve. When the axons of the optic nerve reach the optic chiasma, some of them cross over the median plane to the opposite side (Fig. 12-45). Beyond the chiasma the axons constitute the **optic tracts** which curve towards the superior colliculi, where some of the axons synapse with midbrain neurons involved with optic reflexes. Other axons of the optic nerve continue to the thalamus and synapse there with neurons projecting to the visual cortex in the occipital lobe of the cerebrum where the visual impulses are perceived and interpreted.

The **auditory pathway** originates with the sensory receptors of the spiral organ of Corti in the cochlear duct of the internal ear. The impulses are carried to the brain via fibers of the **cochlear division** of the **vestibulocochlear nerve** (VIII). The nerve cell bodies for these fibers reside in the **spiral ganglion** which lies adjacent to the cochlear duct (Fig. 12-46). When the fibers reach the brain stem they take a variety of routes to participate in complex auditory reflexes. The impulses are ultimately relayed to the temporal lobe of the cerebral hemisphere where auditory perception takes place.

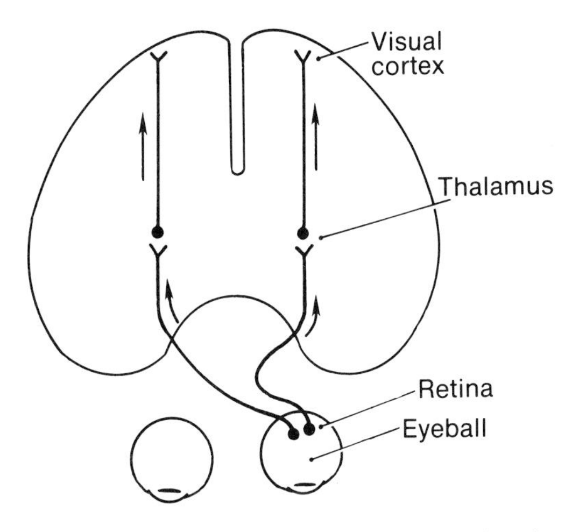

Fig. 12-45. Schematic diagram of the visual pathway from the left eyeball.

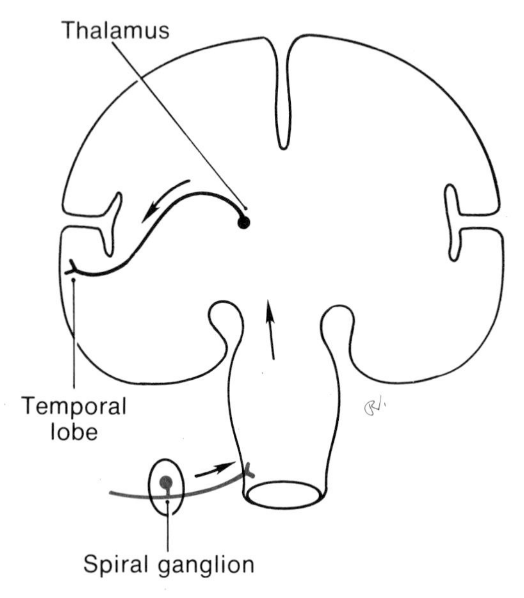

Fig. 12-46. Schematic diagram of the auditory pathway. First order neuron is in red, second order in blue, third order in black.

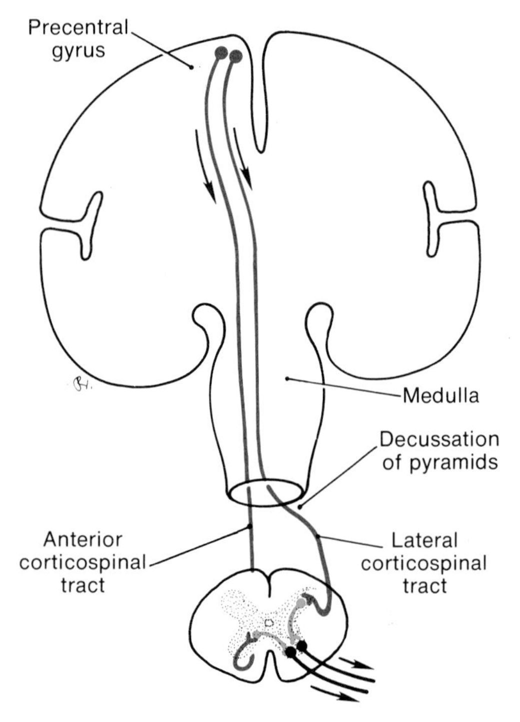

Fig. 12-47. Schematic diagram of the corticospinal pathway. First order neurons are in red, second order in blue, third order in black.

The **vestibular pathway** carries impulses relating to balance and equilibrium. These impulses originate at sensory receptors in the semicircular ducts, utricle, and saccule of the internal ear. The impulses travel to the reticular formation of the brain stem via the **vestibular fibers** of the vestibulocochlear nerve. From the brain stem the impulses are relayed to a variety of regions including the spinal cord and the nuclei of cranial nerves supplying the extrinsic eye muscles. It is believed that many of these impulses travel along central pathways similar to those used by auditory impulses. The widespread connections of the vestibular pathways explain why rapid rotation of the body may produce a broad range of symptoms such as dizziness (vertigo), nausea, and vomiting.

The **olfactory pathway** arises in the olfactory epithelium where gases in the inhaled air become dissolved in the fluid which covers the surface of the epithelial cells. The axons of these olfactory cells constitute the **olfactory nerve** and pass into the cranial cavity to synapse with neurons in the **olfactory bulb** on the underside of the frontal lobe of the cerebrum. The neurons in the olfactory bulb transmit impulses via the **olfactory tracts** which travel to ill-defined areas in the temporal and insular lobes of the cerebrum. The olfactory pathway is linked to a complex series of reflex pathways. An example of such reflexes are the nausea and vomiting which may occur in reaction to unpleasant odors.

The sense of smell dulls gradually with age. Also, repeated bombardment of olfactory impulses can dull one's perception of an odor, so that one becomes acclimated to it. This can be of benefit when one is forced to smell obnoxious odors for an extended period of time, but the danger exists that odors of some potentially lethal gases may be ignored.

The pathway for the sensation of **taste (gustatory sense)** is complex, since taste can actually be combinations of various other senses such as smell and temperature. Taste impulses are initiated when substances dissolved in the watery saliva stimulate taste buds. The impulses from the taste buds in the anterior two-thirds of the tongue are carried via axons in the **facial nerve** (VII), those from the posterior one-third via the **glossopharyngeal nerve** (IX), and those from the laryngeal and pharyngeal regions via the **vagus nerve** (X). The fibers of these nerves enter the medulla and synapse with second order neurons which cross over the median plane to the opposite side and ascend to the thalamus. Third order neurons in the thalamus then transmit the impulses to the lower end of the postcentral gyrus and portions of the temporal and insular lobes of the cerebrum.

Visceral Pain

The type of pain which originates from a visceral organ tends to be diffuse and difficult to localize. It travels into the spinal cord via sensory fibers in the dorsal root of the spinal nerve and synapses with second order neurons, some of whose fibers cross over the median plane and pass upward in the **lateral spinothalamic tract** of the opposite side. Other second order neurons send their fibers upward in the lateral spinothalamic tract of the same side. Since the impulses travel via crossed and uncrossed tracts, the lateral spinothalamic tract would have to be transected on both sides to abolish visceral pain.

The pain generated from visceral organs often is identified as emanating from areas of the body quite distant from the source of pain. This poorly understood phenomenon is known as **referred pain.** For example, pain from the heart may be referred to the left arm. A possible explanation is that the nerves carrying visceral pain from the heart enter the same segment of the spinal cord as do those carrying pain from the left arm, and the brain is unable to discriminate between impulses from these two regions.

Phantom Pain

The inability for the brain to distinguish the exact source of pain is also believed to be responsible for the phenomenon known as phantom pain. If a portion of a limb is amputated, the cut ends of nerves in the stump become irritated and send impulses to the brain. These impulses are interpreted as originating from the original nerve endings in the amputated portion so that the individual experiences pain as if the lost structure were still present. Phantom pain eventually subsides over a period of time.

Motor Pathways

Motor impulses can be initiated from various levels of the CNS, including the cerebral cortex, basal nuclei, cerebellum, brain stem, and spinal cord. Some of these impulses are initiated consciously and are under voluntary control, as when one reaches for a pencil. Other motor impulses originate involuntarily or unconsciously such as those concerned with reflexes, skeletal muscle tone, or smooth muscle activity in visceral organs.

Voluntary movements are initiated by **pyramidal cells** in the precentral gyrus of the cerebrum. The pyramidal cell fibers descend via the internal capsule to the medulla, where they form two bundles of fibers, the **pyramids,** each of which lies alongside the midline. Most of the fibers cross to the opposite side (decussation of the pyramids) and continue down the spinal cord in the **lateral corticospinal tracts** (Fig. 12-47). The latter may synapse directly with motor neuron cell bodies in the anterior horns or with internuncial neurons which in turn synapse with motor neurons. Some pyramidal cell fibers do not decussate in the medulla but instead descend in the **anterior corticospinal tracts** and then synapse with internuncial neurons which cross over in the spinal cord. The anterior horn neurons convey the motor impulses out to the skeletal muscles which respond by contracting. Because of the involvement of pyramidal cells and the lateral corticospinal tracts, this route taken by impulses for voluntary movements is often called the **pyramidal system** or **corticospinal pathway.**

Coordinated voluntary movements also occur via pathways grouped together as the **extrapyramidal system.** These originate in

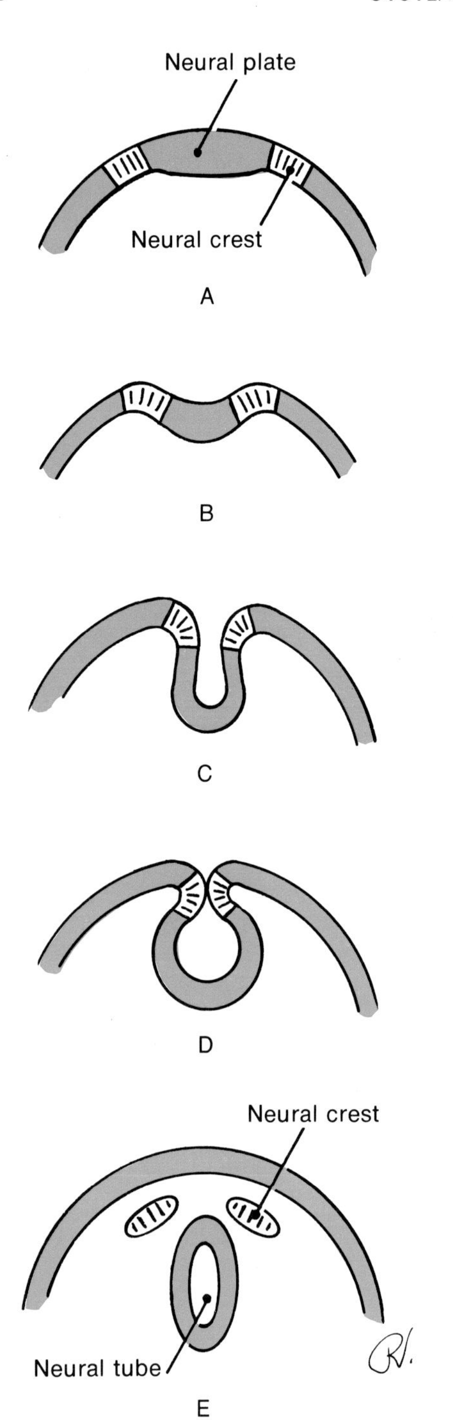

Fig. 12-48. Transverse sections through dorsal regions of embryos showing development of the neural tube.

motor areas (e.g., basal nuclei) of the cerebrum and pass through the internal capsule to synapse with neurons in the brain stem. Fibers from the brain stem nuclei descend in the anterior and lateral funiculi to synapse with anterior horn cells or internuncial neurons. A portion of the extrapyramidal system acts in an inhibitory capacity to regulate the strength of contractions. Damage to these neurons can thus result in exaggerated movements.

Involuntary movements can occur as spinal reflexes or they can be initiated in various regions of the brain (midbrain, pons, medulla, cerebellum) and travel down tracts to reach internuncial neurons and anterior horn neurons in the spinal cord. Involuntary movements concerned with the visceral organs are under control of the autonomic system (sympathetic and parasympathetic).

Neurological Lesions

Lesions in neurological pathways produce varied effects, depending on the location of the damage. If the spinal cord is transected or severely damaged, sensation is lost below the level of the lesion, since ascending sensory pathways are interrupted and cannot carry the impulses to the brain where they are perceived. Motor pathways will also be affected; thus paralysis occurs, since voluntary motor impulses initiated by the brain cannot reach the anterior horn neurons to be transmitted out to the muscles. However, spinal reflexes still remain intact below the lesion since these are not initiated by higher centers. For example, the bladder will empty spontaneously when it reaches a certain degree of distention. This is known as a "cord bladder," and the individual is incontinent due to lack of voluntary control over the act of urination.

DEVELOPMENTAL AND CLINICAL ANATOMY

As indicated in Chapter 5, the nervous system is an ectodermal derivative and is one of the first organ systems to develop in the embryo.

The ectoderm thickens in the midline to form the **neural plate,** and the edges of the neural plate then elevate and fuse dorsally to form the **neural tube** (Fig. 12-48). This fusion begins first in the cervical region and then progresses cranially and caudally (Fig. 12-49).

When the neural tube closes and pulls away from the overlying ectoderm, it leaves behind a cluster of **neural crest cells** lying in a longitudinal band on each side of the neural tube. Some of the neural crest cells form clusters of neurons which develop into the spinal and cranial ganglia. Other neural crest cells migrate ventrally and form the sympathetic ganglia. Still others become aligned alongside nerve cell processes and differentiate into Schwann cells.

Occasionally varying portions of the neural tube fail to close, leading to a group of congenital defects collectively termed **rachischisis.** In many instances the neural tube defect is associated with a gap in the skull or vertebral column, and the meninges and brain or spinal cord may even herniate to the outside. **Spina bifida** represents one of the most common of such defects and shows varying degrees of severity. For example if there is only a slight gap in the vertebra no symptoms may occur. However, cases in which the spinal cord and meninges bulge through the gap and onto the surface of the body result in severe neurological impairment (Fig. 12-50).

At an early phase of development the cranial part of the neural tube displays five vesicles: the **telencephalon, diencephalon, mesencephalon, metencephalon,** and **myelencephalon** (Fig. 12-51). The remainder of the tube becomes the spinal cord. The telencephalon enlarges considerably to form the two **cerebral hemispheres** which eventually comprise the major portion of the human brain. The diencephalon develops into the thalamus, and gives rise to the **pineal gland** superiorly and the **posterior lobe** of the **hypophysis** (pituitary) inferiorly. Laterally the diencephalon gives rise to the two **optic vesicles** which grow outward to form the eyes. The mesencephalon develops into the **superior** and **inferior colliculi** and **tegmentum,** and the metencephalon

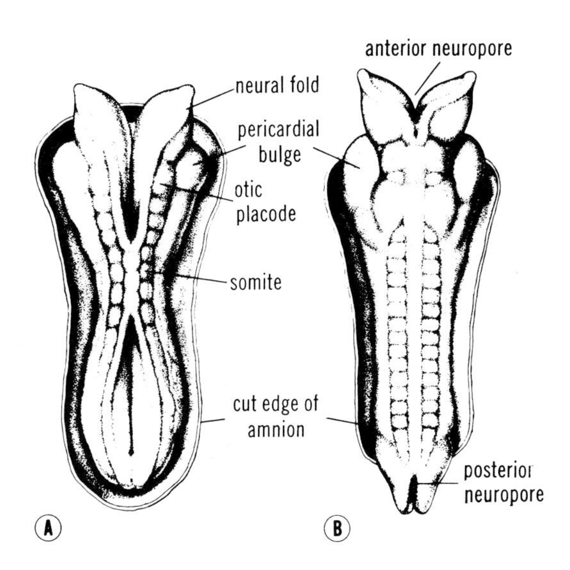

Fig. 12-49. Dorsal views of human embryos: (A) at approximately 22 days of gestation, with partial fusion of neural folds in midline; (B) at approximately 23 days of gestation, with more extensive fusion of neural folds, except at anterior and posterior neuropores. (From J. Langman, *Medical Embryology,* Ed. 3, The Williams & Wilkins Co., Baltimore, 1975.)

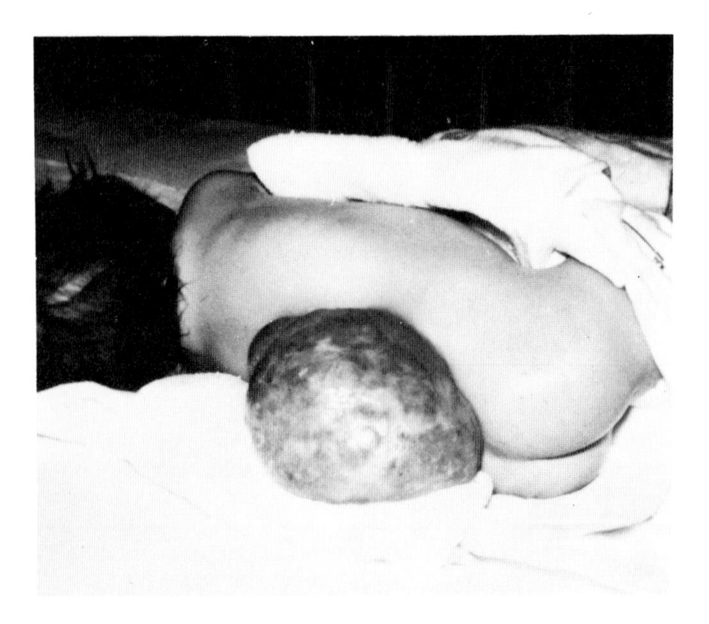

Fig. 12-50. A severe congenital defect involving marked protrusion of meninges and the spinal cord onto the surface of the body. (Reproduced with permission from L. V. Crowley: *An Introduction to Clinical Embryology*. Copyright © 1974 by Year Book Medical Publishers, Inc., Chicago.)

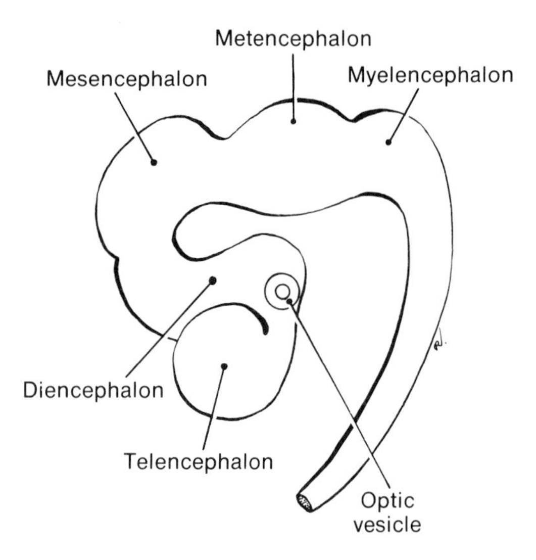

Fig. 12-51. Embryonic development of the brain. During the sixth week of gestation the brain consists of five portions: telencephalon (primitive cerebral hemispheres), diencephalon, mesencephalon, metencephalon, and myelencephalon.

forms the **cerebellum** dorsally and the **pons** ventrally. The myelencephalon becomes the **medulla oblongata** leading into the spinal cord.

The ventricles of the brain are expansions of the hollow interior of the embryonic neural tube. In the early stages of development the cavity within the mesencephalon is quite large but it gradually becomes narrower as the walls of the mesencephalon increase in thickness, until finally only the slender cerebral aqueduct remains. Sometimes this aqueduct becomes completely occluded during development and thus prevents proper flow of cerebrospinal fluid from the first three ventricles to the fourth ventricle. This results in **hydrocephalus** and eventual brain damage because of the severe pressure created by the accumulation of fluid.

As the optic vesicles grow out from the diencephalon, they remain attached to the brain by means of an **optic stalk.** Each vesicle then invaginates to form an **optic cup** (Fig. 12-52). The inner layer of this cup develops into the retina, which sends nerve fibers to the brain via the optic stalk, thereby converting it into the optic nerve. The outer layer of the optic cup becomes the pigment layer of the retina. The

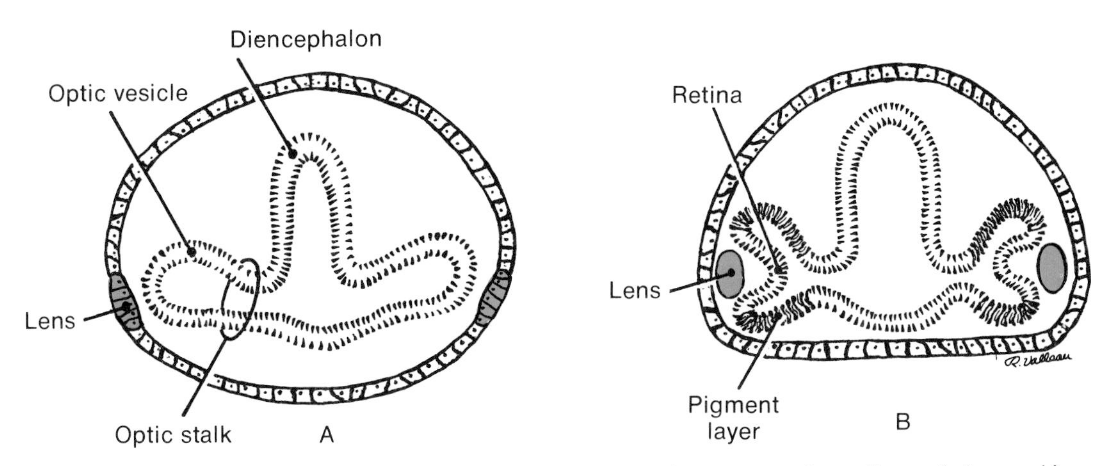

Fig. 12-52. Embryonic development of the eye. (A) Optic vesicles grow out from diencephalon, and lens develops as a thickening (blue) in the epidermal ectoderm. (B) Optic vesicles invaginate to form optic cups, and the lens pinches off from the surface and sinks into the optic cup.

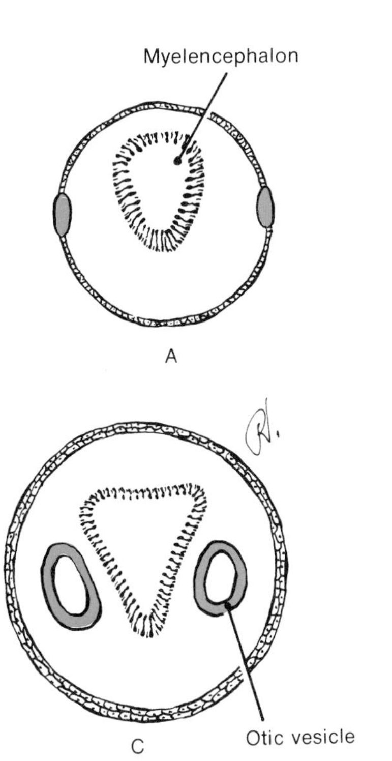

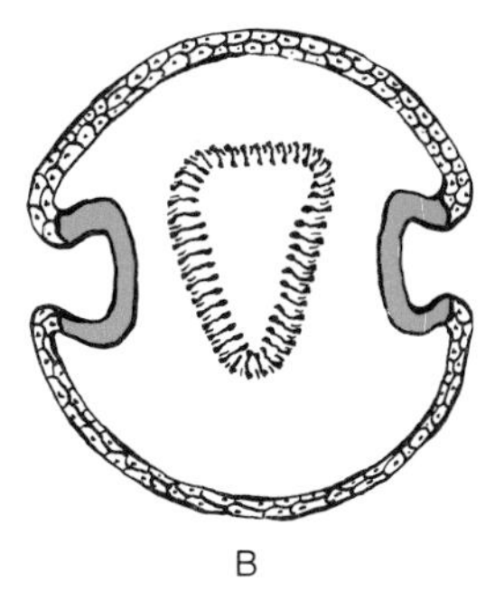

Fig. 12-53. Development of the inner ear from a portion of the surface ectoderm of the embryo. (A) Surface ectoderm thickens lateral to myelencephalon. (B, C) Thickened ectoderm forms otic vesicle which detaches from surface. (Otic vesicle will develop into the membranous labyrinth.)

small slitlike cavity between the retina and pigment layer eventually disappears, although it is possible for the two layers to become separated once again in adult life. This separation is termed a **detached retina.** The **lens** develops from a thickening of the epidermal ectoderm overlying the optic cup. This soon detaches and sinks down into the mouth of the cup. The remaining overlying ectoderm becomes transparent and develops into the **cornea.**

The internal ear originates from a thickening of the surface ectoderm near the myelencephalon (Fig. 12-53). This thickened ectoderm forms the **otic** (**auditory**) **vesicle** which pinches off from the surface and eventually differentiates into the membranous labyrinth. The middle and external ears develop quite independently from other structures in the head. Thus congenital defects may affect only one portion of the ear while leaving the other portions virtually unaffected.

13

The Endocrine System

The endocrine system is composed of specialized glands and groups of cells whose secretions are called **hormones.** Since hormones are secreted directly into the vascular system, the endocrine glands are often referred to as ductless glands, in contrast to the exocrine glands whose secretions are carried via a system of ducts or tubules.

Three of the endocrine glands are unpaired: the pituitary (hypophysis), thyroid, and pineal glands (Fig. 13-1). Three are paired: the superior parathyroid, inferior parathyroid, and suprarenal (adrenal) glands. Other glands contain endocrine components and may thus be classified as endocrine organs: the gonads (ovaries or testes) and the pancreas. In addition, there are endocrine cells in the digestive and urinary systems which secrete hormones into the blood stream. The thymus gland is sometimes also included in the endocrine system, although its immunologic role warrants its inclusion in the lymphatic system (Chapter 10).

Several general principles should be kept in mind as one studies the endocrine system. Endocrine organs are highly vascularized since they depend on the blood to distribute their hormones throughout the body. Despite this extensive area of distribution, most hormones affect only certain target tissues or organs. Also, the quantity of hormone necessary to elicit a response from a target organ is often quite minute. Hormones act as chemical messengers and thus play an important role in regulating various body processes. In this respect the endocrine system shows a similarity to the nervous system, and indeed the interactions of the two warrant their being grouped together as the neuroendocrine system. However, hormonal action lacks the speed of the nervous system, although hormonal effects are often longer lasting.

PITUITARY GLAND

The pituitary gland or hypophysis has often been called the "master gland" because its hormones affect and regulate various other endocrine organs. The pituitary is housed in a hollow depression (the sella turcica) of the sphenoid bone and consists of two portions: the **adenohypophysis (anterior lobe)** and the **neurohypophysis (posterior lobe)** (Fig. 13-2). In the embryo the adenohypophysis develops from the roof of the mouth as a pouch of ectoderm **(Rathke's pouch)** which becomes detached and grows upward toward the developing brain. At the same time a downward growing diverticulum develops from what will be the hypothalamus of the brain. The diverticulum is called the **infundibulum,** and it develops into the neurohypophysis (Fig. 13-2).

The adult adenohypophysis contains several subdivisions: a **pars distalis** which develops from the thickened anterior wall of

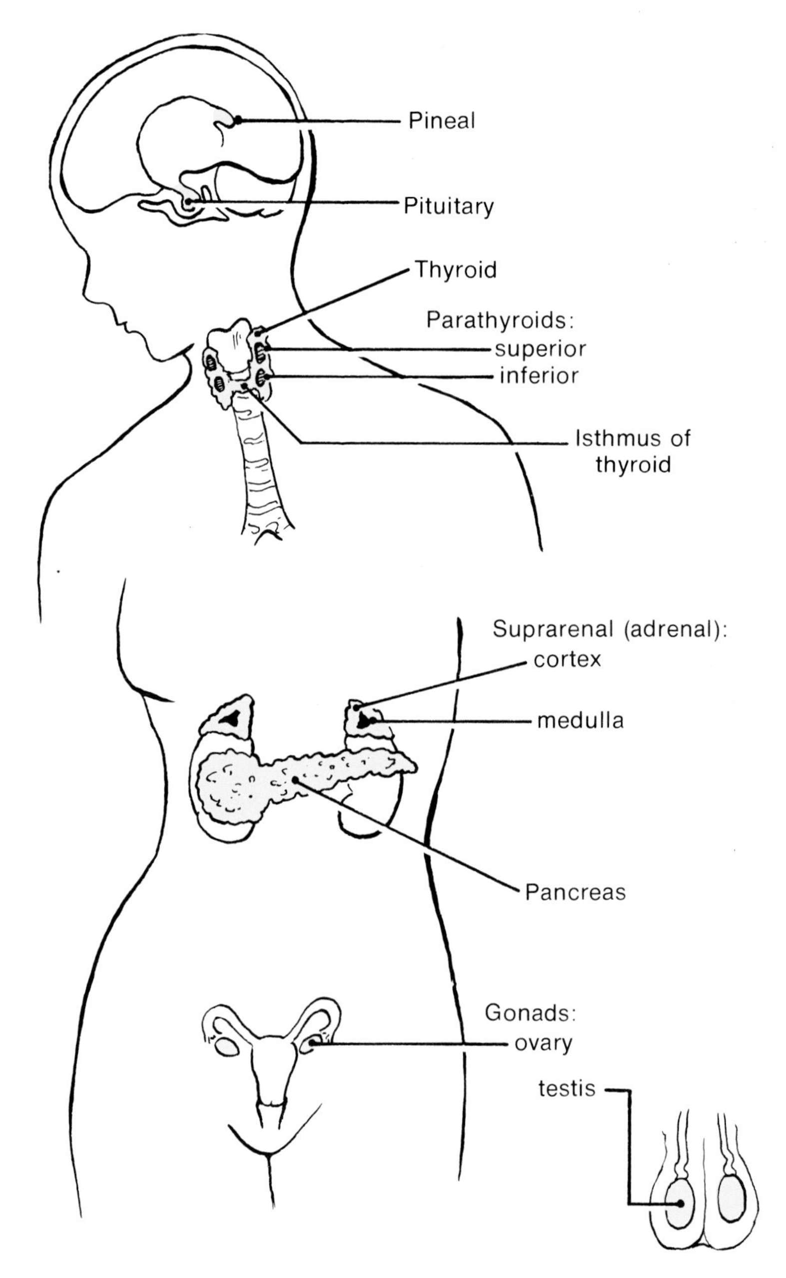

Fig. 13-1. The endocrine organs (in yellow).

Rathke's pouch, a **pars tuberalis** representing an upward extension of the pars distalis surrounding the neurohypophysis, a thin **pars intermedia** which develops from the posterior wall of Rathke's pouch, and a tiny slit representing the lumen of the pouch (Fig. 13-2). The adult neurohypophysis consists of a **neural stalk** and **pars nervosa** derived from the embryonic infundibulum.

Adenohypophysis

The adenohypophysis secretes several hormones which affect the activities of other endocrine glands and are thus termed **trophic**

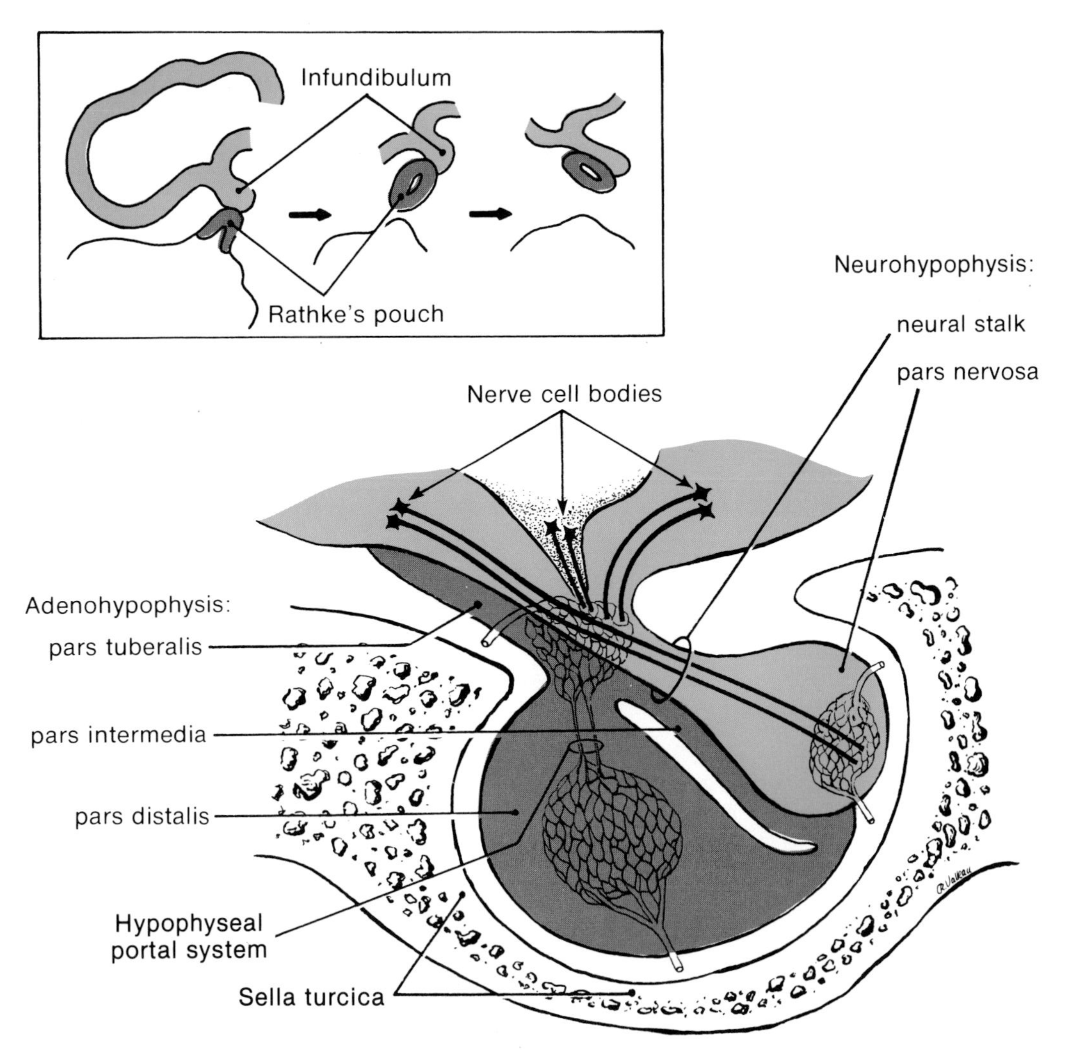

Fig. 13-2. Diagram of a sagittal section through the sella turcica and the pituitary gland (hypophysis), showing the hypophyseal portal system. Red structures are portions of the adenohypophysis (anterior lobe); blue structures represent the neurohypophysis (posterior lobe) and ventral aspect of the brain (hypothalamus). Insert *(upper left)* shows embryonic origins of components of the hypophysis from Rathke's pouch (red) and infundibulum (blue).

hormones. The release of these trophic hormones depends on substances called "releasing factors" produced by cells in the hypothalamus whose axons terminate in the neurohypophysis. The releasing factors reach the adenohypophysis by way of blood vessels (hypophyseal portal veins) which connect the capillary beds of these two regions. This interconnecting vascular network is called the **hypophyseal portal system** (Fig. 13-2).

The pars distalis and pars tuberalis of the adenohypophysis consist of epithelial-like cells arranged in loose cords. These cells have been classified into three types on the basis of their staining characteristics: acidophils, basophils, and chromophobes (Fig. 13-3A).

The **acidophils** comprise about 40% of the cells of the adenohypophysis and are responsible for producing two hormones: growth hormone and lactogenic hormone. **Growth hor-**

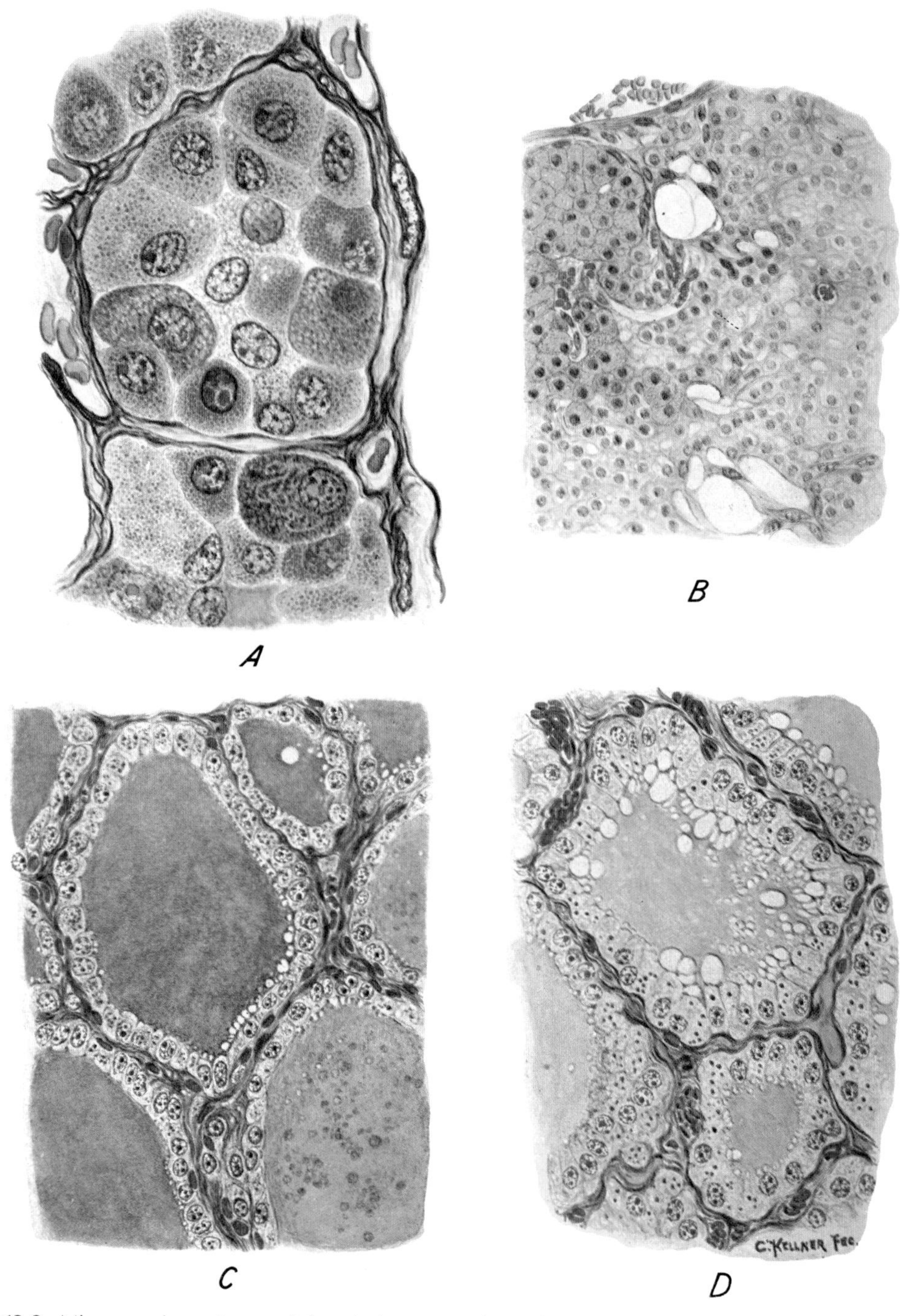

Fig. 13-3. Microscopic anatomy of the pituitary, parathyroid, and thyroid glands. (A) Cords of cells in the pars distalis of the pituitary gland. Acidophils are pink, basophils are blue, and chromophobes are gray. (B) Parathyroid gland showing oxyphil cells (pink) and chief cells (light blue). (C) Normal thyroid gland showing several follicles lined with cuboidal cells and containing colloid (dark blue). (D) Highly activated thyroid gland with tall columnar cells. (From W. M. Copenhaver, R. P. Bunge, and M. B. Bunge, *Bailey's Textbook of Histology,* Ed. 16, The Williams & Wilkins Co., Baltimore, 1971.)

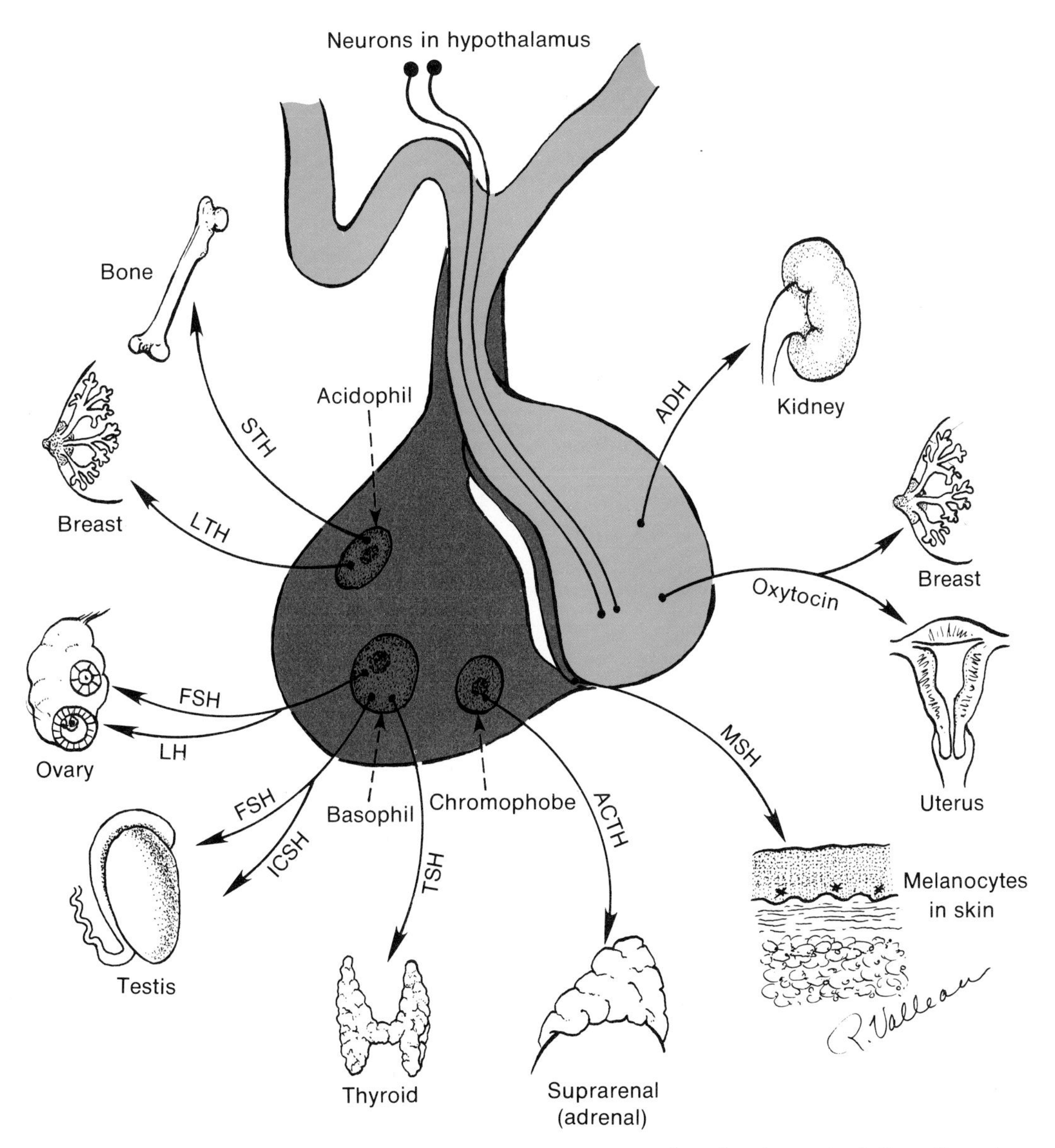

Fig. 13-4. Summary of pituitary hormones and their target organs. The adenohypophysis (in red) produces somatotrophic hormone (STH), luteotrophic hormone (LTH), follicle stimulating hormone (FSH), luteinizing hormone (LH), interstitial cell stimulating hormone (ICSH), thyroid stimulating hormone (TSH), adrenocorticotrophic hormone (ACTH), and melanocyte stimulating hormone (MSH). The neurohypophysis (in blue) produces antidiuretic hormone (ADH) and oxytocin. (After Leeson and Leeson.)

mone (also called **somatotrophic hormone,** or **STH**) has a generalized effect on body growth and a specific effect on bone growth (Fig. 13-4). Deficiency of this hormone results in **dwarfism.** On the other hand, an overabundance of growth hormone in growing children produces **gigantism,** and in adults a thickening of bony structures, especially in the face, hands, and feet. The latter condition is known as **acromegaly.** The **lactogenic hormone** (also called **pro-**

lactin, luteotrophic hormone, or **LTH**) acts specifically on the female breast during pregnancy and is responsible for the production of milk (lactation).

The **basophils** of the pars distalis and tuberalis comprise only about 10% of the total number of cells, but are responsible for producing important **gonadotrophic** and **thyrotrophic hormones.** One of the gonadotrophic hormones is **follicle stimulating hormone (FSH)** which causes growth of the ovarian follicles in females and the production of sperm in males. The other hormone is **luteinizing hormone (LH)** which in the female is necessary for ovulation and corpus luteum growth, and in the male (where it is known as **interstitial cell stimulating hormone,** or **ICSH**) stimulates the testes to produce the male hormone testosterone. The **thyrotrophic hormone (thyroid stimulating hormone, TSH)** acts on the thyroid gland and causes it to produce, store, and release thyroxine.

The **chromophobe cells** are so named because they do not stain well when processed for light microscopy. Many of these cells may actually be precursors or inactive states of acidophils or basophils. However, certain of these chromophobe cells are now known to produce **adrenocorticotrophic hormone (ACTH)** which stimulates the cortex of the suprarenal (adrenal) glands.

The **pars intermedia** of the adenohypophysis is not well-developed in humans and often contains small epithelial-lined vesicles. A hormone, **melanocyte stimulating hormone (MSH),** is produced here and is believed to stimulate pigment formation in the skin.

Neurohypophysis

The **neural stalk** and **pars nervosa** of the neurohypophysis contain nerve endings and fibers extending downward from nerve cell bodies in the hypothalamus (Fig. 13-2). Some of these cell bodies produce releasing factors, which act on the adenohypophysis. Other hypothalamic nerve cell bodies produce the hormones oxytocin and antidiuretic hormone. **Oxytocin** has a stimulatory effect on the smooth muscle of the uterus and also stimulates contraction of myoepithelial cells in the mammary gland to cause milk to be released during lactation. **Antidiuretic hormone (ADH, vasopressin)** acts on the kidney to regulate water balance. The releasing factors and hormones are transported in the axons which make up the neural stalk and are stored in the nerve endings in the pars nervosa, from which they are eventually released into the blood capillary network of the pituitary. In addition to the nerve fibers and their endings, the neurohypophysis contains a population of cells called **pituicytes** which are similar in form and function to the supporting cells (neuroglia) of the central nervous system.

THYROID GLAND

The thyroid gland is located anterior and lateral to the upper part of the trachea and lower part of the larynx (Fig. 13-1). This butterfly-shaped gland consists of two lateral lobes connected by a narrow bridge of tissue, the **isthmus.** An outer capsule of dense connective tissue subdivides the gland into lobules. Each lobule in turn contains numerous closed sacs called **follicles** (Fig. 13-3*C*). The follicles are lined by a simple cuboidal epithelium which produces the hormone **thyroxine.** These cuboidal cells become tall columnar cells in a highly active thyroid gland (Fig. 13-3*D*).

Thyroxine has a generalized effect on the body by accelerating metabolism and increasing heat production. Thyroxine is stored in the form of **thyroglobulin** in the central cavity (lumen) of the thyroid follicles. This storage material is quite thick and viscous and is often referred to simply as **colloid.** The stored thyroglobulin is periodically released after being reconverted to thyroxine which then passes out through the follicle cells and into the blood vessels surrounding the follicle. The synthesis, storage, and release of thyroxine are under control of the thyrotrophic hormone (TSH) from the pars distalis of the pituitary gland.

Hypothyroidism occurs when the thyroid does not produce sufficient amounts of thyrox-

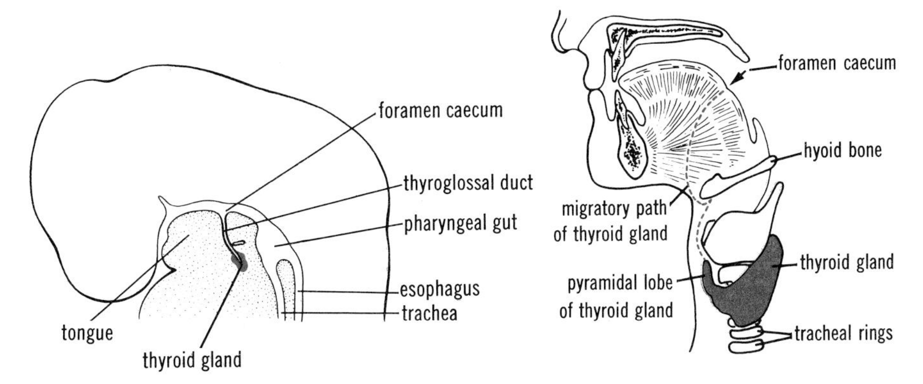

Fig. 13-5. Development of the thyroid gland. *(Left)* The thyroid develops as a ventral diverticulum from the foregut near the developing tongue. *(Right)* The thyroid diverticulum detaches and migrates caudally from its point of origin to its adult position anterior to the larynx and trachea. (From J. Langman, *Medical Embryology,* Ed. 3, The Williams & Wilkins Co., Baltimore, 1975.)

ine. In such individuals there is an overall sluggishness, decreased heat production and sensitivity to cold, and tissue fluid accumulation (referred to as myxedema). An overproduction of thyroxine constitutes **hyperthyroidism.** Such individuals are nervous, and the accelerated body metabolism results in weight loss.

The thyroid can become enlarged due to a variety of factors, and this enlargement is known as **goiter.** One cause of goiter is a lack of iodine, since iodine is important in the synthesis of thyroxine. Most of the iodine ingested in foods becomes concentrated for use in the thyroid gland, and this forms the basis for a clinical diagnostic test in which the uptake of radioactive iodine serves as an indicator of thyroid activity. Thyroxine is also important during prenatal development and childhood, during which time a deficiency can result in a growth lag, dwarfism, edema, and mental retardation. This syndrome is known as **cretinism.**

In addition to thyroxine the thyroid gland also produces a second hormone, **thyrocalcitonin,** which helps to lower the calcium level in the blood by facilitating the deposition of calcium salts in bone tissue. Thyrocalcitonin is produced by parafollicular cells which occur along the base of each follicle but which do not reach the lumen.

The thyroid gland develops embryologically as a ventral median outgrowth from the floor of the embryonic pharynx in the region where the tongue develops. The gland then loses its connection with the pharynx and migrates downward to assume its adult position anterior to the larynx and trachea (Fig. 13-5). Occasionally the thyroid retains its earlier position near the tongue and is thus termed a lingual thyroid. Also, it is possible for a trail of thyroid tissue to be left behind as the thyroid gland migrates downward, and even for a duct to be present connecting the base of the tongue to the thyroid gland. Such anomalies in position are unusual and seldom create difficulties, unless the aberrant thyroid tissue represents the only source of thyroid hormone and is mistakenly removed, thereby depriving the body of its essential supply of thyroxine.

PARATHYROID GLANDS

Four tiny parathyroid glands are situated on the posterior aspect of the thyroid gland. Associated with each lobe of the thyroid are a **superior parathyroid** and **inferior parathyroid gland** (Fig. 13-1). The parathyroids secrete **parathyroid hormone** (parathormone) which raises the level of calcium in the blood by mobilizing calcium from the bones. The action of parathyroid hormone is antagonistic to the action of thyrocalcitonin from the thyroid gland, and the two hormones thus regulate the level of calcium in the blood. Although the parathyroid glands contain two cell types (**chief cells** and **oxyphil cells**), a functional distinction between them has not yet been determined (Fig. 13-3*B*).

Hypersecretion of parathyroid hormone causes an excessive demineralization of the bones. Hyposecretion of the hormone produces a lowering of the calcium level in the blood, thereby affecting muscle contraction so that muscle spasms (tetany) occur. Because the parathyroid glands are essential for life, care must be taken to avoid damaging them during surgery on the thyroid gland.

In the embryo, the parathyroid glands develop as endodermal outpouchings from the lateral aspect of the embryonic pharynx. These endodermal cells then break away and migrate caudally to their final position along the back of the thyroid gland. As in the case of the thyroid gland, tiny nests of parathyroid cells can occasionally remain along their migration pathway.

SUPRARENAL (ADRENAL) GLANDS

The suprarenal or adrenal glands are located near the upper poles of the kidneys and are considered to be retroperitoneal. Each gland consists of a cortex and a medulla (Fig. 13-1).

The **cortex** of the adrenal gland produces several hormones, including glucocorticoids, mineralcorticoids, and small amounts of sex hormones. The **glucocorticoids (cortisone, cortisol, corticosterone)** aid in breaking down body proteins, especially in muscle, and are generally secreted in response to stress. They also help to lessen inflammatory responses, and cortisone is thus often used clinically as an antiinflammatory agent. The synthesis and release of glucocorticoids are under control of adrenocorticotrophic hormone (ACTH) from the anterior pituitary gland. The **mineralcorticoids** produced by the adrenal cortex include the hormone **aldosterone**, which is important in regulating water balance by increasing reabsorption of sodium by the kidney tubules, thereby resulting in water retention as well. (Diuretics, which are used to cause water loss, act by blocking aldosterone activity in the kidney.) Small amounts of male and female sex hormones are also produced by the adrenal cortex in both sexes.

Histologically the adrenal **cortex** consists of three zones (Fig. 13-6). The outermost zone contains numerous nests of cells and is called the **zona glomerulosa.** The middle zone is the largest, consists of straight rows of cells, and is thus termed the **zona fasciculata.** The innermost zone, the **zona reticularis,** is composed of a network of anastomosing cords of cells. Although attempts have been made to assign the secretion of certain hormones to each zone, there is still some debate as to the functional significance of this zonation.

The **medulla** of the suprarenal gland produces the well-known hormone **adrenalin (epinephrine)**, as well as a related hormone **noradrenalin (norepinephrine).** These hormones are released in response to stressful circumstances and produce what is known as the fight or flight reaction, in which the heart beat accelerates, blood is shunted away from visceral structures to skeletal and heart muscles, and the overall metabolic rate is increased. This reaction is similar to that produced by stimulation of the sympathetic nervous system, and indeed the cells of the adrenal medulla are derived embryologically from the same source as the postganglionic sympathetic neurons (i.e., from neural crest cells). The adrenal medulla cells are also termed **chromaffin cells** because of their ability to be stained with chrome salts.

Although an individual could survive quite well without the adrenal medulla, the adrenal cortex is vital. Hypofunction of the cortex produces **Addison's disease** characterized by profound changes in water balance, kidney function, and carbohydrate metabolism. Hyperfunction of the cortex can produce **Cushing's syndrome** consisting of a depletion of body proteins and a masculinization in females because of the increased production of androgens. Hyperfunction of the adrenal medulla results in increased metabolism.

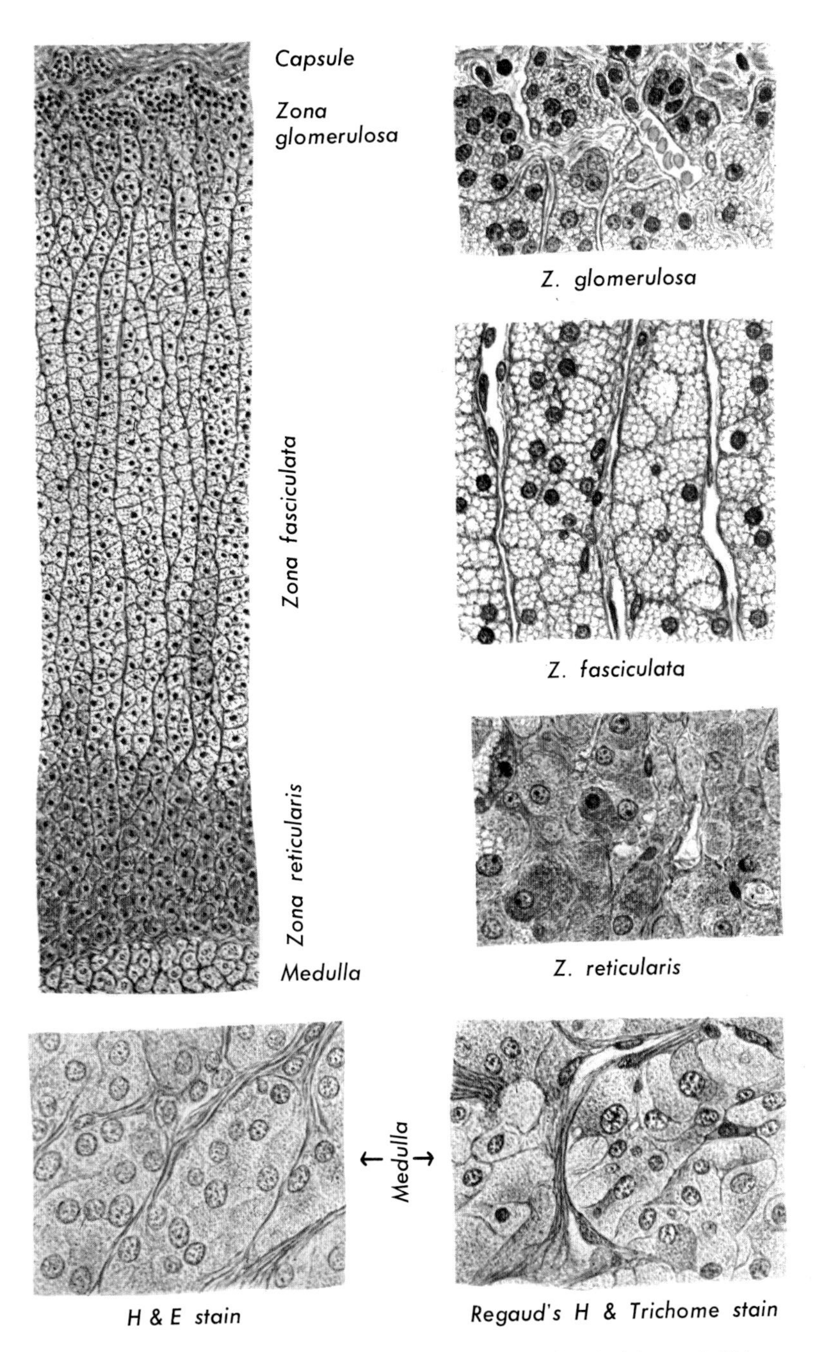

Fig. 13-6. Microscopic sections through the adrenal (suprarenal) gland. *(Upper left)* Low magnification. Other sections show higher magnifications of each zone. (From W. M. Copenhaver, R. P. Bunge, and M. B. Bunge, *Bailey's Textbook of Histology,* Ed. 16, The Williams & Wilkins Co., Baltimore, 1971.)

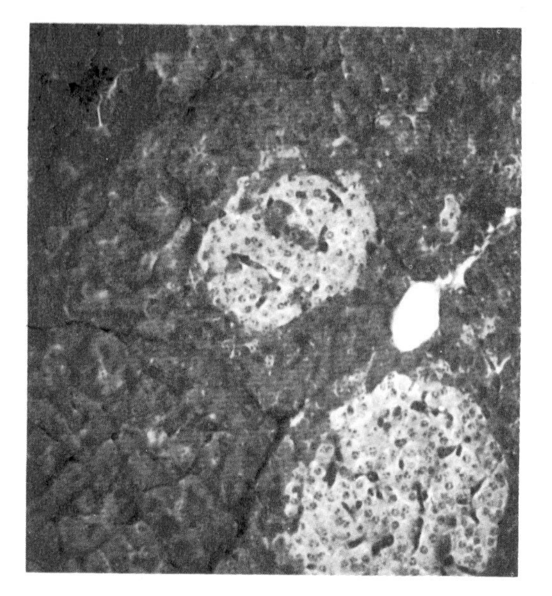

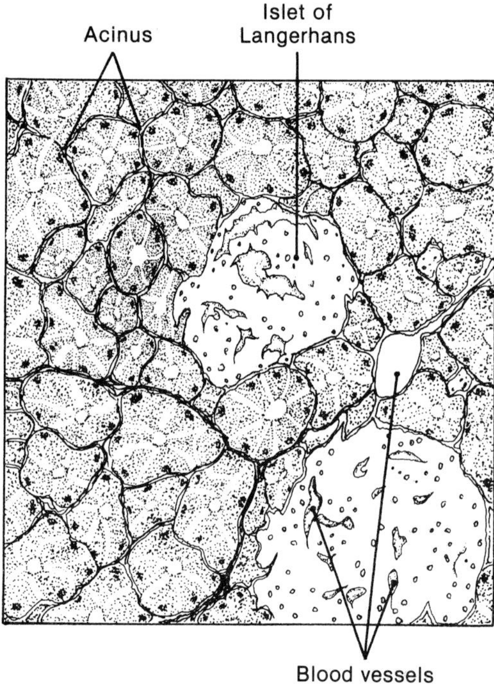

Fig. 13-7. *(Top)* Microscopic section of the pancreas showing the endocrine portion (islets of Langerhans) stained light pink and surrounded by darker staining exocrine portions of the pancreas. The clear areas represent large blood vessels in the tissue. (Courtesy of Dr. Hadley Kirkman, Stanford University.) *(Bottom)* Sketch of section.

PANCREAS

The pancreas is classified as an accessory gland of the digestive system, since it produces several important digestive enzymes which are carried from the gland by way of a system of ducts. The cells which produce these enzymes are thus known as exocrine cells. However, the pancreas also is considered to be an endocrine organ on the basis of cells which secrete their products directly into the blood stream. This endocrine portion of the gland consists of cell clusters known as **islets (of Langerhans)** (Fig. 13-7). The islet cells are of two main types: one produces **insulin** and the other produces **glucagon.** Both hormones regulate the level of glucose in the blood. When glucose levels become too high, insulin is released and causes the glucose to be converted to glycogen for storage. (Insufficient amounts of insulin result in **diabetes,** in which the level of glucose in the blood becomes so high that the sugar is excreted in the urine.) If the blood level of glucose becomes too low, glucagon causes the breakdown of glycogen to glucose.

PINEAL GLAND

The pineal gland (body) can be classified as an endocrine organ, although little is known about its function. The pineal gland projects upward from the roof of the third ventricle of the brain and consists of **pinealocytes** which produce two hormones, **serotonin** and **melatonin.** In some animals such as rats and hamsters the pineal hormones seem to be involved in controlling reproductive cycles, but this function in man has not yet been ascertained. With advancing age the pineal usually contains calcified deposits and is often used as a landmark in skull X-rays.

The gonads also may be properly classified as endocrine organs; their function is discussed in terms of the reproductive system in Chapter 16. Likewise, endocrine cells found in various regions of the urinary and digestive systems are treated with respect to those organ systems.

14

The Digestive System

GENERAL FEATURES

The digestive system extends from the lips of the mouth to the anus and consists of the alimentary canal and accessory glands such as the salivary glands, liver, and portions of the pancreas (Fig. 14-1). The major functions of this system are to ingest food and fluids, break them down both mechanically and chemically so as to enable nutrients to be absorbed, and eliminate the residues of digestion from the body.

The alimentary canal is a hollow tube consisting of the mouth, pharynx, esophagus, stomach, small intestine, and large intestine (including rectum and anal canal). The walls of most of the alimentary canal are composed of four basic layers: the mucosa, submucosa, muscularis externa, and either serosa or adventitia depending on whether the organ is in the abdominal cavity or not (Fig. 14-2).

The **mucosa** is the innermost layer which lines the lumen of the alimentary canal and which contains glandular secretory cells. The mucosa consists of an **epithelium,** a **lamina propria** composed of connective tissue, and in some regions a thin layer of smooth muscle called the **muscularis mucosae** (muscularis interna).

Deep to the mucosa is the **submucosa** consisting of loose connective tissue and containing a **submucosal (Meissner's) plexus** composed of autonomic nerve fibers. (A submucosa is lacking in the mouth and pharynx.)

The **muscularis externa** is located just beyond the submucosa and contains smooth muscle usually arranged in an inner circular layer (which narrows the tube) and an outer longitudinal layer (which shortens the tube). Between these two layers is the **myenteric (Auerbach's) plexus** composed of autonomic nerve fibers.

The **serosa** (visceral peritoneum) is the outermost layer which covers the digestive organs in the abdominal cavity. Serosa consists of a simple squamous epithelium (mesothelium) overlying connective tissue. Digestive organs not located in the abdominal cavity (such as the pharynx, esophagus, lower rectum, and anal canal) are covered with a fibrous connective tissue layer called the **adventitia.**

MOUTH

The mouth is the site where food is ingested, masticated (chewed), moistened, and subjected to mild enzymatic digestion by salivary secretions. The sensation of taste originates here via tiny taste buds on the surface of the tongue. The mouth also plays an important role in speaking, a function discussed more appropriately with the respiratory system.

The entrance to the mouth is surrounded by the upper and lower **lips** containing the **orbicularis oris muscle** as well as the insertions of a number of other facial muscles. The lips are covered externally by skin (containing keratinized stratified squamous epithelium). The internal surface of each lip is lined by a mucous membrane with nonkeratinized stratified squa-

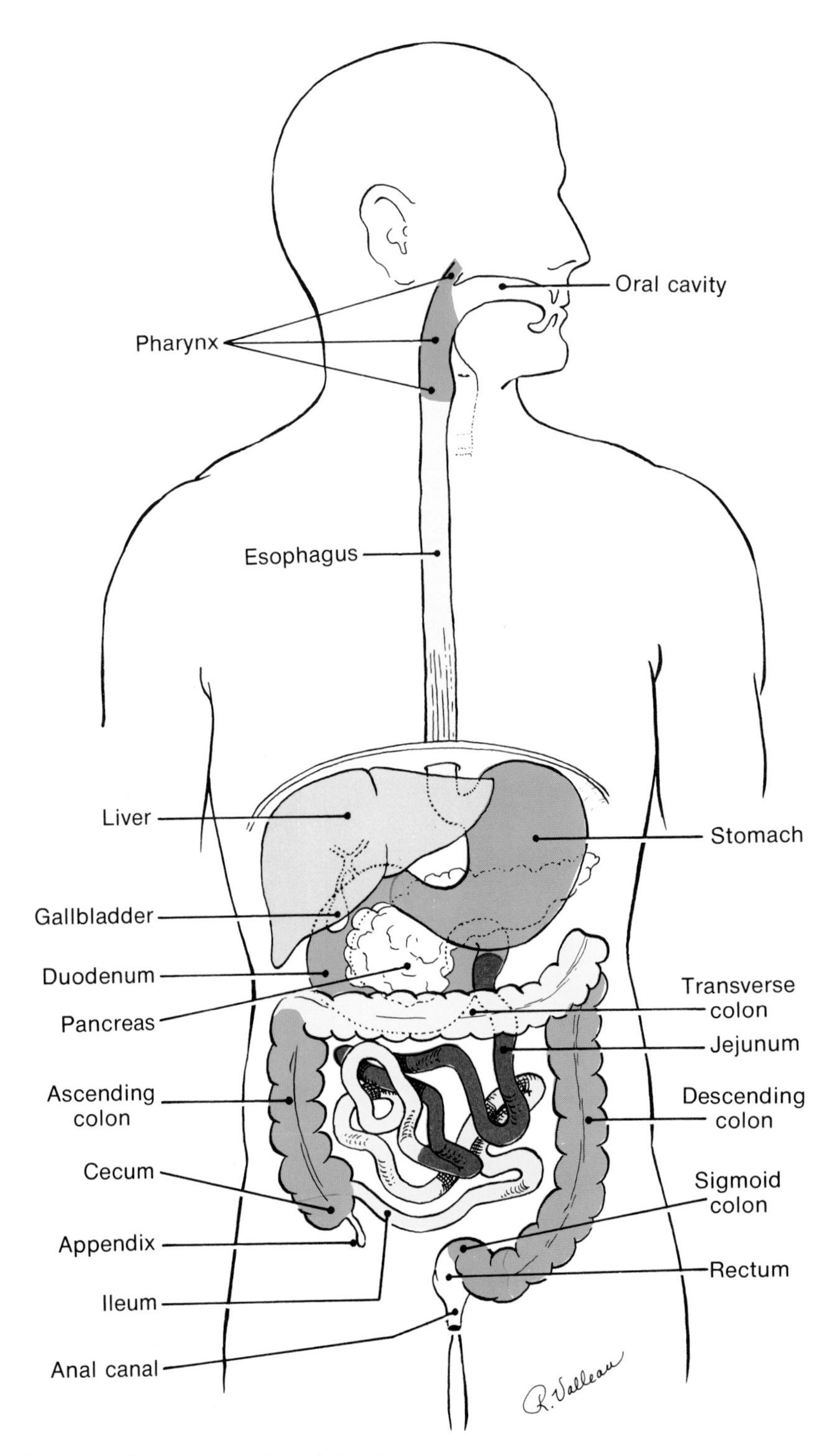

Fig. 14-1. Diagrammatic representation of the digestive system. The coils of the jejunum and ileum are shortened and do not indicate the true length of the small intestine. (Modified after Grant.)

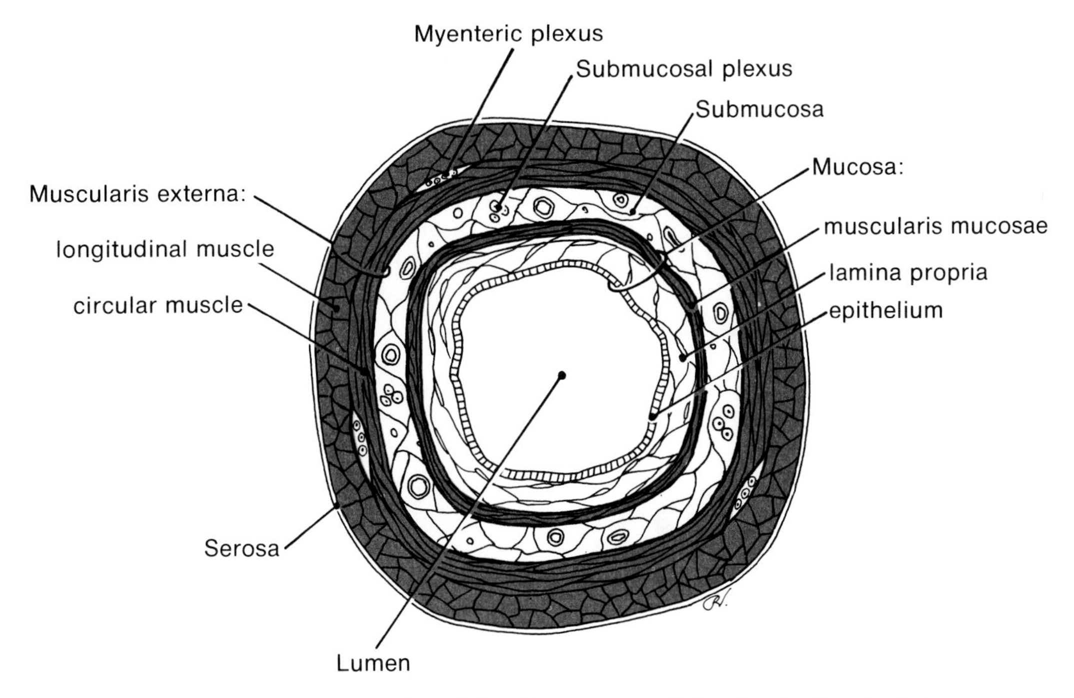

Fig. 14-2 Schematic cross section of the alimentary canal showing the four basic layers.

mous epithelium as well as a number of mucus-secreting labial glands. The border of each lip normally has a reddish color imparted by blood vessels beneath a very thin layer of translucent epidermis. (In cases of cyanosis where the oxygen content of the blood is reduced, the lips may appear bluish).

The mouth is subdivided into two portions: the vestibule and the oral cavity. The **vestibule** is the narrow space bounded by the lips and cheeks externally and by the gums and teeth internally; the remainder of the mouth is the **oral cavity.** The vestibule communicates with the oral cavity by means of a space behind the last molar teeth when the mouth is closed.

The oral cavity contains the teeth, tongue, and openings from three pairs of salivary glands. The **hard** and **soft palate** constitute the roof of the cavity, the **teeth** and **gums** its lateral walls, and the **tongue** occupies its floor. Posteriorly the oral cavity is delimited by a pair of **palatoglossal folds (arches)** which arch downward from the sides of the soft palate to the sides of the tongue (Fig. 14-3). Suspended

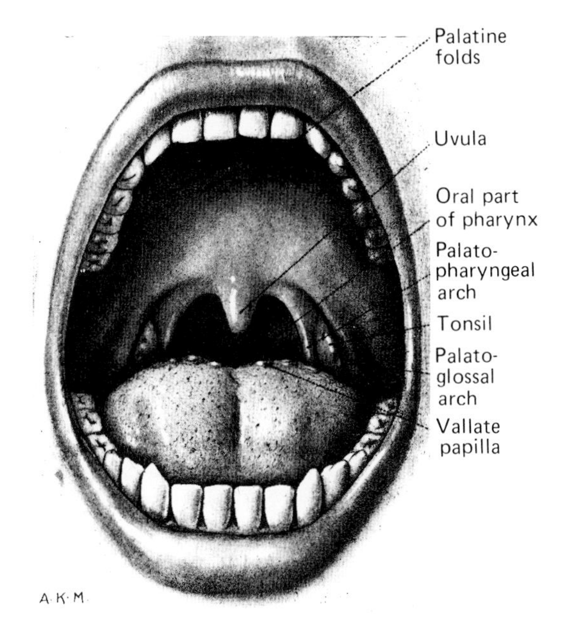

Fig. 14-3. Anterior view of the mouth. (From W. J. Hamilton, G. Simon, and S. G. I. Hamilton, *Surface and Radiological Anatomy,* Ed. 5, The Macmillan Press, London, 1971.)

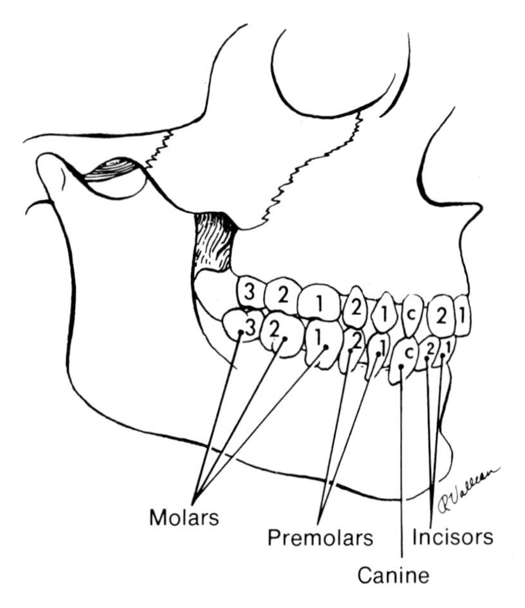

Fig. 14-4. Permanent (adult) dentition. Right upper and lower quadrants, lateral view.

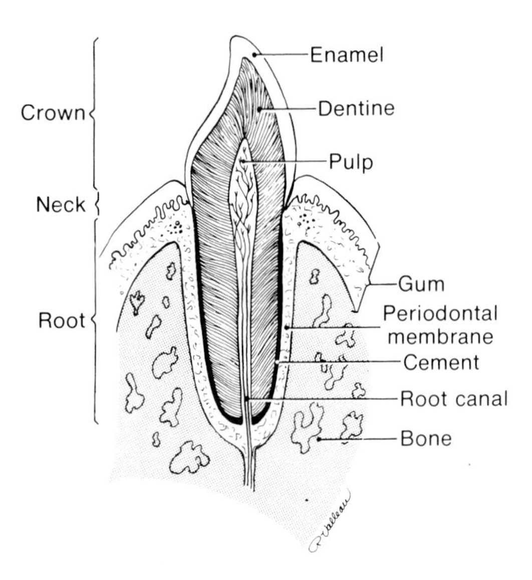

Fig. 14-5. Longitudinal section of a tooth. (Modified after Grant.)

downward from the middle of the free edge of the soft palate is a fleshy projection, the **uvula.** All of these structures, except the teeth, are covered by a mucous membrane containing stratified squamous epithelium and liberally supplied with mucous glands.

In the adult a full set of dentition consists of 32 **teeth** (16 in the maxilla, 16 in the mandible) arranged in four quadrants: upper left, upper right, lower left, and lower right. There are four basic types of teeth in each quadrant: 2 **incisors** for biting, 1 **canine (cuspid)** for tearing, and 2 **premolars (bicuspids)** and 3 **molars (tricuspids)** for grinding (Figs. 14-4 and 14-6). The most posteriorly placed molar (third molar) in each quadrant is commonly called a "wisdom" tooth, but may be lacking.

Each tooth projects upward from an **alveolus** or socket lined with a dense fibrous connective tissue, the **periodontal membrane** (Fig. 14-5). This membrane, along with a calcified substance called **cementum (cement)**, helps to anchor the tooth. The portion of the tooth within the socket is the **root,** whereas the part which projects above the socket is the **crown.**

Each tooth has three basic components: (1) the **pulp** which contains numerous vessels and nerves, (2) the harder **dentine** surrounding the pulp, and (3) an outer covering of extremely hard **enamel** found only on the surface of the crown. A **root canal** transmits vessels and nerves into the pulp. Although the enamel is relatively insensitive to pain, the pulp and dentine are extremely pain sensitive.

The **gums (gingivae)** are composed of fibrous connective tissue covered by mucous membrane. The gingivae cover the base of the crown at a region termed the **neck** of the tooth. The gingivae tend to recede slightly from the neck with increasing age, and can also become inflamed (gingivitis).

There are two sets of teeth: the deciduous (primary) teeth and the permanent teeth. Both sets develop before birth but do not erupt from the surface of the gum until after birth. The **deciduous** ("baby") **teeth** begin to erupt at approximately 6 months after birth and continue to appear until about 2½ years of age. In all, 20

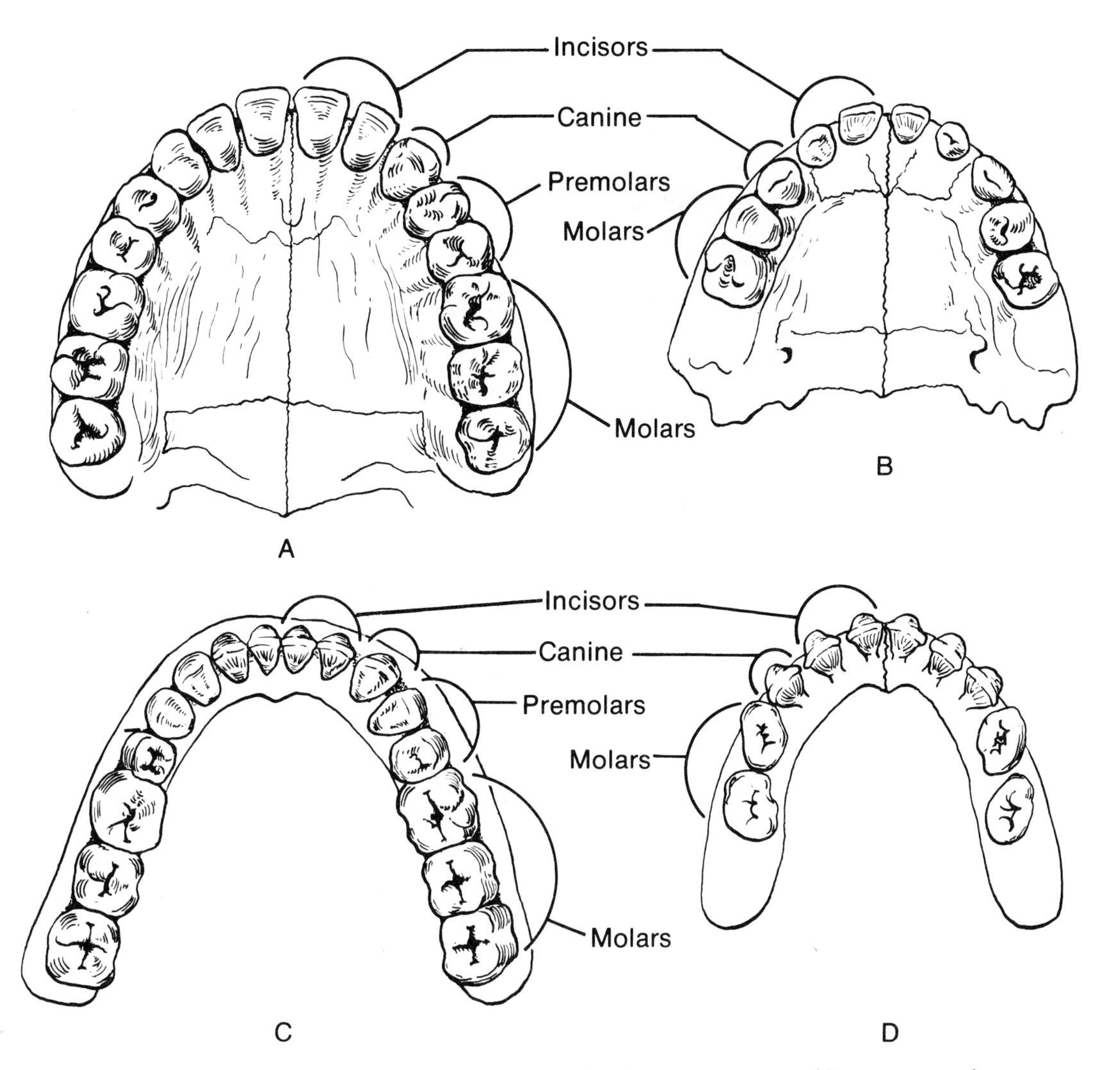

Fig. 14-6. The dentition. (A) Permanent, upper jaw; (B) deciduous, upper jaw; (C) permanent, lower jaw; (D) deciduous, lower jaw.

deciduous teeth appear (with 5 in each quadrant: 2 incisors, 1 canine and 2 molars) (Fig. 14-6). After approximately 6 years of age the deciduous teeth are gradually lost and replaced by the **permanent teeth.** Since the permanent molars are not preceded by deciduous counterparts, there are 12 additional permanent teeth bringing the total to 32.

The **tongue** is a highly versatile muscular organ which helps to macerate food by pushing it against the teeth, palate, and gums. The tongue also participates in the act of swallowing and in speech. It is composed of a mass of **intrinsic muscles** consisting of interlacing skeletal muscle fibers which allow considerable mobility and changes in shape. **Extrinsic muscles** attach the tongue to the mandible, styloid process, and hyoid bone (Fig. 14-7) and to the wall of the pharynx laterally. The tongue is connected to the floor of the mouth by means of a midline fold of mucous membrane termed the *frenulum* (Fig. 14-8). (A shortened frenu-

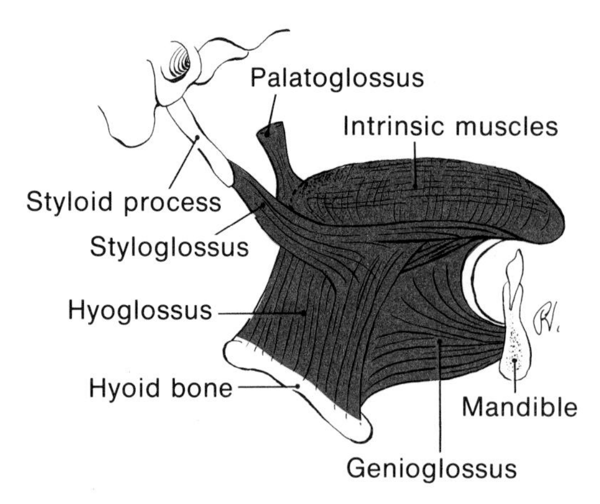

Fig. 14-7. Lateral view of the tongue and its extrinsic and intrinsic muscles.

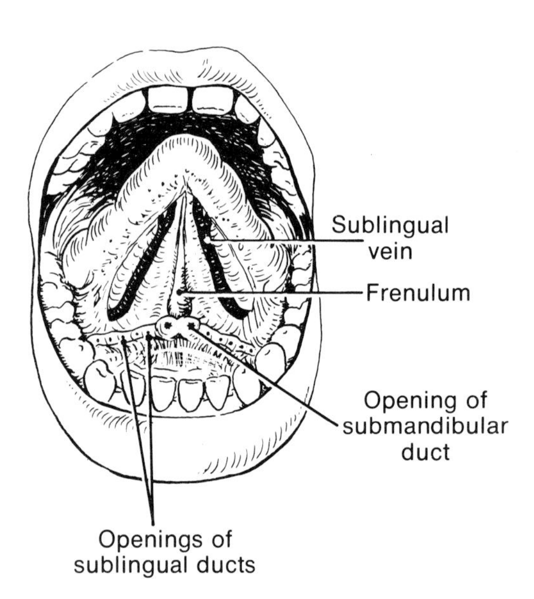

Fig. 14-8. Anterior view of the mouth with the tongue elevated.

lum results in a condition termed "tongue-tied.") In the midline a fold of mucous membrane also attaches the tongue to the epiglottis of the larynx (Fig. 14-9).

The dorsum of the tongue is covered by mucous membrane with a series of small projections termed papillae. The most prominent of these are **vallate (circumvallate) papillae** arranged in a V-shaped line which demarcates the anterior two-thirds of the tongue from the posterior third (Fig. 14-9). The anterior two-thirds contains additional types of papillae **(fungiform, filiform,** and rudimentary **foliate)**; the posterior third lacks papillae but contains masses of lymphoid tissue termed **lingual tonsils.** (The lingual tonsils and palatine tonsils are discussed more fully with the lymphatic system in Chapter 10.)

Specialized structures called **taste buds** are scattered in the mucosa on the dorsal surface of the tongue and are particularly numerous in the vallate papillae (Figs. 14-9 and 14-10). Sensory nerve endings convey taste impulses from the taste buds to the central nervous system. The sensation of taste is to some degree dependent on the ability to perceive odors (olfaction), and for this reason one's sense of taste is often dulled when a common cold congests the nasal passages. The senses of taste and smell also become less acute with advancing age.

The mucous membrane of the oral cavity is well endowed with mucous glands which contribute to the saliva and aid in moistening and swallowing the ingested food as well as providing a liquid medium in which taste can be perceived. Much of the saliva consists of watery secretions from three pairs of **salivary glands:** the parotid, submandibular, and sublingual glands. The saliva also contains an enzyme **(salivary amylase)** which begins to break down starches.

Of the paired salivary glands, the **parotid** is the largest and lies beneath the skin just anterior and inferior to the external ear (Fig. 14-11). (This region is often termed the parotid region.) The **parotid duct** extends from the gland across the external surface of the masseter muscle and then pierces the cheek to open

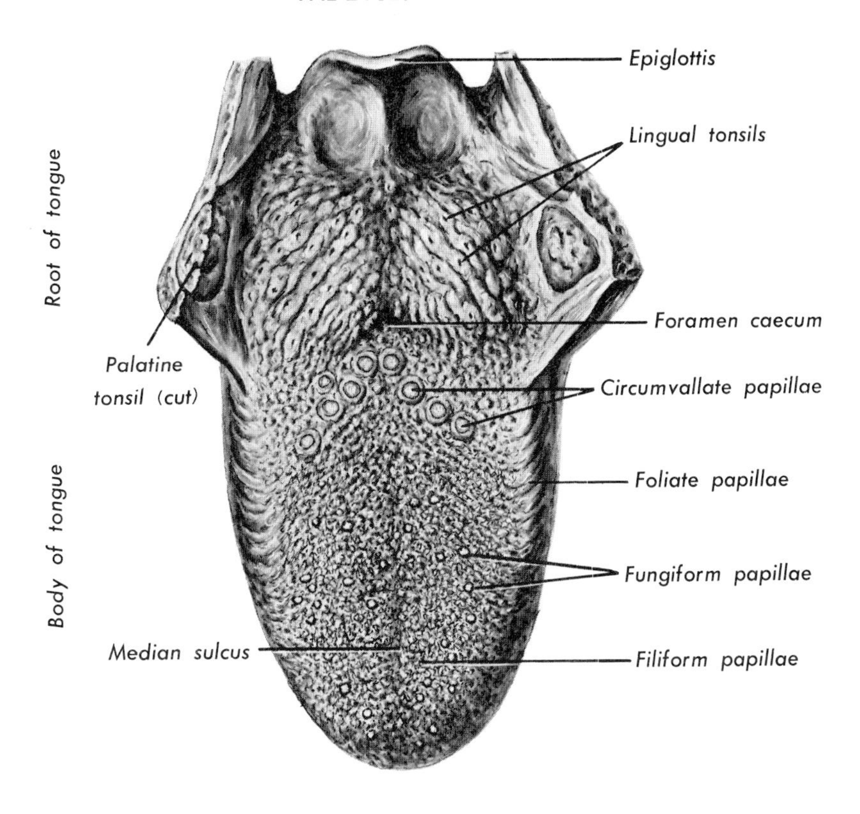

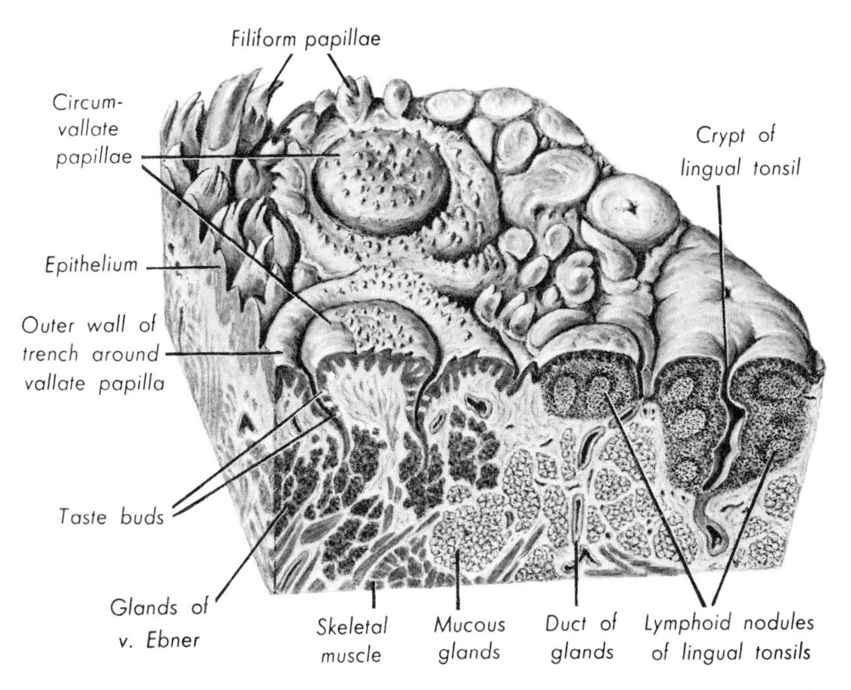

Fig. 14-9. The tongue. *(Top)* Surface view of dorsum, (*bottom*) three dimensional view, showing higher magnification of papillae, taste buds, and lingual tonsils. (From W. M. Copenhaver, R. P. Bunge, and M. B. Bunge, *Bailey's Textbook of Histology,* Ed. 16, The Williams & Wilkins Co., Baltimore, 1971.)

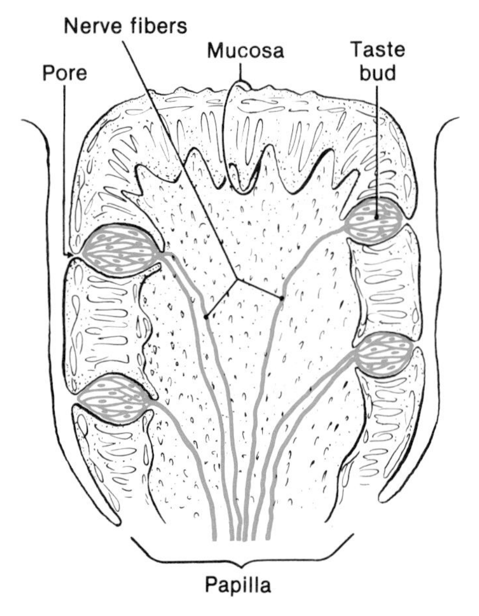

Fig. 14-10. Diagram of a section through a papilla of the tongue showing the location of taste buds.

into the vestibule of the mouth at the level of the upper second molar. The parotid gland is considered to be entirely serous, i.e., its secretions are watery and proteinaceous in nature.

The **submandibular gland** is located below the body of the mandible and curves around the mylohyoid muscle in the floor of the mouth. The **submandibular duct** empties into the mouth at the side of the frenulum beneath the tongue (Fig. 14-9). The **sublingual gland** is small and slender and lies under the mucous membrane in the floor of the mouth. It opens by means of a series of small ducts along the side of the frenulum near the opening of the submandibular gland. The submandibular and sublingual glands are both considered to be mixed, i.e., their secretions are mucous as well as serous in nature.

PHARYNX

The pharynx is a muscular tube which serves both the digestive and respiratory systems. It consists of three portions: the nasopharynx, oropharynx, and laryngopharynx (Fig. 14-12). The **nasopharynx** lies above the soft palate and communicates in front with the posterior region of the nasal cavities. The **oropharynx** is located below the soft palate and contains the **palatine tonsils** which are lodged in a depression between the palatoglossal folds in front and the palatopharyngeal folds behind (Fig. 14-3). The **laryngopharynx** is situated behind the larynx and ends near the lower border of the lowermost laryngeal cartilage (cricoid cartilage) to become continuous with the esophagus (Fig. 14-8). The nasopharynx belongs to the respiratory system and is lined by a ciliated mucous membrane characteristic of the respiratory tract, whereas the oropharynx and laryngopharynx are lined mainly with stratified squamous epithelium similar to that in the mouth.

Once the various structures of the mouth have mechanically macerated and moistened the food, it is called a **bolus** and is ready to be swallowed. During the act of **swallowing (deglutition)** the tongue pushes the bolus back-

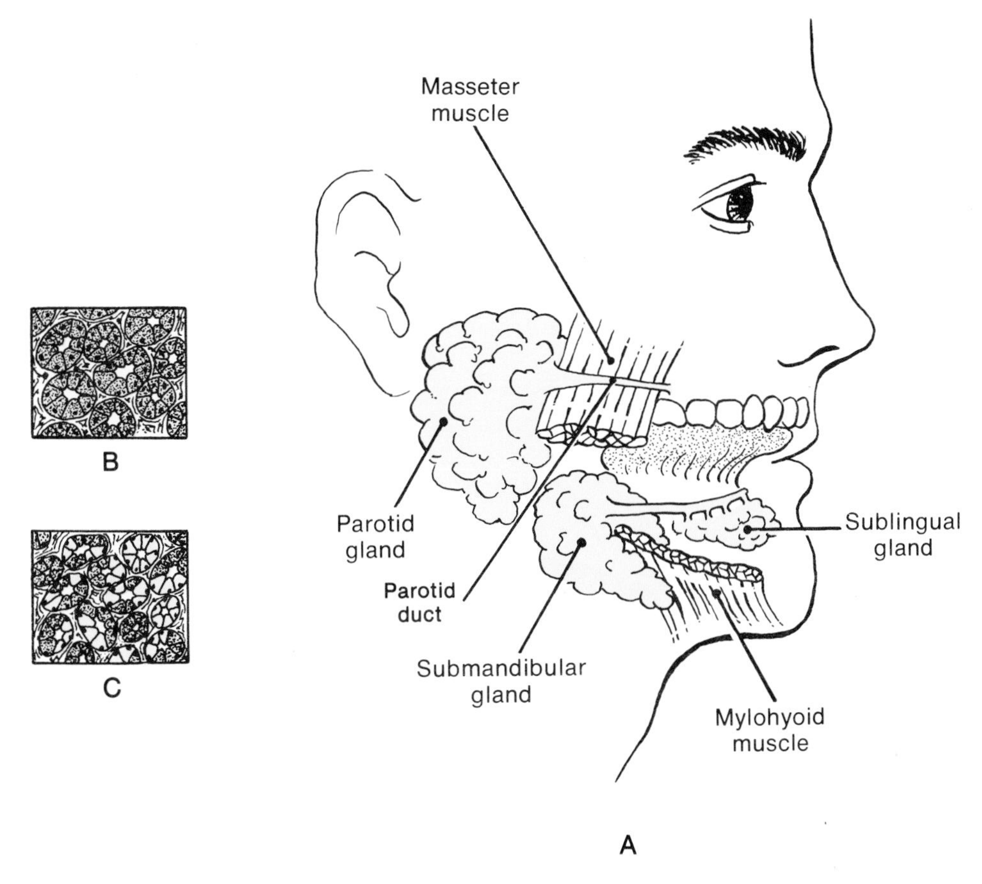

Fig. 14-11. (A) The salivary glands, lateral view. The masseter and mylohyoid muscles have been cut, and the mandible has been removed. (B) Diagram of a microscopic section characteristic of parotid gland and (C) of sublingual and submandibular glands.

ward, and the hyoid bone and larynx are elevated by suprahyoid muscles, thereby pushing the larynx against the epiglottis. This closes off the larynx from the laryngopharynx and prevents the bolus from entering the lower respiratory passages. The soft palate likewise elevates and shuts off the oropharynx from the overlying nasopharynx in order to prevent the bolus from entering the upper respiratory passages.

ESOPHAGUS

The esophagus is a slender easily distensible tube which transmits the bolus of food and liquids from the laryngopharynx to the stomach. Most of the esophagus lies in the thorax except for a short upper part in the cervical region and a short lower portion in the abdominal cavity (Fig. 14-1).

Microscopic Anatomy

In the collapsed state, the mucous membrane contains folds (Fig. 14-13), which disappear as the esophagus becomes distended by a passing bolus of food. The mucous membrane is composed of stratified squamous epithelium overlying a lamina propria with some mucous glands. The muscularis mucosae is particularly

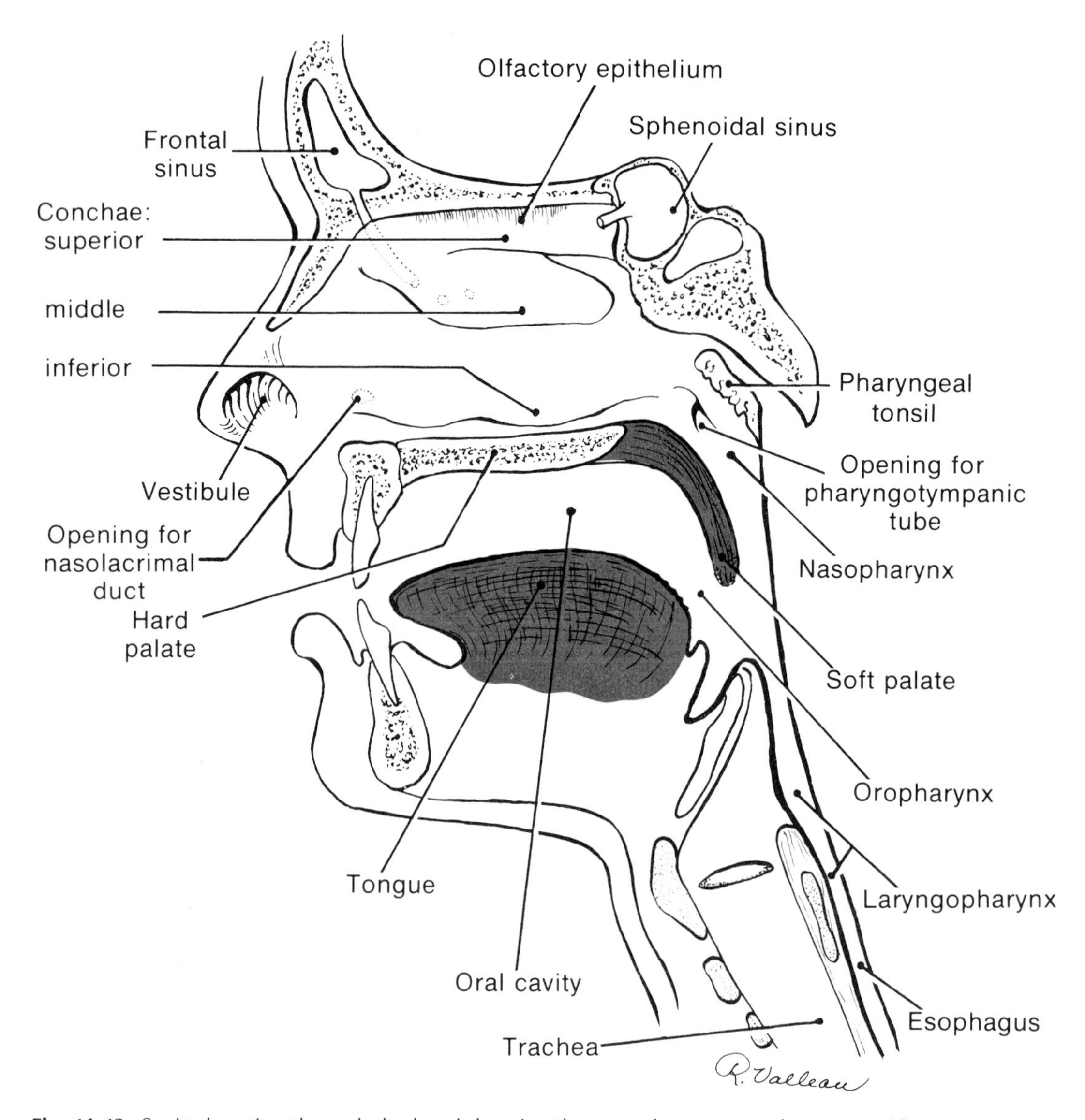

Fig. 14-12. Sagittal section through the head showing the nasopharynx, oropharynx, and laryngopharynx.

well developed (Fig. 14-14). The submucosa contains mucous glands which empty their secretions into ducts passing upward through the mucosa.

The muscularis externa is composed of skeletal muscle fibers in the upper portion of the esophagus but gradually changes to smooth muscle in its lower portion. Thus the middle region contains both skeletal muscle and smooth muscle. The muscularis externa shows an arrangement typical of the alimentary canal with an inner circular and outer longitudinal layer. The outermost covering of the cervical and thoracic portions of the esophagus is an adventitia of loose connective tissue; the abdominal portion contains a covering of visceral peritoneum (serosa).

The blood supply for the esophagus comes largely by way of esophageal branches from the aorta and is returned via esophageal veins emptying into the azygous system of veins. Since the esophageal veins also communicate with veins of the hepatic portal system, increased pressure in this system (due to a blockage or an enlarged liver) can cause the esophageal veins to enlarge greatly and even burst, resulting in a serious and sudden loss of blood. These enlarged veins are termed **esophageal varices.**

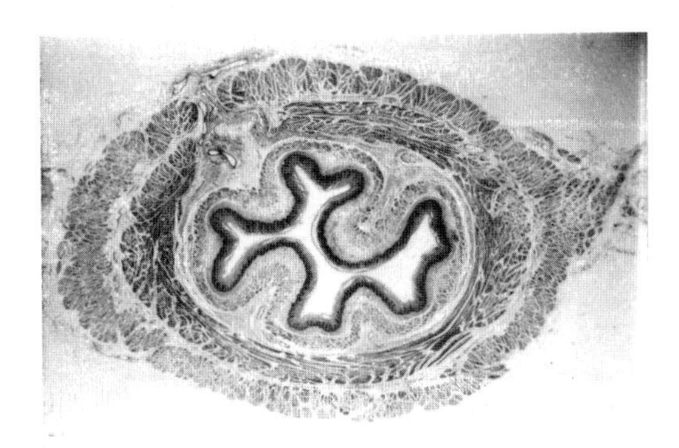

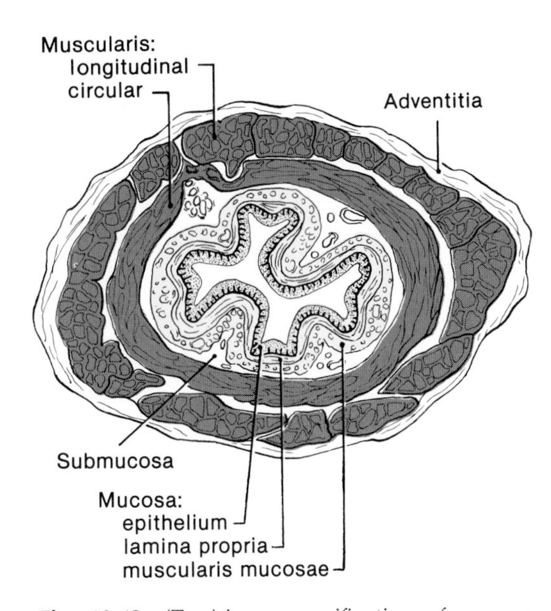

Fig. 14-13. *(Top)* Low magnification of a cross section through the esophagus. (Courtesy of Dr. Hadley Kirkman, Stanford University.) *(Bottom)* Sketch of the section, with the mucosa shown in yellow.

GASTROINTESTINAL TRACT

The digestive organs below the diaphragm can conveniently be called the gastrointestinal tract, and it is here that digestion, absorption, and excretion take place. The gastrointestinal tract consists of the stomach, small intestine (duodenum, jejunum, ileum), and large intestine (cecum, appendix, ascending colon, transverse colon, descending colon, sigmoid colon, rectum, anal canal) (Fig. 14-1). Most of the gastrointestinal tract lies in the abdominopelvic cavity (the body cavity below the diaphragm and above the pelvic inlet). However, the lowermost portions of the gastrointestinal tract (rectum and anal canal) are situated below the pelvic inlet.

The walls of the gastrointestinal tract contain the four basic layers characteristic of the alimentary canal, including the submucosal and myenteric autonomic nerve plexuses. The **blood supply** to the gastrointestinal tract is as follows: the stomach and part of the duodenum are supplied by the celiac artery, the rest of the duodenum, jejunum, ileum, cecum, appendix, ascending colon, and proximal portion of the transverse colon by the superior mesenteric artery, the distal part of the transverse colon, the descending colon, sigmoid colon, rectum, and upper part of the anal canal by the inferior mesenteric artery, and the lower part of the anal canal by branches from the internal iliac artery. Venous drainage occurs via the portal system (see Chapter 9).

Peritoneum

The peritoneum is a serous membrane which lines the abdominal cavity and consists of a me-

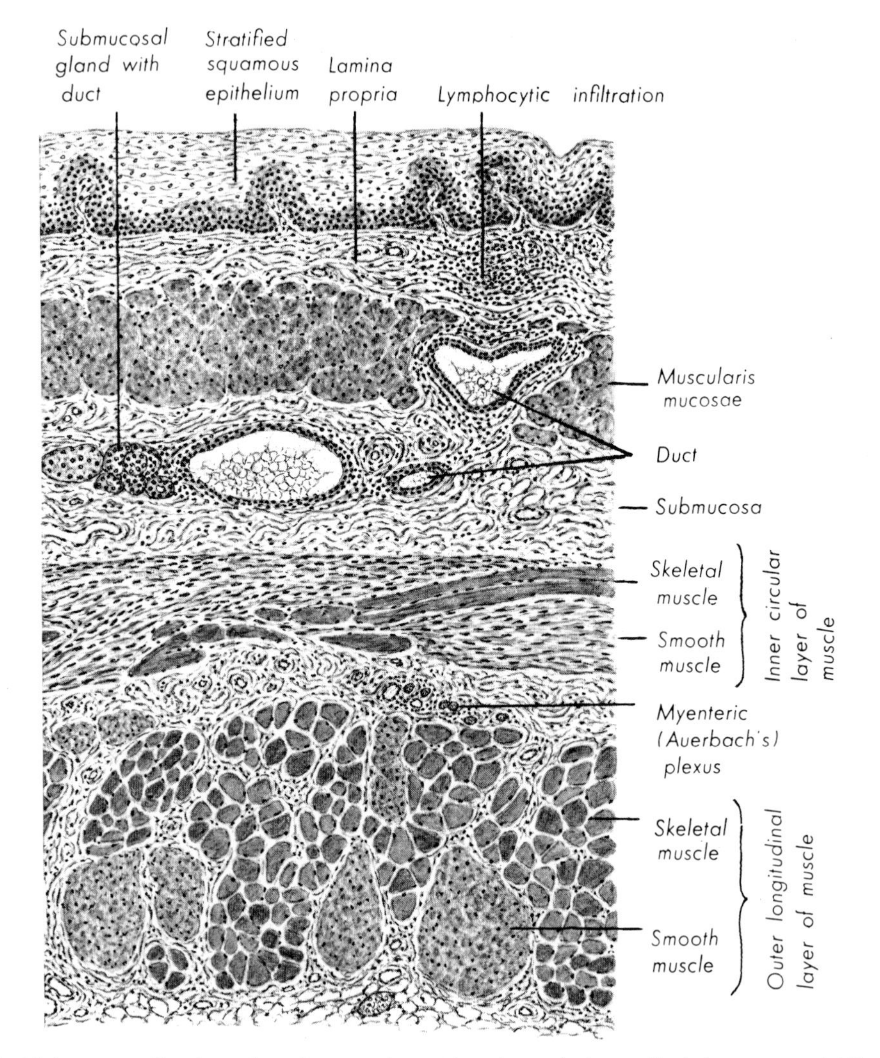

Fig. 14-14. Higher magnification of a microscopic section through the wall of the upper middle region of the esophagus. (From W. M. Copenhaver, R. P. Bunge, & M. B. Bunge, *Bailey's Textbook of Histology,* Ed. 16, The Williams & Wilkins Co., Baltimore, 1971.)

sothelium (simple squamous epithelium) overlying a small amount of connective tissue. The peritoneum which lines the body wall is termed **parietal peritoneum;** that which is found on the surfaces of various abdominal viscera (organs) is **visceral peritoneum** (Fig. 14-15). Extending from the parietal to the visceral peritoneum are double layered sheets of peritoneum called **mesenteries** which transmit vessels and nerves to and from the various organs. These organs are so closely packed together that only a narrow fluid-filled space known as the **peritoneal cavity** occurs between them. The fluid, along with the slippery nature of the peritoneum, enables the viscera to slide easily over one another.

There are some abdominal organs which are not completely encompassed by visceral peritoneum and which lack a mesenteric attachment to the body wall. These organs (such as the kidneys) are said to be **retroperitoneal,** *i.e.*, behind the peritoneum.

Stomach

The stomach receives the bolus of food from the esophagus, continues the process of digestion, begins a limited amount of absorption, and passes the food (now known as **chyme**) to the small intestine. The size, position, and shape of the stomach vary among different individuals and also in the same individual depending on the stomach's fullness or the position of the body.

The stomach shows two curvatures: the **lesser curvature** along its right margin and the **greater curvature** along its left margin (Fig. 14-16). There are four general regions of the stomach: the **cardiac portion** occurs near the

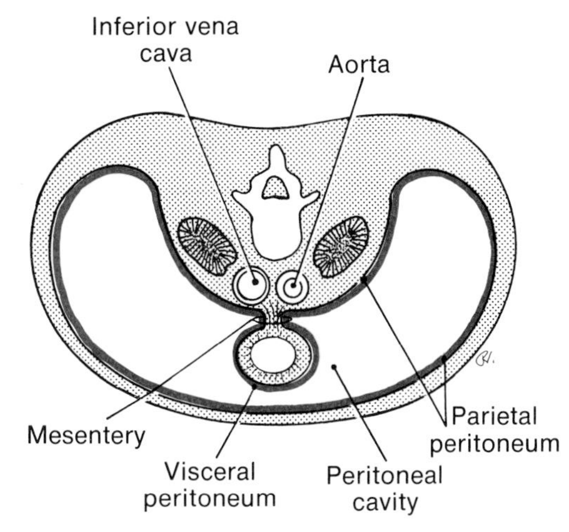

Fig. 14-15. Schematic representation of a transverse section of the abdominal cavity, with the peritoneum depicted in red. (The size of the peritoneal cavity is greatly exaggerated.)

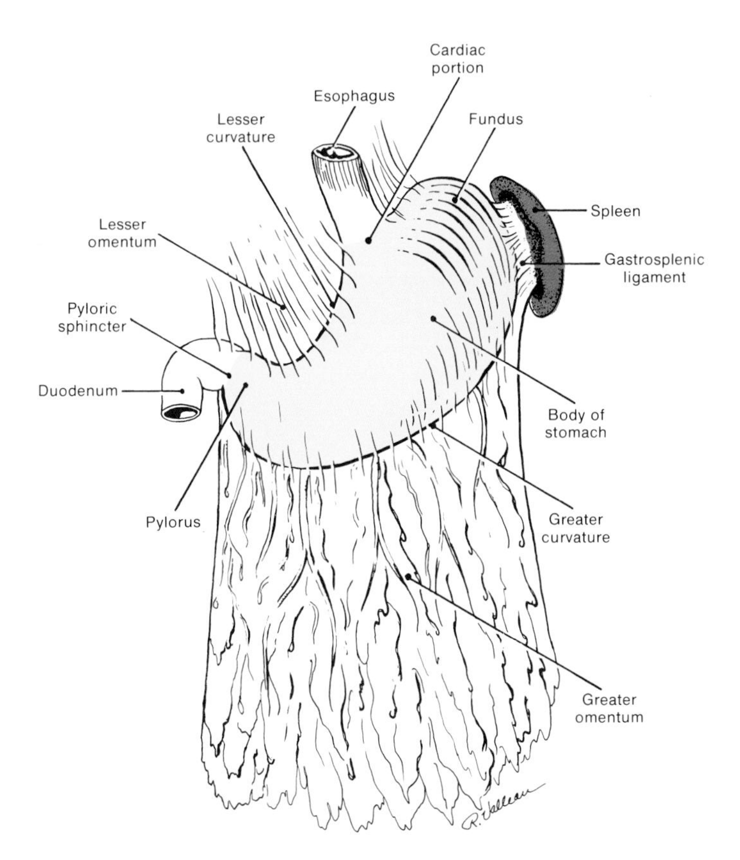

Fig. 14-16. Anterior view of the stomach (in yellow) with associated mesenteries and organs.

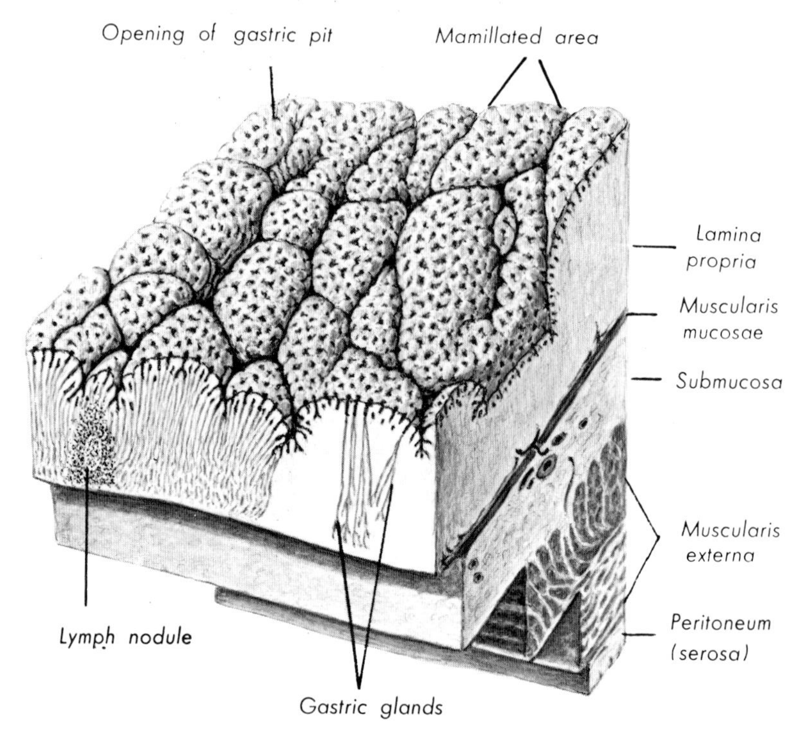

Fig. 14-17. A three dimensional scheme of the wall of the stomach. (From W. M. Copenhaver, R. P. Bunge, and M. B. Bunge, *Bailey's Textbook of Histology,* Ed. 16, The Williams & Wilkins Co., Baltimore, 1971.)

opening of the esophagus, the **fundus** is the region of the stomach which bulges upward above the level where the esophagus enters, the **body** is the major central portion of the stomach, and the **pylorus** is the narrower lower region which communicates with the duodenum (the first portion of the small intestine) at a constriction, the **pyloric sphincter.**

A number of mesenteries are associated with the stomach, of which the largest is the **greater omentum,** a sheet of tissue hanging downward like an apron from the lower portion of the greater curvature and covering many of the abdominal viscera anteriorly (Fig. 14-16). Another mesentery, the **lesser omentum,** extends from the lesser curvature of the stomach to the liver. To the left and somewhat behind the stomach is the spleen (an organ belonging to the lymphatic system), which is suspended from the upper portion of the greater curvature of the stomach by means of a mesentery called the **gastrosplenic "ligament."**

Microscopic Anatomy

At the junction between the esophagus and stomach the stratified squamous epithelium of the esophagus changes abruptly to simple columnar epithelium, which typifies most of the remainder of the gastrointestinal tract. The lining of the stomach contains a series of gastric pits, and numerous **gastric glands** extend downward from these pits into the lamina propria (Figs. 14-17 and 14-18). The epithelium of these glands contains two basic cell types. The **chief cells** secrete the digestive enzymes **pepsin** and **rennin** to break down (hydrolyze) proteins; the **parietal cells** secrete **hydrochloric acid** which promotes the release of pepsin into

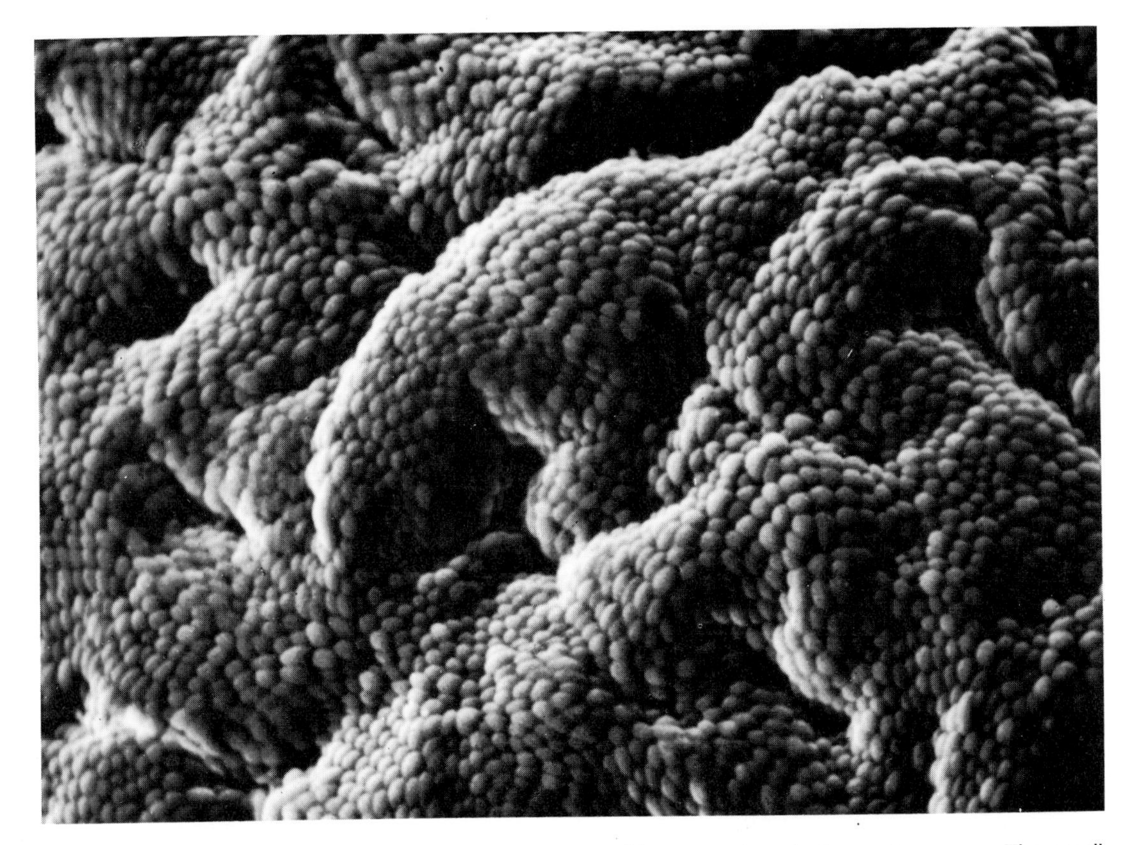

Fig. 14-18. The surface of the stomach lining as seen with a scanning electron microscope. The small beadlike projections represent the rounded contours of the surface cells. (Courtesy of J. Riddell, from W. Bloom and D. W. Fawcett, *A Textbook of Histology,* Ed. 10, W. B. Saunders Co., Philadelphia, 1975.)

the lumen of the stomach (Fig. 14-19). Numerous mucus-secreting goblet cells occur along the surface of the epithelium and help to lubricate and moisten the stomach contents.

A limited amount of absorption (particularly of alcohol and water) takes place in the stomach. Also, the pyloric portion of the stomach produces a hormone, **gastrin,** which is released into the blood stream and then acts on the gastric glands, especially the parietal cells, to stimulate their digestive secretions. The stomach (and small intestine as well) contains a small number of other hormone-producing cells known collectively as enterochromaffin cells.

The thin muscularis mucosae, as well as the loose underlying submucosa, enable the mucosa of the stomach to be elevated into temporary ridges termed **rugae** which disappear as the stomach becomes distended. Shadows of these ridges can often be seen on an X-ray after ingestion of barium (Fig. 14-20).

The churning movements of the stomach are due in large part to the circular and longitudinal layers of smooth muscle in the muscularis externa. Since the arrangement of these layers tends to be somewhat oblique, the stomach can undergo a variety of squeezing and wringing motions which help to mix the stomach contents and to macerate and liquify them. The outer covering of the stomach is the serosa (visceral peritoneum).

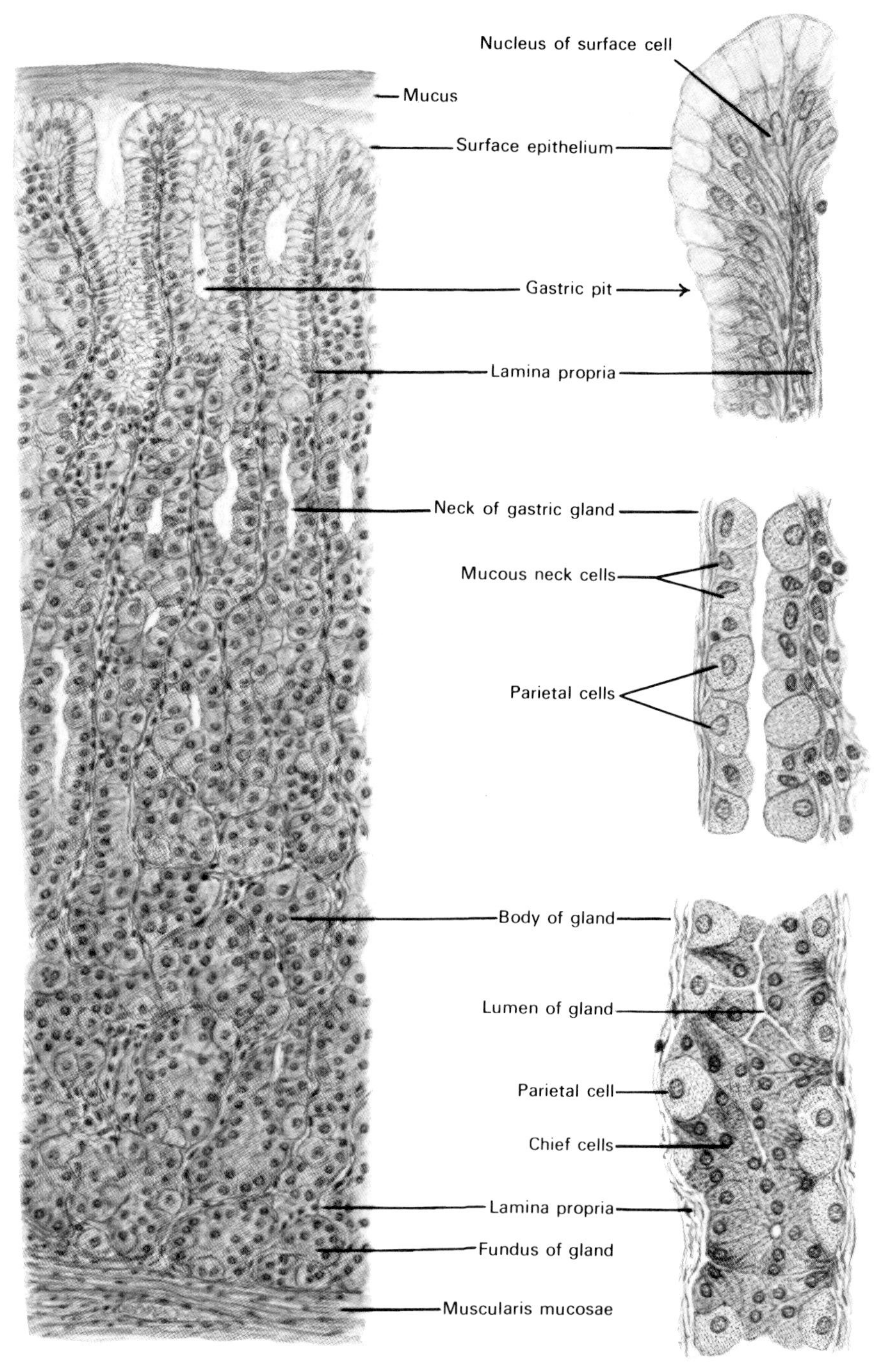

Fig. 14-19. Section through the mucosa of the stomach. At left, low magnification; at right, higher magnification. (From W. M. Copenhaver, R. P. Bunge, and M. B. Bunge, *Bailey's Textbook of Histology,* Ed. 16, The Williams & Wilkins Co., Baltimore, 1971.)

Small Intestine

The small intestine is the major site of digestion and absorption. For this reason it is a long tube (approximately 5–8 meters long) with a highly developed internal surface area. It secretes digestive enzymes and receives secretions from the liver and pancreas. The small intestine also produces a number of hormones, including **secretin** and **pancreozymin** (which stimulate secretion of enzymes from the pancreas) and **cholecystokinin** (which stimulates release of bile from the gallbladder). There are three subdivisions of the small intestine: the duodenum, jejunum, and ileum. (The special gross features of each region will be discussed later.)

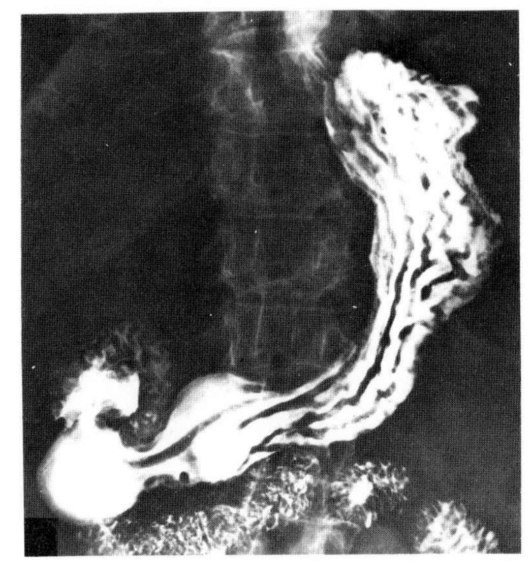

Fig. 14-20. An X-ray of the stomach after swallowing barium. Note the outlines of ridges (rugae). (From E. D. Gardner, D. J. Gray, and R. O'Rahilly, *Anatomy,* Ed. 4, W. B. Saunders Co., Philadelphia, 1975.)

Microscopic Anatomy

The small intestine shows the four basic layers of the alimentary tract. However, the mucosa and submucosa are elevated into permanent folds called **plicae circularis,** upon which are found an abundance of long finger-like **intestinal villi** (Fig. 14-21). The mucosal epithelium consists of simple columnar cells among which are interspersed numerous

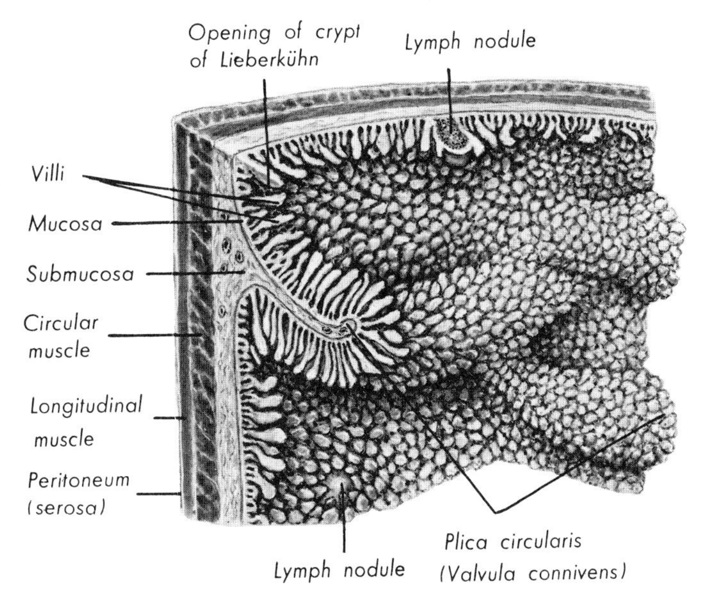

Fig. 14-21. Diagram of a portion of the wall of the small intestine. (Modified after Braus, from W. M. Copenhaver, R. P. Bunge, and M. B. Bunge, *Bailey's Textbook of Histology,* Ed. 16, The Williams & Wilkins Co., Baltimore, 1971.)

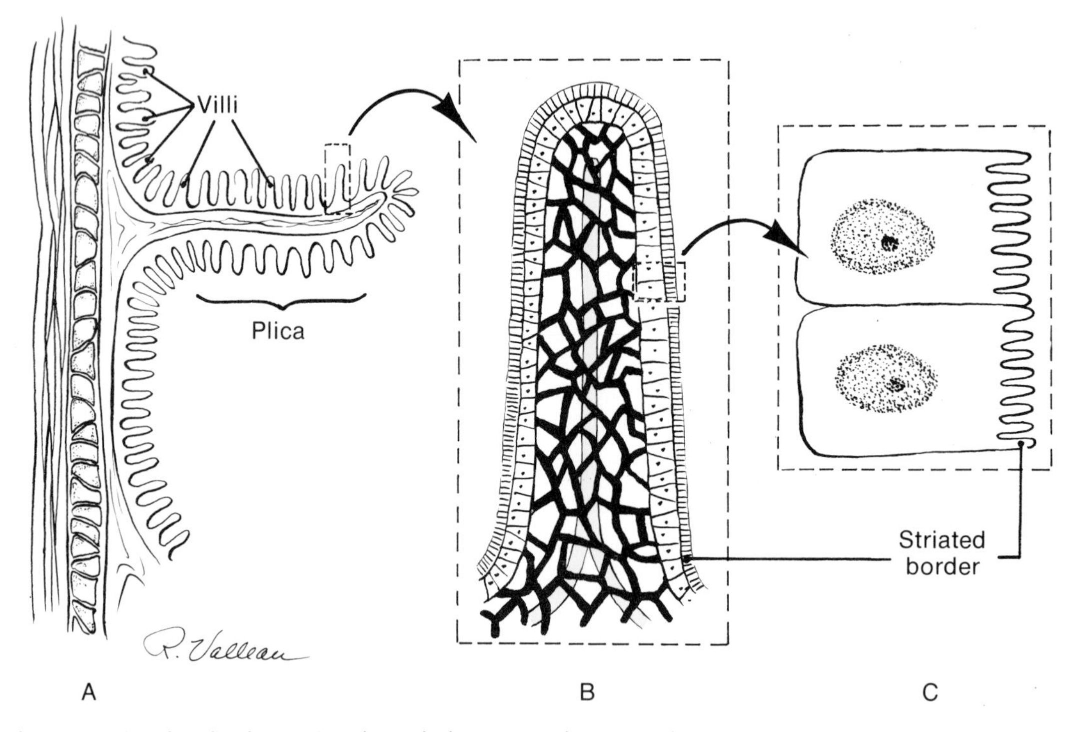

Fig. 14-22. (A) Sketch of a section through the intestinal mucosa showing a plica and villi. (B) Higher magnification of the villus outlined in the rectangle in A. The lacteal (yellow) is centrally located and surrounded by a blood capillary plexus. (C) Higher magnification of two epithelial cells showing the striated border consisting of microvilli.

mucus-secreting goblet cells. **Intestinal glands** (of Lieberkuhn) extend downward into the lamina propria and contain the epithelial cells which produce the digestive enzymes. These enzymes complete the digestion of proteins, fats, and carbohydrates and reduce them to smaller molecules so as to be absorbed.

Absorption of the end products of digestion takes place via the intestinal villi, each of which contains a central connective tissue core with blood capillaries (which absorb amino acids and simple sugars) and with lymphatic capillaries known as **lacteals** (which absorb fat, mainly in the form of fatty acids and glycerol) (Fig. 14-22). Around this connective tissue core are simple columnar epithelial cells with an elaborate system of microvilli which provide increased surface area for absorption along their luminal borders. These microvilli appear as a **striated border** with the light microscope; with the electron microscope the microvilli show a particularly prominent covering of carbohydrate, known as a fuzzy coat or **glycocalyx.**

Duodenum

The duodenum is largely retroperitoneal (i.e., it is fixed against the posterior abdominal wall and lacks a mesentery). It is a C-shaped tube (about 25 cm long) which begins at the pyloric sphincter and ends by merging with the jejunum. The pancreatic duct (from the pancreas) and bile duct (from the liver and gallbladder) empty by means of a common opening into the middle part of the duodenum. In the submucosa of the duodenum are a special group of **duodenal (Brunner's) glands** which secrete an alkaline serous fluid so as to neutral-

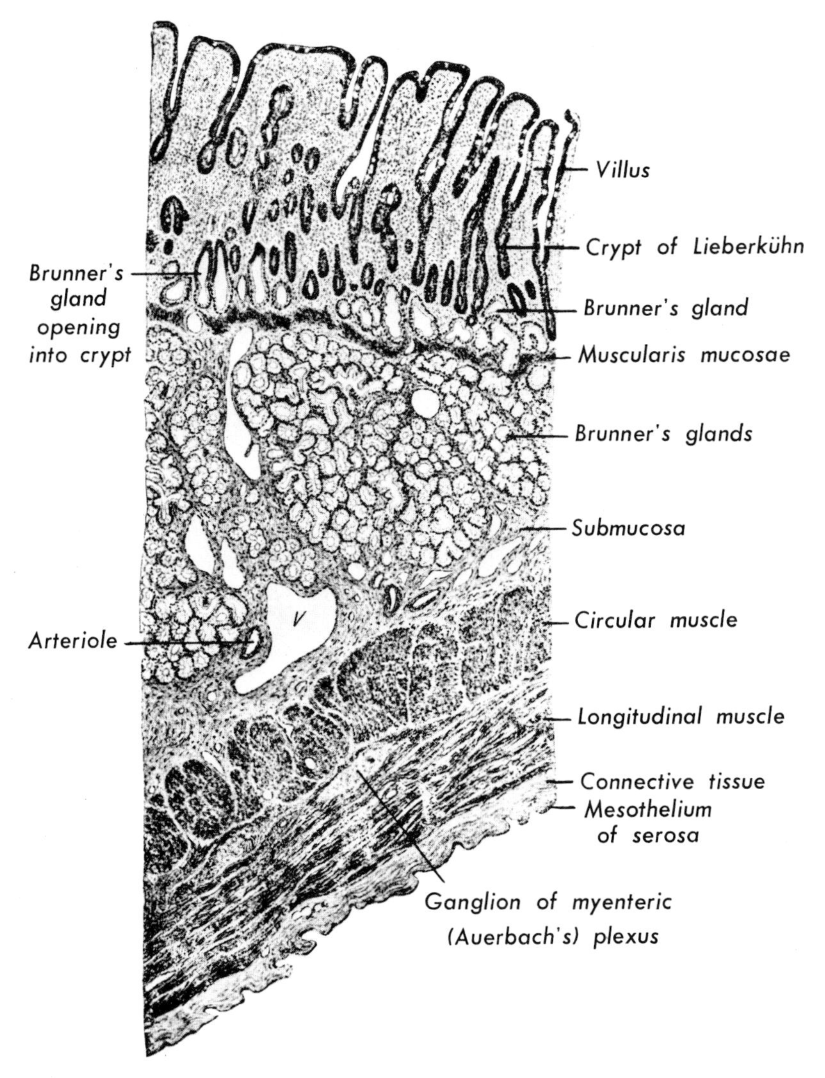

Fig. 14-23. Microscopic section through the wall of the duodenum showing duodenal (Brunner's) glands in the submucosa. (From W. M. Copenhaver, R. P. Bunge, and M. B. Bunge, *Bailey's Textbook of Histology,* Ed. 16, The Williams & Wilkins Co., Baltimore, 1971.)

ize the acidity of the chyme after it enters the duodenum (Fig. 14-23). These submucosal glands send ducts upward to communicate with the intestinal glands of the mucosa and thereby discharge their secretions into the lumen of the gut.

Jejunum and Ileum

The jejunum and ileum together comprise a long segment of the small intestine which is highly coiled and suspended by means of a fan-shaped mesentery from the posterior body wall. The jejunum represents roughly two-fifths of this segment, while the ileum comprises the remainder of it. Although it is difficult to distinguish the jejunum from the ileum on the basis of their gross appearance, microscopically the ileum shows distinctive concentrations of lymph nodules known as **Peyer's patches** in the mucosa and submucosa (Fig. 14-24). The

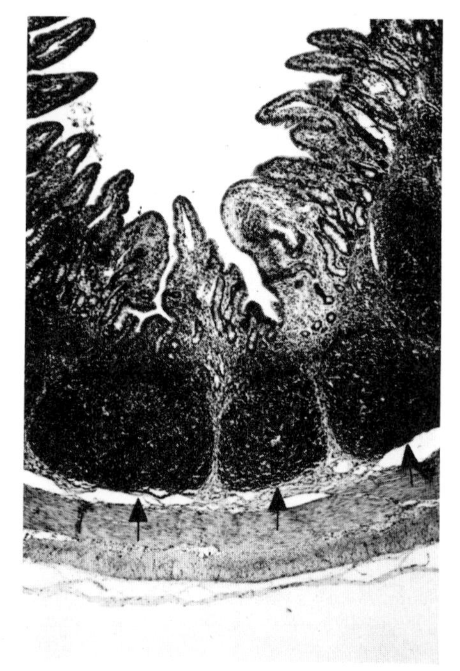

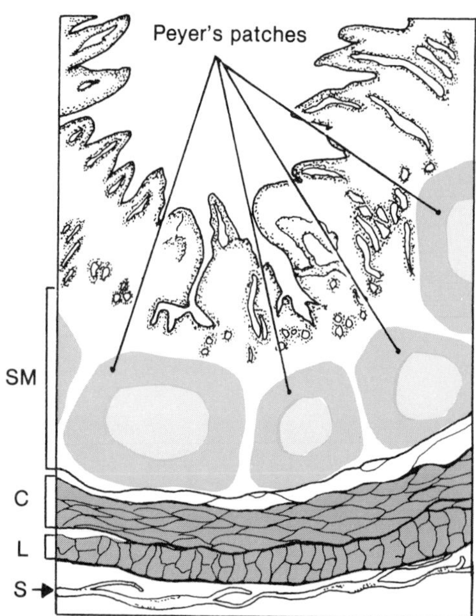

Fig. 14-24. *(Top)* Microscopic section through the wall of the ileum. The *arrows* indicate three lymph nodules (Peyer's patches) in the mucosa and submucosa. (From W. J. Banks, *Histology and Comparative Organology,* The Williams & Wilkins Co., Baltimore, 1974.) *(Bottom)* Sketch of the microscopic section. *SM,* submucosa; *C,* circular layer of muscle; *L,* longitudinal layer of muscle; *S,* serosa.

ileum communicates with the large intestine at the **ileocecal orifice** where two flaps of tissue project into the lumen and constitute the **ileocecal valve.** It is questionable whether or not this valve actually guards the orifice.

Large Intestine

The large intestine includes the cecum and appendix, colon, rectum, and anal canal (Fig. 14-25). In the large intestine fluid is absorbed as the residues of digestion become converted into feces. The feces thus become increasingly solid and hard, unless they are transported too rapidly and not enough water is absorbed, in which case diarrhea results. If fecal matter remains too long in the colon, then excessive water resorption results in constipation.

Cecum and Appendix

The cecum is a short pouch (about 6 cm long) which projects downward from the area where the ileum joins the large intestine (Fig. 14-25). The slender appendix is suspended from the apex of the cecum and is attached by means of a small mesentery (mesoappendix) to the mesentery of the ileum. The cecum and appendix contain the typical four layers of the gastrointestinal tract; however, the mucosa and submucosa of the appendix are crowded with lymphatic tissue (lymph nodules).

Colon, Rectum, and Anal Canal

The colon is comprised of four portions: the ascending, transverse, descending, and sigmoid colon. The **ascending colon** is continuous with the cecum below and passes upward along the right side of the abdomen to the **right colic flexure** where it becomes continuous with the transverse colon. The **transverse colon** extends across the abdomen to the left and lies under cover of the first part of the greater omentum which is actually fused to its anterior surface. The transverse colon becomes the descending colon at the **left colic flexure.** (The left colic flexure is usually higher than the right one.) The **descending colon** passes downward along

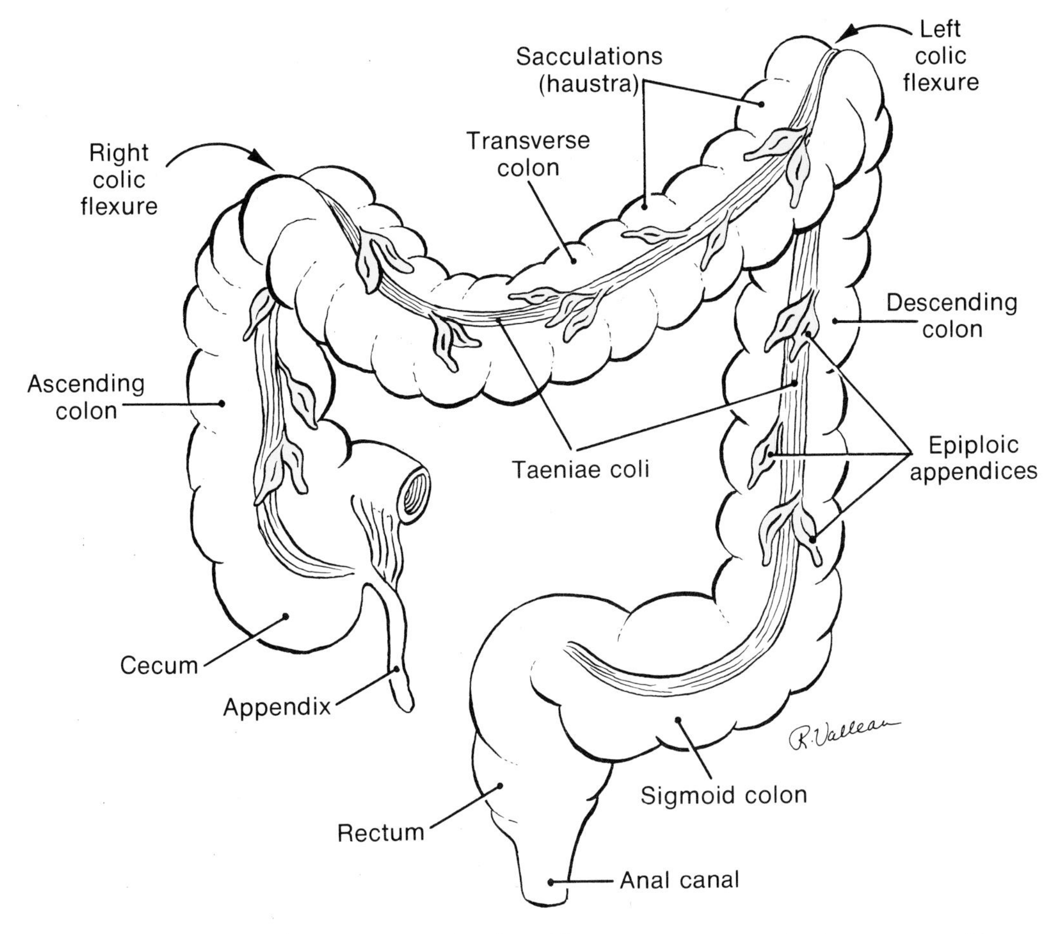

Fig. 14-25. The large intestine, anterior view. (The greater omentum has been removed.)

the left side of the abdomen and reaches the pelvic inlet to become the sigmoid colon. The **sigmoid** (S-shaped) **colon** arches backward along the sacrum and becomes continuous with the rectum at the midsacral region. The **rectum** follows the curvature of the lower sacrum and coccyx and then passes through the pelvic diaphragm and narrows to become the anal canal. The **anal canal** ends at the anal opening.

The transverse colon and sigmoid colon are suspended from the posterior abdominal wall by mesenteries (transverse mesocolon and the sigmoid mesocolon, respectively). The ascending colon, descending colon, and rectum lack a mesentery and are thus considered retroperitoneal. However, they may vary in their degree of immobility and fixation against the posterior abdominal wall.

In much of the cecum and colon the outer longitudinal layer of the muscularis externa shows three thickened longitudinal bands called **taeniae coli.** These bands are slightly shorter than the length of the intestine and produce a puckering effect so that **sacculations** or **haustra** are formed (Fig. 14-25). On the surface of the colon are little fat-filled tags of peritoneum called **epiploic appendices.** Since the taeniae coli and epiploic appendices are associated only with the colon these features are of

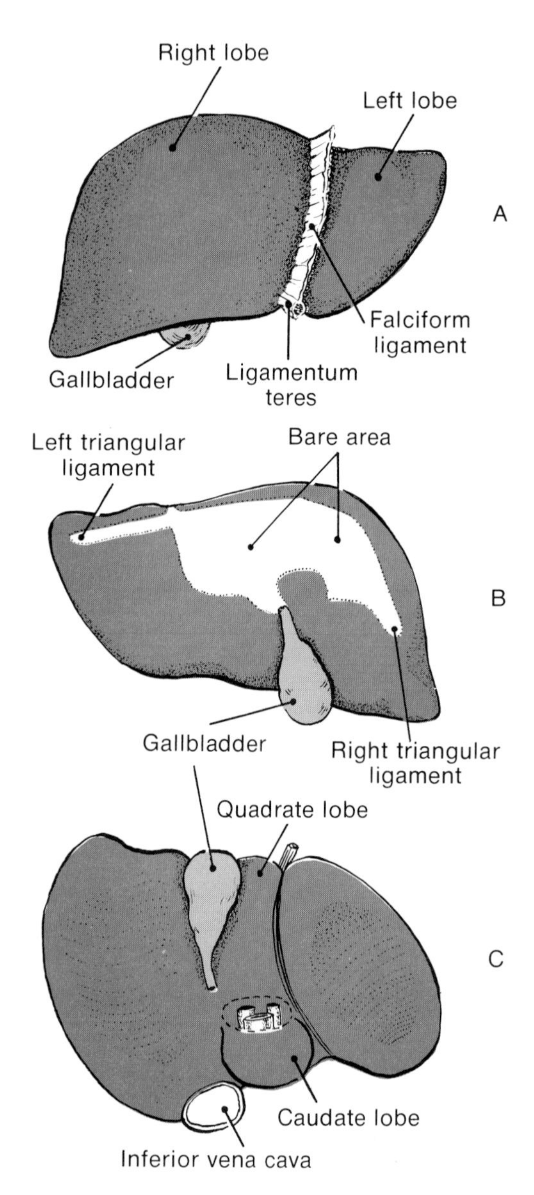

Fig. 14-26. The liver and gallbladder. (A) Anterior view, (B) posterior view. *Dotted line* represents coronary ligament forming the boundary of the bare area. (C) Inferior view. The *broken line* demarcates the porta hepatis.

use, particularly during surgery, in distinguishing the large intestine from the small intestine.

Microscopic Anatomy

The mucosa of the colon lacks villi or plicae but contains columnar epithelial cells with microvilli. Extending downward from the surface are tubular glands studded with numerous goblet cells whose mucous secretions form a protective coating for the mucosa, as well as lubrication for propelling the feces. At the anal opening (anus) the lining of the anal canal changes from simple columnar to stratified squamous. The anus is surrounded by a sphincter consisting of smooth muscle (internal anal sphincter) and skeletal muscle (external anal sphincter). The walls of the anal canal also contain a rich venous plexus which can become painfully enlarged and result in the formation of **hemorrhoids.**

Peristalsis

The transport of materials through the alimentary canal depends on waves of contraction known as peristalsis. Both the circular and longitudinal layers of muscle participate in this action. The muscularis mucosae also helps to propel material by producing a localized churning action.

The fecal material in the colon is periodically transported by means of mass movements to the sigmoid colon where storage occurs. The rectum usually does not contain feces until a bowel movement (defecation) occurs. **Defecation** is initiated by a mass movement which sends the feces from the sigmoid colon into the rectum, and the rectal smooth muscle contracts to expel the feces through the anal canal and anal opening. Evacuation of the bowel requires a relaxation of the external and internal anal sphincters. Contraction of the abdominal musculature and diaphragm also aids in evacuation by increasing the intra-abdominal pressure.

ACCESSORY ORGANS OF THE DIGESTIVE SYSTEM

Although the liver, gallbladder, and pancreas are often considered as accessory organs of the

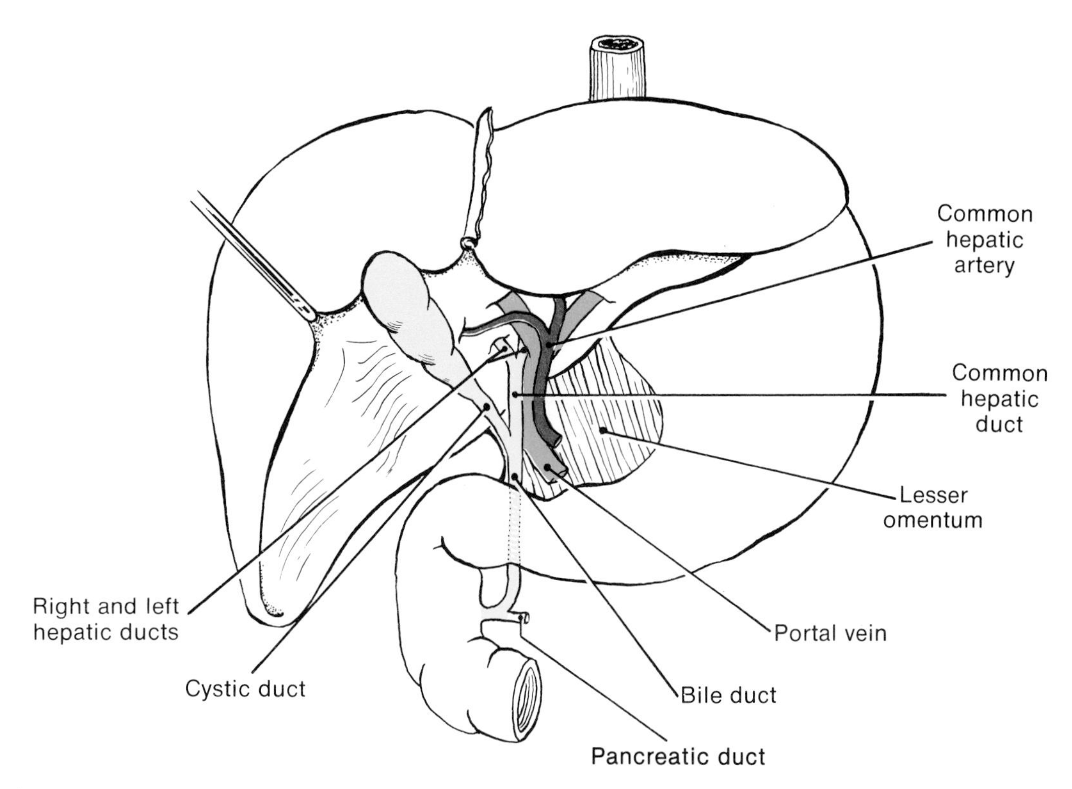

Fig. 14-27. Anterior view of the liver reflected upward to show the major blood vessels and biliary ducts. A portion of the lesser omentum has been removed in the region of the bile duct. (Modified after Grant.)

digestive system, they play a vital role in the process of digestion. In addition, the liver performs a variety of other metabolic activities, and the pancreas also functions as an endocrine organ. The salivary glands (described with the mouth) are also classified as accessory organs.

Liver and Gallbladder

The liver is the largest gland in the body and occupies a considerable portion of the abdominal cavity. It shows a multitude of functions, including the production of bile which emulsifies fats so that they can be acted upon by enzymes (lipases) from the pancreas and small intestine. The liver also synthesizes various proteins and serves as a storage site for glucose which has been converted to glycogen. The liver detoxifies harmful substances and converts metabolic waste products such as ammonia to urea for eventual excretion by the kidneys.

The liver is situated on the right side of the abdomen under cover of the lower thoracic cage and is attached to the underside of the diaphragm, with which it moves during respiration. The liver also is attached to the anterior body wall by means of a double layered sheet of peritoneum called the **falciform ligament** (Fig. 14-26). The lower free edge of the falciform ligament contains a fibrous band of tissue, the **ligamentum teres,** representing the obliterated umbilical vein of the fetus. The liver is covered with visceral peritoneum except for a region on its posterior surface called the "bare area." This bare area is bounded by the **coronary ligament** which consists of peritoneum reflected from the posterior surface of the liver upward and onto the surface of the diaphragm (Fig. 14-26). (The coronary ligament is tapered

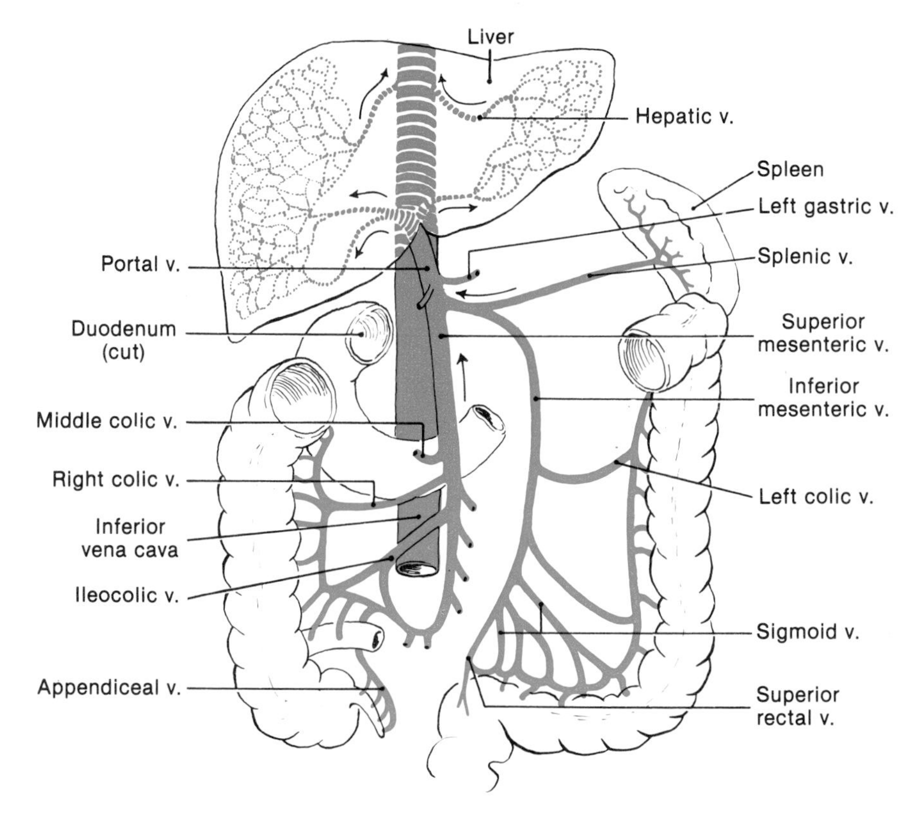

Fig. 14-28. The hepatic portal circulation. *Arrows* indicate the direction of flow.

laterally to form **right** and **left triangular ligaments.**)

The falciform ligament demarcates the two major lobes of the liver: a large **right lobe** and a smaller **left lobe.** On the inferior surface of the liver the right lobe shows two smaller portions, the **caudate lobe** posteriorly and the **quadrate lobe** anteriorly (Fig. 14-26). The inferior surface of the right lobe also contains the **gallbladder,** a pear-shaped sac nestled in its own fossa. Between the caudate and quadrate lobes is a depression called the **porta hepatis** ("door of the liver") which serves as an entrance or exit for blood vessels and for the hepatic ducts (see below). The **inferior vena cava,** however, occupies its own depression along the posterior aspect of the liver.

Bile is produced by hepatic cells and transported via a system of bile passages which eventually unite to form **right** and **left hepatic ducts** draining the right and left lobes, respectively (Fig. 14-27). The right and left ducts unite to form the **common hepatic duct** which in turn joins the **cystic duct** from the gallbladder to form the **bile duct** (sometimes called the common bile duct). The bile duct travels downward in the free edge of the lesser omentum and eventually enters the duodenum.

Before the bile reaches the duodenum, it passes from the lower end of the common hepatic duct upward through the cystic duct and into the gallbladder to be concentrated and stored until it is needed for digestion. When fats enter the duodenum, the duodenum secretes the hormone **cholecystokinin** into the blood stream. Cholecystokinin causes the gallbladder to contract and send the bile back down the cystic duct and through the bile duct

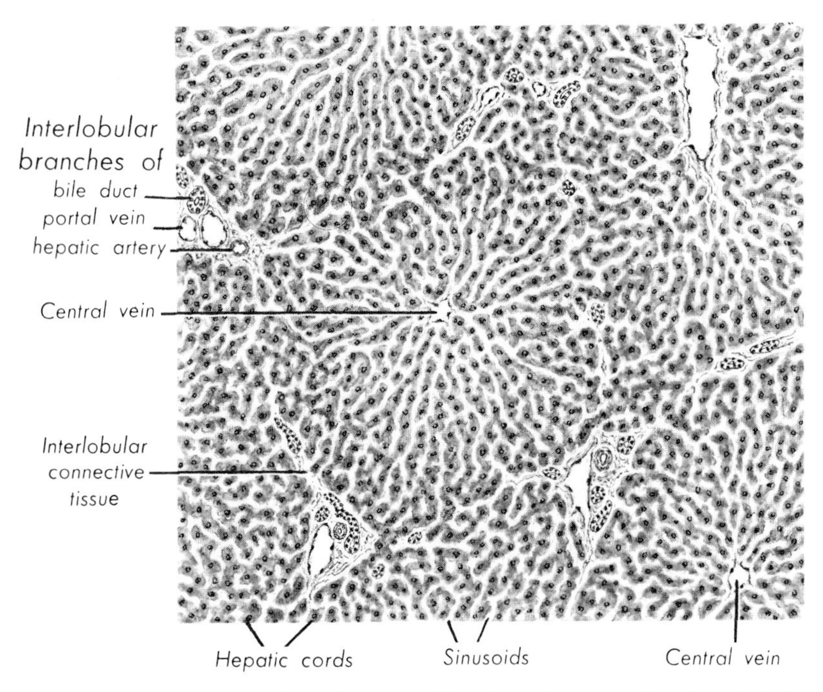

Fig. 14-29. Microscopic section of the liver, low magnification. One complete lobule is in the center of the photograph. (From W. M. Copenhaver, R. P. Bunge, and M. B. Bunge, *Bailey's Textbook of Histology,* Ed. 16, The Williams & Wilkins Co., Baltimore, 1971.)

to the duodenum where the bile emulsifies fats and facilitates their digestion by intestinal and pancreatic enzymes.

The liver receives a dual blood supply from the common hepatic artery and the hepatic portal vein. The **common hepatic artery** is a branch of the celiac artery and lies alongside the bile duct in the lesser omentum (Fig. 14-27). When the common hepatic artery reaches the liver, it divides into **right** and **left hepatic arteries** for the right and left lobes, respectively. The **portal vein** lies behind the common hepatic artery and bile duct in the lesser omentum and is formed by the union of various venous tributaries from the gastrointestinal tract (Fig. 14-28). The portal vein carries venous blood to be processed by the liver. After entering the liver the portal vein divides into a series of interlobular branches, each of which is accompanied by a biliary duct and a branch of the hepatic artery. The vein, duct, and artery together constitute a **portal triad.**

Microscopic Anatomy

The liver consists of interconnecting cords of hepatic cells arranged in a system of **lobules** (Fig. 14-29). Around the periphery of each lobule are several portal triads. The vein and artery of each triad empty their blood into a system of irregular vessels called **sinusoids.** The sinusoids carry the blood from the periphery of each lobule to a **central vein** located in the center of the lobule, and each central vein in turn joins with other central veins to form the **hepatic veins** which ultimately empty into the inferior vena cava near the upper border of the liver.

The liver sinusoids pass between radially arranged sheets of **hepatic cells,** which often are referred to as **hepatic cords** because of their appearance in histological sections. The hepatic cells act on various substances brought to the liver by the portal blood, and the blood in turn picks up substances produced by the he-

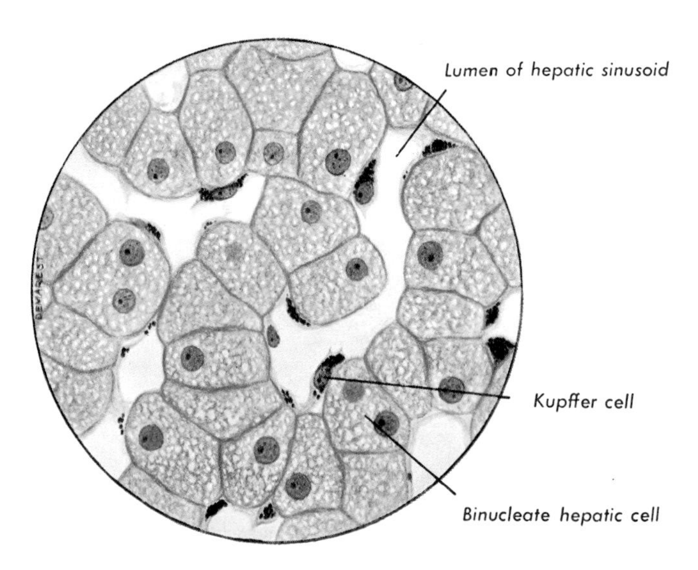

Fig. 14-30. Microscopic section of the liver showing Kupffer cells which have ingested dye particles by phagocytosis. (From W. M. Copenhaver, R. P. Bunge, and M. B. Bunge, *Bailey's Textbook of Histology*, Ed. 16, The Williams & Wilkins Co., Baltimore, 1971.)

patic cells. A series of special phagocytic cells called **Kupffer cells** is also situated along the sinusoids, and these cells operate as part of the body's defense mechanism by engulfing bacteria and other foreign substances (Fig. 14-30).

Bile is manufactured by the hepatic cells and is conveyed from the liver via biliary passages which begin as tiny slits called **bile canaliculi** between adjacent hepatic cells. The canaliculi unite to form the **interlobular biliary ducts** of the portal triad which eventually empty into the right and left hepatic ducts.

The gallbladder is lined with simple columnar epithelium. The mucosa is folded and has a honeycombed appearance (Fig. 14-31). The muscularis consists of circular and oblique muscle fibers which contract to propel the bile down the cystic duct and into the bile duct.

Pancreas

The pancreas contains both exocrine and endocrine components. The **exocrine portion** produces the digestive enzymes **trypsin, pancreatic amylase,** and **pancreatic lipase.** These pass to the small intestine where they break down proteins, carbohydrates, and fats, respectively. (Pancreatic secretion is under the influence of two hormones produced by the small intestine: 1) pancreozymin, which stimulates the output of the pancreatic digestive enzymes, and 2) secretin, which stimulates bicarbonate secretion for pH regulation.) The **endocrine portion** of the pancreas produces the hormones **insulin** and **glucagon** which regulate the level of glucose in the blood.

The pancreas consists of a **head** which fits into the C-shaped concavity on the outside of the duodenum, a **body** extending to the left, and a **tail** ending near the spleen (Fig. 14-32). Most of the pancreas is fixed against the posterior abdominal wall as a retroperitoneal organ, and it is richly supplied by arterial branches from the celiac and superior mesenteric arteries. A main **pancreatic duct** runs the length of the gland and joins the duodenum along with the bile duct, which lies behind the pancreas. At their entrance to the duodenum the pancreatic duct and bile duct together form a swelling, the **hepatopancreatic ampulla,**

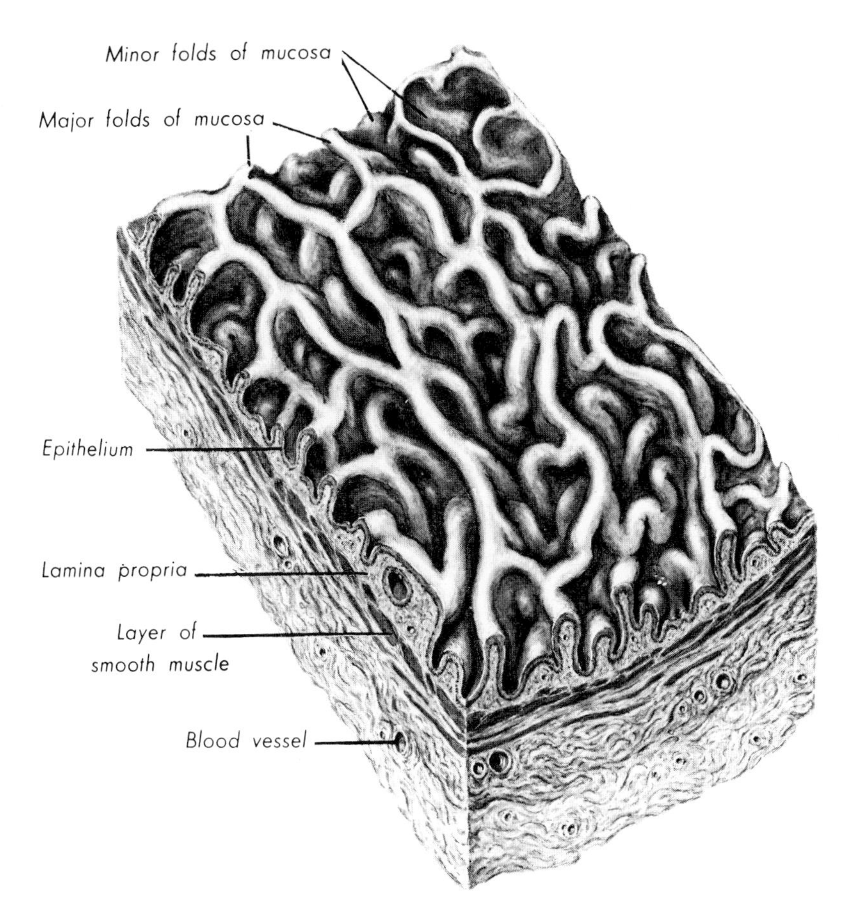

Fig. 14-31. Three dimensional view of the wall of the gallbladder. (From W. M. Copenhaver, R. P. Bunge, and M. B. Bunge, *Bailey's Textbook of Histology,* Ed. 16, The Williams & Wilkins Co., Baltimore, 1971.)

which also creates an elevated papilla on the inner surface of the duodenum. An **accessory pancreatic duct** is sometimes present in the head of the pancreas and empties by itself into the duodenum.

Microscopic Anatomy

The exocrine portion of the pancreas is composed of little sacs called acini, each of which contains **pancreatic acinar cells** arranged around a small central lumen. The digestive enzymes produced by these cells pass into the lumen and then into an anastomosing system of ducts, eventually emptying into the main pancreatic duct.

The endocrine cells of the pancreas are arranged in clusters called **islets (of Langerhans)** (Fig. 14-33). The islet cells consist of two types, one producing **insulin** and one producing **glucagon**. Both hormones are released into the blood which passes via the pancreatic veins to the portal system of the liver.

DEVELOPMENTAL AND CLINICAL ANATOMY

The digestive system develops from the **primitive gut** of the embryo. The primitive gut consists of a longitudinal tube which develops initially from endoderm and acquires an outer coat of splanchnic mesoderm (Chapter 5). The endodermal cells become the epithelial lining

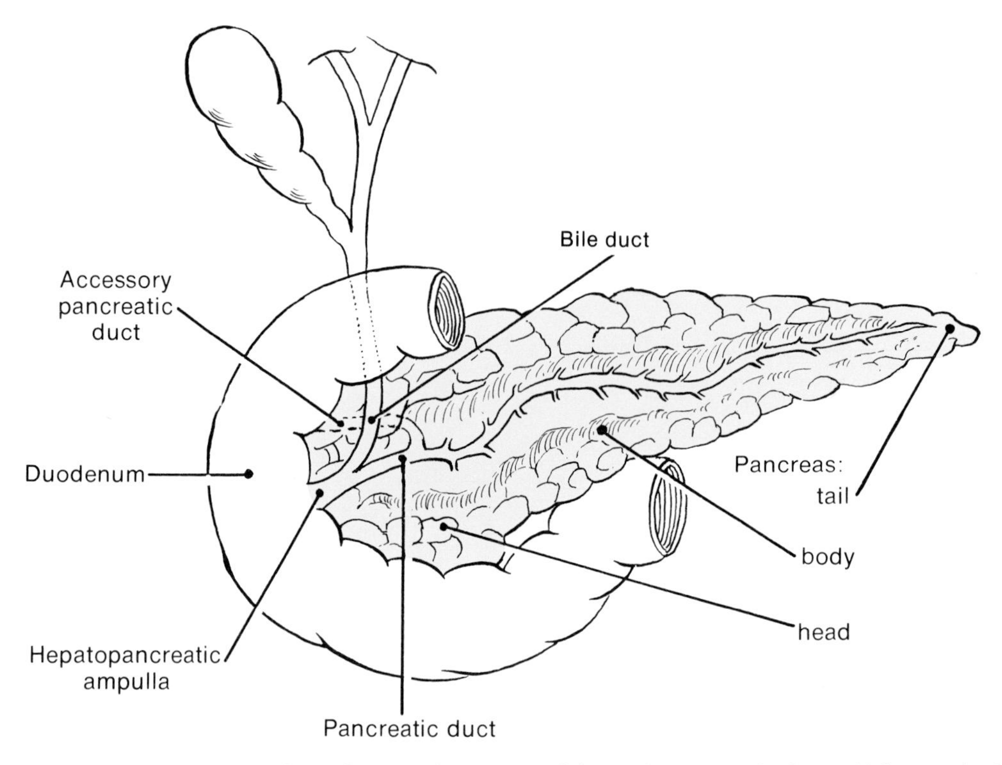

Fig. 14-32. The pancreas (in yellow) showing the course of the main pancreatic duct which joins the bile duct (from gallbladder and liver) at the hepatopancreatic ampulla.

and glands of the tube, while the splanchnic mesoderm differentiates into the various other components of the wall, including the lamina propria, muscularis mucosae, submucosa, and muscularis externa. The serosa or adventitia covering the outer surface of the tube likewise develops from the splanchnic mesoderm.

The primitive gut consists of three parts: **foregut, midgut** (which communicates with the yolk sac), and **hindgut** (Fig. 14-34A). The midgut gradually becomes cut off from the yolk sac, except at the attachment of the narrow **vitelline duct** which serves as a connection between the yolk sac and the midgut. Another extraembryonic structure, the **allantois,** also communicates with the hindgut.

The endoderm at the cranial end of the foregut initially is in contact with the **stomodeum,** an ectodermal depression on the ventral surface of the embryonic head. This area of contact between endoderm and ectoderm is called the **oral (buccopharyngeal) membrane.** The caudal end of the hindgut is known as the **cloaca.** Here the endoderm comes in contact with the **proctodeum,** an ectodermal depression on the ventral surface in the caudal region of the body. The fused ectoderm and endoderm are termed the **cloacal membrane.** The oral and cloacal membranes eventually disappear, and the primitive gut then communicates with the amniotic cavity via the oral cavity and anal opening, respectively.

The upper part of the foregut develops into the **pharynx** which in turn leads downward into the esophagus (Fig. 14-34B). The caudal portion of the foregut expands to form the stomach and then abruptly narrows again to become the duodenum. From the upper part of the duodenum a number of outgrowths (diverticula) appear. An **hepatic diverticulum** projects ventrally and becomes the liver and gallbladder, both of which retain their common communication with the duodenum by means of the bile duct. A **ventral pancreas** grows out in common with the hepatic diverticulum from the duodenum. From the opposite side of the duodenum a **dorsal pancreas** develops. The ventral and dorsal pancreas eventually unite to form the adult pancreas. In most individuals the duct of the embryonic ventral pancreas is retained as the main pancreatic duct of the adult, while the dorsal pancreatic attachment to the duodenum is lost. However, in some instances the dorsal pancreatic duct may be retained as an accessory pancreatic duct.

The midgut elongates considerably and forms the caudal part of the duodenum, jejunum, ileum, cecum, appendix, ascending colon, and proximal part of the transverse colon. The hindgut develops into the distal part of the transverse colon, descending colon, sigmoid colon, rectum and the upper part of the anal canal.

Each portion of the embryonic gut receives its own arterial supply as follows. The caudal part of the foregut is supplied by the celiac artery, the midgut by the superior mesenteric artery, and the hindgut by the inferior mesenteric artery.

The primitive gut is suspended from the posterior abdominal wall by a two-layered sheet of mesoderm called the **dorsal mesentery** (Figs. 14-34 and 14-35). In the region of the stomach, the dorsal mesentery provides the ligaments associated with the spleen, which develops as a condensation of mesodermal cells between the two layers of the mesentery. A less extensive **ventral mesentery** attaches the embryonic stomach and duodenum to the anterior abdominal wall. When the hepatic diverticulum grows into the ventral mesentery, the mesentery becomes converted into the **falciform ligament** (attaching liver to anterior abdominal wall) and the **lesser omentum** (attaching liver to stomach and duodenum).

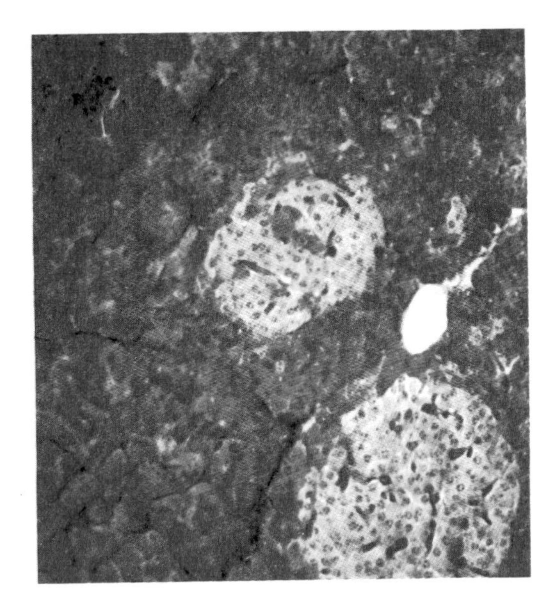

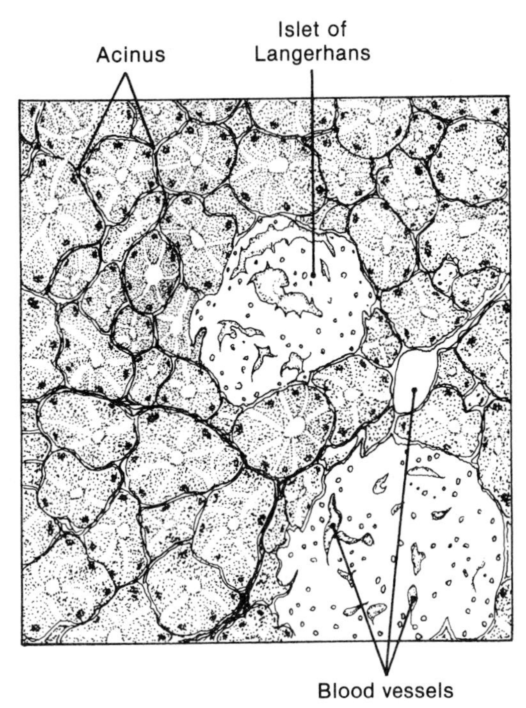

Fig. 14-33. *(Top)* Microscopic section of the pancreas showing endocrine islets of Langerhans (pale pink) and exocrine acinar cells (dark red). (Courtesy of Dr. Hadley Kirkman, Stanford University.) *(Bottom)* Sketch of microscopic section.

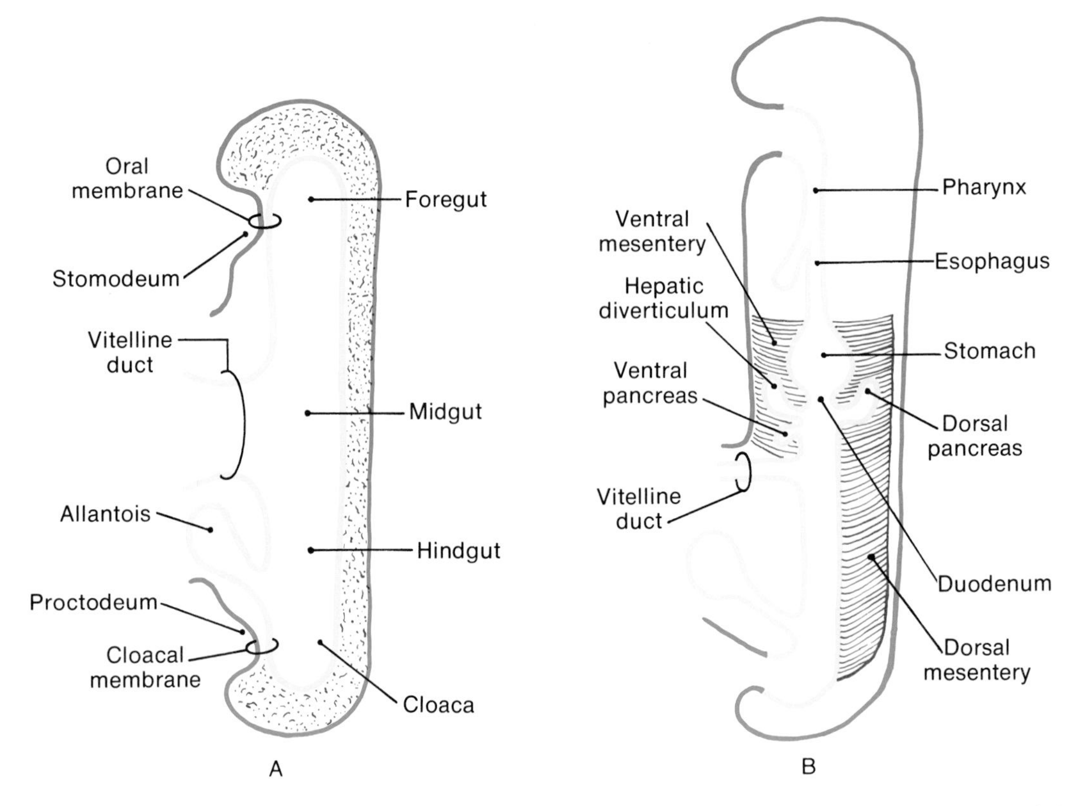

Fig. 14-34. Development of the digestive system. (A) Left lateral view at approximately 3 weeks, (B) left lateral view at approximately 4 weeks. Dorsal and ventral mesenteries (in red) suspend the gut from the body wall.

The embryonic gut continues to elongate and undergoes a complex rotation whereby the liver eventually becomes located on the right side of the abdominal cavity and the stomach is shifted over to the left. The lower portions of the gut form a loop which temporarily herniates out into the umbilical cord (Fig. 14-35). When the loop withdraws back into the abdominal cavity, the ascending colon comes to lie on the right side and the descending colon on the left. The cecum and appendix are initially located in the upper right quadrant of the abdomen but gradually migrate downward and can end up at various levels along the right side. After birth the highly variable position of the appendix can create difficulties in distinguishing the pain of appendicitis from other disorders in the abdominal cavity.

As the gut rotates and elongates, various organs adhere to and fuse with the posterior abdominal wall and lose their dorsal mesentery, thus becoming fixed in a retroperitoneal position. These organs include the duodenum, pancreas, ascending colon, and descending colon. Other portions of the gut retain their dorsal mesenteric attachments. These mesenteries are often given special names such as the transverse mesocolon and sigmoid mesocolon. The rectum, however, does not have any mesenteric attachment.

In the region of the stomach, the dorsal mesentery pushes forward and downward to

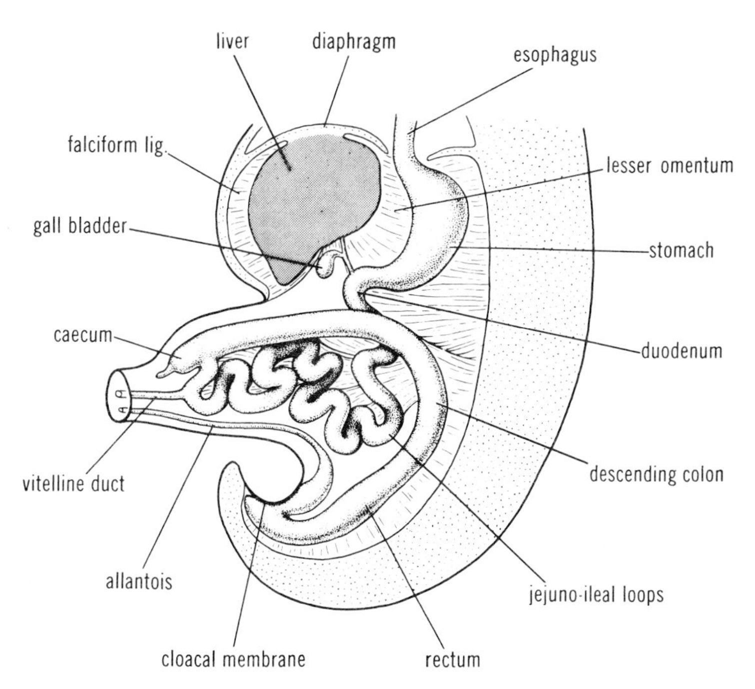

Fig. 14-35. The gastrointestinal tract of an embryo at approximately eight weeks' gestation, left lateral view. Note the temporary herniation of the intestinal loops into the umbilical cord. (From J. Langman, *Medical Embryology*, Ed. 3, The Williams & Wilkins Co., Baltimore, 1975.)

form a four-layered apron in front of the coils of the intestines. This is the **greater omentum** which also eventually fuses with the anterior surface of the transverse colon.

The yolk sac is attached to the portion of the gut which will become the ileum. This attachment, the **vitelline duct,** ordinarily degenerates before birth, but in some individuals it may be retained after birth as a blind-ending sac called **Meckel's diverticulum.** The diverticulum sometimes becomes inflamed and produces symptoms similar to those of appendicitis.

In some instances embryonic intestinal loops fail to withdraw completely from the umbilical cord, and the intestine can be seen protruding into the umbilicus at the time of birth (Fig. 14-36). This condition is known as an **omphalocele** and usually can be corrected surgically. Various other congenital anomalies can also occur, such as malrotation, whereby the intestine may fail to form a loop or may rotate incompletely.

Occasionally a portion of the peritoneum may adhere to adjacent regions of peritoneum, resulting in **adhesions.** These can also occur postnatally subsequent to surgical procedures or inflammations of the peritoneum **(peritonitis).** Also, a failure of the intestinal loops to slide freely over one another and along the body wall may produce a kink and lead to **obstruction** of the lumen. **Strangulation,** an impairment of an organ's blood supply, may also occur.

The lining of the alimentary canal is susceptible to damage, as may occur from hyperacidity. An erosion which extends through or beyond the mucosa is known as an **ulcer,** and

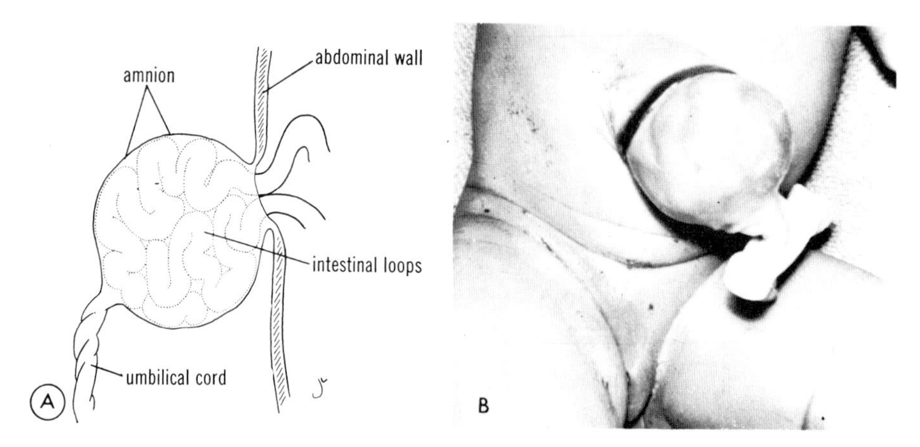

Fig. 14-36. Omphalocele, a failure of the intestinal loops to withdraw from the umbilical cord. (A) Drawing (left lateral view), (B) photograph of newborn (anterior view). (Courtesy of Dr. A. Shaw, Dept. of Surgery, University of Virginia, from J. Langman, *Medical Embryology,* Ed. 3, The Williams & Wilkins Co., Baltimore, 1975.)

these most commonly occur in the stomach and duodenum. Such ulcers may erode the blood vessels and cause blood to be released into the lumen. A particularly dangerous situation occurs when an ulcer perforates through the entire thickness of the wall and allows digestive contents to seep into the peritoneal cavity, thereby leading to peritonitis.

Inflammation of the liver is termed **hepatitis.** The pancreas also may become inflamed **(pancreatitis)**. Chronic damage to liver cells results in the formation of fibrous scar tissue, known as **cirrhosis. Gallstones** are frequently present in the gallbladder but are not particularly dangerous unless they become lodged in the bile duct, obstructing the flow of bile from the liver to the duodenum and leading to **jaundice.**

15

The Urinary System

The urinary system consists of two kidneys, two ureters, the urinary bladder, and the urethra (Fig. 15-1). A primary function of the kidneys is to excrete metabolic wastes, such as urea, which have accumulated in the blood. The kidneys also regulate fluid and acid-base balance.

Urine is formed in the kidneys and passes by means of the ureters to the urinary bladder, where it is stored until urination occurs. The bladder then contracts, and the urine is expelled through the urethra. The urinary organs are the same in both sexes, except for the urethra which is longer in the male and which serves also as the channel for sperm transport during ejaculation.

KIDNEYS

Gross Anatomy

The kidneys are located in the upper lumbar region of the posterior abdominal wall on each side of the vertebral column. Each kidney contains a medial concave border, a lateral convex border, superior and inferior poles, and anterior and posterior surfaces. Since the kidney is nestled close to the curved bodies of the vertebrae, the medial border of the kidney projects slightly anteriorly, and the lateral border projects posteriorly; therefore, the anterior and posterior surfaces actually slope obliquely (Fig. 15-2). The kidneys may change position with each respiratory movement or with changes in body position, and in most individuals the right kidney is slightly lower than the left one.

The kidneys lie behind the parietal peritoneum of the abdomen and are considered as retroperitoneal structures. Surgical procedures can thus be done on the kidney without entering the peritoneal cavity. In such cases an oblique incision is made through the posterolateral abdominal wall usually midway between the twelfth rib and iliac crest. This approach can also be used to drain pus from a retroperitoneal abscess.

Each kidney is covered by a tough connective tissue **capsule,** which is surrounded with varying amounts of **perirenal fat** (Fig. 15-2). The fat is held in place by a sheet of extraperitoneal connective tissue which has split to form an **anterior** and **posterior layer** of **renal fascia.** The anterior layer of renal fascia lies immediately behind the parietal peritoneum; the posterior layer is in contact with posterior abdominal muscles (primarily the psoas major, quadratus lumborum, and transversus abdominis) and with the diaphragm. Superior to each kidney is a suprarenal (adrenal) gland, which is also enclosed within the renal fascia. Since the lower ribs pass obliquely downward, the suprarenal glands and upper poles of the kidneys are somewhat protected by these bony structures; the lower portions of the kidneys, however, are more vulnerable to injury.

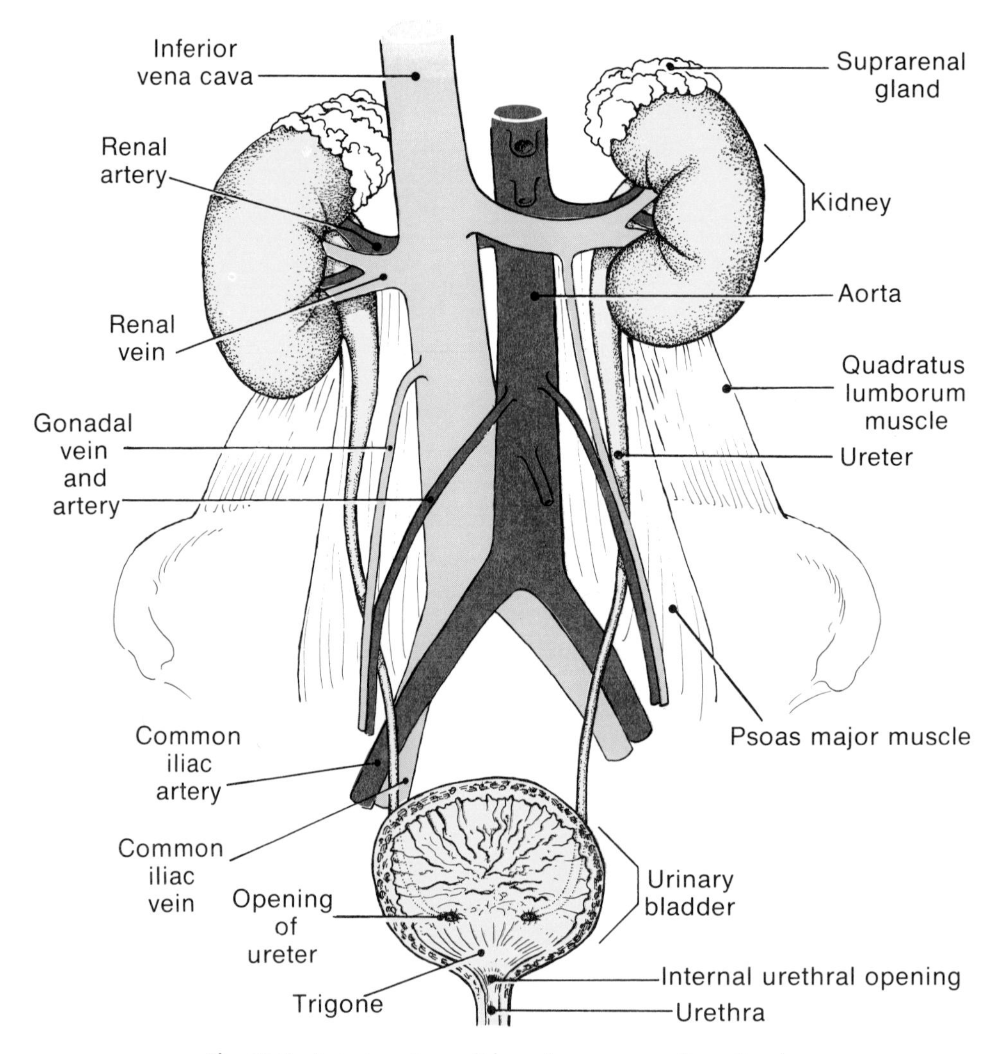

Fig. 15-1. Anterior view of the urinary organs (in yellow).

The ureter, renal artery and vein, lymphatic vessels, and autonomic nerves leave and enter each kidney at a fissure, the **hilus,** along its medial border. The upper end of the ureter is expanded into a funnel-shaped structure, the **renal pelvis** (Fig. 15-3). Surrounding the renal pelvis and the renal vessels is a fat-filled depression, the **renal sinus.**

The substance of the kidney shows two general regions: an inner **medulla** and an outer **cortex.** The medulla is composed of pyramid-shaped blocks of tissue, **renal pyramids,** whose bases face peripherally toward the cortex whereas the apices project centrally toward the hilus. The cortex lies peripheral to the medulla but sends strands of cortical tissue, the **renal columns,** between the pyramids of the medulla. (Conversely, the medulla sends medullary tissue, the **medullary rays,** outward into the cortex.)

The apex of each renal pyramid fits into a **minor calyx** which is a cup-shaped projection of a major calyx. Each **major calyx** in turn communicates with the renal pelvis. These

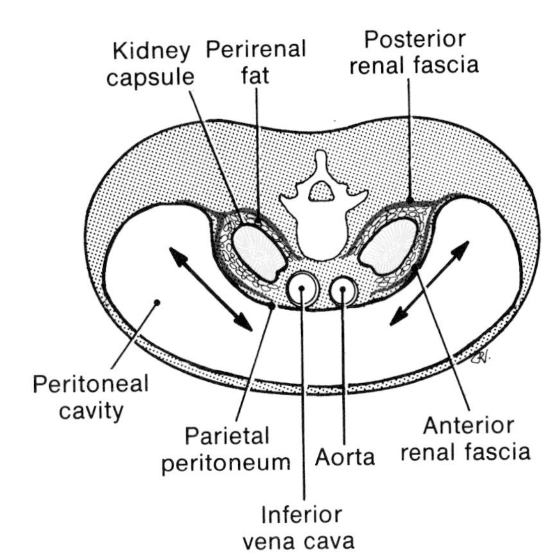

Fig. 15-2. Cross section through the lumbar region of the body showing kidneys and perirenal structures. *Arrows* indicate oblique orientation of the kidneys. The renal fascia is indicated in red. (Digestive organs are not included in the diagram.)

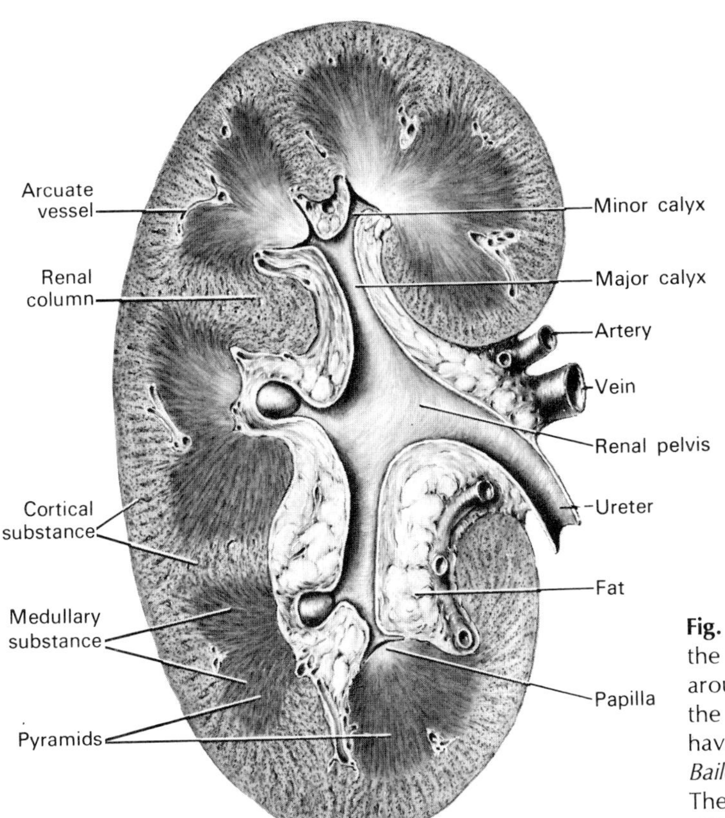

Fig. 15-3. Longitudinal section through the kidney. The fat-containing area around the renal pelvis and calyces is the renal sinus. (From W. M. Copenhaver, R. P. Bunge, and M. B. Bunge, *Bailey's Textbook of Histology,* Ed. 16, The Williams & Wilkins Co., Baltimore, 1971.)

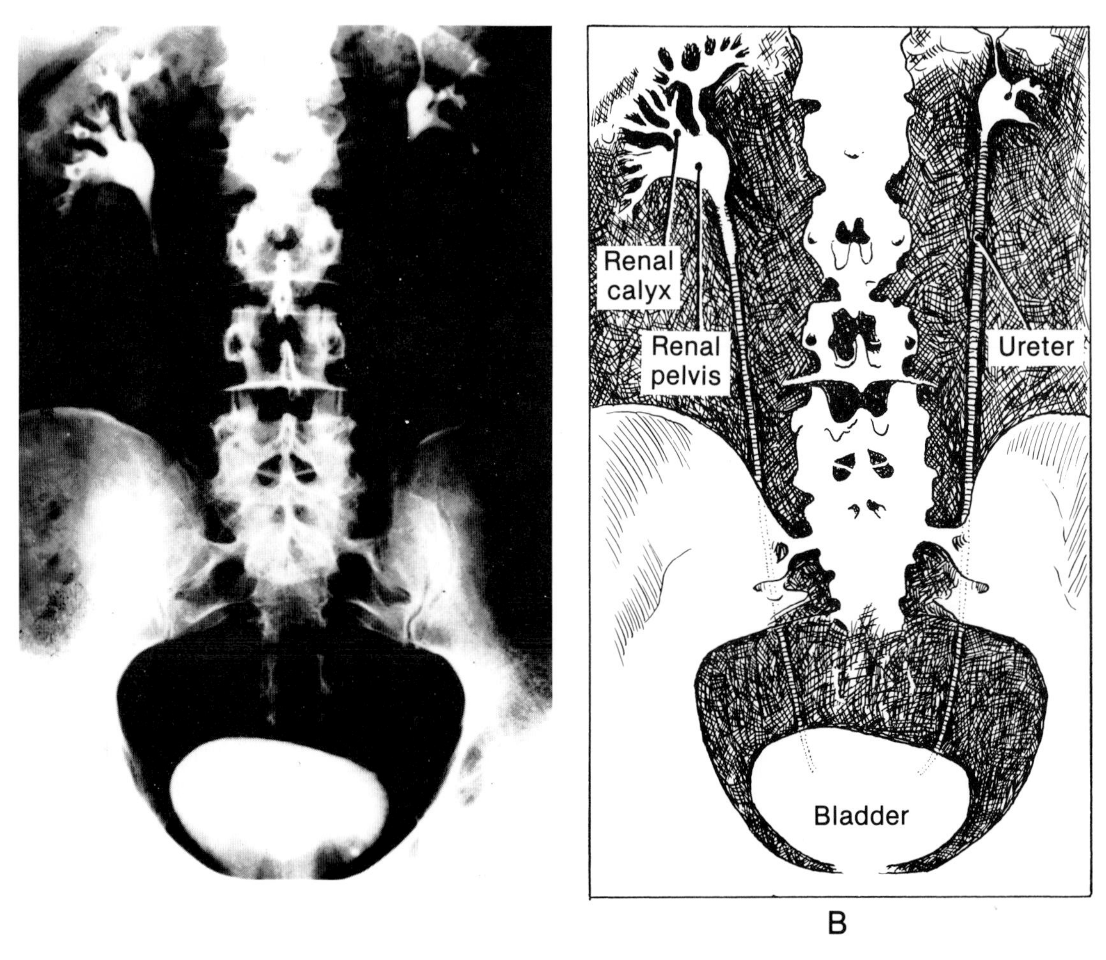

Fig. 15-4. (A) X-ray (intravenous pyelogram) taken after an intravenous injection of an opaque dye. The dye is being excreted by each kidney. Note the slightly lower position of the right kidney. (From E. D. Gardner, D. J. Gray, and R. O'Rahilly, *Anatomy,* Ed. 4, W. B. Saunders Co., Philadelphia, 1975.) (B) Sketch of X-ray. *Dotted lines* represent the course of the ureters, which are not clearly visible in A.

structures can be visualized radiologically in an **intravenous pyelogram,** which capitalizes on the kidney's ability to excrete and concentrate contrast media injected into the blood stream (Fig. 15-4).

The kidneys are richly supplied with blood by a pair of renal arteries which are branches of the abdominal aorta. Each **renal artery** enters the kidney at the hilus and breaks up into a number of **interlobar arteries** which pass radially through the medulla (Fig. 15-5). The interlobar arteries then branch into a number of **arcuate arteries** arching over the bases of the renal pyramids, much like the spokes of an umbrella. The arcuate arteries give rise to a series of straight **interlobular arteries** which pass radially through the cortex. Each interlobular artery in turn supplies numerous **afferent arterioles** to small balls of capillaries called **glomeruli** (Fig. 15-6). **Efferent arterioles** pass away from the glomeruli and break up into a second capillary network (the **peritubular capillary plexus**) which eventually connects with **interlobular veins** running parallel to the in-

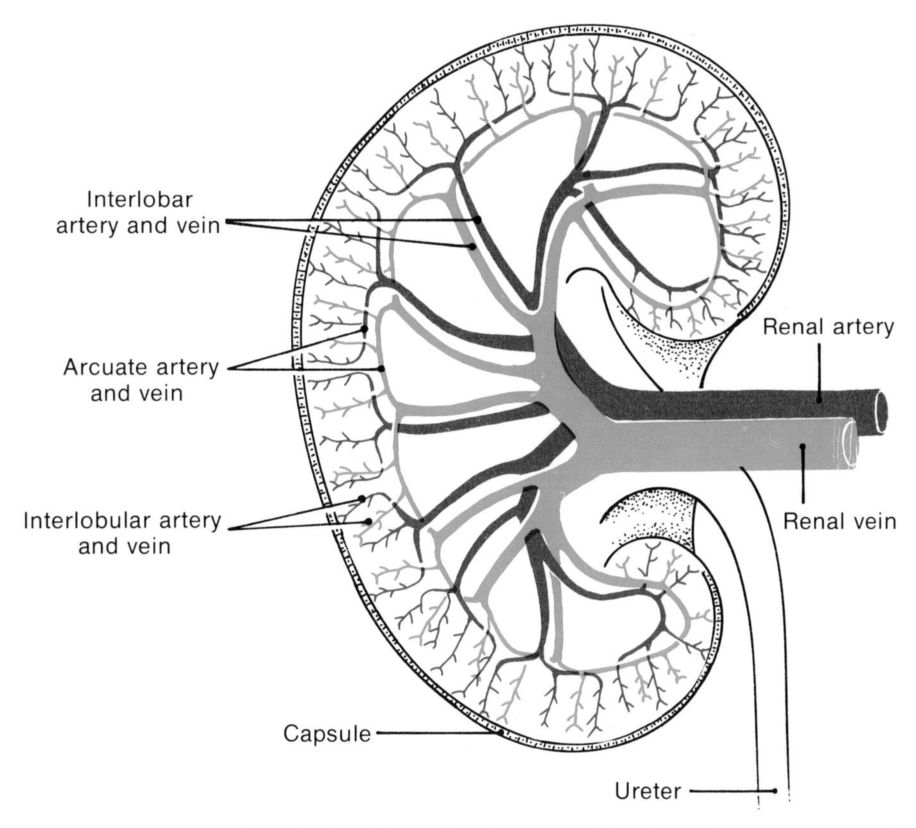

Fig. 15-5. Longitudinal section through the kidney showing major blood vessels and upper portion of the ureter.

terlobular arteries. The interlobular veins then join **arcuate veins** which in turn connect with **interlobar veins.** The interlobar veins unite to form the **renal vein** passing to the inferior vena cava.

Microscopic Anatomy

Each kidney is composed of approximately one million functional units called **nephrons.** Each nephron begins in the cortex and consists of a long hollow tube, one end of which is a thin-walled sac invaginated by a ball of capillaries (the glomerulus) (Fig. 15.6). The invaginated portion of the nephron is the **glomerular (Bowman's) capsule.** The glomerulus and glomerular capsule together constitute a **renal corpuscle.** Beyond the glomerular capsule the nephron becomes highly coiled and is called the **proximal convoluted tubule.** The tubule then leads to a hairpin-shaped structure, the **loop of Henle,** which consists of a descending limb and an ascending limb. The **descending limb** has a short thick-walled segment and a long thin-walled segment and passes from the cortex into the medulla. The **ascending limb** has a short thin-walled segment and a long thick-walled segment and passes back into the cortex where the tubule once again becomes coiled and is termed the **distal convoluted tubule.** In the cortex the distal convoluted tubule empties into a **collecting tubule** which extends through the medulla to the apex of the renal pyramid. (Groups of collecting tubules in the cortex constitute the thin strands of medullary tissue, the medullary rays.)

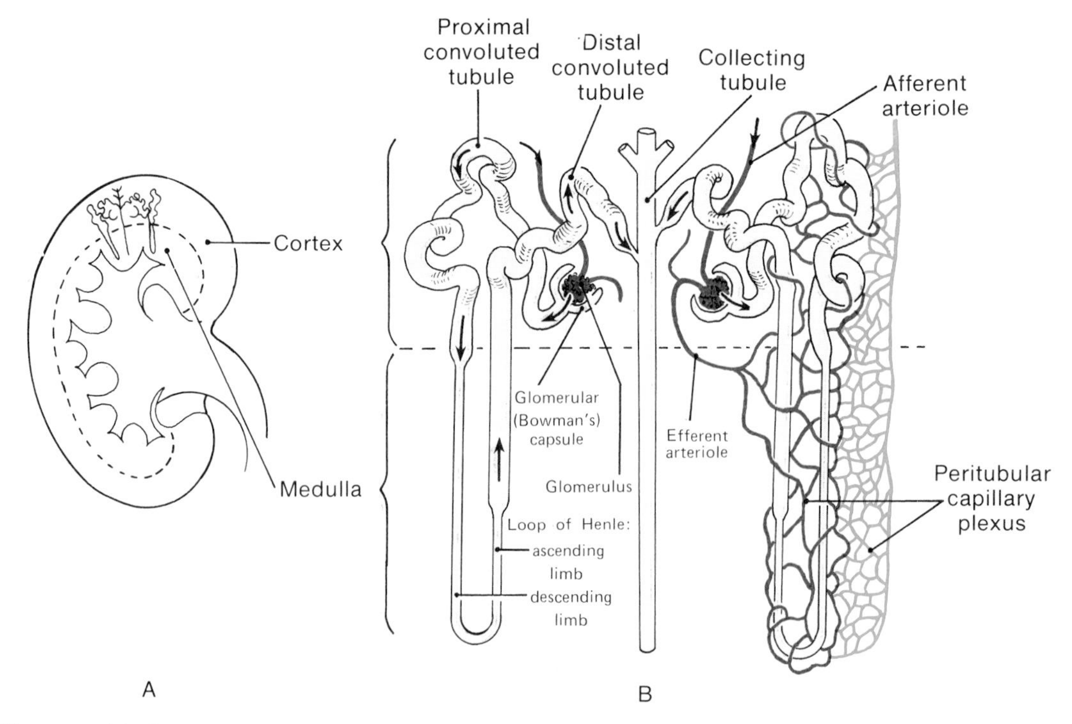

Fig. 15-6. (A) The course of two nephrons (highly magnified) relative to the cortical and medullary portions of the kidney. (B) Details of two nephrons. *Arrows* indicate the pathway of substances which form the urine. (The peritubular capillary plexus is shown only on the nephron on the right.)

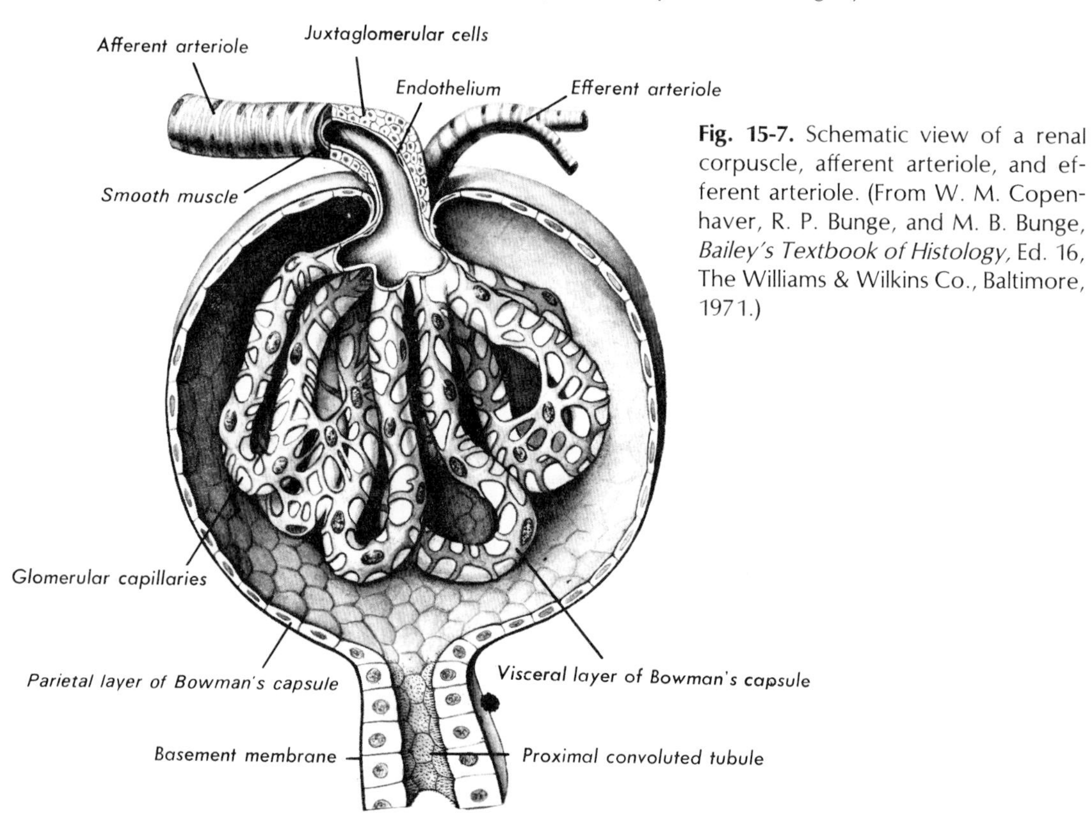

Fig. 15-7. Schematic view of a renal corpuscle, afferent arteriole, and efferent arteriole. (From W. M. Copenhaver, R. P. Bunge, and M. B. Bunge, *Bailey's Textbook of Histology,* Ed. 16, The Williams & Wilkins Co., Baltimore, 1971.)

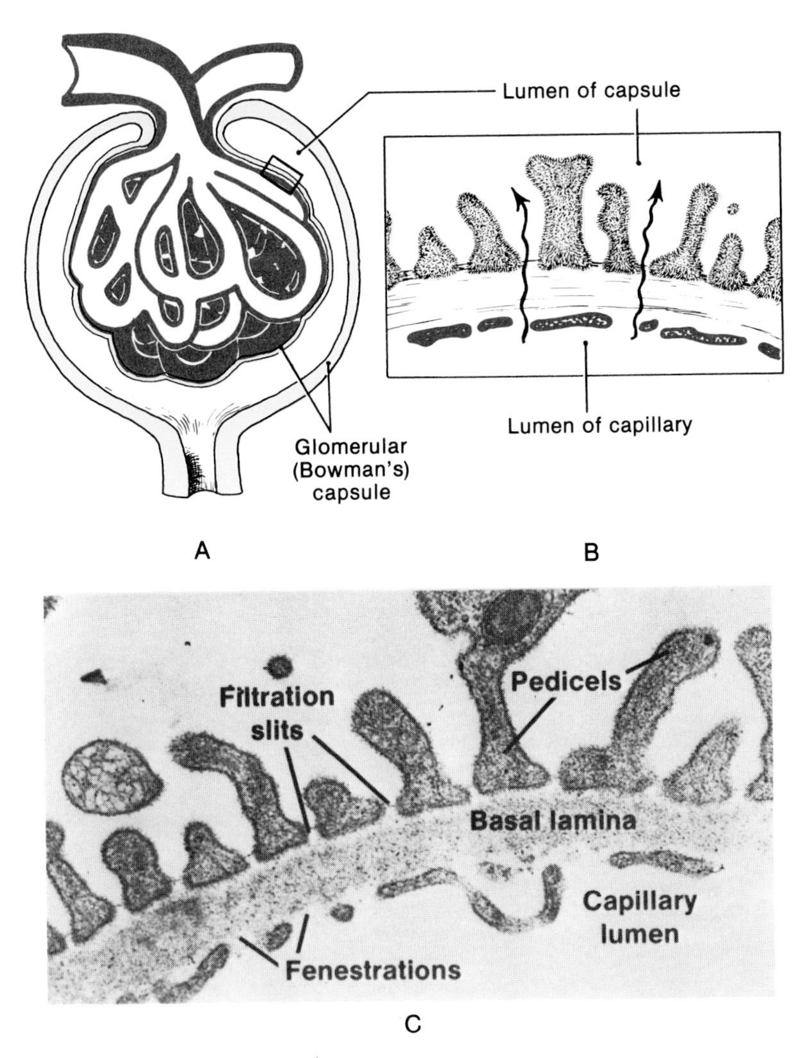

Fig. 15-8. The filtration membrane in the kidney. (A) The glomerulus (red) projects into the glomerular (Bowman's) capsule (yellow). The rectangle represents an area of the filtration membrane shown at higher magnification in B. *Arrows* indicate direction of filtration flow across the filtration membrane from capillary lumen to lumen of glomerular capsule. (C) Electron micrograph of the filtration membrane showing pedicels of capsule cells, basal lamina, and the capillary endothelium. (From R. G. Kessel, and R. H. Kardon, *Tissues and Organs: A Text-Atlas of Scanning Electron Microscopy,* W. H. Freeman and Company. Copyright © 1979.)

The capillaries of the glomerulus are supplied by an afferent arteriole and are drained by an efferent arteriole, which leads into the peritubular capillary plexus surrounding the various tubular portions of the nephron (Fig. 15-6). The afferent arteriole brings blood under pressure to the glomerulus. The glomerular capillaries are covered by a thin layer of epithelium (simple squamous) representing the **visceral layer** of the glomerular (Bowman's) capsule (Fig. 15-7). (The remainder of the capsule is termed the **parietal layer.**) Large amounts of fluid pass by pressure filtration from the blood in the glomerular capillaries across a filtration membrane (composed of the capillary wall and epithelium of the glomerular capsule) into the lumen of the capsule (Fig. 15-8). The endothelial cells of the capillaries lie

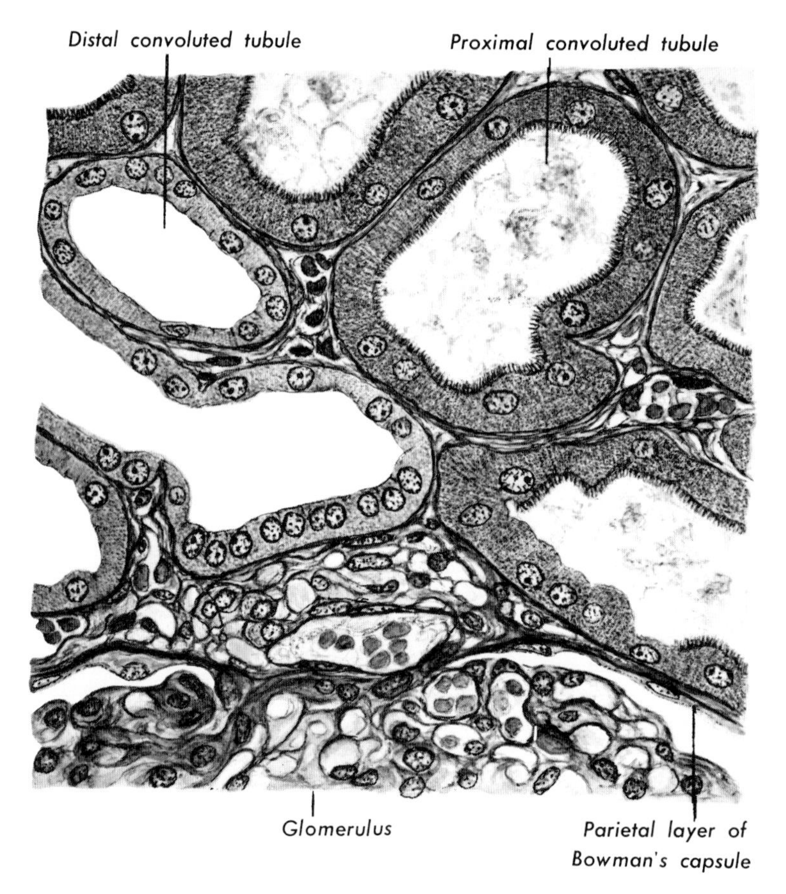

Fig. 15-9. Cross section of portion of a glomerulus, as well as proximal convoluted tubules and distal convoluted tubules in the cortex of the kidney. (From W. M. Copenhaver, R. P. Bunge, and M. B. Bunge, *Bailey's Textbook of Histology,* Ed. 16, The Williams & Wilkins Co., Baltimore, 1971.)

against a basal lamina and contain fenestrations or pores. The basal lamina in turn lies adjacent to foot processes (pedicels) from the specialized cells (podocytes), which represent the visceral layer of the glomerular capsule.

The filtrate is actually similar in composition to blood plasma; hence, fluid and substances vital to the welfare of the body must be selectively resorbed and returned to the peritubular capillary plexus. This selective resorption is carried out in the remainder of the nephron and depends partly on an efficient but energy-requiring process of active transport as well as on passive transport.

In the proximal convoluted tubule the cuboidal epithelial cells are characterized by a well developed "brush" border consisting of microvilli (Fig. 15-9). These microvilli actively resorb some of the fluid, as well as glucose and various ions such as sodium, from the lumen of the tubule. The energy for this active resorption is provided by large numbers of mitochondria in the base of each cell (Fig. 15-10). The epithelial cells pass these substances back to the blood in the peritubular capillary plexus. The remaining fluid in the kidney tubule then flows into the loop of Henle, where large amounts of water continue to be resorbed. The thin segments of the loop are lined by squamous (flattened) cells, whereas the cells lining the thick segments are low cuboidal (Fig. 15-11).

In the distal convoluted tubule the cells are

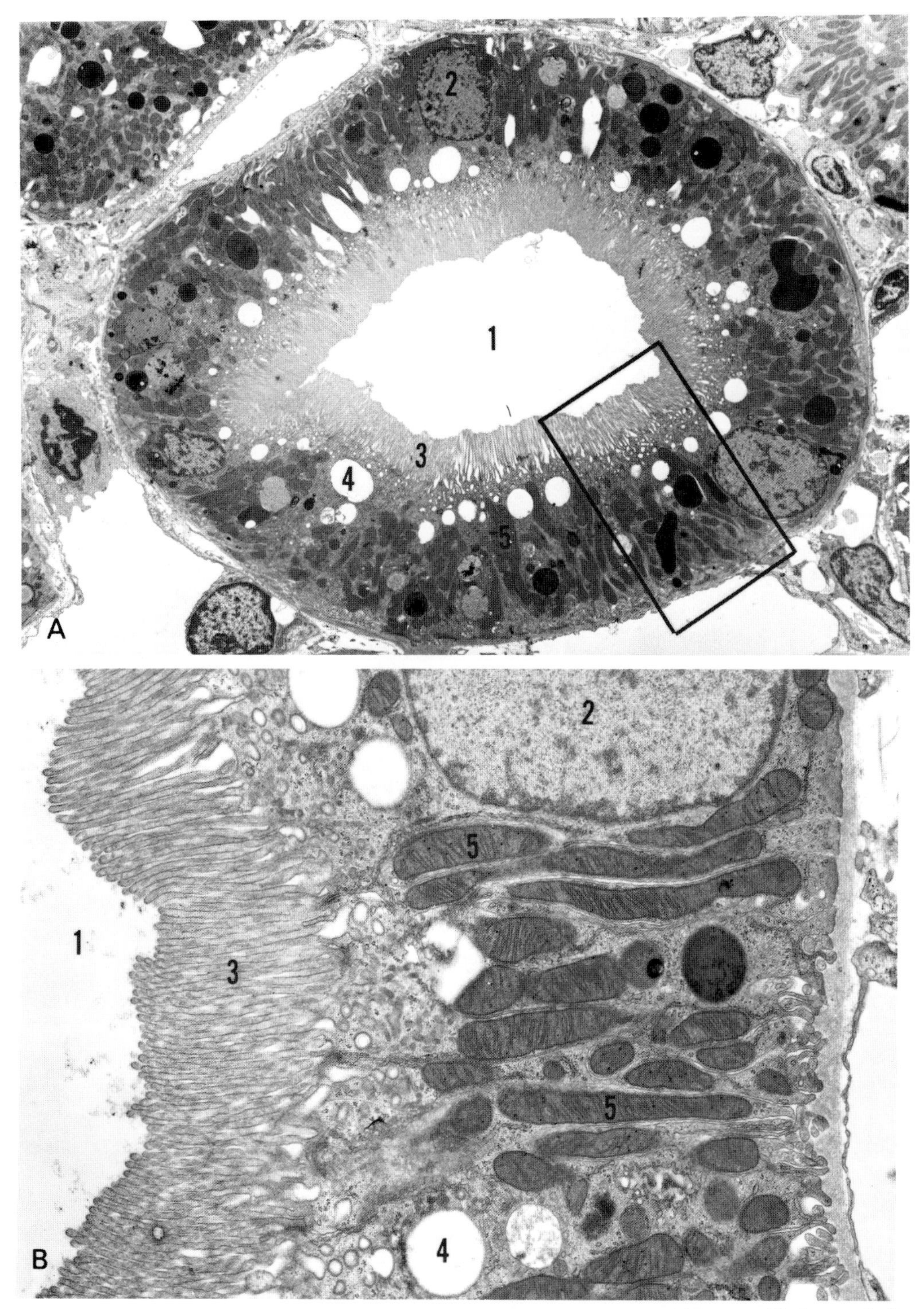

Fig. 15-10. (A) Cross section through a proximal convoluted tubule. (B) Highly magnified area similar to that represented by the rectangle in A. *1*, Lumen of tubule; *2*, nucleus; *3*, microvilli; *4*, vacuole; *5*, mitochondria. (From *Histology: A Text and Atlas* by Johannes A. G. Rhodin. Copyright © 1976 by Johannes A. G. Rhodin. Reprinted by permission of the author and Oxford University Press, Inc.)

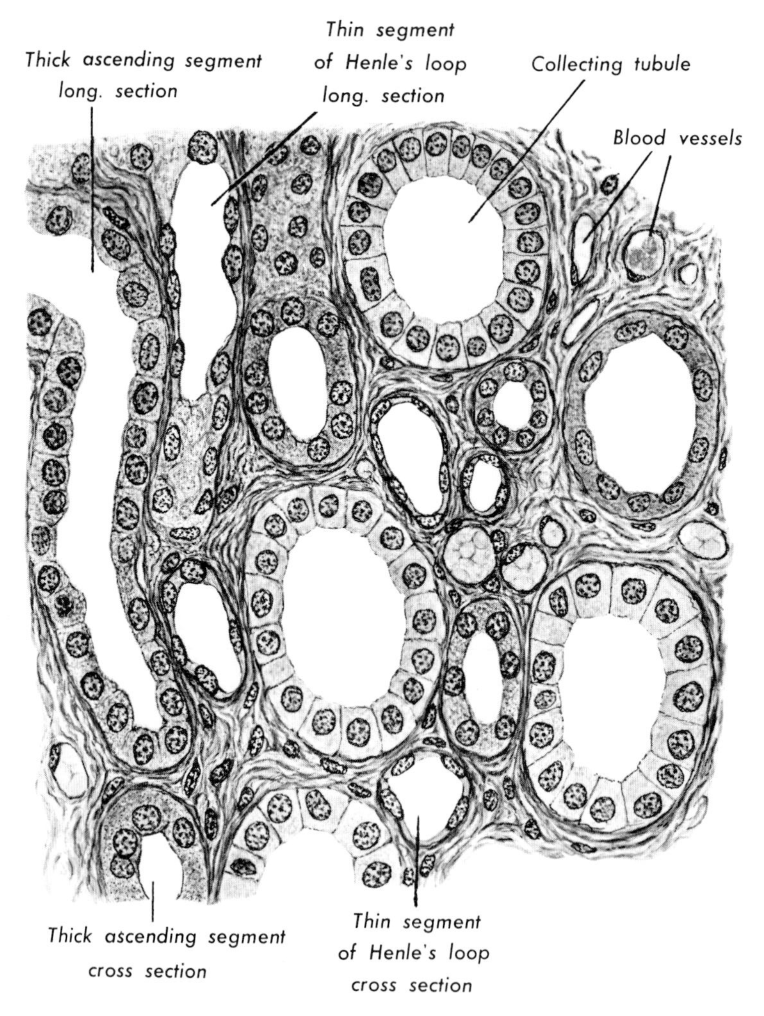

Fig. 15-11. Cross section through the medulla of the kidney. (From W. M. Copenhaver, R. P. Bunge, and M. B. Bunge, *Bailey's Textbook of Histology,* Ed. 16, The Williams & Wilkins Co., Baltimore, 1971.)

cuboidal but have fewer microvilli and mitochondria than is the case in the proximal convoluted tubule. However, as the distal convoluted tubule passes in the vicinity of the afferent and efferent arterioles, it exhibits a localized area of tall columnar epithelial cells which lie against specialized smooth muscle fibers known as **juxtaglomerular cells** in the wall of the afferent arteriole (Fig. 15-7). These juxtaglomerular cells secrete into the blood stream an enzyme, **renin,** which participates in a complex series of reactions producing **angiotensin.** Since angiotensin constricts blood vessels and thereby elevates the blood pressure, hyperactivity of the juxtaglomerular cells can lead to a form of high blood pressure known as **renal hypertension.** Angiotensin also triggers the release of **aldosterone** from the adrenal gland, which increases sodium and water resorption from the distal convoluted tubule, thus making the urine more concentrated. The amount of water resorbed is under the control

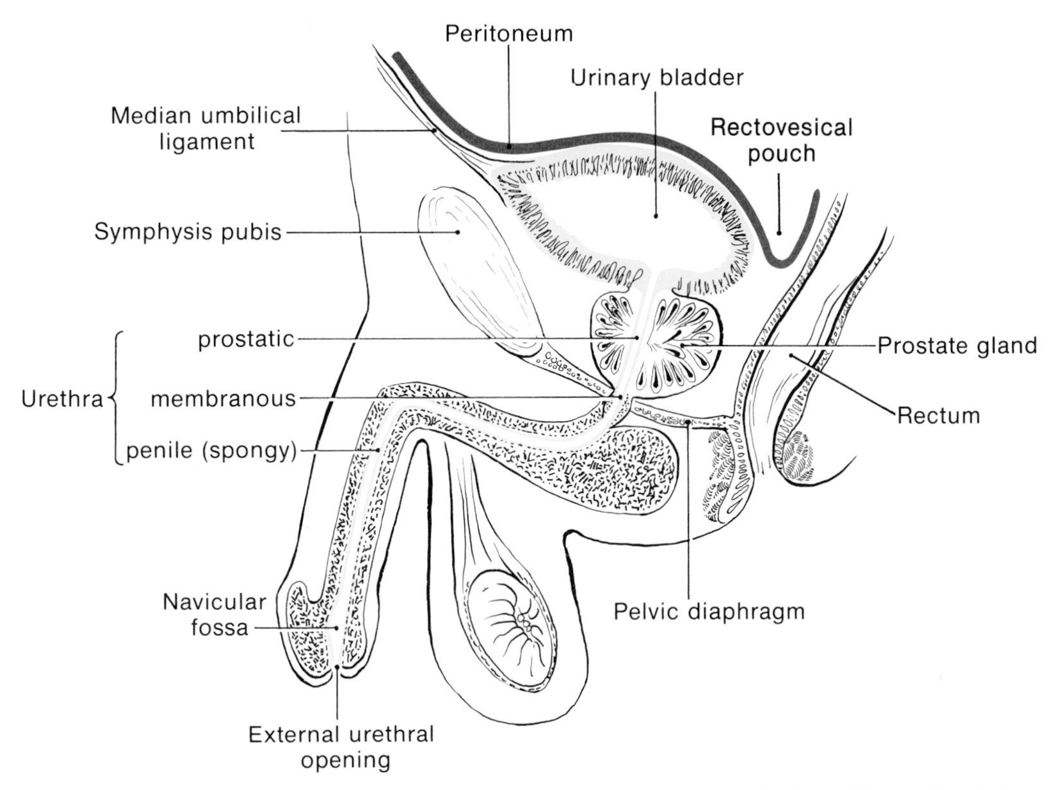

Fig. 15-12. Median section of the male pelvis showing pelvic urinary organs (yellow). The red line indicates the reflection of the peritoneum onto the upper surface of the urinary bladder.

of the **antidiuretic hormone (ADH)** released by the neurohypophysis. (ADH also acts on both the distal convoluted tubule and collecting tubule.)

In addition to the process of resorption, the distal convoluted tubule is also engaged in secretion. For example, hydrogen ions are secreted from the blood in the peritubular capillaries into the lumen of the distal convoluted tubule so as to regulate acid-base balance.

The highly concentrated urine passes from the distal convoluted tubule into a collecting tubule which receives urine from several nephrons and transmits it to the apex of the renal pyramid. At the apex each collecting tubule empties the urine into a minor calyx, which transmits it to a major calyx and then to the renal pelvis.

URETERS, URINARY BLADDER, AND URETHRA

Gross Anatomy

The function of the **ureter** is to receive urine from the renal pelvis and transport it to the urinary bladder. As each ureter passes caudally, it lies behind the parietal peritoneum of the posterior abdominal wall. In the vicinity of the pelvic brim the ureter crosses anterior to the common iliac artery, travels along the lateral wall of the pelvis, and then turns anteromedially to enter the posterior wall of the bladder (Fig. 15-1). Urine is transmitted to the bladder by means of peristaltic waves of contraction which occur along the length of the ureter.

The **urinary bladder** lies in the pelvic cavity but gradually bulges into the lower abdominal cavity as urine accumulates. A fibrous band of tissue, the **median umbilical ligament,** extends from the apex of the bladder to the umbilicus and represents a remnant of the allantois of the embryo (Fig. 15-12). Peritoneum covers only the superior portion of the bladder whereas the remainder is surrounded by pelvic fibrous connective tissue. In the male, a deep **rectovesical pouch** occurs posterior to the bladder where the peritoneum is reflected posteriorly onto the rectum. In the female, the peritoneum is reflected onto the uterus, thus forming the **vesicouterine pouch** (Fig. 16-16).

The interior of the bladder is smooth when the bladder is filled with urine. As the bladder empties, the lining is thrown into temporary folds, except for a triangular area between the openings of each ureter **(ureteral orifices)** and of the urethra **(internal urethral orifice)**. This smooth area is called the **trigone** (Fig. 15-1).

In both sexes the **urethra** extends from the inferior portion (neck) of the bladder to the **external urethral opening (orifice)**. During its course, the urethra passes through the **pelvic diaphragm**, a slinglike sheet of skeletal muscle, and the **urogenital diaphragm,** both of which constitute an **external urethral sphincter.** This sphincter is under voluntary control and prevents the passage of urine until the time of urination.

The female urethra is short and lies anterior to the vagina. In the male, the urethra is longer and consists of three consecutive regions: the prostatic, membranous, and penile (spongy) portions (Fig. 15-12). The **prostatic portion** passes through the prostate gland, the **membranous portion** pierces the pelvic diaphragm, and the **penile portion** passes through a mass of erectile tissue, the corpus spongiosum of the penis. At the distal end of the penis the urethra expands to form the **navicular fossa**.

Parasympathetic nerve fibers from the lower segments of the spinal cord innervate the ureters, bladder, and urethra, as do sympathetic fibers. However, it is the parasympathetic fibers which are involved in the control of bladder and urethral contractions during **urination.** As the bladder fills with urine, receptor cells in the wall of the bladder are stimulated. This initiates a reflex whereby impulses travel along sensory nerves to the lower spinal cord, and motor (parasympathetic) nerves carry impulses back to the bladder to elicit an involuntary contraction of its smooth muscle (the **detrusor muscle**). This reflex can be suppressed by higher centers of the central nervous system which maintain contraction of the external urethral sphincter (pelvic diaphragm). At the time of urination the external sphincter relaxes, the abdominal muscles and thoracic diaphragm contract, the neck of the bladder moves downward, the urethra shortens and widens, and the detrusor muscle of the bladder contracts. Although the bladder normally can accommodate volumes up to 500 ml, the sensation of fullness is usually elicited with volumes of 200–300 ml. The ureters, bladder, and urethra are also richly innervated by pain fibers; thus urinary infections or occlusions may be extremely distressing and painful.

Microscopic Anatomy

The renal pelvis, ureters, and bladder are all lined by a mucosa (mucous membrane) consisting of transitional epithelium which overlies connective tissue. The epithelium varies in thickness according to the degree of distention, particularly in the bladder. When the bladder is in the contracted state the epithelial cells are rounded and arranged in 6–8 layers, whereas in the distended bladder the cells are flattened and arranged in only 2–3 layers. Beneath the epithelium is a layer of loose connective tissue, deep to which is a mass of smooth muscle (the detrusor muscle) arranged in three ill-defined layers. The ability of the renal pelvis, ureters, and bladder to change shape and accommodate increases and decreases in volume can be attributed to the special properties of transitional epithelium and to the underlying loose connective tissue which allows the mucous membrane to be thrown into folds.

When the ureter is in the contracted condition, its mucosa also is thrown into deep folds (Fig. 15-13). The smooth muscle is arranged in an inner longitudinal and outer circular layer, except for the lower third of the ureter where an additional outer longitudinal layer is added.

The proximal portion of the female urethra is lined with transitional epithelium which gradually changes to a stratified squamous epithelium in the distal third of the urethra. The male urethra likewise is lined by transitional epithelium which becomes stratified squamous in the distal region of the penile portion. In both sexes the urethra contains mucous glands.

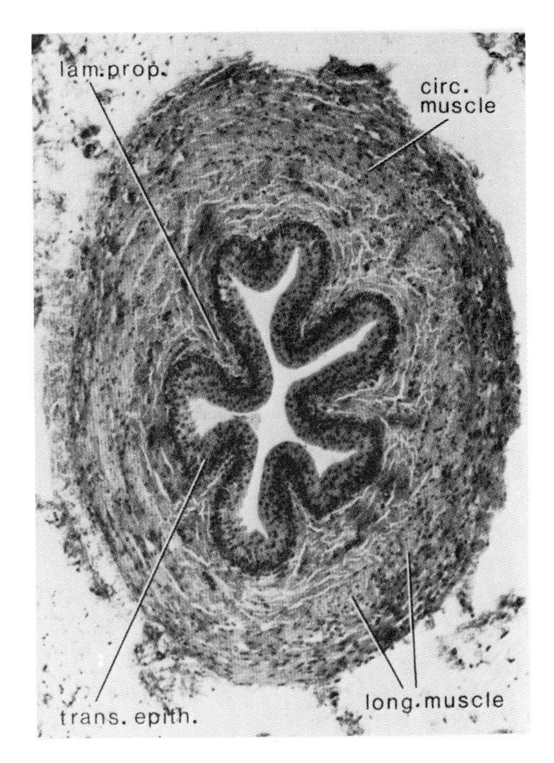

Fig. 15-13. Cross section of the ureter, low magnification, showing folds in the mucous membrane. (From A. W. Ham and D. H. Cormack, *Histology,* Ed. 8, J. B. Lippincott Company, Philadelphia, 1979.)

DEVELOPMENTAL AND CLINICAL ANATOMY

The urinary system shows a variety of congenital defects which occur during prenatal development. Much of the urinary system is derived from intermediate mesoderm, which lies between the somites and the lateral plate mesoderm (Chapter 5). During normal embryonic development three pairs of kidneys develop from the intermediate mesoderm: the pronephros, mesonephros, and metanephros. Each pair develops consecutively in terms of time and position within the body. Thus the pronephros is the first to develop and is most cranial in position, whereas the metanephros is the last to develop and is most caudal (Fig. 15-14).

The **pronephros** is rudimentary and nonfunctional in human embryos. It disappears prenatally by the end of the first month; however, its duct is transformed into the mesonephric duct. The **mesonephros** develops a few urinary tubules which apparently function temporarily but involute by the end of the fourth month. These tubules empty into the **mesonephric (Wolffian) duct,** which passes caudally from the mesonephros and eventually communicates with the caudal portion of the hindgut (cloaca).

Just before entering the cloaca the mesonephric duct gives rise to a small outgrowth, the **ureteric bud,** which grows cranially. The distal portion of the ureteric bud expands and induces the intermediate mesoderm to condense around it to form **metanephric tissue caps.** These two components (the ureteric bud

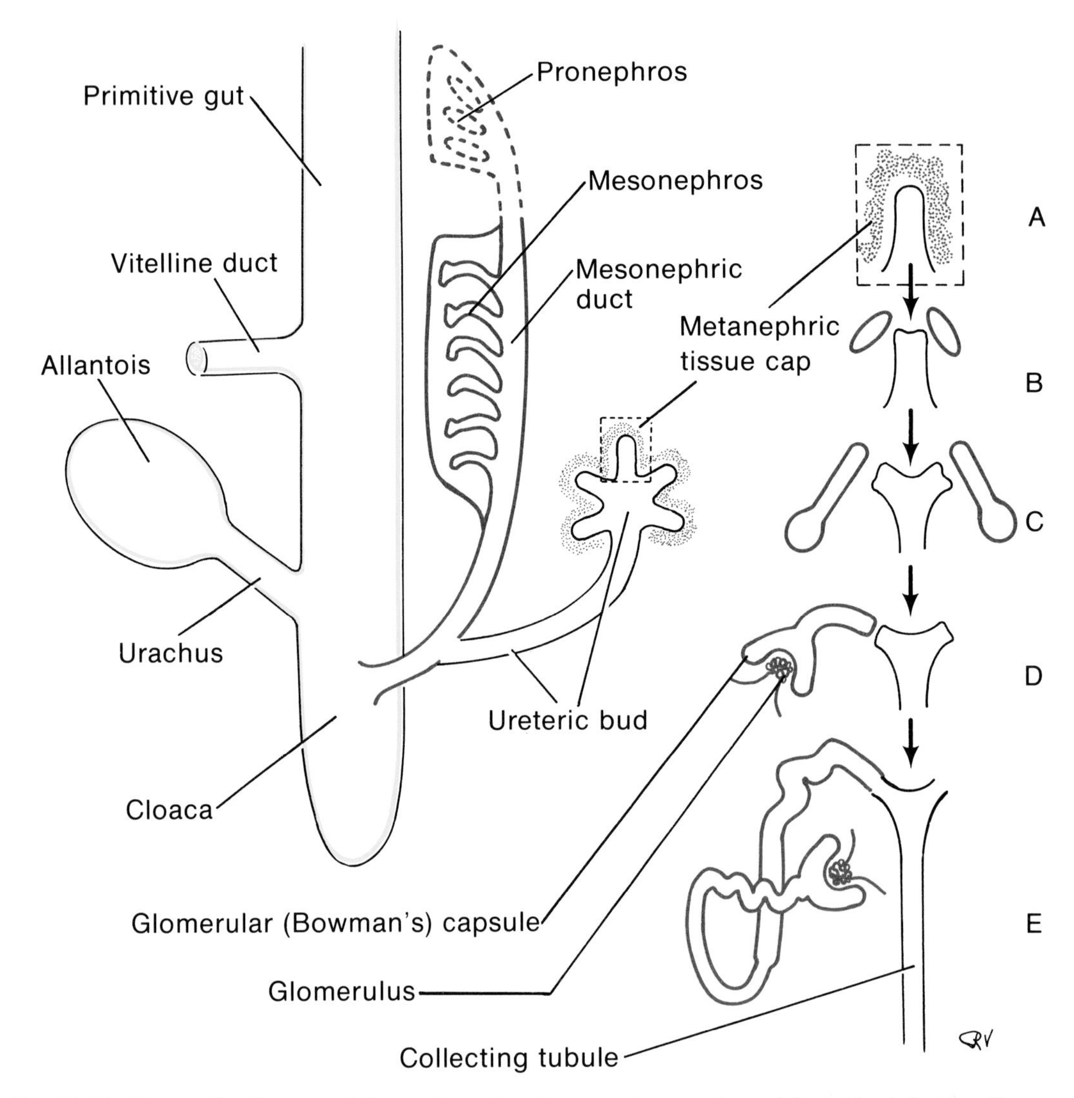

Fig. 15-14. Composite diagram of the embryonic urinary system as viewed from the left side. The pronephros is depicted here even though it degenerates early during embryonic development. The *broken-line* rectangle represents a portion of the metanephros shown chronologically in diagrams A through E. (A) Metanephric tissue cap (red) has condensed around a projection from the ureteric bud (black). (B) Hollow vesicles develop from the tissue cap. (C) Vesicles elongate and form tubules; one end of each tubule expands. (D) The expanded portion is invaginated by the glomerulus. The opposite end is in contact with a projection from the ureteric bud. (E) Tubules elongate and various portions become distinct. Tubules communicate with the collecting tubule which has developed from projections of the ureteric bud.

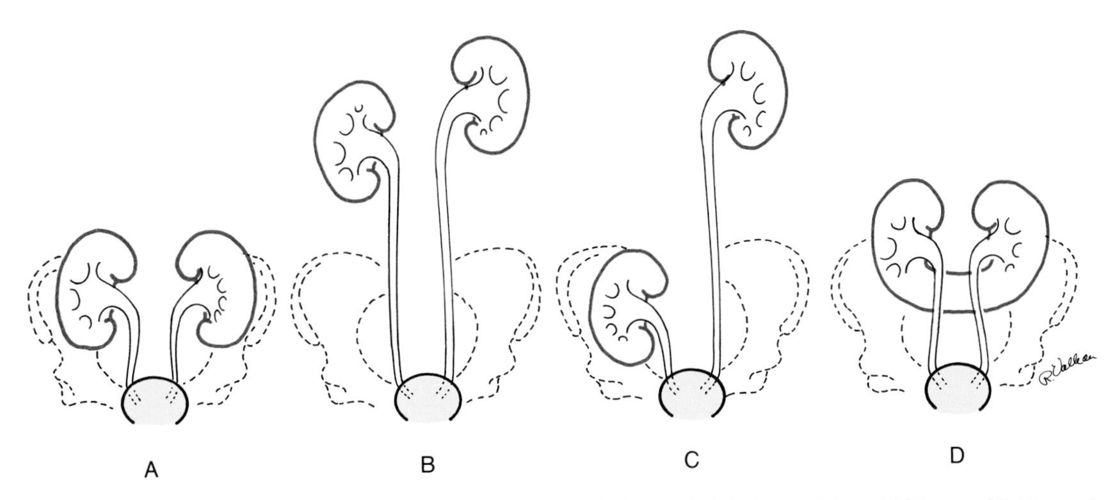

Fig. 15-15. Anterior views showing the ascent of the kidneys. (A) Pelvic origin of kidneys. (B) Normal ascent to the upper lumbar region, 8 weeks. (C) Failure of the right kidney to ascend (right pelvic kidney). (D) Fusion of lower poles of the kidneys (horseshoe kidney).

and tissue caps) represent the **metanephros** which will be the adult kidney. The expanded portion of the ureteric bud develops into the renal pelvis and calyces, from which collecting tubules extend outward toward the tissue caps. The tissue caps differentiate into the glomerular capsules, proximal convoluted tubules, loops of Henle, and distal convoluted tubules. At first, the collecting tubules and distal convoluted tubules do not communicate with one another, but eventually they unite to provide a passageway for urine to leave the kidney. Should this union fail to occur, the blind-ending convoluted tubules gradually accumulate urine and eventually may become cystic.

The narrow proximal portion of the ureteric bud becomes the ureter which elongates as the kidney migrates upward from the pelvic region to the upper lumbar region. Occasionally a kidney may fail to ascend and will remain as a **pelvic kidney** in the adult (Fig. 15-15). The two kidneys are normally in close proximity during their ascent; consequently, the lower poles of the kidneys may sometimes fuse to produce a **horseshoe kidney.** The ascent of a horseshoe kidney tends to be incomplete since a median branch of the abdominal aorta (the inferior mesenteric artery) prevents its upward migration.

The urinary bladder develops from the cloacal region of the embryo and is thus an endodermal derivative. The **cloaca** is the caudalmost portion of the hindgut and receives the two embryonic mesonephric (Wolffian) ducts. The cloaca is also the region from which the allantois, an extraembryonic membrane sac, projects anteriorly.

The cloaca soon becomes subdivided into an anterior and a posterior region by means of a crescent-shaped mass of tissue known as the **urorectal septum,** which develops posterior to the entrances of the mesonephric ducts (Fig. 15-16). The anterior region of the cloaca is called the **urogenital sinus** and becomes associated with the urinary and genital systems. The posterior region of the cloaca becomes the **anorectal canal,** which is a part of the digestive system. If the urorectal septum is defective, it is possible for a **fistula** (abnormal opening) to occur between the lower ends of the digestive tract and urinary and genital systems. This can create serious difficulties, particularly if the urinary system becomes contaminated with fecal material.

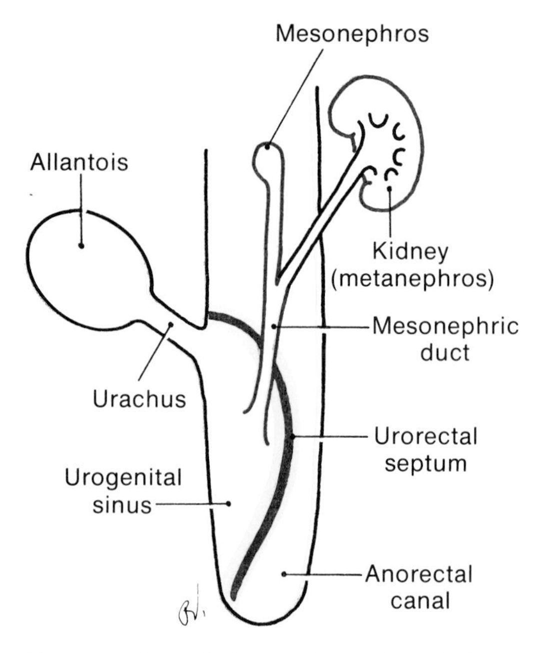

Fig. 15-16. Lateral view of the embryonic hindgut as seen from the left side. The cloaca becomes subdivided by the urorectal septum to form the urogenital sinus and anorectal canal.

The upper portion of the urogenital sinus will develop into much of the bladder while the lower portion becomes the urethra. The ureter initially communicates with the bladder by way of the lower portion of the mesonephric duct. Eventually this portion of the duct is absorbed into the wall of the bladder so that the ureter then empties directly into it. During early stages of development the apex of the bladder communicates with the allantois by means of a narrow channel (the **urachus**). When the allantois degenerates the urachus becomes occluded by a band of fibrous connective tissue. The urachus then is termed the **median umbilical ligament** which extends from the apex of the adult bladder to the umbilicus. In some instances the urachus may abnormally remain open, resulting in the congenital defect known as **patent urachus** and characterized by the seepage of urine outward through the umbilicus.

In addition to congenital defects, the urinary system is subject to a variety of disorders which can occur postnatally. Various mineral salts such as calcium phosphate, calcium oxalate, and magnesium ammonium phosphate occasionally precipitate in the urine and form **kidney stones (renal calculi)**. Small stones may be passed during urination, but larger ones tend to become trapped in such locations as the calyces, renal pelvis, ureter, bladder, or urethra. If the stone is large enough to obstruct a narrow structure such as the ureter, this will result in extreme pain known as **renal colic**. The movement of sharp stones along the urinary tract may also damage the mucous membrane, causing blood to be released into the urine.

An inflammation of the kidney is referred to as **nephritis,** which may result from a variety of causes. **Glomerulonephritis** is an inflammation of the glomeruli, whereas **tubular nephritis** affects the tubular portions of the nephron. In both types of nephritis, red blood cells and large protein molecules may pass into the urine, and excretory functions of the kidneys are impaired.

Urinary incontinence (the involuntary release of urine from the urinary bladder) may result from damage to various portions of the nervous system. For example, if the spinal cord is transected above the sacral region, voluntary control over the bladder is abolished, and urination occurs whenever the bladder becomes sufficiently distended to initiate the emptying reflex, which remains unaffected by the transection. However, if the sacral nerves are damaged, then the emptying reflex is impaired and the bladder becomes overly distended.

In both sexes the urinary bladder and urethra are subject to damage when the pelvic bones are fractured. In the adult female, the urethra also can be injured during childbirth because of the close proximity of the urethra to the vagina. The prostatic portion of the male urethra can become occluded by an enlarged prostate gland. Urine then accumulates and eventually distends the bladder, ureters, renal pelves, and calyces. If this condition goes untreated, the increased pressure in the tubule system may cause degeneration in the kidneys and eventual renal failure.

16

The Reproductive System

The organs of the reproductive (genital) system are often grouped together with the urinary organs to constitute the urogenital (genitourinary) system. Whereas the urinary organs are similar in both sexes (except for the urethra which is longer in males), the reproductive organs show distinctive differences.

The reproductive system consists of internal and external genital organs and certain features which constitute the secondary sexual characteristics, such as the distribution of hair and body fat, the pitch of the voice, and the development of the breasts. The **internal genital organs (internal genitalia)** consist of a pair of gonads (testes or ovaries), genital ducts, and various accessory glands. The **external genital organs (external genitalia)** are located in the **perineal region (perineum)**, a diamond shaped area below the pelvic diaphragm and extending from the symphysis pubis to the coccyx (Fig. 16-1). The anterior portion of this region is the **urogenital triangle**; the posterior portion is the **anal triangle**.

MALE REPRODUCTIVE SYSTEM

Gross Anatomy

External Genital Organs

The external genital organs of the male are the scrotum and penis. The **scrotum** is a pouch suspended below the symphysis pubis and anterior to the anal opening. The scrotum is subdivided into two compartments, with the left one usually slightly lower than the right (Fig. 16-2). Each compartment contains a testis (plural: testes), epididymis, and portion of the spermatic cord (to be described later). The wall of the scrotum consists of skin and a mass of smooth muscle fibers (the **dartos muscle**) which contracts in response to cold and thus pulls the scrotum upward and closer to the body. Warmth causes the scrotum to relax and become more pendulous. These changes are important in maintaining a scrotal temperature slightly lower than body temperature, since sperm production in the testis is adversely affected by heat.

The **penis** consists of two portions: the **root** which is bound to the fascia of the urogenital region, and the **body** which hangs freely (Fig. 16-3). The root of the penis contains three cylinders of **erectile tissue** (venous sinuses which become engorged with blood for erecting the penis). These cylinders are the two **crura** (singular: crus, each of which is attached to the inferior ramus of the pubic bone), and the single **bulb** (situated between the two crura and containing the penile portion of the urethra). Each crus is covered by a skeletal muscle, the **ischiocavernosus muscle**, which is involved in maintaining erection of the penis, whereas the bulb is covered by a pair of **bulbospongiosus muscles** which also help to maintain erection as

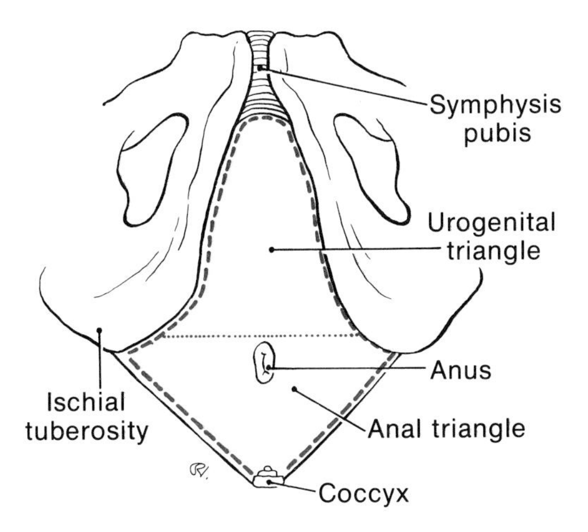

Fig. 16-1. The perineal region viewed from below. *Broken red lines* represent boundaries of the perineal region; *transverse dotted red line* represents boundary between urogenital triangle and anal triangle.

well as to expel urine and semen from the urethra. Both the bulb and crura continue into the body of the penis.

The body of the penis is suspended from the front of the symphysis pubis. In the flaccid condition the dorsal surface (dorsum) of the penis faces anteriorly, and the ventral surface posteriorly. In the erected penis the dorsum faces upward and posteriorly. The body of the penis contains a continuation of the three cylindrical masses of erectile tissue from the root. In the body of the penis these erectile masses constitute two **corpora cavernosa** and the **corpus spongiosum.** The distal end of the penis contains a slight enlargement, the **glans,** with the urethral opening (external urethral orifice) at its tip. The **prepuce (foreskin)** is a double fold of skin extending forward over the glans (Fig. 16-2). (Circumcision involves removal of the prepuce.)

Internal Genital Organs

The internal genitalia of the male are the testis, epididymis, ductus (vas) deferens, ejaculatory duct, seminal vesicle, urethra, prostate gland, and bulbourethral gland (Fig. 16-4). All of these are paired structures except the urethra and prostate gland.

Each **testis** is a somewhat flattened oval organ housed in the scrotum. The left testis usually lies lower than the right one. The testis

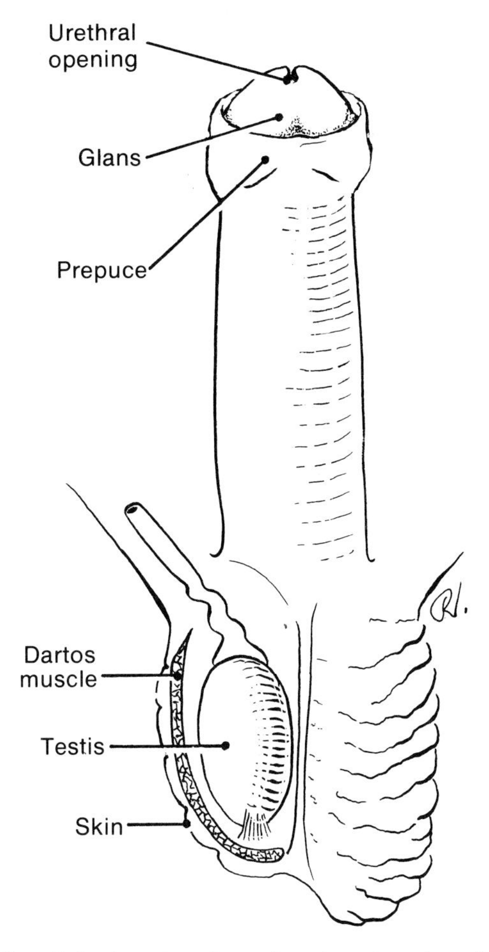

Fig. 16-2. Anterior view of male external genitalia. The penis has been elevated, and the anterior wall of the right side of the scrotum removed to reveal the testis.

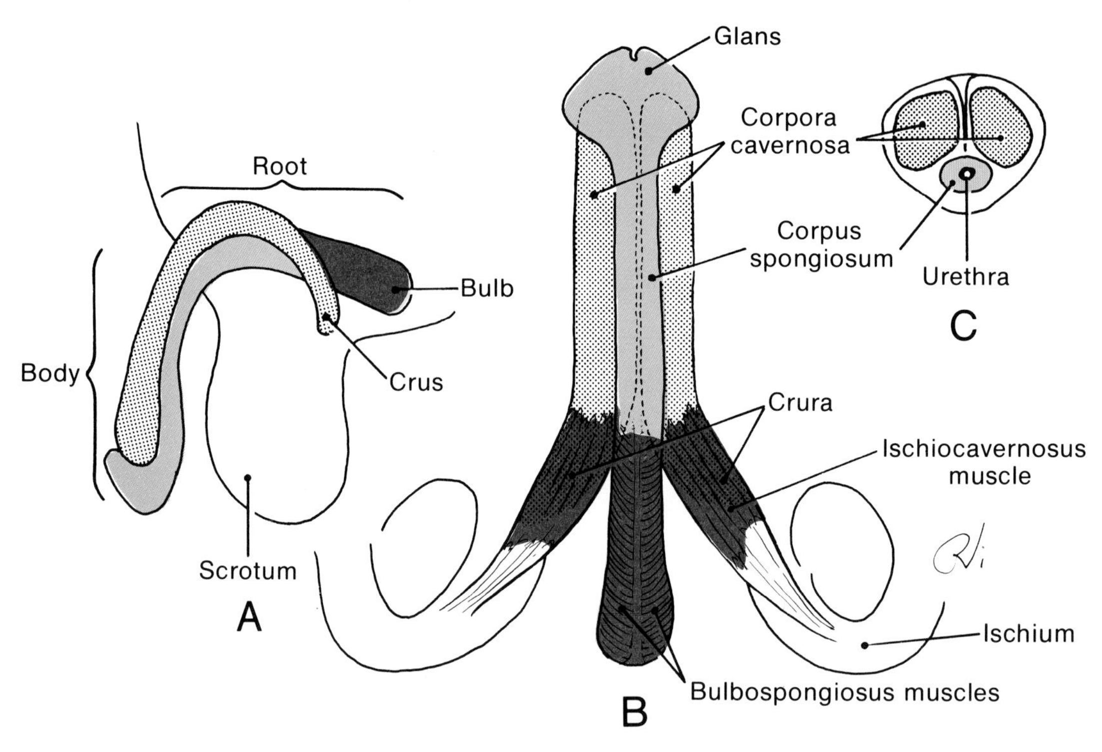

Fig. 16-3. Penis, with skin removed. (A) Lateral view, showing body, root, bulb, and left crus. (B) Inferior view (magnified) with the body of the penis elevated. *Broken lines* show outline of corpora cavernosa dorsal to the corpus spongiosum of the bulb. (C) Cross section of the body of the penis.

is anchored in the scrotum by a short connective tissue band called the **gubernaculum.** The testes produce the male gametes (sperm, spermatozoa) as well as the male hormone **testosterone.** The sperm are transmitted to the **epididymis,** a highly coiled C-shaped structure lying along the posterior border of each testis. The sperm complete their maturation in the epididymis which consists of a **head** (the upper expanded portion), followed by a narrower **body** and **tail** (Fig. 16-5).

The tail of the epididymis leads into the **ductus (vas) deferens** which passes upward along the posterior wall of the testis and then from the scrotum to the pelvis via a narrow channel, the **inguinal canal.** As the ductus deferens leaves the epididymis it is accompanied by a mass of veins (the pampiniform plexus), arteries, nerves, and lymphatics. These structures collectively constitute the **spermatic cord.** The testis, epididymis, and spermatic cord are covered by several layers of connective tissue as well as delicate strands of skeletal muscle (the **cremaster muscle**) which can contract reflexively to draw the testis upward.

In the pelvis the ductus deferens passes medially and then downward behind the urinary bladder where each ductus lies medial to a seminal vesicle. Each **seminal vesicle** is a mass of convoluted sacs and tubes adjacent to the posterior aspect of the bladder. The duct from the seminal vesicle travels downward and joins the ductus deferens to form the **ejaculatory duct,** which in turn passes through the prostate gland to empty into the prostatic part of the urethra.

The **prostate gland** is a bulbous structure surrounding the urethra as the latter emerges

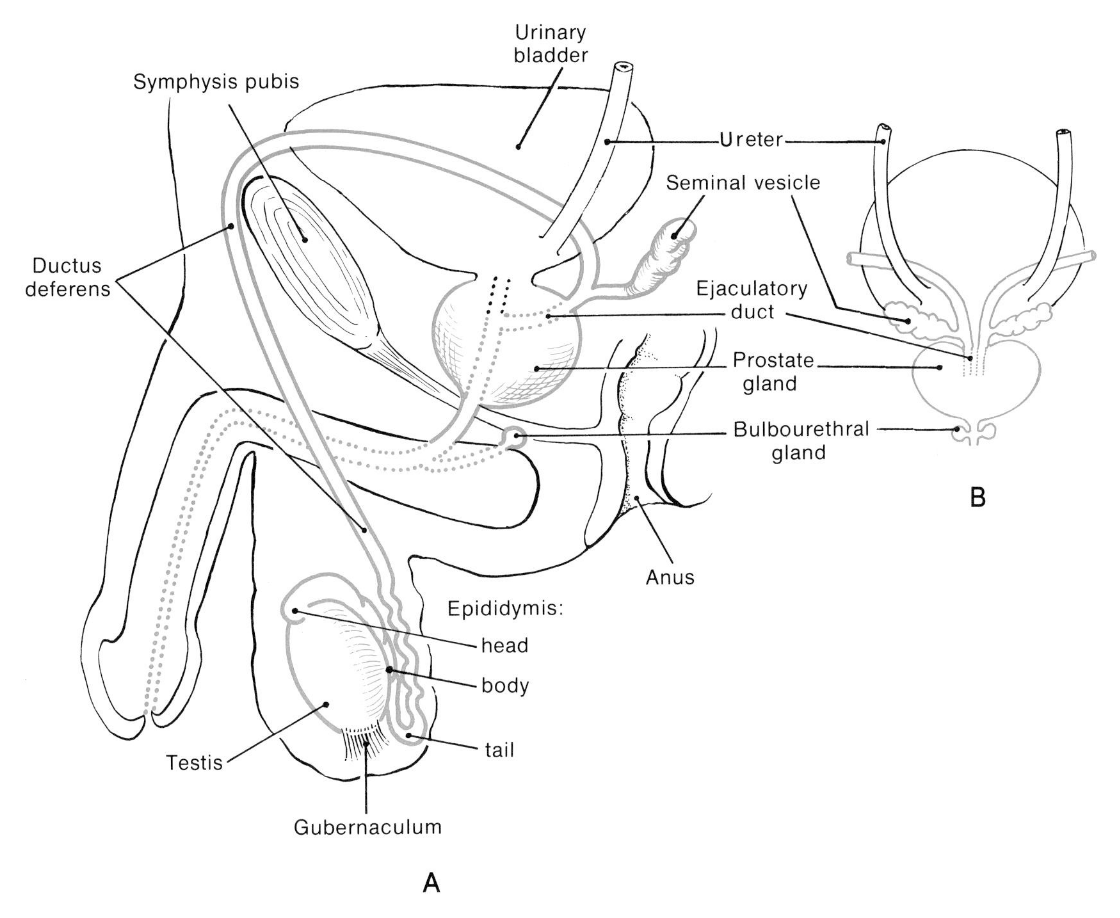

Fig. 16-4. Male genital organs. (A) Lateral view, (B) posterior view.

from the urinary bladder. Since the prostate gland lies just anterior to the rectum, the size and consistency of the gland can be examined clinically via the rectum. The **prostatic urethra** becomes the **membranous urethra** as it passes through the pelvic diaphragm and urogenital diaphragm. Here are located a pair of tiny **bulbourethral (Cowper's) glands**. The urethra then enters the bulb of the penis, becomes the **penile** or **spongy (cavernous) urethra**, receives the ducts from the bulbourethral glands, and extends through the corpus spongiosum.

At the time of ejaculation the sperm are rapidly transported through the ductus deferens, ejaculatory ducts, and urethra. Secretions from the testes, epididymes, seminal vesicles, prostate gland, and bulbourethral glands contribute to the seminal fluid which, along with the sperm, is emitted as semen from the end of the penis.

Microscopic Anatomy

Testis

The surface of the testis contains a layer of simple squamous epithelium (mesothelium), called the **tunica vaginalis,** beneath which lies dense connective tissue, the **tunica albuginea** (Fig. 16-5). Within the testis are masses of coiled **seminiferous tubules** leading into a system of **straight tubules,** which in turn join an

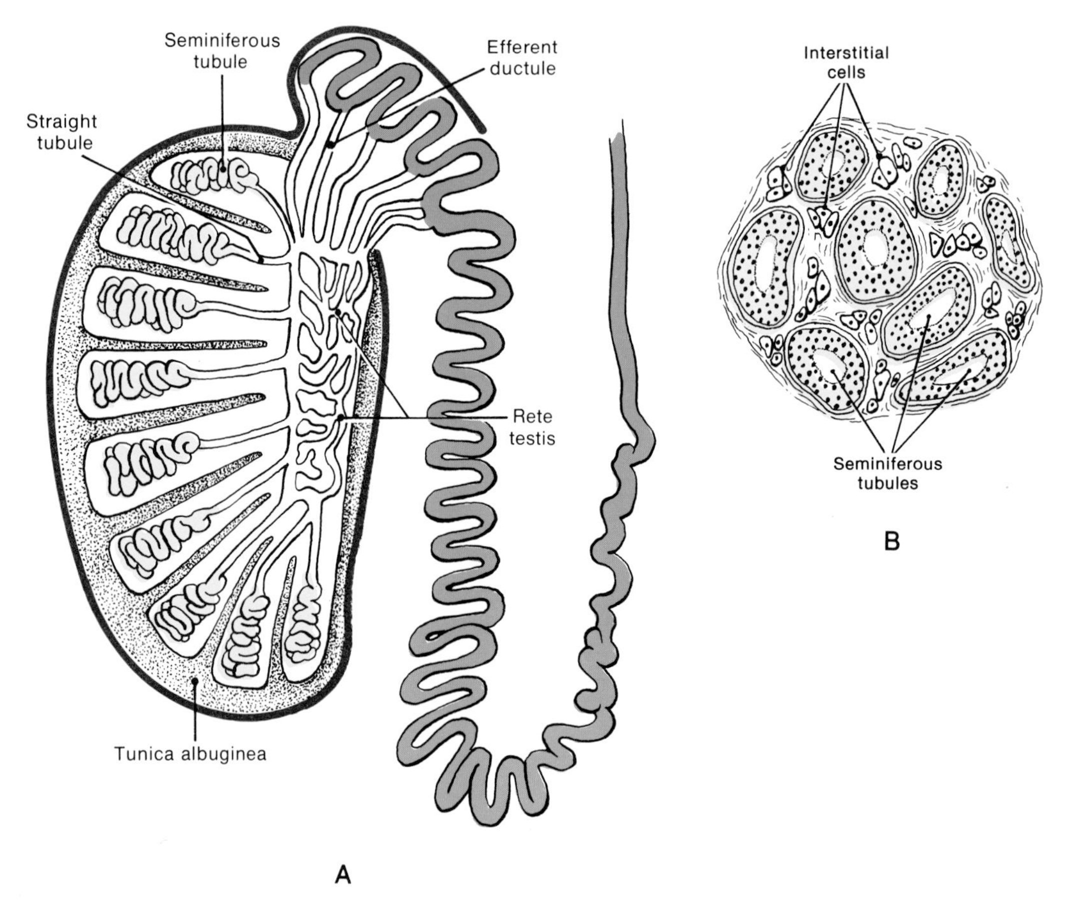

Fig. 16-5. (A) Diagram of a sagittal section through the testis. The red line represents the tunica vaginalis. The epididymis and ductus deferens are shown in blue; seminiferous tubules are in yellow. (B) Diagram of a microscopic section through the seminiferous tubules.

interconnecting network of spaces termed the **rete testis.** A radiating system of **efferent ductules** then passes from the rete testis to the epididymis.

The seminiferous tubules are lined with an epithelium containing two basic cell types (Figs. 16-6 and 16-7). One type produces sperm cells, while the other type serves as supporting or **sustentacular** (**Sertoli, nurse**) **cells**. Throughout the reproductive life of a man the precursors of the sperm cells are the **spermatogonia** (singular: **spermatogonium**), a mitotically active group of cells located along the basement membrane of the epithelium (Fig. 16-7). Some of these spermatogonia grow extensively and are transformed into **primary spermatocytes** which have 46 double-stranded chromosomes. Other spermatogonia are retained as stem cells to generate new spermatogonia. A primary spermatocyte completes the first meiotic division to become 2 **secondary spermatocytes,** each with 23 double-stranded chromosomes. These secondary spermatocytes undergo the second meiotic division to form 4 **spermatids,** each with 23 single-stranded chromosomes (Figs. 16-7 and 16-8). The spermatids then become transformed into spermatozoa (sperm) by a process known as **spermiogenesis.**

During spermiogenesis the spermatid loses

much of its cytoplasm and becomes a streamlined, highly specialized sperm cell. While undergoing this process the developing sperm invaginate the surfaces of the large sustentacular (Sertoli) cells (Fig. 16-9). The mature sperm cell contains three regions: the **head, middle piece** (neck), and **tail piece (flagellum)**. The head region is formed when the Golgi complex becomes molded into a caplike **acrosome** covering the anterior two-thirds of the nucleus. The nucleus becomes quite dense, and the cytoplasm tapers into the middle piece. Numerous mitochondria are retained to provide energy for sperm movement. The flagellum grows from the centrioles at the base of the head through the middle piece region to form the tail piece of the spermatozoan.

The total time required for mature sperm to be formed from spermatogonia is about 2 months. At maturity the sperm detach from

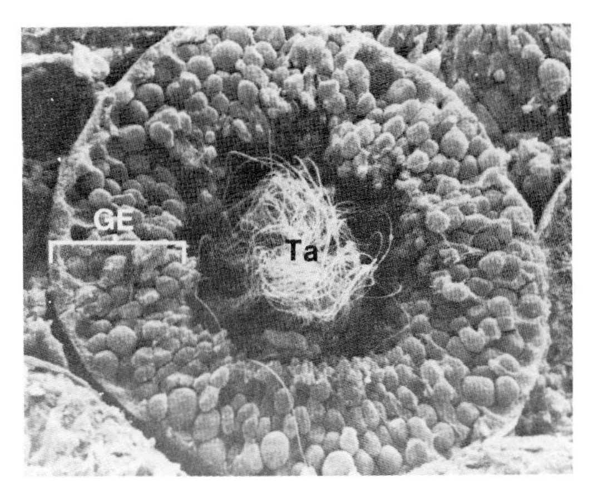

Fig. 16-6. A scanning electron micrograph of a seminiferous tubule, showing the tails (*Ta*) of sperm in the lumen of the tubule. *GE*, germinal epithelium. (From R. G. Kessel and R. H. Kardon, *Tissues and Organs: A Text-Atlas of Scanning Electron Microscopy*, W. H. Freeman and Company. Copyright © 1979.)

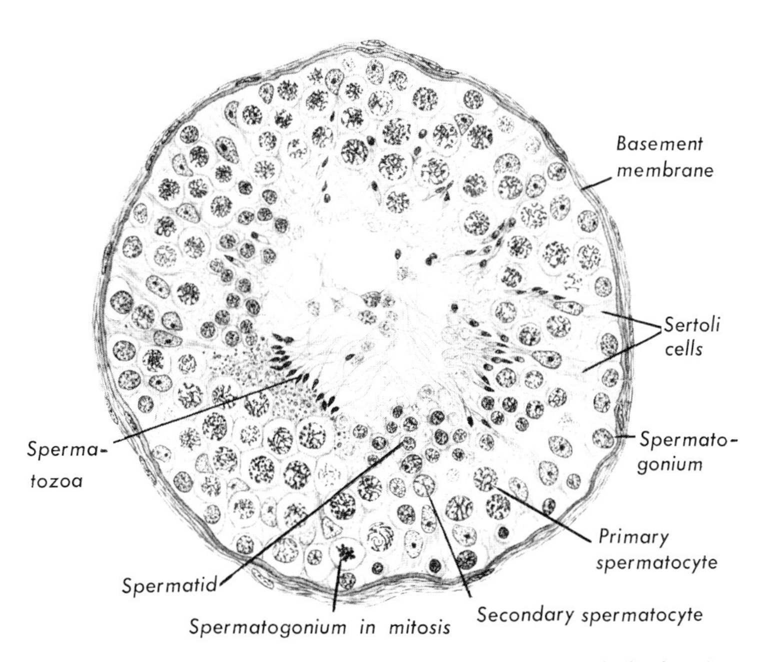

Fig. 16-7. Diagram of a highly magnified section through a seminiferous tubule showing various stages of spermatogenesis. (From W. M. Copenhaver, R. P. Bunge, and M. B. Bunge, *Bailey's Textbook of Histology*, Ed. 16, The Williams & Wilkins Co., Baltimore, 1971.)

Fig. 16-8. Scheme of spermatogenesis, including spermiogenesis.

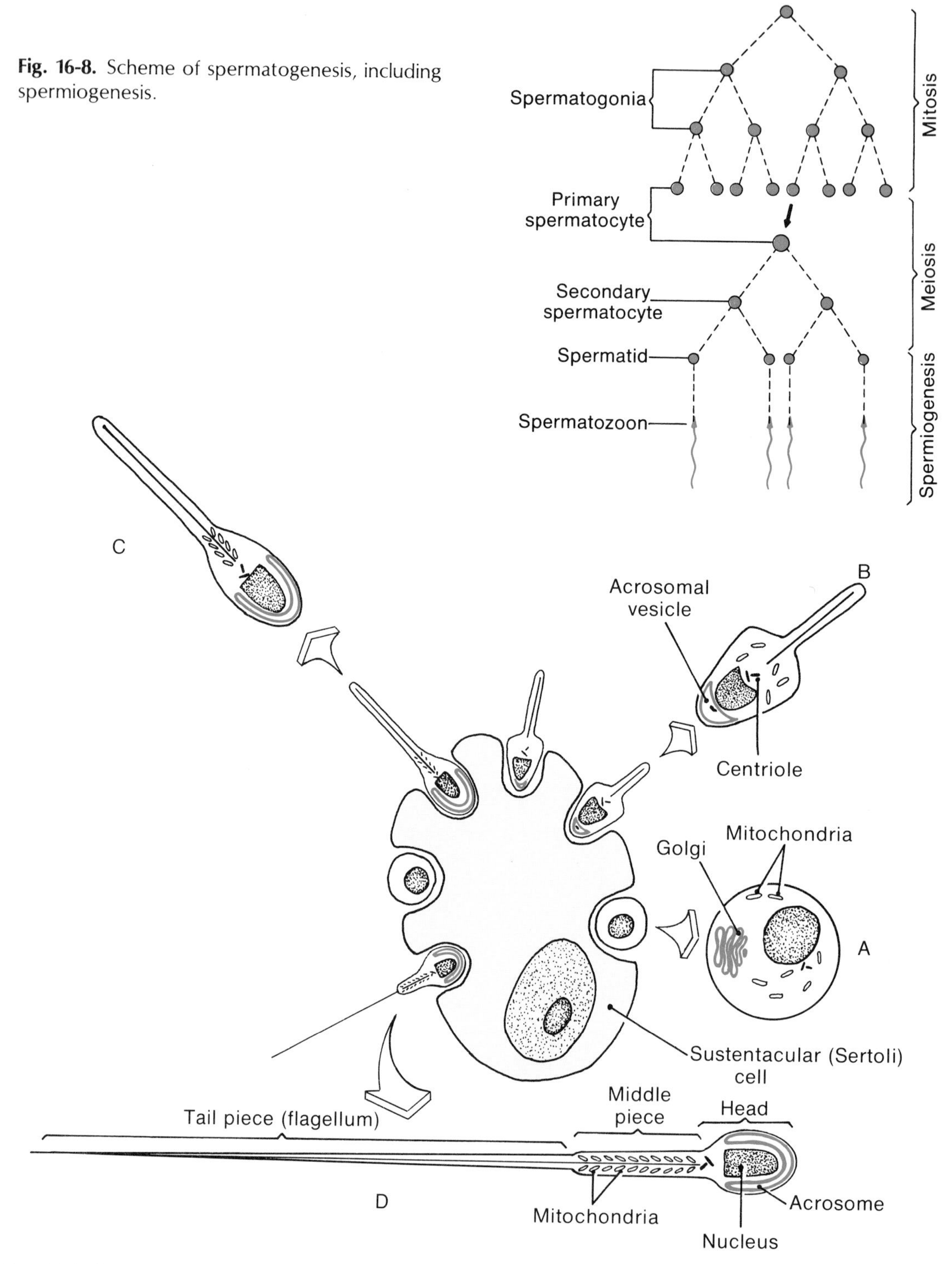

Fig. 16-9. Spermiogenesis. In the center of the diagram is a sustentacular (Sertoli) cell (in yellow) in which are embedded several cells in various stages of spermiogenesis. Higher magnifications of some of these are indicated in A–D. (A) A spermatid, (B, C) maturing sperm, (D) mature sperm at the time of detachment from the sustentacular cell.

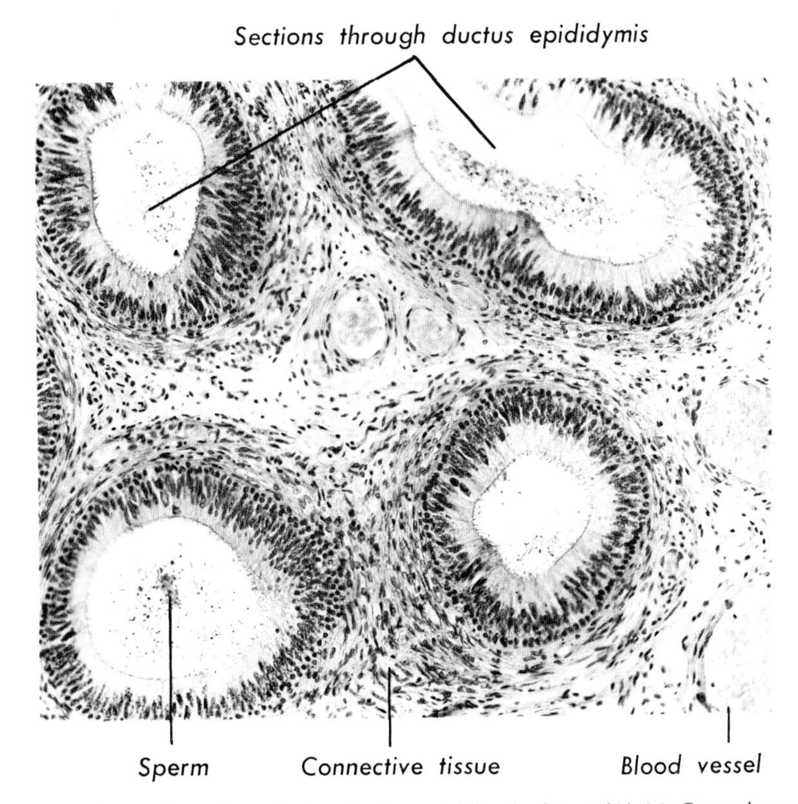

Fig. 16-10. Microscopic sections through the ductus epididymis. (From W. M. Copenhaver, R. P. Bunge, and M. B. Bunge, *Bailey's Textbook of Histology,* Ed. 16, The Williams & Wilkins Co., Baltimore, 1971.)

the sustentacular cells and are transported along with fluid from the seminiferous tubules toward the upper pole of the testis, first along the straight tubules and then into the rete testis.

In between the seminiferous tubules of the testis are **interstitial (Leydig) cells.** These cells produce the male hormone **testosterone** which is secreted into the vascular system and helps to maintain functional accessory glands and genital ducts as well as the sex urge (libido). The secretion of testosterone is particularly important at puberty in order to produce and maintain the various male secondary sexual characteristics such as a deep voice, growth of beard, and male distribution of fat. The interstitial cells are under control of the **interstitial cell stimulating hormone (ICSH),** whereas the process of spermatogenesis depends on **follicle stimulating hormone (FSH).** Both ICSH and FSH are produced by the anterior lobe of the pituitary gland and are carried to the testis via the blood stream.

Efferent Ductules and Epididymis

After the sperm have been brought to the rete testis, they pass into the epididymis via the **efferent ductules.** These ductules are lined with alternating groups of cuboidal and columnar cells, many of which are ciliated. The ciliary action plus the contractions of smooth muscle fibers outside of the basement membrane help to propel the sperm and seminiferous fluid into the ductus epididymis.

The **ductus epididymis** is a single highly coiled tube lined with a pseudostratified columnar epithelium (Fig. 16-10). The luminal

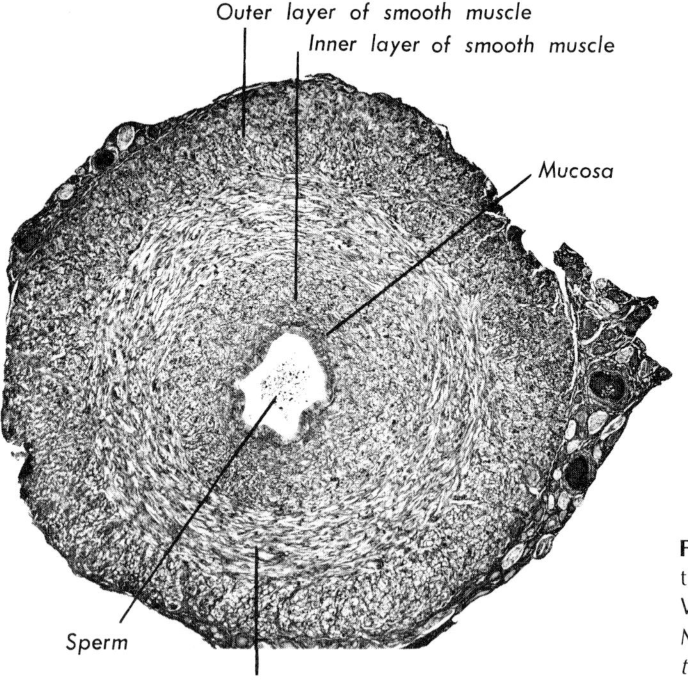

Fig. 16-11. A transverse section cut through the ductus deferens. (From W. M. Copenhaver, R. P. Bunge, and M. B. Bunge, *Bailey's Textbook of Histology,* Ed. 16, The Williams & Wilkins Co., Baltimore, 1971.)

surfaces of these epithelial cells show long nonmotile cytoplasmic processes (called **stereocilia**) which increase the surface area. Both absorption and secretion occur in the ductus epididymis, and it is here that the sperm acquire motility.

Ductus Deferens and Urethra

The ductus (vas) deferens is a highly muscular tube containing smooth muscle arranged in inner longitudinal, middle circular, and outer longitudinal layers (Fig. 16-11). The duct is lined by a mucous membrane (mucosa) which is thrown into folds and which consists of pseudostratified columnar cells overlying a lamina propria composed of connective tissue. Sperm are stored in the lower end of the ductus deferens near the epididymis until ejaculation occurs, when muscular contractions propel the sperm through the ductus and ejaculatory duct into the prostatic urethra.

The **prostatic urethra** contains transitional epithelium. In passing from the **membranous urethra** through the **penile (spongy) urethra,** the epithelium gradually becomes stratified columnar, stratified cuboidal, and eventually stratified squamous.

Accessory Glands

The **seminal vesicles** are composed of highly convoluted sacs lined with a pseudostratified epithelium. These epithelial cells secrete an alkaline fluid rich in fructose which serves as an energy source for the sperm after they have been deposited in the female genital tract. The seminal vesicles contain smooth muscle which contracts at the time of ejaculation to expel their secretions into the urethra via the ejaculatory ducts.

The **prostate gland** is well supplied with fibromuscular tissue which, like that in the seminal vesicles, helps to expel its secretions during ejaculation. The gland is actually a conglomeration of numerous tiny glands, many of which empty their secretions directly into the prostatic urethra (Fig. 16-12A). The glands contain sacs lined with cuboidal or columnar epithelial cells whose function is to secrete a milky fluid containing acid phosphatase. In addition, the lumen of a sac may contain a hardened mass of material called an **amyloid body** (Fig. 16-12B). These masses tend to increase with age. The prostate gland as a whole may undergo a benign increase in size (hypertrophy) with age, particularly its middle (median) lobe (Fig. 16-12A), which may then obstruct the outlet of the urinary bladder into the prostatic urethra and impede the flow of urine.

The paired **bulbourethral (Cowper's) glands** consist of many tiny sacs which secrete a mucouslike lubricating substance into the penile urethra. Since these glands are embedded in the urogenital diaphragm, they contain an outer covering of skeletal muscle fibers in addition to some smooth muscle fibers within the gland.

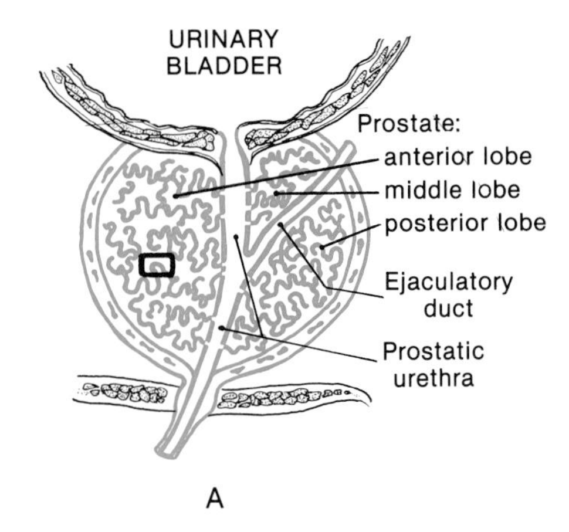

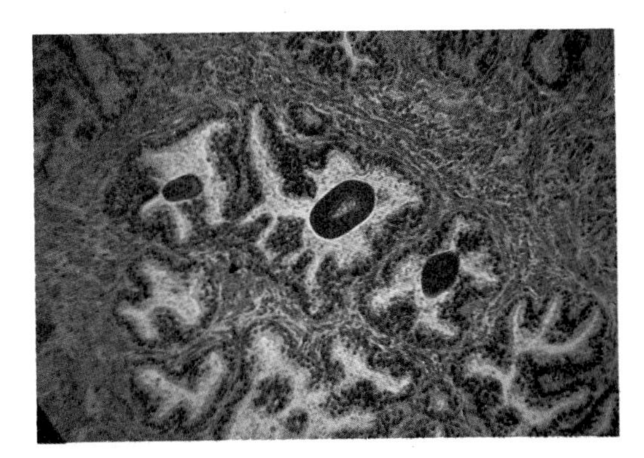

Fig. 16-12. (A) Sagittal section of prostate gland showing its three lobes and the entrance of the prostatic ducts directly into the prostatic urethra. (B) Microscopic section of the area indicated by the rectangle in A. Note the presence of dense, brown, oval amyloid bodies. (From the teaching collection, Department of Anatomy, College of Physicians and Surgeons, Columbia University.)

Erection and Ejaculation

Erection is under control of the parasympathetic pathways of the autonomic nervous system. In the flaccid or nonerected state, the venous sinuses in the corpora cavernosa of the penis are collapsed because of the contraction of smooth muscle fibers in the surrounding connective tissue. Erotic stimulation causes a relaxation of these fibers and of the smooth muscle fibers in the walls of arteries supplying the cavernous spaces. Additional blood thus suddenly rushes into the sinuses, and the corpora cavernosa become turgid. This stiffening also compresses the veins situated around the periphery of the corpora cavernosa and impairs venous drainage from the area. The walls of the arteries supplying the cavernous spaces eventually contract and decrease the flow of blood into the sinuses. The sinus walls then collapse, and the blood is gradually pushed from the spaces, thereby returning the penis to the flaccid condition.

In contrast to erection, ejaculation is under control of sympathetic pathways of the autonomic nervous system. Ejaculation occurs with the contraction of smooth muscle fibers in the

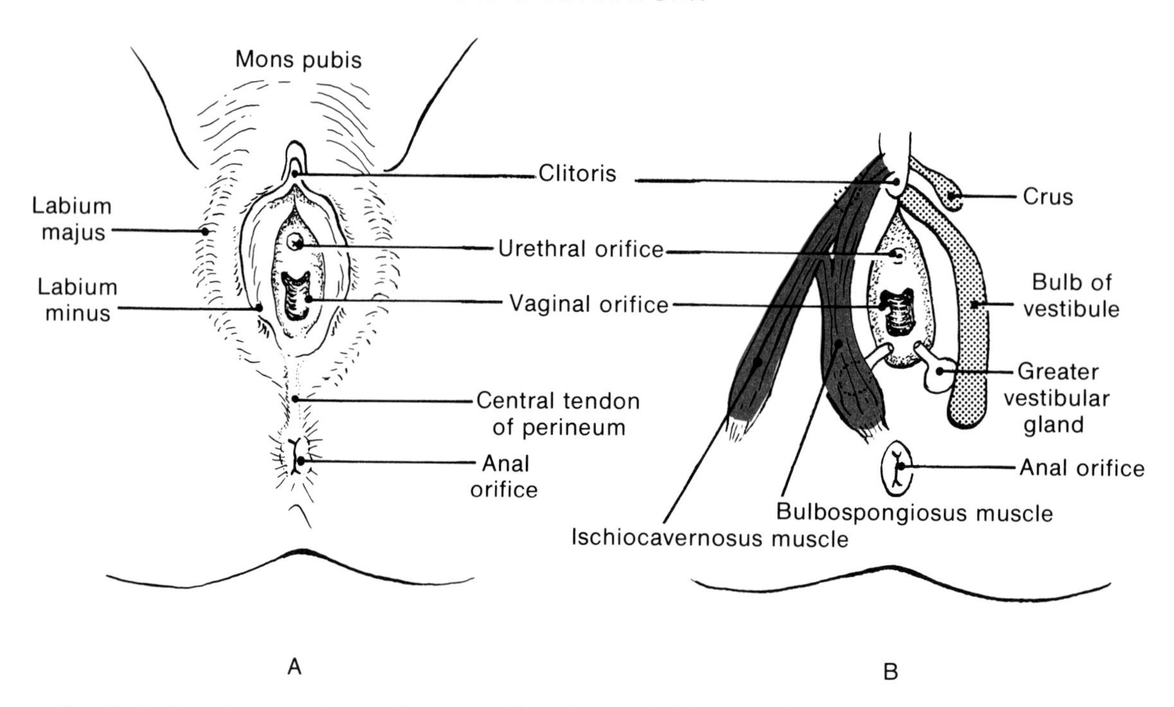

Fig. 16-13. Female external genitalia, viewed from below. (A) Superficial view, (B) deeper structures. On the left side of the diagram are two muscles of the urogenital triangle which have been removed on the right to show the bulb and greater vestibular gland.

walls of the genital ducts aided by skeletal fibers of the bulbospongiosus muscles at the root of the penis. The seminal fluid containing the sperm is rapidly propelled through the ducts and out the external urethral opening. The volume of a single ejaculate ranges from 2 ml to 5 ml and contains roughly 200 million to 600 million sperm.

During ejaculation a sphincter at the neck of the bladder also contracts, thereby preventing sperm from entering the bladder and urine from leaving it. Meanwhile, the ductus deferens, seminal vesicles, prostate gland, and bulbourethral (Cowper's) glands contract and pump their secretions into the urethra. The first part of the ejaculate contains mainly sperm and fluid from the epididymis, ductus deferens, and bulbourethral glands, whereas subsequent portions of the ejaculate contain greater proportions of secretions from the seminal vesicles and prostate gland.

FEMALE REPRODUCTIVE SYSTEM
Gross Anatomy

External Genital Organs

The external genital organs of the female are sometimes termed the **vulva** and include the mons pubis, clitoris, labia majora, labia minora, vestibule, and a pair of greater vestibular glands. The female external genitalia are located in the perineal region between the symphysis pubis and the coccyx. Two pairs of labia (lips) surround the genital and urinary openings of the female (Fig. 16-13). The larger and outermost are the **labia majora** (singular: **labium majus**). These are covered externally with pubic hair and contain a substantial amount of subcutaneous fat. Anteriorly the labia majora become continuous with a mound of fatty tissue (the **mons pubis**) overlying the anterior part of the symphysis pubis. Posteriorly the labia majora unite indistinctly and

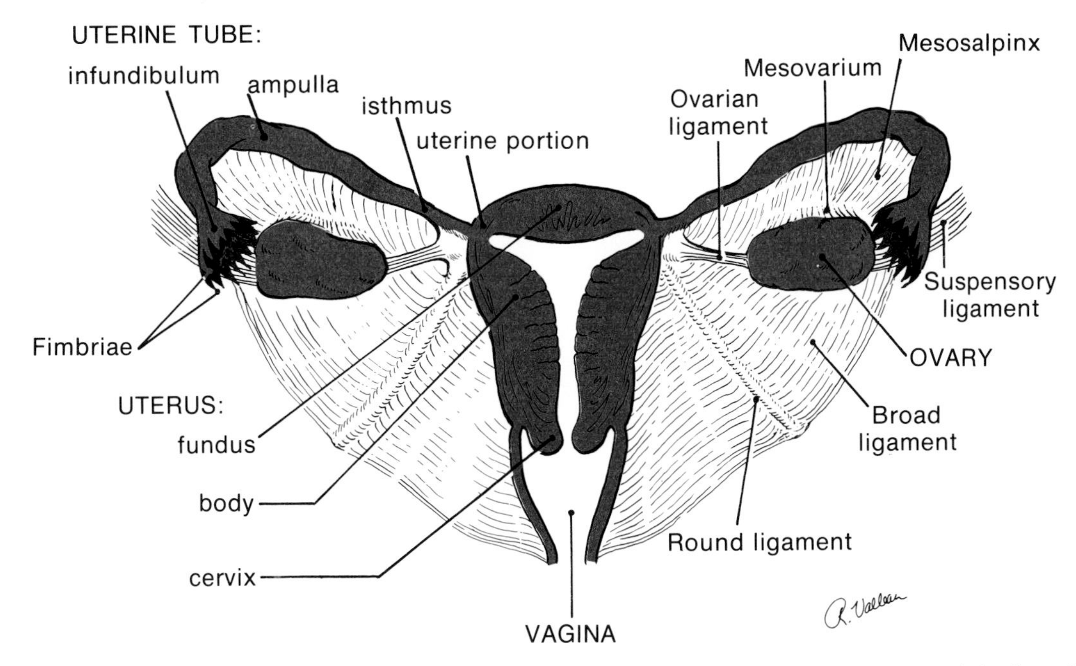

Fig. 16-14. Posterior view of the female internal genital organs (in red). The lower edges of the broad ligaments have been cut.

blend with the **central tendon of the perineum** (also called the **perineal body**). The latter is a midline fibromuscular mass of tissue which extends backward to the anal opening. Since it is possible for the central tendon of the perineum to become torn during childbirth, a surgical incision is sometimes made downward from the vagina to allow the infant to be born more easily without risk of damage to the surrounding tissues, particularly the anal sphincter muscle. This procedure is termed an **episiotomy.**

The **labia minora** (singular: **labium minus**) are small inner folds which lack hair and subcutaneous fat. The labia minora come together anteriorly to overlap the **clitoris.** The clitoris is the counterpart of the penis, although it is much smaller and does not contain the urethra. However, the clitoris does contain two cylindrical masses of erectile tissue, the **corpora cavernosa,** which cause the clitoris to become erected in response to erotic stimulation.

The two labia minora enclose a shallow area termed the **vestibule** which contains the **urethral orifice** (external urethral opening) anteriorly and the **vaginal orifice** posteriorly. The vaginal orifice is surrounded by a variable amount of mucous membrane, the **hymen**. Once the hymen is torn (as after sexual intercourse), discontinuous tags of tissue remain around the vaginal opening. A mass of erectile tissue, the **bulb of the vestibule**, lies on each side of the vagina and is covered by the **bulbospongiosus muscle**. Near the lower end of each bulb is the **greater vestibular (Bartholin's) gland** which, during sexual excitement, secretes a mucous lubricant through a minute opening on each side of the vaginal orifice.

Internal Genital Organs

The internal genital organs of the female are located in the pelvis and consist of two ovaries, two uterine tubes, the uterus, and the vagina (Fig. 16-14). A double layered sheet of

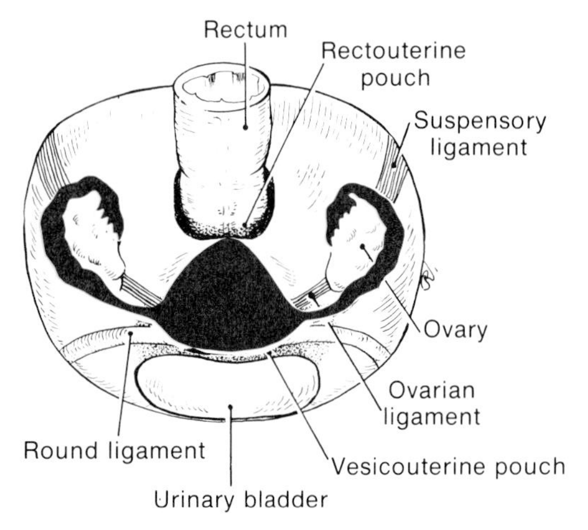

Fig. 16-15. Superior view of female pelvic organs.

peritoneum, the **broad ligament**, extends upward from the floor and lateral walls of the pelvis to the uterus and uterine tubes and envelops these organs.

Each **ovary** is attached to the lateral wall of the pelvic cavity by a short **suspensory ligament** (Figs. 16-14 and 16-15). The ovary is also suspended from the posterior portion of the broad ligament by means of the **mesovarium** and from the uterus via the **ovarian ligament.** These attachments are fairly loose so that the ovaries can be displaced, particularly during pregnancy when the pelvic region becomes filled with the expanding uterus.

Each **uterine tube (oviduct, Fallopian tube)** extends from ovary to uterus and consists of four regions: the infundibulum, ampulla, isthmus, and uterine portion. The **infundibulum** is the funnel-shaped portion at the ovarian end of each tube. It opens into the peritoneal cavity and shows long fingerlike projections **(fimbriae)**, one of which often attaches to the surface of the ovary. However, there is no direct communication between the ovary and the opening of the uterine tube, and at ovulation the egg must break through the ovarian surface and traverse the small peritoneal space before being collected into the opening of the tube. The **ampulla** is the longest portion of the uterine tube, which narrows to become the **isthmus** and then passes through the wall of the uterus as the **uterine portion.** The portion of the broad ligament between the uterine tube and the mesovarium is termed the **mesosalpinx** (Fig. 16-14). (The root word salpinx means "trumpet" and refers to the shape of the uterine tube; the medical term **salpingitis** denotes an inflammation of the tube.)

The **uterus** is a pear-shaped muscular organ specialized for housing the growing embryo during pregnancy. The uterus is situated in the pelvis between the rectum and sigmoid colon posteriorly and the urinary bladder anteriorly (Figs. 16-15 and 16-16). The portion of the peritoneal cavity between the rectum and uterus is the **rectouterine pouch**, whereas that portion between the bladder and uterus is the **vesicouterine pouch.** The uterus is normally

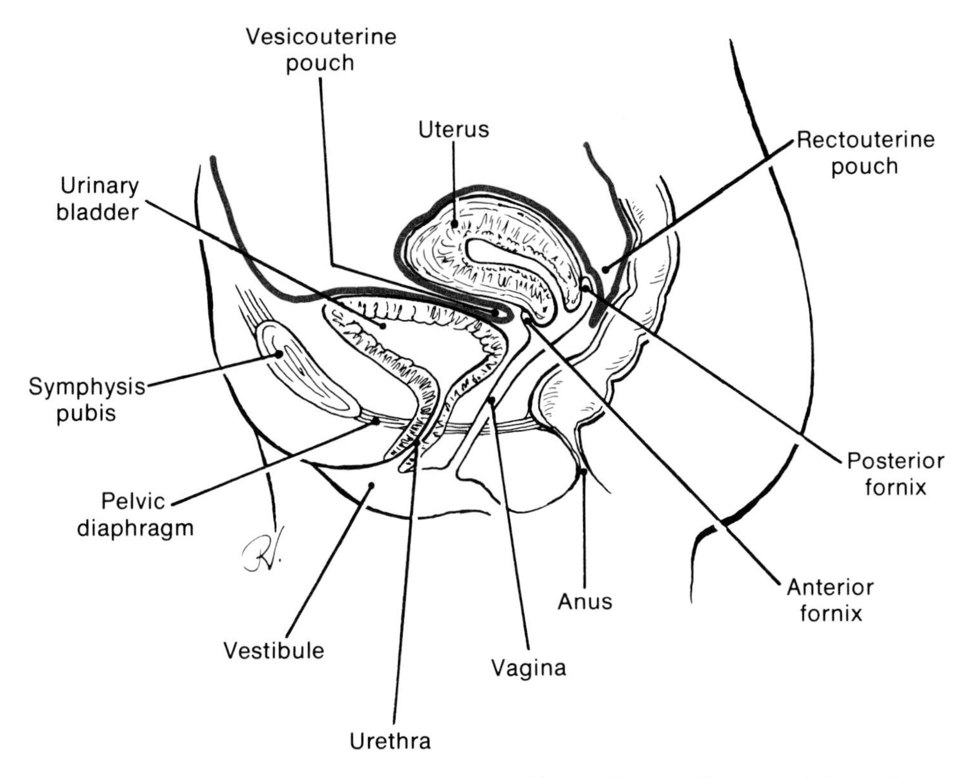

Fig. 16-16. Sagittal section of female pelvis. The red line indicates reflections of the peritoneum.

anteflexed, i.e., it tilts slightly forward and forms a right angle with the vagina.

The major portion of the uterus is the **body,** whereas the upper region which projects above the entrances of the uterine tubes is the **fundus.** The lower part of the uterus narrows to become the **cervix** which projects downward and into the vagina.

The body and fundus of the uterus are highly mobile regions which change position readily when the urinary bladder becomes distended or during pregnancy when the uterus enlarges with the growing fetus. The body and fundus are slightly stabilized by the broad ligament and by two **round ligaments**, the latter arising from the lateral uterine wall just below the entrances of the uterine tubes and passing obliquely downward and forward between the two layers of the broad ligament and then via the inguinal canal to insert into the labia majora. The cervix of the uterus is relatively more stable and is supported by some dense fibrous connective tissue passing from the pelvic diaphragm and sacrum to the cervix and upper vagina.

The **vagina** slants obliquely downward and forward from the cervix of the uterus to the vestibule (Fig. 16-16). The vagina and uterus together are sometimes called the "birth canal" since they provide the pathway along which the infant passes at the time of birth (parturition). The vagina also conducts menstrual fluid from the uterus to the vestibule and receives the penis during intercourse.

In the region where the cervix projects into the vagina, a recess occurs between the walls of the vagina and the vaginal portion of the cervix. This recess is the **fornix** which consists of posterior, anterior, and lateral portions. The posterior fornix is important clinically, since slender instruments can be passed upward in the vagina and through the wall of the fornix

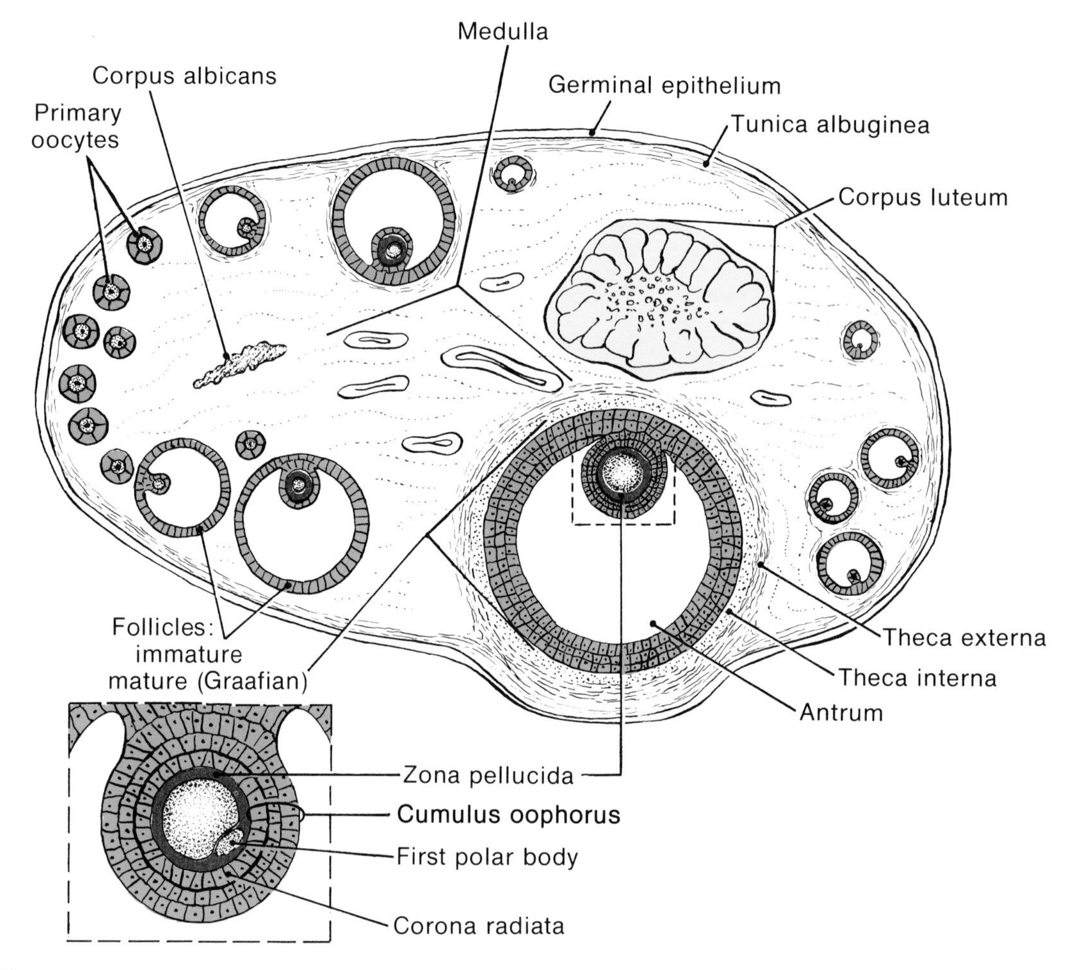

Fig. 16-17. Diagrammatic representation of a sagittal section through the ovary. Blue represents the follicle cells. *Broken-line* box is more highly magnified in diagram at lower left, showing formation of the first polar body just before ovulation.

and into the rectouterine pouch to drain pus or blood which may accumulate in the peritoneal cavity as a result of infection or injury. Such a procedure is called **culdocentesis.**

Microscopic Anatomy

Ovary

The ovary is the site where **eggs (ova, oocytes)** are produced. It is also the source of the female hormones **estrogen** and **progesterone.** The surface of the ovary contains a thin layer of modified epithelial cells called the **germinal epithelium**, beneath which is a variable amount of dense connective tissue, the **tunica albuginea** (Fig. 16-17). The ovary contains two regions: an extensive peripheral area (the **cortex**) where the oocytes develop, and a smaller centrally located area (the **medulla**) which is characterized by numerous vessels, nerves, lymphatics, and by connective tissue.

At the time of birth the ovaries in a female infant contain thousands of **primary oocytes** located in follicles consisting of a single layer of epithelial cells. These oocytes originated prenatally from mitotically dividing cells called **oogonia** (Fig. 16-18). In contrast to their male counterparts (spermatogonia), the oogonia disappear before birth. The primary oocytes do not divide but instead remain dormant until puberty, after which several primary oocytes begin to mature each month until menopause occurs.

The maturation of a primary oocyte involves an increase in size and the acquisition of several layers of follicle cells. A gelatinous substance, the **zona pellucida** is layed down between the oocyte and follicle cells, and a cavity (antrum) forms within the follicle. The cavity grows in size, and the oocyte becomes pushed to one side of the follicle but is still surrounded by several layers of follicle cells, termed the **cumulus oophorus**, of which the innermost layer is often termed the **corona radiata cells.**

As the follicle grows, the nearby connective tissue becomes arranged into two layers around the outside of the follicle cells. The inner layer is the **theca interna**, which secretes the hormone **estrogen** into the vascular system. Estrogen has many effects, including maintenance of the female secondary sex characteristics. The outer layer of connective tissue is the fibrous **theca externa**.

Although several follicles grow each month, ordinarily only one of these reaches full maturity and is then called a **Graafian follicle.** Just before ovulation the primary oocyte of the Graafian follicle undergoes the first meiotic division to form a large **secondary oocyte** and a small **first polar body.** When ovulation occurs the secondary oocyte along with its polar body, zona pellucida, and corona cells are expelled as a unit through the surface of the ovary. In the sexually mature human female, usually only one oocyte fully develops and is ovulated from the ovary each month; the other partially developed oocytes and follicles remain in the ovary and eventually become atretic and degenerate.

The ovulated oocyte and associated cells are collected into the infundibulum of the uterine tube, where fertilization can occur if sperm

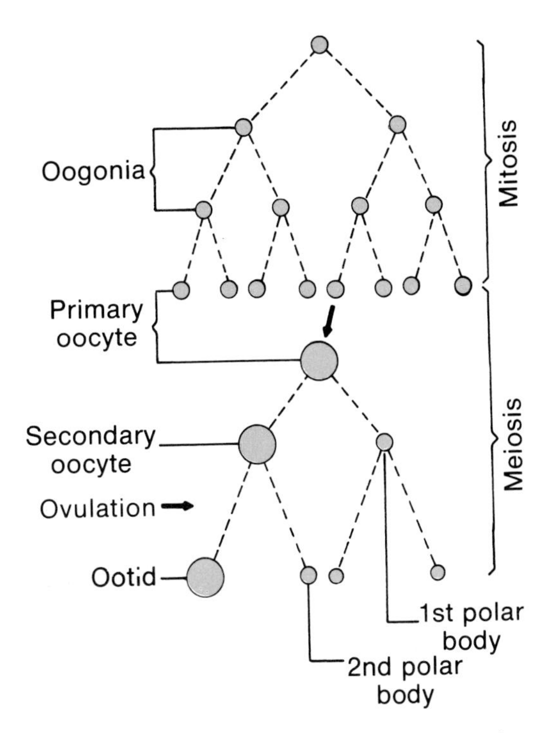

Fig. 16-18. Schematic diagram of oogenesis. The horizontal arrow indicates the point at which ovulation occurs. (Note that the first polar body is given off just before ovulation; the second polar body is given off only if the secondary oocyte is fertilized.

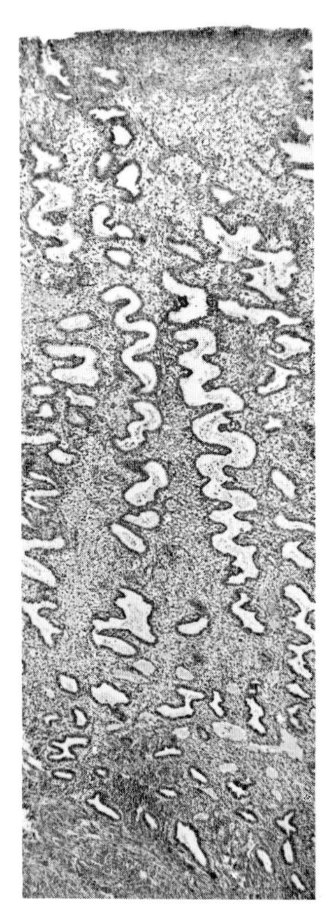

Fig. 16-19. Microscopic section of the uterus showing the endometrium (with highly developed uterine glands). (From W. M. Copenhaver, R. P. Bunge, and M. B. Bunge, *Bailey's Textbook of Histology,* Ed. 16, The Williams & Wilkins Co., Baltimore, 1971.)

are present. Just after sperm entry, the secondary oocyte completes the second meiotic division and gives off a **second polar body** (Fig. 16-18). If the oocyte fails to be fertilized it soon degenerates, as do the corona cells, polar body, and zona pellucida.

Meanwhile the remaining cells of the Graafian follicle in the ovary become the **corpus luteum** and begin to secrete the hormone **progesterone** which has a stimulating effect on the uterus to prepare it for implantation. If fertilization occurs the corpus luteum continues to function for about 4 months, or until such time as the placenta can take over the hormone-producing functions. If fertilization does not occur, the corpus luteum begins to degenerate about 10 days after ovulation, and the remains of the corpus luteum become a fibrous mass of connective tissue, the **corpus albicans** (Fig. 16-17).

Uterine Tube

The wall of the uterine tube is lined by a mucosa consisting of simple columnar epithelial cells, some of which are ciliated, overlying a small amount of connective tissue. The cilia beat toward the uterus and thus create a current along which the ovulated oocyte or fertilized egg may pass on its way to the uterus. The mucosa is in the form of long folds, particularly in the ampulla, but these folds gradually diminish toward the uterine portion of the tube. The smooth muscle is arranged in an inner circular and outer longitudinal layer, with decreasing amounts of muscle toward the ovarian end of the tube. When sperm have been deposited in the female tract, wavelike contractions of the muscular walls propel the sperm upward toward the infundibulum and against the ciliary current. The outermost layer of the uterine tube is the serosa (mesothelium and connective tissue).

Uterus

The adult uterus in a premenopausal woman normally shows cyclic changes in structure and function as well as extensive modifications during pregnancy. The wall of the uterus is composed of three layers: the endometrium, myometrium, and perimetrium. The **endometrium** lines the uterine cavity and is basically a highly modified mucous membrane containing simple columnar epithelial cells overlying a thick connective tissue **stroma** which is highly vascular (Fig. 16-19). Numerous mucus-secreting (uterine) glands extend downward from the epithelium into the stroma. The **myometrium** is a thick layer of interlacing smooth muscle fibers whose contractions are particularly important during childbirth. The **perimetrium** is the outer covering (serosa) consisting of mesothelium and connective tissue. The cyclic changes which the uterus undergoes will be described later in terms of the reproductive cycle.

The cervix is lined by simple columnar epithelium and contains cervical mucous glands as well. Cells are constantly being shed from this region and can thus be easily obtained and examined for early signs of malignancy by means of a "**Pap smear**" (named after Papanicolaou who first perfected the technique).

Vagina

The vaginal lining is normally thrown into ridges and consists of stratified squamous epithelium overlying a thin layer of connective tissue. The epithelial cells contain large amounts of glycogen which may serve as a nutrient source for sperm when they are deposited there. Since there are virtually no glands in the vagina, it depends upon mucus secreted from the uterine and cervical glands for its lubrication. The smooth muscles of the vaginal wall run primarily in a longitudinal direction. Skeletal muscle fibers of the bulbospongiosus muscles occur near the vaginal opening.

Mammary Glands

The two mammary glands or breasts are considered accessory organs to the female reproductive system. They are present in both sexes, but usually become highly developed only in the female in response to estrogen stimulation from the ovaries.

The breasts are located just anterior to the pectoralis major muscle and consist mainly of glandular tissue and fat (Fig. 16-20). At the apex of each breast is a slight elevation, the **nipple**, surrounded by a ring of pigmented skin, the **areola.** The glandular tissue is grouped into lobes and smaller lobules which are separated from one another by strands of dense connective tissue. In the inactive (nonlactating) gland there is a predominance of connective tissue in each lobule, while the glandular elements consist only of a system of ducts lined with a simple cuboidal epithelium (Fig. 16-21*A*). These ducts merge with one another as they pass radially toward the nipple, where they join larger **lactiferous ducts**. There are approximately 10–20 lactiferous ducts, each of which opens separately by means of a small pore on the surface of the nipple.

During pregnancy the glandular tissue increases, and little sacs (alveoli) of cuboidal cells develop at the ends of the smallest ducts. There is also a relative decrease in the amount of connective tissue (Fig. 16-21*B*). Initially after parturition the alveoli secrete **colostrum**, a thin fluid rich in protein. Within a few days the secretion changes to milk containing fats, sugars, and protein. The expulsion of milk is triggered by the release of the hormone **oxytocin** from the neurohypophysis, which in turn causes contraction of slender myoepithelial cells interspersed among the alveoli and ducts. Although the initial development of the breasts at puberty depends on estrogen stimulation, further development during pregnancy requires **progesterone** produced by the placenta, as well as **lactogenic hormone (LTH, prolactin)** secreted by the anterior pituitary gland.

Female Reproductive Cycle

A major difference between female and male reproductive physiology is the cyclic nature of the female system. This cyclic activity is basically under control of the hypothalamic region of the brain, but it also involves complex interactions among the anterior lobe of the pituitary gland, ovaries, uterus, and breasts. The dura-

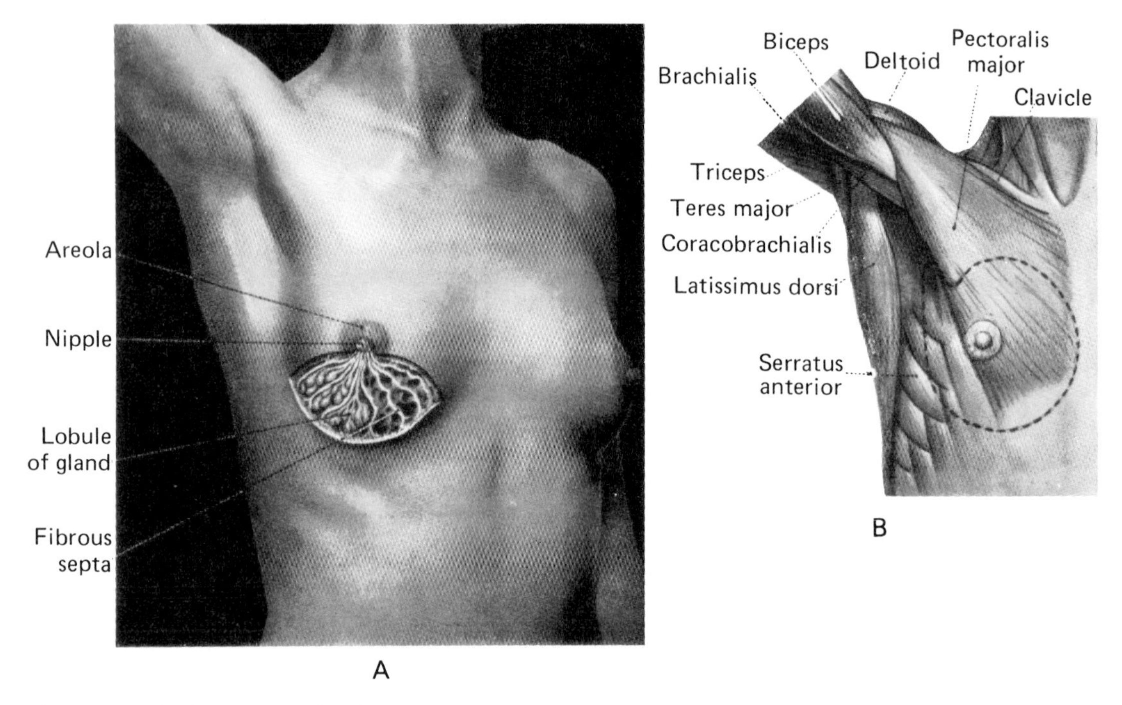

Fig. 16-20. The breast. (A) The skin has been removed from the lower half of the right breast to show lobular structure. (B) The position of the breast *(broken line)* anterior to the pectoral muscles. (From W. J. Hamilton, G. Simon, and S. G. I. Hamilton, *Surface and Radiological Anatomy,* Ed. 5, The Macmillan Press, London, 1971.)

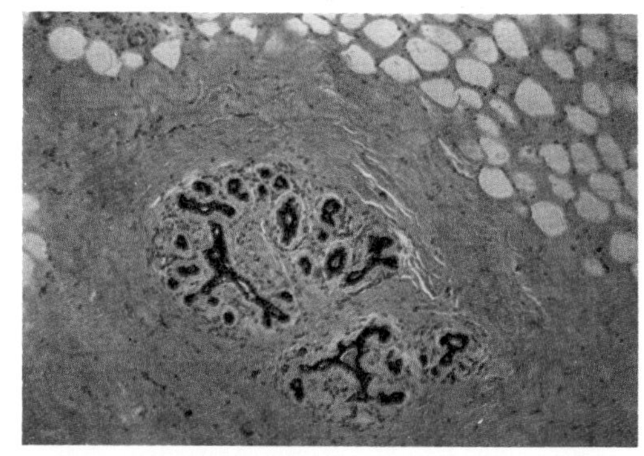

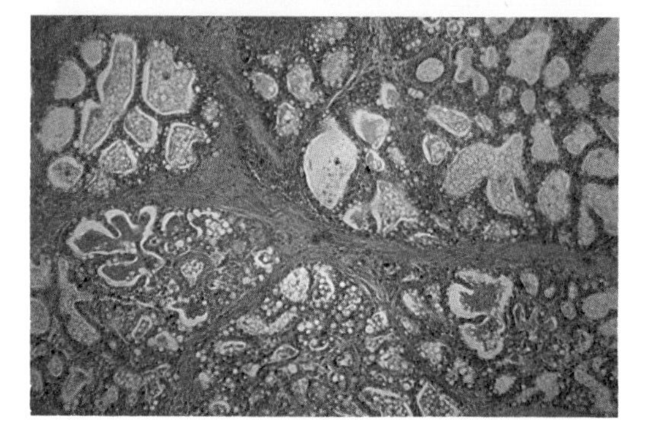

Fig. 16-21. Microscopic sections through the mammary gland. *Above,* inactive (nonlactating) gland. *Below,* active (lactating) gland. (From the teaching collection, Department of Anatomy, College of Physicians and Surgeons, Columbia University.)

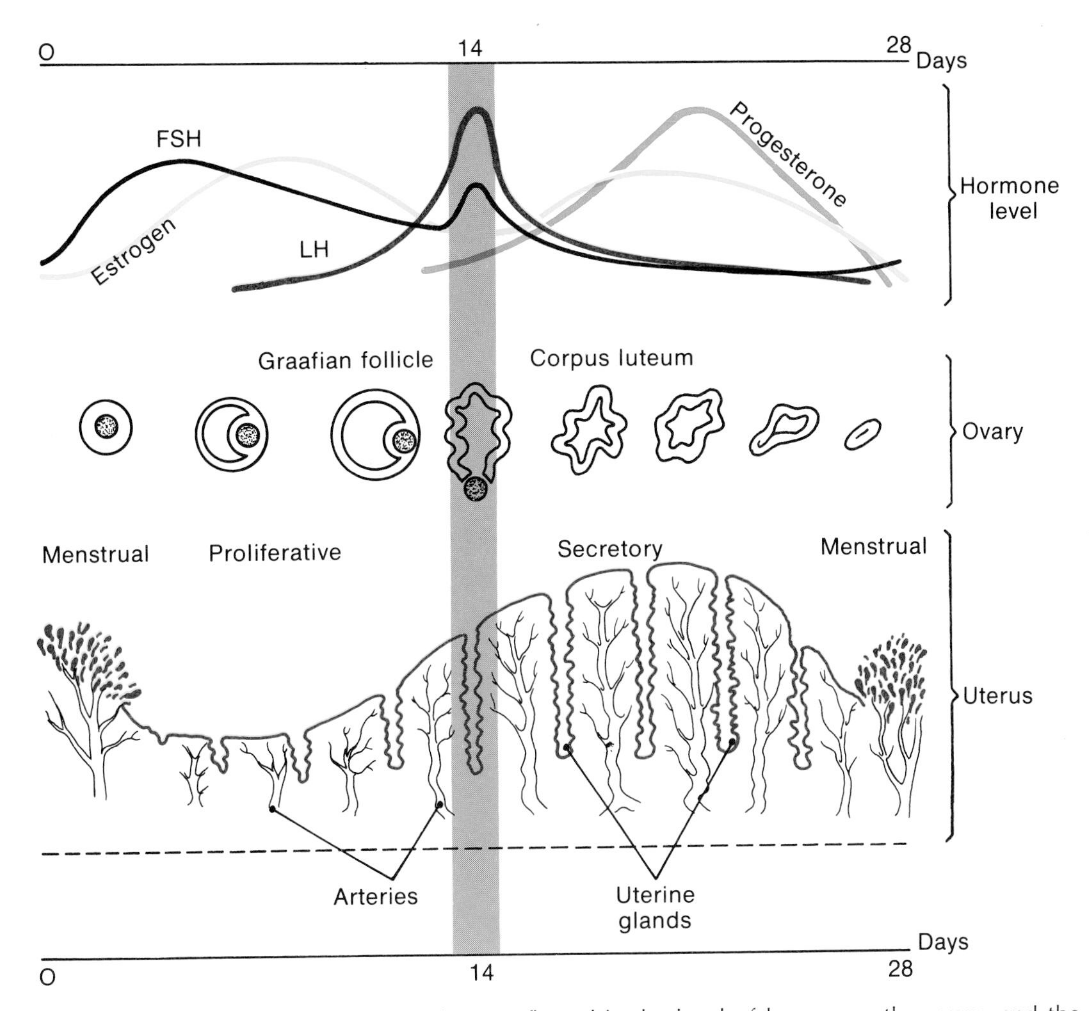

Fig. 16-22. The female reproductive cycle, as reflected in the level of hormones, the ovary, and the uterus. The vertical red band represents ovulation.

tion of the reproductive (menstrual) cycle usually ranges from 20 to 35 days (28 days being average) and can vary from individual to individual and at different times in the same individual. The onset of menstruation each month can arbitrarily be considered as the beginning of each cycle.

At the beginning of the cycle the hypothalamus produces a releasing factor which acts on the anterior lobe of the pituitary gland and causes it to release **follicle stimulating hormone (FSH)** (Fig. 16-22). As the cycle proceeds, FSH stimulates the growth of several follicles in the ovaries and also stimulates the secretion of **estrogen** from the theca interna cells surrounding the follicles. The estrogen in turn acts on the uterine endometrium, causing it to proliferate. This phase of the uterine cycle is appropriately designated as the **proliferative phase** and lasts for a variable period of time.

The rising estrogen level in the blood stream acts on the hypothalamus which in turn allows **luteinizing hormone (LH)** to be released from the anterior pituitary. The increased estrogen level eventually suppresses the output of FSH. A brief surge in the release of LH, and to a lesser extent of FSH, causes the wall of the follicle in the ovary to weaken and

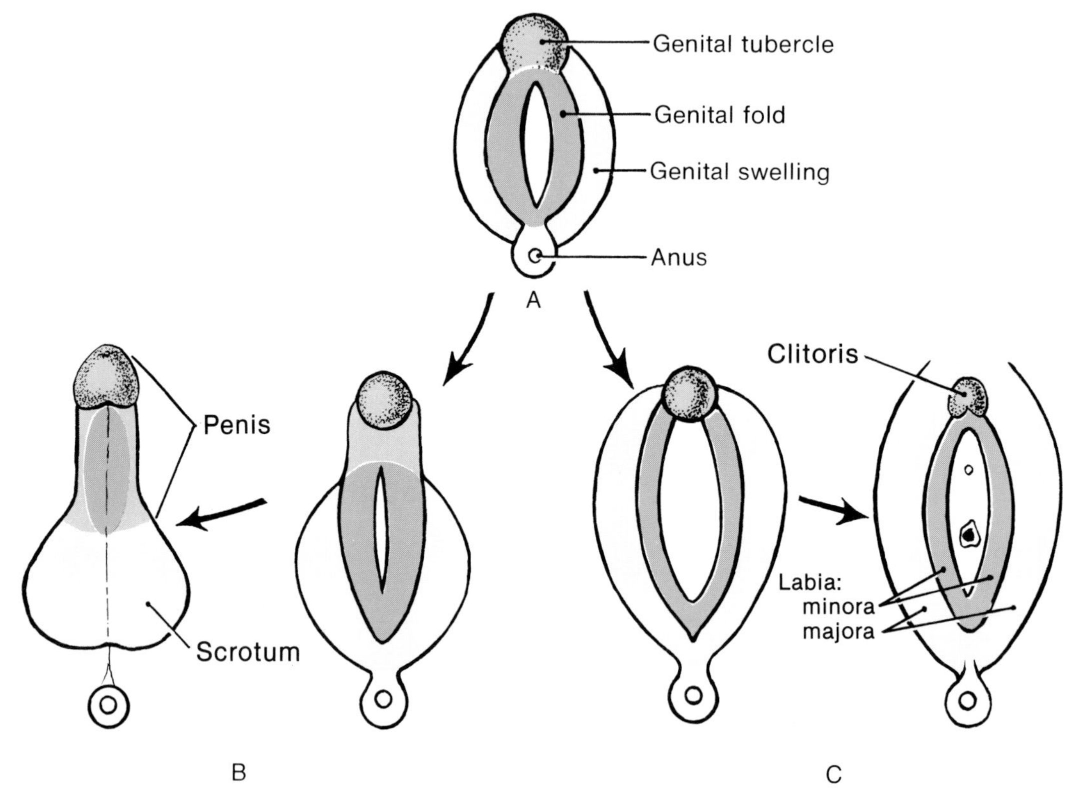

Fig. 16-23. Development of the external genitalia. (A) Indifferent stage, (B) differentiation in the male, (C) differentiation in the female.

to permit the mature egg to be released at ovulation. LH also causes the mature follicle to transform into the corpus luteum. The growing corpus luteum secretes increasing amounts of **progesterone,** as well as estrogen, which prepare the uterus for implantation by effecting an increase in the thickness and vascularity of the endometrium and stimulating the growth of the uterine glands (Fig. 16-22). The epithelial cells of these glands secrete mucus, glycogen, and lipids, thereby creating a hospitable environment for implantation to occur. In the uterus this phase is termed the **secretory phase;** in the ovary it is called the **luteal phase.** Progesterone also suppresses the flow of LH from the pituitary gland and has a slight stimulatory effect on the ducts of the mammary glands.

If fertilization does not occur, the corpus luteum begins to regress about 10 days after ovulation, and the level of progesterone falls. There is also a drop in the estrogen level. This sudden withdrawal of progesterone and estrogen initiates **menstruation** as the uterine endometrium begins to break down.

Just prior to menstruation the arterioles in the endometrium contract and shut off the flow of blood to the cells in the superficial layers of the endometrium. These cells then start to degenerate, and menstruation begins when the walls of the capillaries break open. The upper layers of the endometrium are shed during the subsequent 3–5 days, with the release of an average of 300 ml of menstrual fluid consisting of epithelial and stromal cells, blood, and secretions of the uterine glands. The deeper regions of the endometrium are not lost but instead remain to provide the basis for regeneration of the endometrium during the next proliferative phase.

The variability in the length of the menstrual cycle reflects the variability in the proliferative phase; the secretory phase lasts two weeks and ordinarily does not vary much in length. Should fertilization and implantation occur, however, the implanted blastocyst secretes human chorionic gonadotrophin (HCG) which is transmitted to the ovary and which maintains the corpus luteum, so that the latter continues to secrete progesterone. The thickened secretory uterine endometrium is thus maintained for its role in the nourishment and sustenance of the developing embryo. (The presence of HCG in the maternal blood and/or urine is used as the basis for pregnancy tests.)

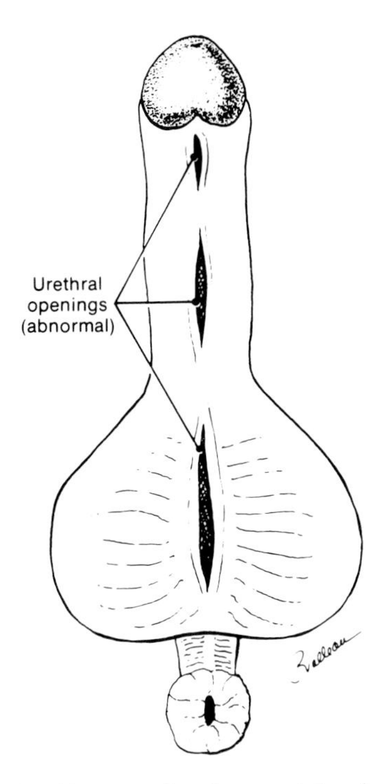

Fig. 16-24. Hypospadias (incomplete closure of the genital folds resulting in one or more gaps along the ventral midline.) (Modified after Langman.)

DEVELOPMENTAL AND CLINICAL ANATOMY

Human embryos go through a stage of development during which their genital organs (both external and internal) show the same characteristics in both sexes. This period is known as the **indifferent stage** and lasts until approximately the end of the second month of prenatal life. The indifferent external genital organs (external genitalia) consist of a median projection (the **genital tubercle**), and two small **genital folds** flanked by a pair of larger **genital swellings** (Fig. 16-23).

In the male embryo the genital tubercle elongates to become the penis, the two genital folds fuse to enclose the urethra within the penis, and the genital swellings unite and form the scrotum. Occasionally the closure of the genital folds is incomplete, resulting in the condition known as **hypospadias** and characterized by abnormal openings of the urethra (Fig. 16-24).

In the female, the genital tubercle becomes the clitoris, and the two genital folds remain open as the labia minora which flank the vestibule. The labia majora develop from the genital swellings and are thus counterparts of the scrotum.

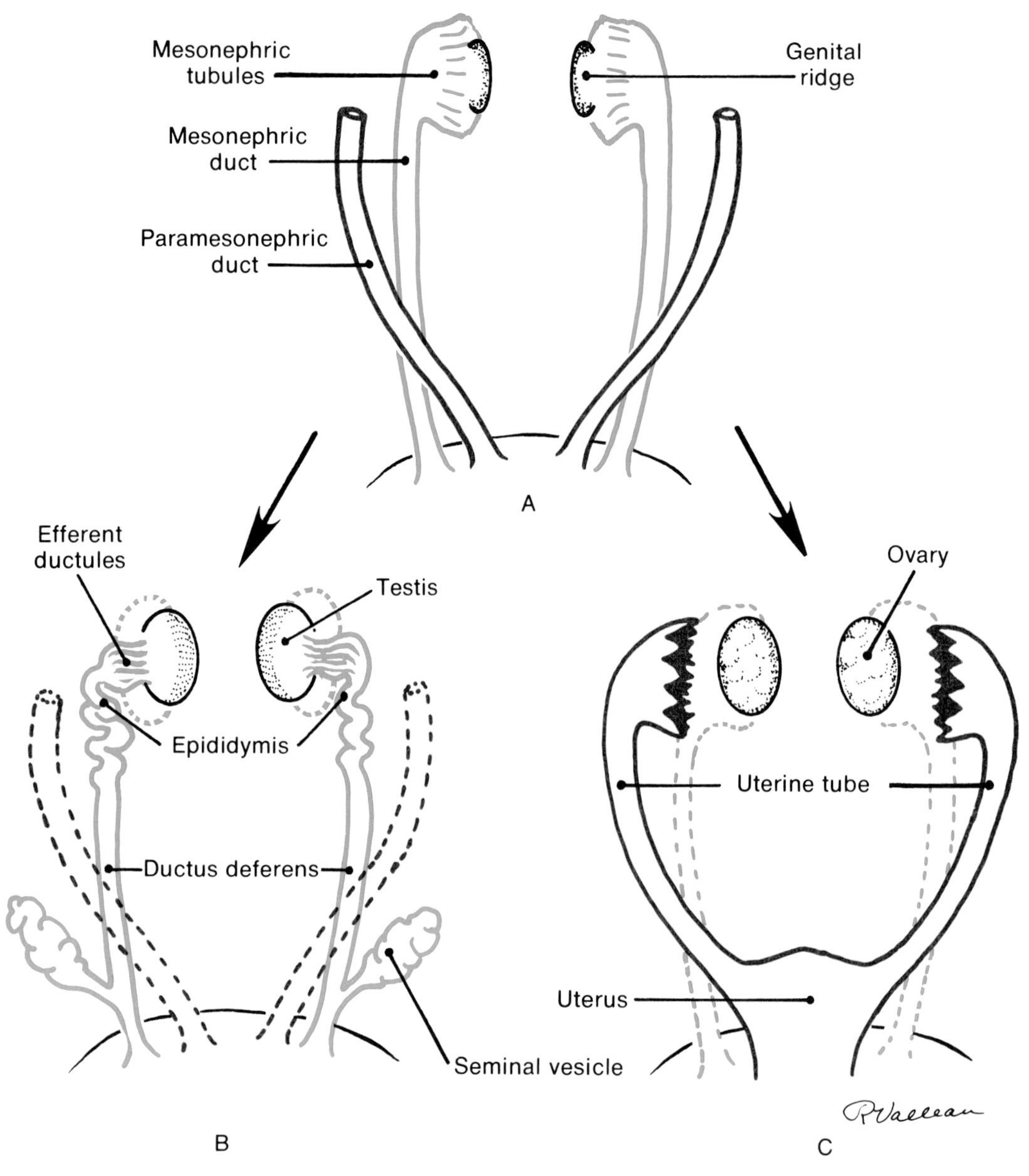

Fig. 16-25. Anterior views of developing internal genital organs. (A) Indifferent stage, (B) male organs (before descent of testes), (C) female organs. *Broken lines* represent structures which degenerate.

The indifferent internal genital organs (internal genitalia) include three paired structures: the gonads, the mesonephric ducts, and paramesonephric ducts (Fig. 16-25). Each **gonad** develops from the **genital ridge,** a thickening of the mesothelium lining the body cavity (coelom) along the medial aspect of the **mesonephros** (the second pair of embryonic kidneys, see Chapter 15). The mesonephric tubules in each mesonephros communicate with a **mesonephric (Wolffian) duct** which passes downward to enter the anterior portion of the urogenital sinus (anterior portion of the cloaca). A second duct develops from the mesothelium

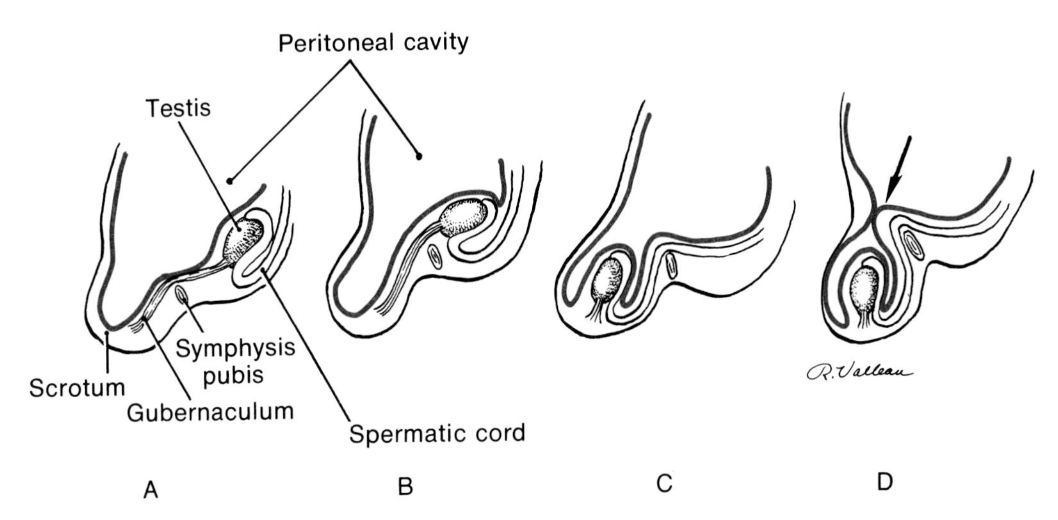

Fig. 16-26. Descent of the testis, lateral view. (A) The testis develops behind the peritoneum (red line) and the scrotum pushes forward from the peritoneal cavity. The gubernaculum extends from the testis to the scrotum. (B, C) As the testis descends into the scrotum, the gubernaculum shortens. The testis invaginates the scrotal cavity. (D) The scrotal cavity pinches off from the peritoneal cavity (*at arrow*).

just lateral to each mesonephric duct and is called a **paramesonephric (Mullerian) duct**, which likewise passes downward to join the urogenital sinus.

If the embryo is a male, by the end of the third month of gestation the gonad differentiates into a fetal testis containing interstitial (Leydig) cells and seminiferous tubules, which contain the precursors of sustentacular (Sertoli) cells and spermatogonia. The seminiferous tubules eventually communicate with some of the mesonephric tubules, which then become converted into efferent ductules. (The remaining mesonephric tubules which do not become efferent ductules will degenerate.) The mesonephric duct becomes the ductus epididymis and ductus deferens, from which a seminal vesicle originates inferiorly (Fig. 16-25). (The prostate gland and bulbourethral glands differentiate as endodermal outpouchings from the urethra.) Meanwhile the paramesonephric ducts degenerate, except for some remnants which can occasionally be identified in the adult.

In the third month of prenatal life, two fetal hormones essential for male development have been identified: paramesonephric (Mullerian)-inhibiting substance and fetal testosterone. **Paramesonephric (Mullerian)-inhibiting substance** is produced by the seminiferous tubules. It causes the regression of the paramesonephric ducts and eventually plays a role in the descent of the testes into the scrotum. **Fetal testosterone** is produced by the interstitial cells and is necessary for the maturation of the seminiferous tubules and for further development of the male reproductive tract.

If the embryo is a female, the gonad differentiates into an ovary with follicle cells and oogonia. By the end of the second trimester of gestation, the oogonia have ceased mitosis and have already developed into primary oocytes which remain dormant until puberty, when certain of these oocytes begin to mature each month. In the female, the mesonephros and mesonephric duct disappear completely except for some atrophied remnants (Fig. 16-25). Each paramesonephric duct, however, becomes fully developed and fuses inferiorly with its counterpart to form the uterus and upper part of the vagina, although there is some evidence that the entire vagina may be derived from the urogenital sinus. The cranial ends of the paramesonephric ducts become the uterine tubes, which remain in open communication with the peritoneal cavity.

It is of interest that if a female embryo is exposed to androgens (male hormones) during gestation, the genitalia of the female embryo become masculinized. Conversely, if a male embryo is exposed to insufficient amounts of androgens its genitalia will exhibit female characteristics.

In male embryos, the testes descend during the last 2 months before birth. During their descent the caudal end of each testis is attached to a band of connective tissue, the **gubernaculum,** which extends down into the scrotum and shortens as the testis descends (Fig. 16-26). Once the testes have reached their final position the communication between the scrotum and peritoneal cavity is obliterated. However, physical stress in the adult can sometimes reopen this communication, in which case an **inguinal hernia** develops. This can be particularly serious if an intestinal loop pushes into the canal and becomes strangulated. Failure of the testes to descend is known as **cryptorchidism.** This leads to sterility unless as soon as possible after birth the testes are surgically brought downward into the scrotum where the temperature is slightly lower than body temperature.

Although the ovaries do not descend as much, they become attached to a gubernaculum which passes from the caudal end of each ovary to the lateral wall of the uterus and then to the genital swelling (labium majus). The portion of the gubernaculum between ovary and uterus becomes the ovarian ligament, whereas the portion between uterus and labium majus becomes the round ligament. The communication between the peritoneal cavity and the genital swelling is not as large in female embryos as in male embryos, since the ovaries do not descend into the swellings. Consequently, when the communication is obliterated, it is not likely to reopen again, and so females are less susceptible to inguinal hernias.

The relatively superficial location of the proximal portion of each adult ductus (vas) deferens makes them readily accessible for **vasectomy,** the contraceptive technique whereby tiny slits are made in the scrotum and each ductus deferens is ligated and cut so as to prevent sperm from leaving the testes and epididymes. In the female the uterine tubes are located deep within the pelvis but can be approached by means of a tiny incision in the umbilical area. The tubes are then tied off so as to prevent sperm from meeting the ovulated egg.

III

REGIONAL ANATOMY

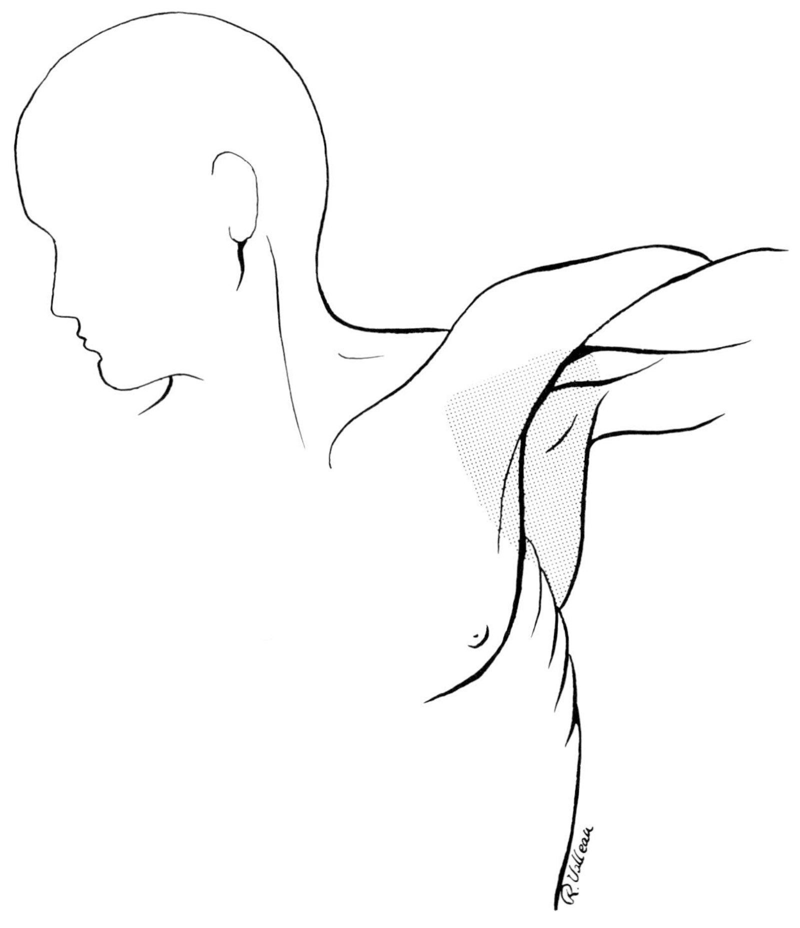

The preceding chapters have dealt with the structural and functional aspects of organs and organ systems. The following chapters summarize and review these structures in terms of their anatomical relationships and clinical significance from a regional point of view. These regions are: the head and neck, the thorax and abdomen (including the pelvis), and the limbs (upper and lower).

17

The Head and Neck

The head and neck are extremely complex regions of the body. The head lodges the body's control center (brain), and also contains an important endocrine organ, the pituitary gland (often called the "master gland"). The head is also the site where food is ingested, and air inspired and expired. It also contributes importantly to one's capacity for communication, not only through speech but also by means of facial expressions which convey one's emotions.

The neck serves as a support for the head and enables it to undergo a certain degree of movement. It also transmits food downward through the esophagus and air downward and upward through the larynx and the trachea. The neck contains important endocrine organs such as the thyroid and parathyroid glands and acts as a conduit for vessels and nerves passing to and from the head.

Blood Vessels and Lymphatics

The various structures of the head and neck region are supplied primarily by branches from the common carotid and subclavian arteries. Venous drainage occurs via the internal and external jugular veins which empty into the brachiocephalic veins. Lymphatic vessels from the left side of the head and neck empty into the thoracic duct; those from the right side empty into the right lymphatic duct. Clusters of lymph nodes occur in a ringlike area where the head joins the neck and also along the course of the internal jugular veins. Infections and inflammations in the head and neck can cause these lymph nodes to become enlarged (commonly called "swollen glands").

Nerves

Structures in the head and neck are supplied by the 12 cranial nerves and the 8 cervical spinal nerves. The parasympathetic portion of the autonomic nervous system sends fibers out via cranial nerves III, VII, IX, and X; the sympathetic portion consists of the cervical sympathetic trunk from which a plexus of fibers travels along with blood vessels to various regions of the head and neck.

THE HEAD

Superficial Structures

The scalp overlies the calvaria (skull-cap) and contains five layers: (1) skin (with long hairs), (2) a highly vascularized subcutaneous layer which bleeds profusely if cut, (3) a fibrous **epicranial aponeurosis (galea aponeurotica),** which is continuous anteriorly with the frontalis muscle and posteriorly with the occipitalis muscle, (4) a loose subaponeurotic layer of connective tissue which allows the upper three layers to be freely movable but which is also a "dangerous area" since it permits scalp infections to spread easily, and (5) the periosteum (pericranium) of the skull (Fig. 17-1).

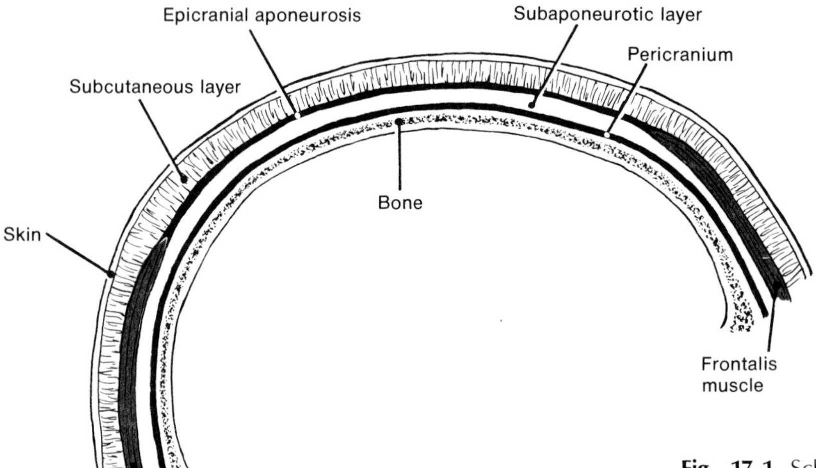

Fig. 17-1. Schematic diagram of the layers of the scalp as seen in sagittal section.

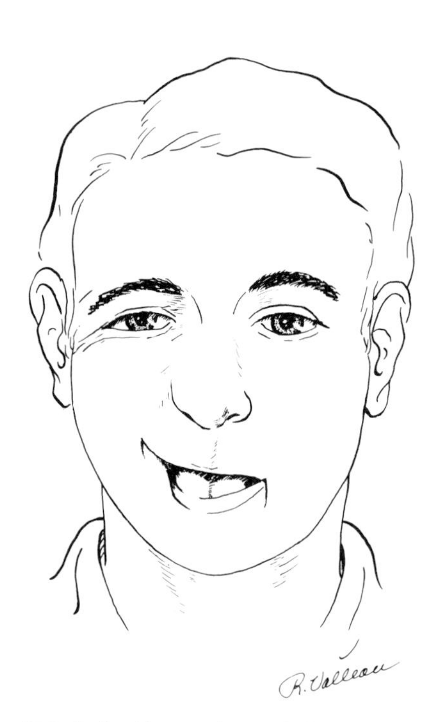

Fig. 17-2. Left side paralysis of the face due to damage to the left facial nerve. When the mouth is opened the unopposed muscles on the right side pull the mouth to the right.

The superficial structures of the face include the outer portions of the eyes (and eyelids), nose, lips, and muscles of facial expression. The skin of the face is relatively thin and is well endowed with sensory nerve fibers, particularly in the oral region. The muscles of facial expression have their origins on the facial bones, tend to lie in the subcutaneous layer of tissue (superficial fascia), and insert in the dermis of the skin. The facial muscles on opposite sides of the face oppose one another. Thus if the muscles on one side become paralyzed (as occurs if cranial nerve VII is damaged), then the unopposed muscles on the opposite side contort the face by pulling such mobile structures as the lips toward the unaffected side (Fig. 17-2).

Cranium

The cranium consists of the skull which serves as a protective covering for the brain. The meninges and cerebrospinal fluid also help to protect and cushion the brain. Nevertheless, serious brain damage can occur should bone fragments from a skull fracture penetrate the nervous tissue or lacerate an intracranial blood vessel. Moreover, an accumulation of fluid from ruptured vessels or in response to inflammatory conditions can compress and damage

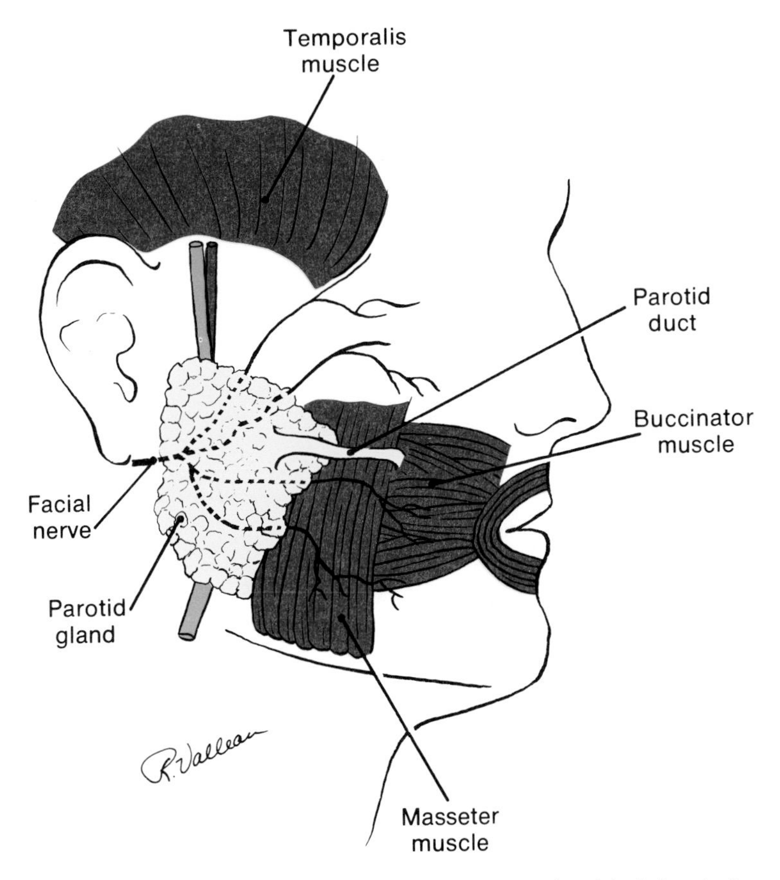

Fig. 17-3. The parotid region and temporal region, lateral view. *Broken black lines* indicate the course of the facial nerve through the substance of the parotid gland (yellow).

the brain, since the rigid skull cannot expand to accommodate the increased pressure.

The superior and lateral regions of the skull are rather thin and fairly smooth, whereas the inferior region is thicker and contains irregular ridges and projections. Despite its thicker bones, the inferior region is quite susceptible to fracture because of the numerous foramina for the entrance or exit of vessels and nerves. Although the cerebrospinal fluid provides some cushioning support for the brain, a sudden sharp blow to the head may cause the brain to crash against jagged projections along the cranial floor.

The paranasal sinuses are often involved in skull fractures and hence may be the source of bleeding into the mouth, nose, or orbits. Severe fractures may also create a communication between the subarachnoid space and the sinuses, resulting in a seepage of cerebrospinal fluid into the sinuses and eventually from the nose.

Parotid Region

The parotid region is located just in front of the lobule (lobe) of the ear and superficial to the ramus of the mandible. It contains the parotid gland whose duct passes forward across the masseter muscle, pierces the buccinator muscle, and enters the mouth (Fig. 17-3). The parotid gland can become painfully enlarged during a mumps infection. Also since the facial nerve (cranial nerve VII) and its branches run through the substance of the gland on their way to the muscles of facial expression, it is

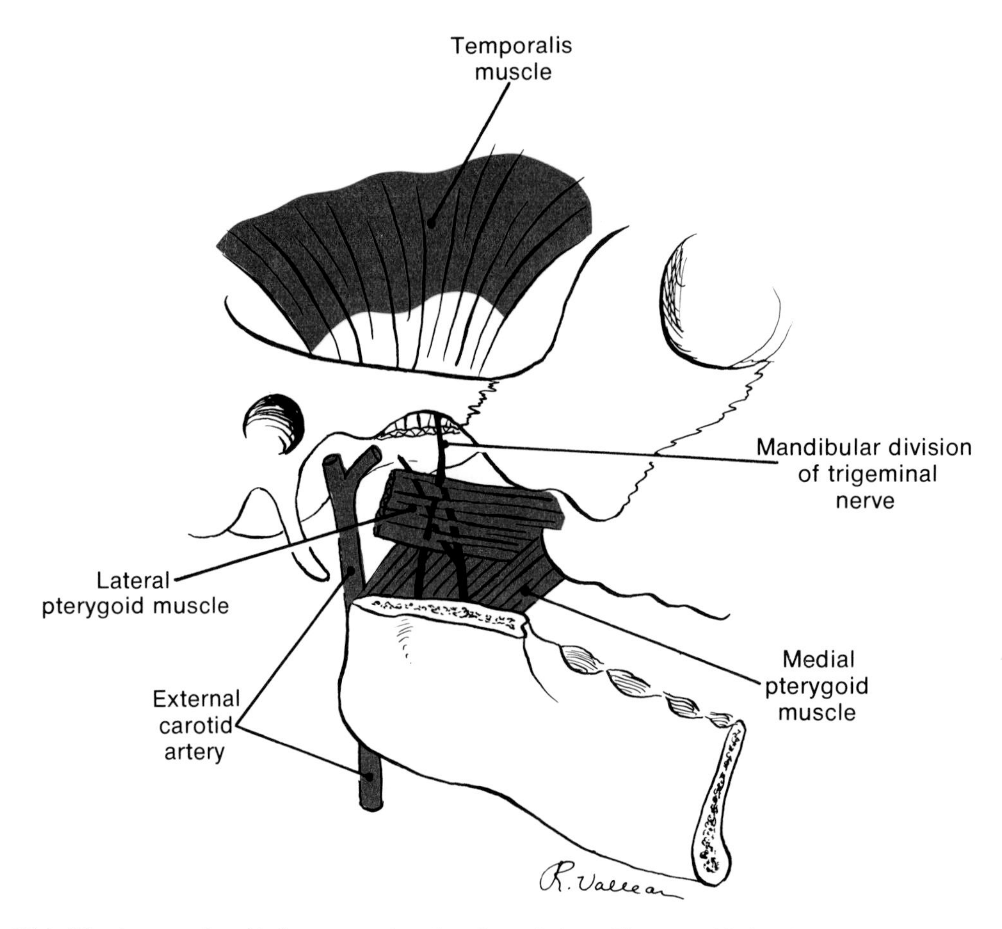

Fig. 17-4. The temporal and infratemporal region, lateral view. The parotid gland and ramus of the mandible have been removed. The pterygoid plexus of veins is not shown.

possible for these fibers to be damaged by cancerous growths or during surgical procedures on this gland, thereby resulting in varying degrees of facial muscle paralysis. The upper part of the external carotid artery as well as tributaries to the external jugular veins also pass through the parotid gland.

Temporal and Infratemporal Regions

The temporal region occurs on the side of the head just above the zygomatic arch (Fig. 17-4). It is largely occupied by the temporalis muscle whose movement can be felt when the jaws are opened and closed. A blow to the temporal region of the head can be particularly dangerous because of potential damage to the internal and middle ear which are situated within the petrous portion of the temporal bone.

The infratemporal region lies inferior to the zygomatic arch and deep to the ramus of the mandible (Fig. 17-4). It contains the lower part of the temporalis muscle and the lateral and medial pterygoid muscles, as well as branches of the mandibular division of the trigeminal nerve (cranial nerve V). The blood vessels in both the temporal and infratemporal regions include branches of the external carotid artery and a group of veins termed the pterygoid venous plexus. This plexus not only drains into

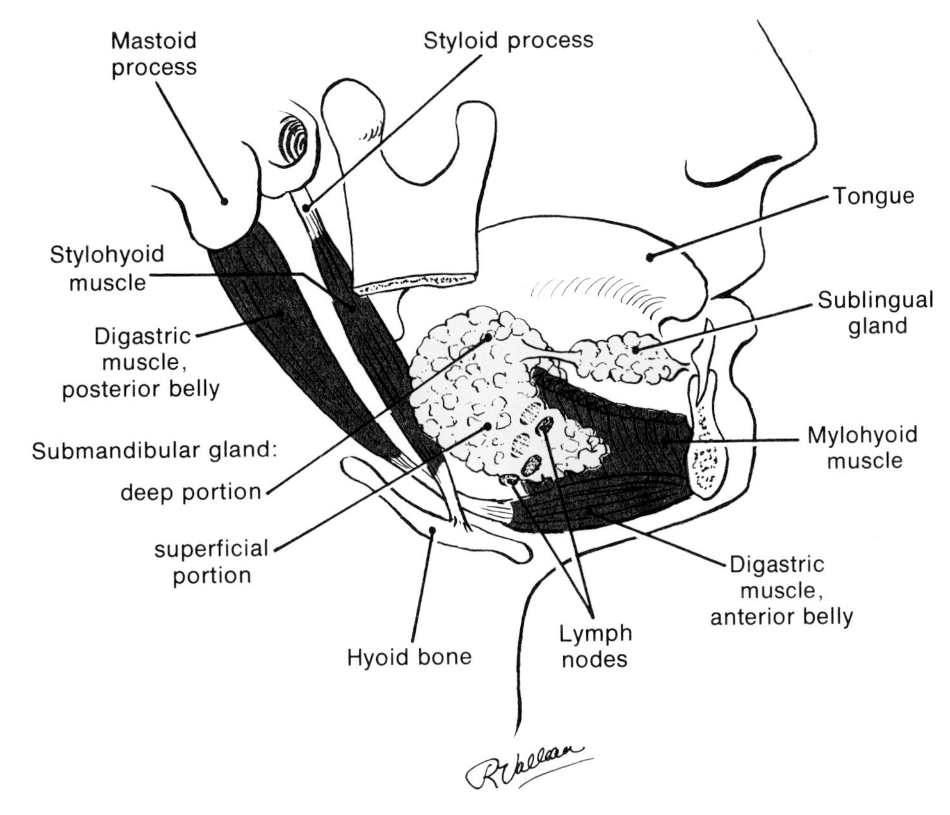

Fig. 17-5. The submandibular region, lateral view. A portion of the mandible has been removed to reveal the sublingual gland and deep portion of the submandibular gland.

tributaries of the internal jugular vein but also communicates with a venous plexus within the cranial cavity, unfortunately enabling infections to spread from the facial region of the head inward to the brain.

Submandibular Region

This region is located between the body of the mandible on each side and is bounded by the tongue above and the hyoid bone below (Fig. 17-5). It contains the suprahyoid muscles (digastric, stylohyoid, mylohyoid, and geniohyoid) and extrinsic muscles of the tongue. Two pairs of salivary glands (the submandibular and sublingual) are also located here, as are numerous submandibular lymph nodes, some of which are embedded in the substance of the submandibular gland.

THE NECK

Surface Anatomy

In most individuals the spinous process of the lowermost cervical vertebra (C7) can be palpated in the midline of the posterior surface of the neck. (Even more prominent is the spinous process of the first thoracic vertebra immediately below it.) Along each side of the midline is the trapezius muscle and the deeper cervical portions of the postural muscles extending upward from the back.

Near the midline of the anterior surface of the neck, the following structures can be felt from above downward: the hyoid bone, the larynx (including the thyroid cartilage and cricoid cartilage), and the cartilaginous rings of the trachea. Pulsations can be detected in each

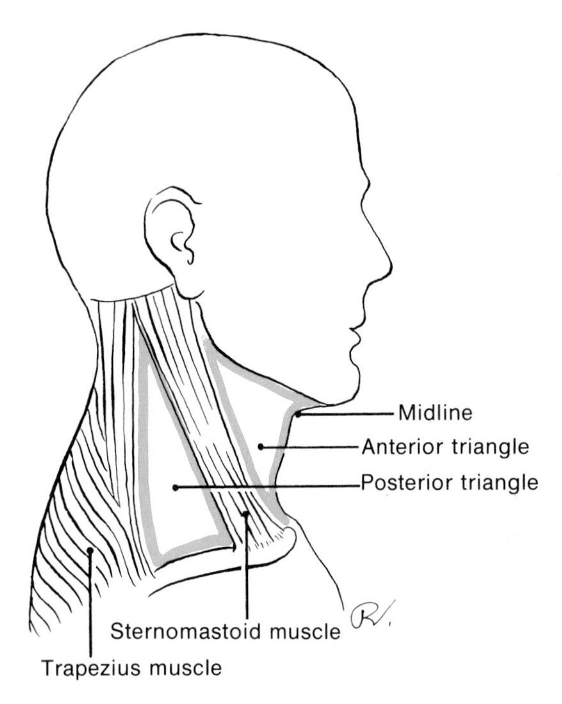

Fig. 17-6. The anterior and posterior triangles of the neck (outlined in blue).

common carotid artery by gently pressing one's fingers just lateral to the thyroid cartilage. The external jugular veins travel in the superficial fascia and may be observable in some individuals.

The muscles on the anterior and lateral surfaces of the neck can also be easily identified. The platysma lies in the superficial fascia and becomes visible when the jaws are clenched. The sternomastoid (sternocleidomastoid) muscle on each side is also visible and becomes particularly prominent when the chin is turned toward the opposite shoulder. This muscle also serves as a line of demarcation between the anterior and posterior triangles in the neck. The **anterior triangle** is bounded posteriorly by the sternomastoid muscle, superiorly by the mandible and anteriorly by the midline (Fig. 17-6). The **posterior triangle** is bounded posteriorly by the trapezius muscle, inferiorly by the clavicle, and anteriorly by the sternomastoid muscle.

Thyroid Gland, Larynx, and Trachea

These three structures show important anatomical relationships to one another and to nearby structures in the neck. The thyroid gland lies partially under cover of the sternohyoid and sternothyroid muscles which are in turn partially overlapped by the sternomastoid muscle (Fig. 17-7). Each of the two lateral lobes of the gland lies alongside the thyroid cartilage, cricoid cartilage, and upper trachea. The isthmus connecting the two lobes overlies the second, third, or fourth tracheal rings. Each lateral lobe of the thyroid gland overlaps a tubular mass of connective tissue, the **carotid sheath,** which encloses three structures: the common carotid artery, internal jugular vein, and vagus nerve (Figs. 17-8 and 17-9). Just behind the carotid sheath is the cervical portion of the sympathetic trunk.

The larynx and trachea are situated in front of the laryngopharynx and esophagus, respectively. Right and left recurrent laryngeal nerves travel upward along a groove between the trachea and esophagus on their way to the larynx, where they innervate muscles control-

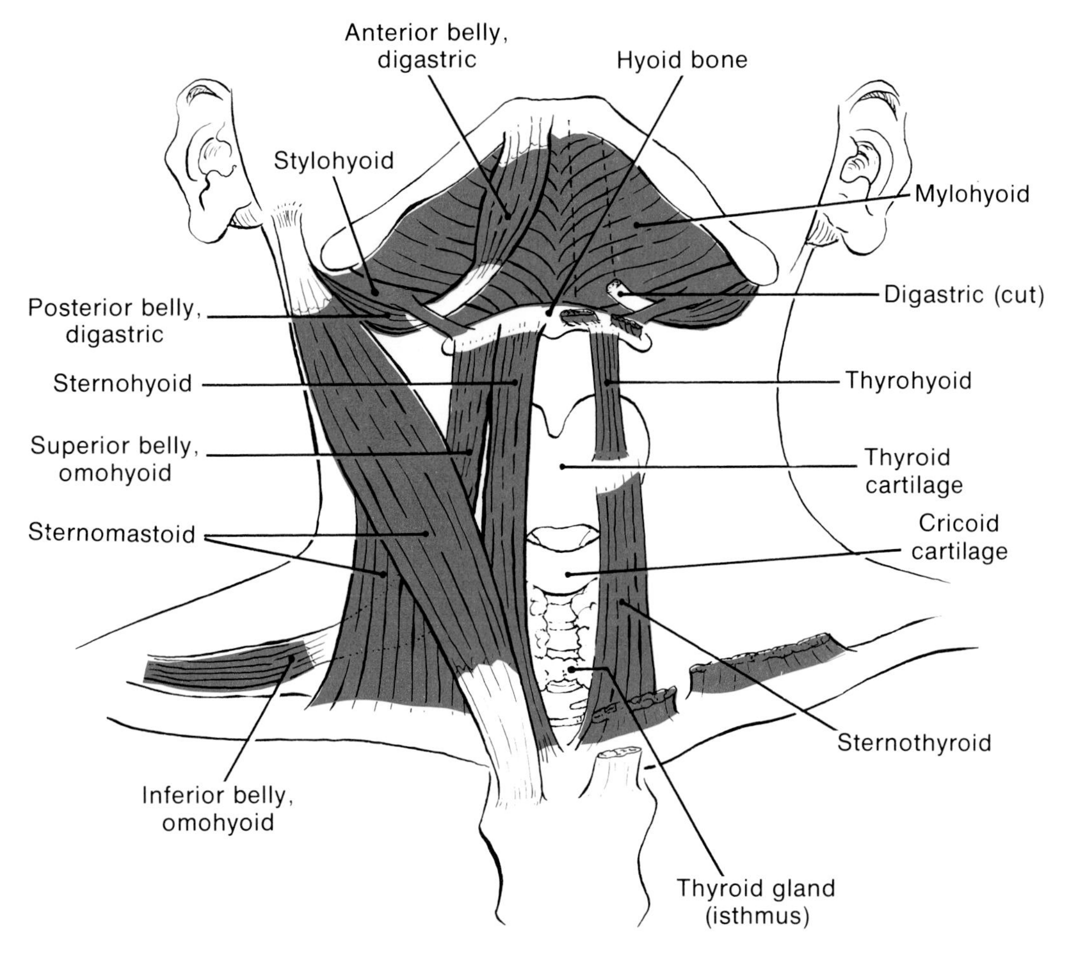

Fig. 17-7. Anterior relationships of the thyroid gland.

ling the position and tension of the vocal folds. For this reason hoarseness may occur if either or both of these nerves are damaged, as from an enlargement of the thyroid gland, trachea, or esophagus or during surgery on the thyroid gland, such as a thyroidectomy. An enlargement of the thyroid gland, trachea, or esophagus may also produce difficulty in swallowing or in breathing, and structures within the carotid sheath may likewise be compressed, as well as the sympathetic trunk. Damage to the sympathetic trunk may produce symptoms known collectively as **Horner's syndrome.** These symptoms reflect the effects of sympathetic deficits in the head and include constriction of the pupil (due to unopposed action of the parasympathetics), ptosis or drooping of the upper eyelid, flushing (because of a lack of sympathetic vasoconstriction), and dryness of skin (failure of the sympathetics to stimulate the sweat glands). Horner's syndrome may also be produced by an aneurysm (ballooning out) of the common carotid artery.

If the larynx should become obstructed so that breathing is impaired, a tracheotomy (tracheostomy) may be performed, consisting of an incision in the trachea to permit air to enter below the obstruction. The procedure can be

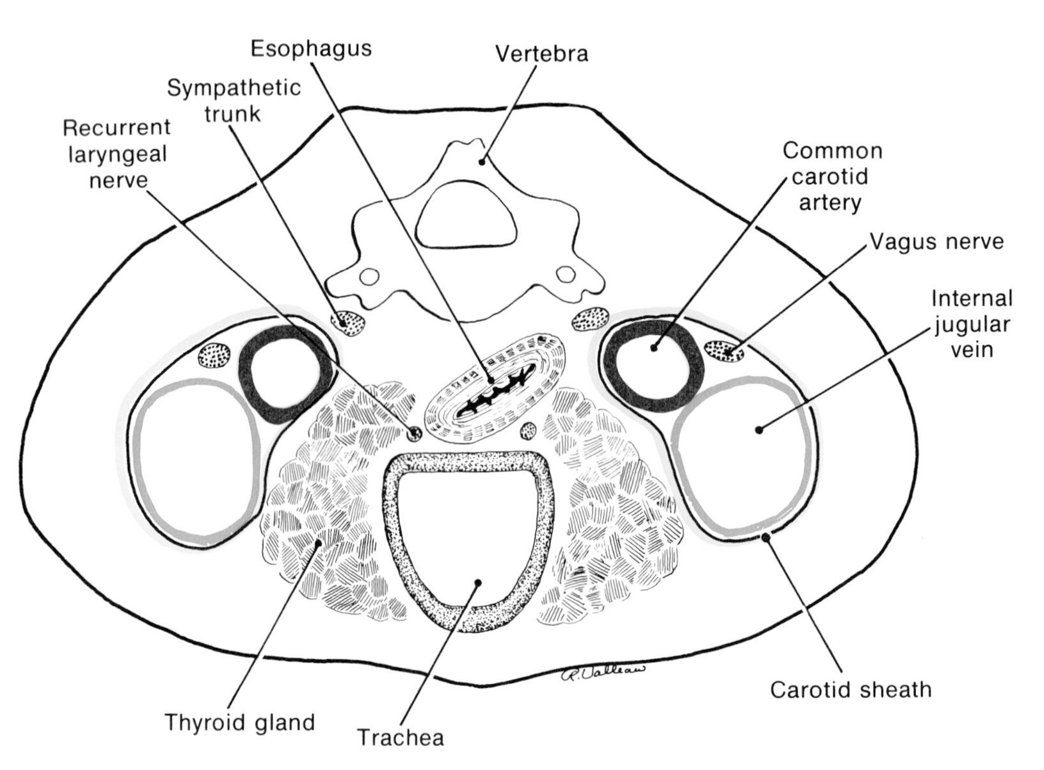

Fig. 17-8. Cross section of the neck through the region of the thyroid gland and trachea, showing the carotid sheath (yellow) and its contents.

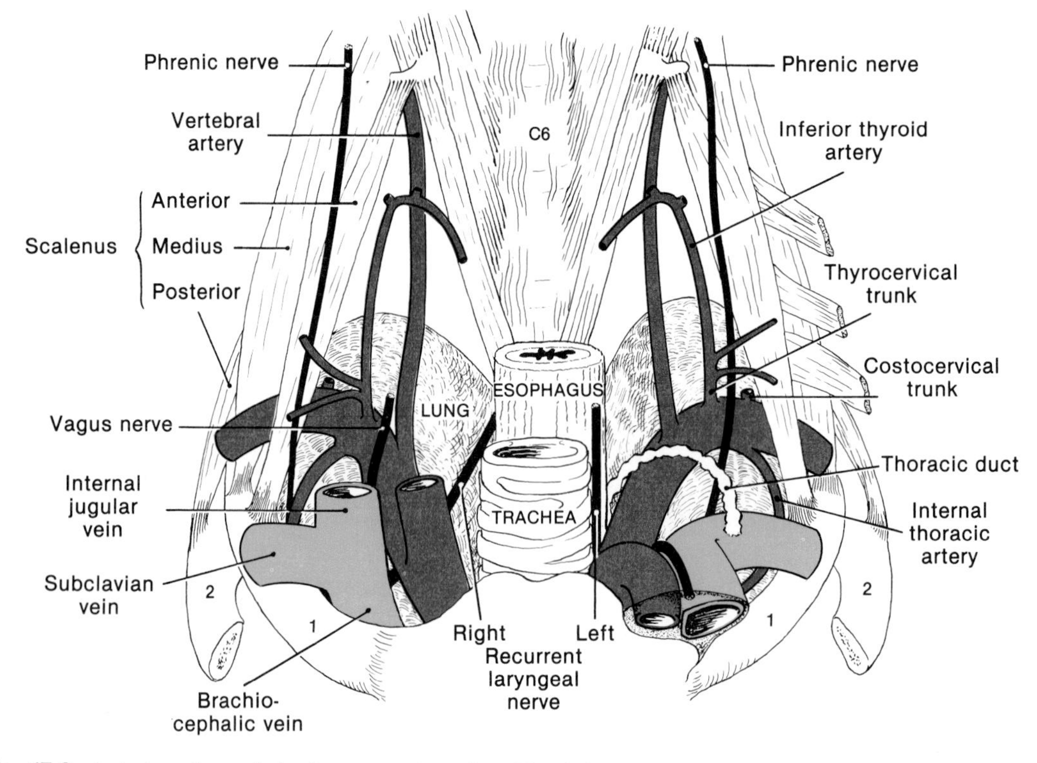

Fig. 17-9. Anterior view of the lower neck region. The left carotid sheath and its contents have been pulled forward to reveal the thoracic duct. (Modified after Grant.)

quite hazardous and requires an exact understanding of anatomical relationships in the neck. It is important that the incision be confined to the midline so as to avoid damage to the laterally situated jugular veins and common carotid arteries. The incision also must not penetrate too deeply, thereby passing through the back of the trachea and damaging the esophagus.

Behind and lateral to the sympathetic trunk and carotid sheath are the scalenus muscles which flex the cervical vertebral column laterally and also aid in respiratory movements. The phrenic nerve runs downward across the scalenus anterior muscle and can be approached surgically in this region (Fig. 17-9). Damage or compression of the nerve results in paralysis of the diaphragm on one side.

The prevertebral muscles of the neck are deeply situated posterior to the esophagus and laryngopharynx and anterior to the cervical vertebral column. These muscles flex the head.

18

The Thorax and Abdomen

Although the thorax and abdomen are often considered separately in regional studies of anatomy, it is well to keep in mind that the diaphragm represents the lower boundary of the thorax and the upper boundary of the abdomen; thus the dimensions of the thorax and abdomen change reciprocally with each respiratory movement of the diaphragm. The upper boundary of the thorax is at the thoracic inlet, which is demarcated by the first thoracic vertebra, the first ribs, and the manubrium of the sternum. The lower boundary of the abdomen (including the pelvis), is the pelvic diaphragm.

THORAX

The walls of the thorax consist of the bony thoracic cage and its associated muscles. The size and shape of the thorax vary from childhood to adulthood and also from person to person. An important surface landmark is the **sternal angle** where the manubrium joins the body of the sternum and where the second costal cartilages join the sternum laterally. Since the sternal angle can be palpated externally, it is often used as a starting point for counting the ribs and intercostal spaces. The level at which the angle occurs (approximately between the bodies of the fourth and fifth thoracic vertebrae) is also roughly the region where the trachea bifurcates into the two bronchi (Fig. 18-1).

In males the nipple lies usually at the level of the fourth intercostal space and lateral to the midclavicular line (Fig. 18-1). In females the breast extends from the second to the sixth ribs; however, since the size and shape of the breast are variable, the position of the nipple is not constant.

The soft organs of the thorax (heart, great vessels, lungs, bronchi, trachea, esophagus) are protected by the bony thoracic cage, which also protects some of the upper abdominal organs. The thoracic cage likewise serves as a point of attachment for the shoulder girdle (scapula and clavicle) which in turn articulates with the upper limbs. Muscles such as the pectoralis major, trapezius, rhomboid major and minor, latissimus dorsi, and serratus anterior are associated with the thorax but actually are concerned with movements of the scapula and humerus. Some muscles which support and move the head (for example, the sternomastoid muscle) also are associated with the upper portion of the thorax. Consequently, those surgical procedures which affect the thoracic wall may likewise affect the functioning of the upper limb, head, and neck.

An anterior view of the thorax shows important relationships among the lungs, pleural cavities, and heart (Fig. 18-2). Of particular importance is the position of the ribs and intercostal spaces relative to underlying structures, since diagnostic and therapeutic procedures require an exact knowledge of these relation-

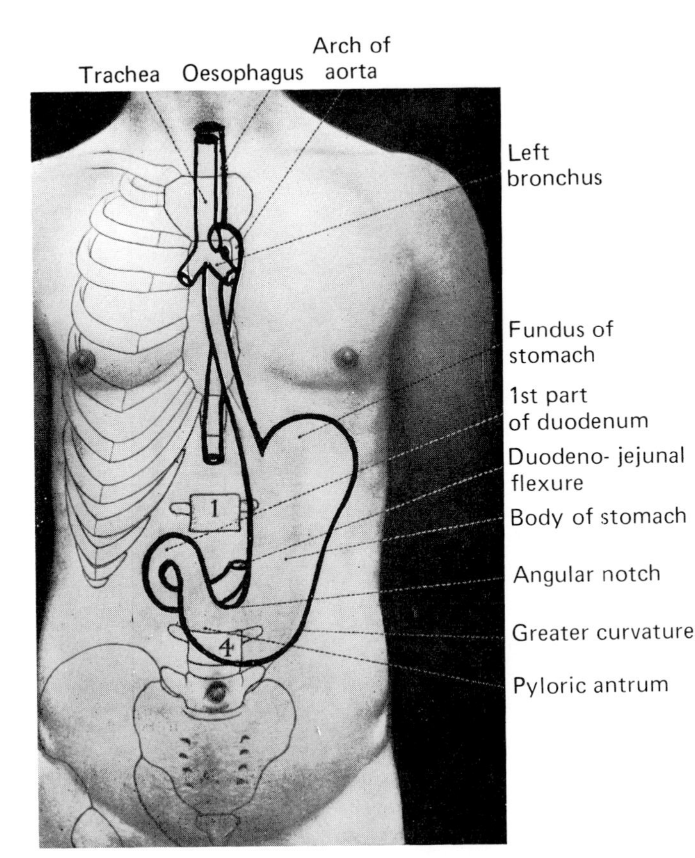

Fig. 18-1. Anterior view of the thorax and abdomen showing surface projections of the underlying organs. (From W. J. Hamilton, G. Simon, and S. G. I. Hamilton, *Surface and Radiological Anatomy,* Ed. 5, The Macmillan Press, London, 1971.)

ships. For example, if one wishes to enter the pleural cavity (thoracentesis) to remove fluid, it is necessary to choose the correct intercostal space so as to avoid puncturing the lungs, pericardial structures, diaphragm, or even the upper abdominal viscera such as the liver and spleen which are protected by the lower portion of the thoracic cage. When a hypodermic needle is inserted into an intercostal space, the intercostal nerves and vessels can be avoided by inserting the needle along the superior border of a rib, since the neurovascular bundle travels along the inferior border. The major layers of tissue through which the needle would pass successively are: skin (epidermis and dermis), superficial fascia (subcutaneous tissue), deep fascia, intercostal muscles, and parietal pleura.

Mediastinum

The mediastinum (Figs. 9-1 and 11-9) contains the trachea, the heart within its pericardial sac, the great vessels, and remnants of the thymus gland. In addition, the mediastinum serves as a passageway for structures which extend between the neck and abdomen. These structures include the esophagus, thoracic duct, and vagus and phrenic nerves.

It is useful to keep in mind the depth at which various mediastinal structures are located. For example, just posterior to the manubrium there are the brachiocephalic (innominate) veins and the superior vena cava. Posterior to this venous plane is a plane which contains the large arteries (arch of the aorta

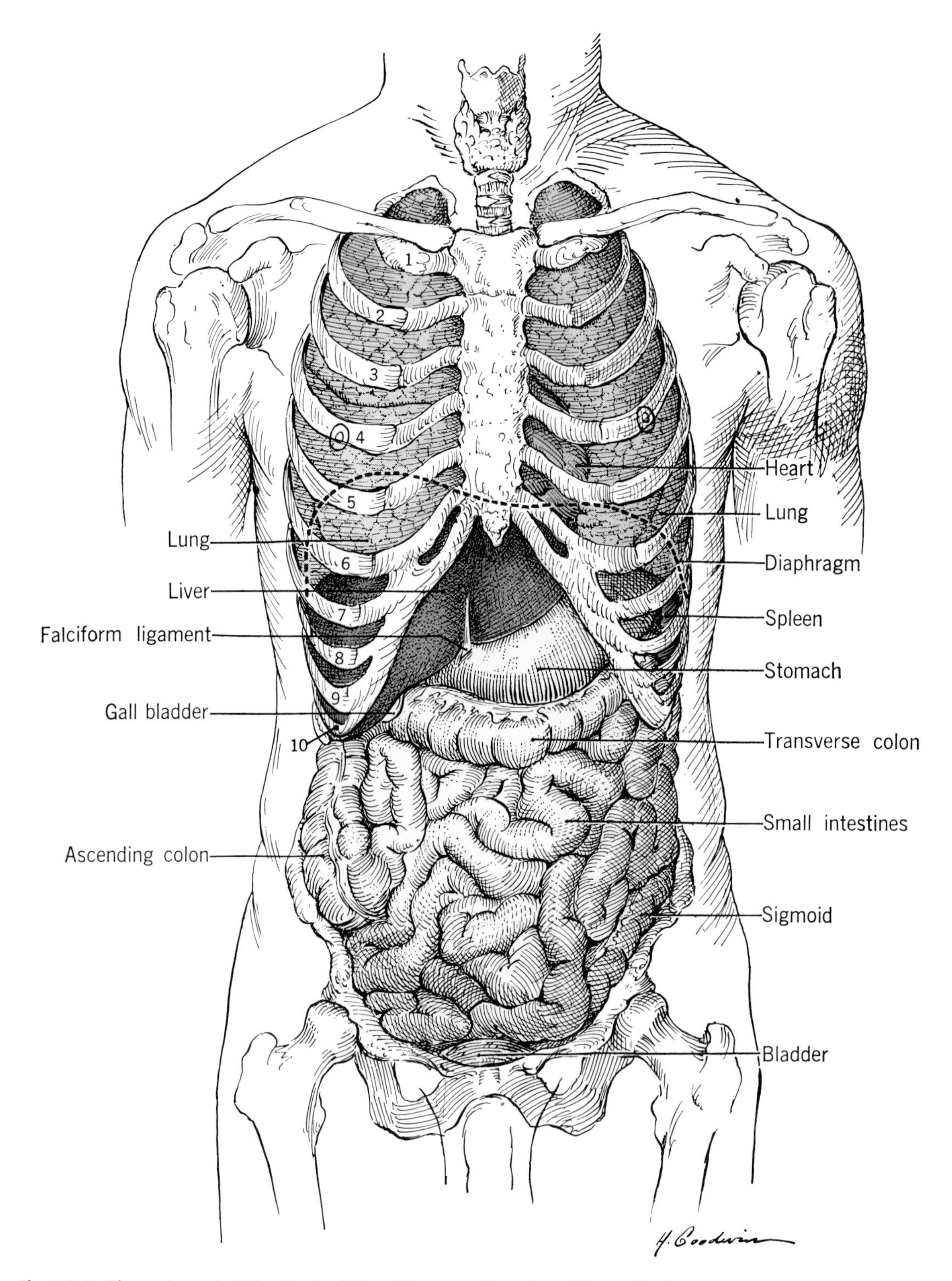

Fig. 18-2. Thoracic and abdominal relationships, anterior view. (From *Stedman's Medical Dictionary*, Ed. 23, The Williams & Wilkins Co., Baltimore, 1976.)

and its branches). Posterior to the arterial plane lie consecutively the trachea, esophagus, thoracic duct, and vertebrae.

The mediastinum consists of four regions: superior, anterior, middle (occupied by the pericardial sac), and posterior. The superior, middle, and posterior mediastinum are regions of motion due to respiratory movements of the trachea, pulsations of the heart and great vessels, and the periodic passage of food and liquids through the esophagus. The mediastinum is able to accommodate and adjust to these movements because of the resiliency of its loosely arranged connective tissue and fat.

Since the mediastinal structures show close spatial relationships to one another and to the vertebral bodies, disease or injury to one organ may adversely affect nearby structures. For example, in the mediastinum the thoracic duct travels along the anterior surface of the vertebral bodies and intervertebral discs. Fractures of the vertebrae may thus cause a tear in the thoracic duct resulting in a leakage of its contents. Also, if one accidentally swallows a sharp object which pierces the walls of the esophagus, it is possible that such nearby structures as the trachea, thoracic duct, aorta, or recurrent laryngeal branch of the vagus nerve may be traumatized (Fig. 18-3). Moreover, contamination of the mediastinum with food and liquids from the esophagus poses a particularly serious threat of infection. There is also a close spatial relationship between the arch of the aorta and the trachea. For this reason a ballooning out of the aortic wall (aortic aneurysm) may encroach upon and displace the trachea and left bronchus.

The spread of lung cancer to lymph nodes of the mediastinum also illustrates important anatomical relationships of various mediastinal structures. For example, the left recurrent laryngeal nerve curves around the arch of the aorta and then passes upward along the trachea (Fig. 18-3). If lymph nodes near the left recurrent laryngeal nerve become affected and enlarged by cancerous cells from the lung, the left vocal cord will not function and hoarseness will result. Complete loss of vocal functions will not

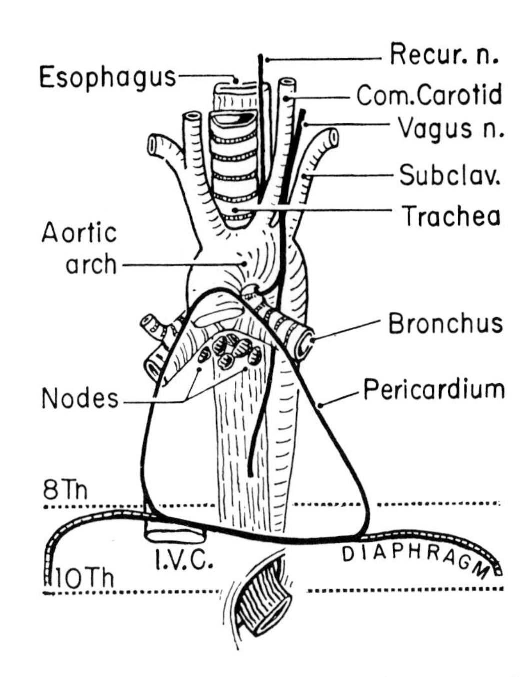

Fig. 18-3. Relationships of the esophagus viewed anteriorly. *Recur. n.,* recurrent laryngeal branch of vagus nerve; I.V.C., inferior vena cava; *8Th, 10Th,* thoracic vertebrae 8 and 10. (From J. V. Basmajian, *Grant's Method of Anatomy,* Ed. 9, The Williams & Wilkins Co., Baltimore, 1975.)

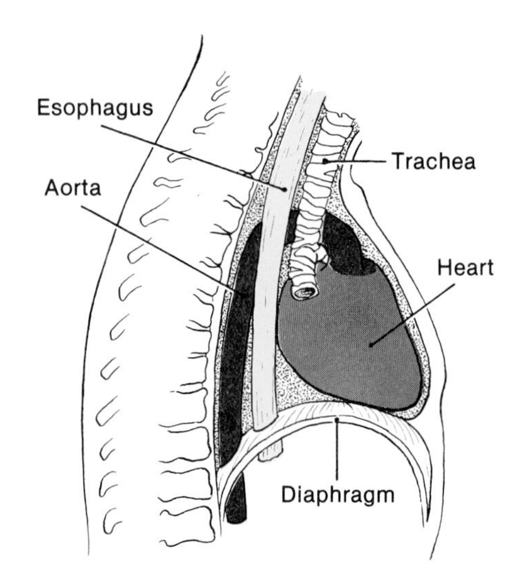

Fig. 18-4. Right lateral view of the esophagus, its relationships, and its course through the thoracic region. Note the proximity of the esophagus to the atrial region of the heart. (Modified after Basmajian.)

occur, however, since the right recurrent laryngeal nerve will remain intact. This is because the right recurrent laryngeal nerve curves around the right subclavian artery at a much higher level and is not involved with mediastinal structures. The phrenic nerves also may be affected by cancerous nodes, and movements of the diaphragm may be impaired. Moreover, enlargement of lymph nodes at the bifurcation of the trachea may lead to an increase in the angle of bifurcation, and the functioning of the esophagus may likewise be affected.

The course of the esophagus changes as it passes through the thorax. The esophagus shows a slight convex curvature to the right, and its uppermost and lowermost portions lie slightly to the left of the midline, while the midportion of the esophagus lies in the median plane. At various levels during its course through the thorax, the esophagus travels posterior to the trachea, left bronchus, and left atrium, but anterior to the thoracic duct, vertebrae, and azygous veins. In the region of the diaphragm the esophagus lies anterior to the aorta. These relationships are of significance in diagnostic radiological procedures, since a swallow of an opaque substance such as barium will pass through the esophagus and reveal its shape as well as encroachments caused by adjacent structures such as an enlarged left atrium (Fig. 18-4).

Cancer of the esophagus often involves the trachea because of the proximity of these two organs. An esophageal tumor may compress the trachea and prevent adequate amounts of oxygen from getting to the lungs. Penetration of the tumorous mass into the trachea or a bronchus may lead to hemorrhages into the conducting passageways and to bronchopneumonia. The left bronchus usually becomes involved more frequently than the right one, since it is more closely related to the esophagus. The left recurrent laryngeal nerve supplying the left vocal fold often becomes compressed, resulting in hoarseness. If the wall of the aorta is penetrated by the tumor, severe and fatal hemorrhage may occur.

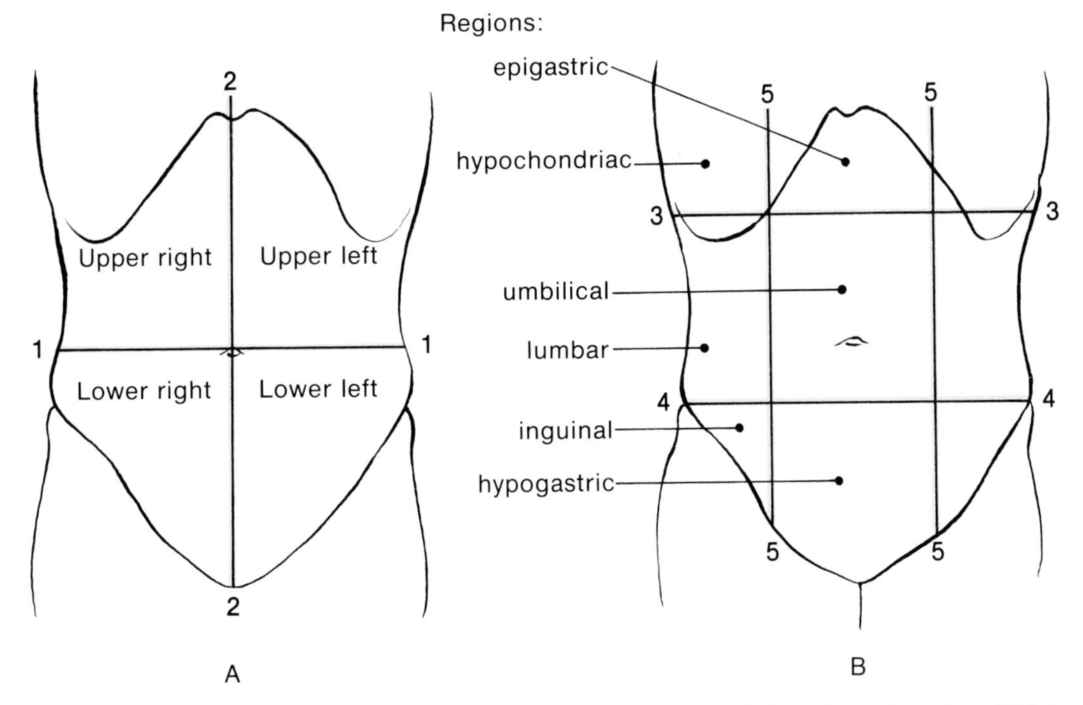

Fig. 18-5. (A) Subdivisions of the abdomen into quadrants: 1, supracristal plane; 2, median plane. (B) Subdivision into nine regions: 3, transpyloric plane; 4, transtubercular plane; 5, lateral planes. (Modified after Gardner, Gray, and O'Rahilly.)

ABDOMEN

The abdomen is separated from the thorax above by the diaphragm; below it is continuous with and includes the pelvis. The upper portion of the abdomen is somewhat protected by the thoracic cage, whereas those portions which lack bony structures are more vulnerable to injury.

Abdominal Wall

The anterior surface of the abdomen contains a fibrous band of connective tissue, the **linea alba,** which extends along the midline from the xiphoid process to the symphysis pubis. The linea alba serves as a point of attachment for the abdominal musculature.

Anteriorly on either side of the midline are the rectus abdominis muscles. In muscular individuals the segmental character of these muscles can be seen; likewise their lateral borders are demarcated by a curved depression, the **semilunar line** (linea semilunaris). Laterally the anterior superior iliac spine is easily palpated, as is the superior border of the ilium, the iliac crest. The lowest point of the inferior border of the thoracic cage is actually rather close to the iliac crest; thus the lateral aspect of the abdomen is better protected than the anterior aspect.

Perpendicular to the midline is the **supracristal plane,** an imaginary line passing transversely across the highest points of the iliac crests (Fig. 18-5A). The intersection of the supracristal plane and median plane occurs roughly at the level between the third and fourth lumbar vertebrae. The umbilicus (navel) is often situated at this intersection, although the position of the umbilicus may vary, particularly in individuals with flabby abdominal muscles.

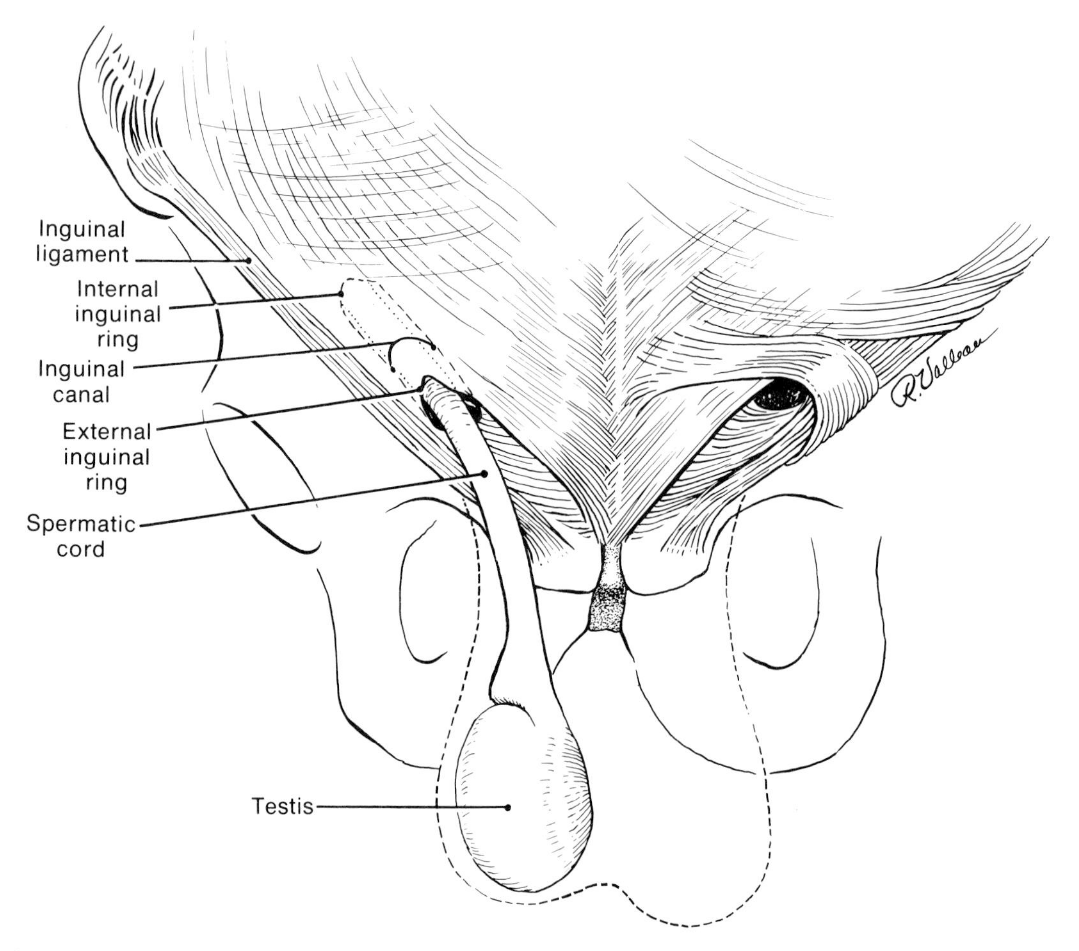

Fig. 18-6. The hypogastric and inguinal regions, anterior view. The testis and spermatic cord have been removed on the left side of the body.

The median plane and supracristal plane subdivide the abdomen into four quadrants: upper right, upper left, lower right, and lower left (Fig. 18-5*A*). The upper right quadrant contains the gallbladder and much of the liver. The upper left quadrant contains the spleen and stomach, although the position of the stomach may shift considerably depending on its degree of fullness. The appendix and ascending colon are located in the lower right quadrant, whereas the descending colon and sigmoid colon lie in the lower left quadrant. A knowledge of the relative positions of these organs can aid in diagnosing various disorders. For example, severe pain in the lower right quadrant suggests appendicitis, whereas pain in the upper right quadrant may be due to gallbladder disease.

The abdomen can also be subdivided into nine regions by two horizontal and two vertical lines (Fig. 18-5*B*). The lower horizontal (transtubercular) line passes across the tubercles of the iliac crests; the upper horizontal (transpyloric) line passes roughly midway between the inferior end of the body of the sternum and the umbilicus. The vertical lines occur approximately halfway between the anterior superior iliac spines and symphysis pubis. The nine regions thus delineated are composed of three unpaired median regions (epigastric, umbilical, and hypogastric) and three paired lateral regions (hypochondriac, lumbar, and inguinal).

The **inguinal region** is of particular importance as an area of weakness in the anterior abdominal wall because of the inguinal canal, which lies superior and parallel to the inguinal ligament (Fig. 18-6). In males the inguinal canal transmits the spermatic cord consisting of the ductus deferens, testicular vessels and nerves, and lymphatics. The coverings of the cord represent various layers of the abdominal wall which are carried downward when the fetal testis descends from the abdominal cavity to the scrotum. In females, the inguinal canal transmits the relatively thin round ligament; hence this region tends to be stronger and less subject to inguinal hernias than is the case in males.

Abdominal incisions are placed so as to allow the maximum amount of room for the surgical procedure while producing the least amount of damage to the abdominal muscles. A midline incision along the linea alba is often used because it passes between the rectus muscles and also avoids the blood vessels and nerves of the abdominal wall. If abdominal muscles must be cut, they are frequently split in the direction of their fibers (rather than transversely across the belly of the muscle) so as to preserve muscle action.

The posterior wall of the abdomen is thicker and less vulnerable than the anterior wall. The posterior wall consists of skeletal elements (vertebrae, lower ribs, and pelvic bones) and muscles (erector spinae, quadratus lumborum, iliopsoas, and posterior portions of the oblique abdominal muscles). Incisions are often made through the posterior wall to approach retroperitoneal structures (such as the kidneys and ureters) in order to avoid entering the peritoneal cavity.

Abdominopelvic Cavity

The abdominopelvic cavity consists of abdominal and pelvic portions and extends from the diaphragm (thoracic diaphragm) above to the pelvic diaphragm below (Fig. 18-7). The pelvic

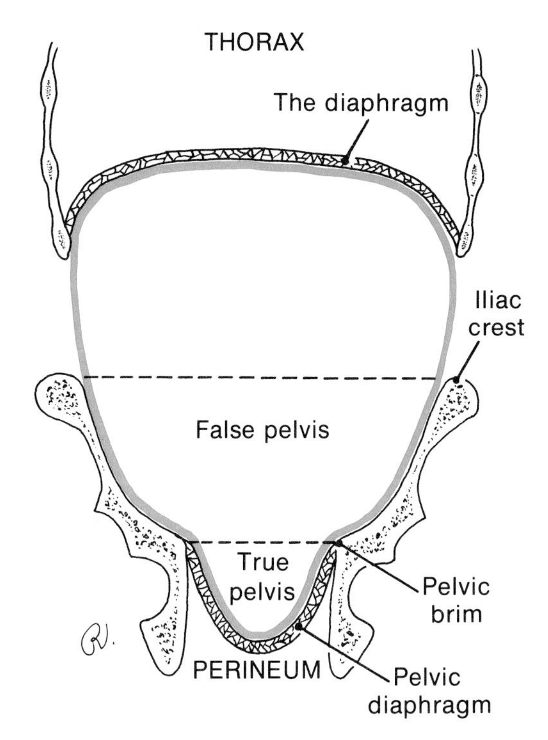

Fig. 18-7. The abdominopelvic cavity (outlined in blue) and its relations to the thorax above and perineum below. The *broken lines* represent subdivision of the pelvis into false and true regions. (Modified after Grant.)

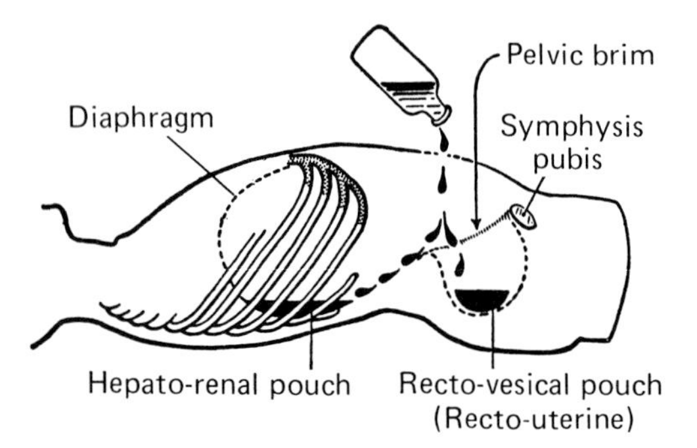

Fig. 18-8. The lowest regions of the abdominopelvic cavity in the supine position, as indicated by the accumulation of fluid. (From J. V. Basmajian, *Grant's Method of Anatomy,* Ed. 9, The Williams & Wilkins Co., Baltimore, 1975.)

portion of the cavity lies between the pelvic bones and consists of the **false (greater) pelvis** and the **true (lesser) pelvis.** The false pelvis is contained between the wings of each ilium (**iliac fossae**) and is usually considered as the lower part of the abdominal cavity. It is demarcated inferiorly by the pelvic brim, beneath which is the true pelvis containing the lower portions of the urinary and digestive tracts and the internal reproductive organs (except for the testes which lie in the scrotum). The cavity of the true pelvis is a curved canal which is quite deep posteriorly because of the curved contour of the sacrum. When one lies in the supine position the posterior portions of the abdominal and pelvic cavities are at the lowest level. Therefore these are often the sites in which blood or pus may accumulate in the event of injury to or disease of the abdominopelvic organs (Fig. 18-8).

The walls of the abdominopelvic cavity are lined by the parietal peritoneum which is reflected onto various organs as the visceral peritoneum. The peritoneal cavity consists of a narrow fluid-filled space between the parietal and visceral layers. The peritoneal cavity is completely closed in males, but in females it communicates with the lumen of each uterine tube. Hence infections such as gonorrhea may be carried upward via the vagina, uterus, and uterine tubes into the peritoneal cavity.

The superior boundary of the peritoneal cavity is the parietal peritoneum of the diaphragm. Inferiorly the peritoneal cavity is bounded by reflections of the peritoneum over upper portions of the urinary bladder, uterus (in the female), and rectum. Some organs (stomach, spleen, jejunum, ileum, transverse colon, and sigmoid colon) are suspended from the body wall by sheets of peritoneum (mesenteries). Other organs (kidneys, ureters, suprarenal [adrenal] glands, pancreas, duodenum, ascending and descending colon, and rectum) are variably fixed against the posterior wall and covered only anteriorly with peritoneum; they are thus considered retroperitoneal. Still other organs (urinary bladder, uterus) are partially draped with peritoneum.

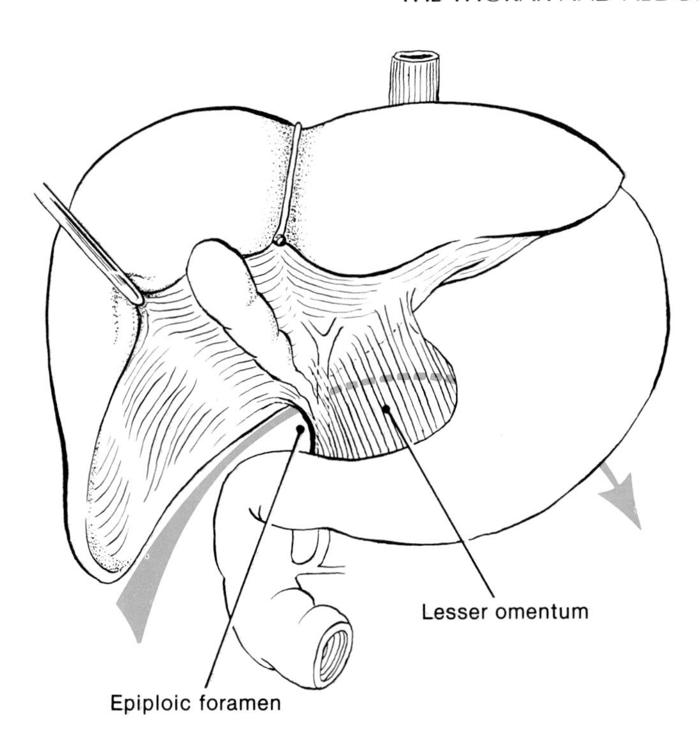

Fig. 18-9. Anterior view of the liver, gallbladder, stomach, duodenum, and lesser omentum. The *arrow* is passing via the epiploic foramen from the peritoneal cavity into the lesser sac behind the stomach. (Modified after Grant.)

The peritoneal cavity contains a number of **fossae** or **recesses** in which blood or an abscess of pus can accumulate. Several of these occur below the liver **(subhepatic)**, between the liver and diaphragm **(subphrenic)**, and between the liver and the kidney **(hepatorenal)**. A relatively large saclike pocket of the peritoneal cavity also lies behind the stomach and is known as the **lesser sac** (or **omental bursa**). It communicates with the remainder of the peritoneal cavity (sometimes referred to as the **greater sac**) via a foramen (the **epiploic foramen**) at the free border of the lesser omentum (Fig. 18-9).

The peritoneal cavity also contains channels known as **paracolic gutters** which occur on each side of the ascending and descending colon (Fig. 18-10). These gutters can act as pathways for the spread of fluids or infection from one region of the peritoneal cavity to another. Abscesses can also occur between retroperitoneal organs and their peritoneal coverings or between the organs and the body wall.

The visceral contents of the abdominopelvic cavity are arranged in a rather complex fashion. The proximity of certain groups of organs has clinical significance, since disturbances in one organ may produce a syndrome of symptoms involving several other organs and organ systems.

In the upper abdomen there is a close relationship among the stomach, spleen, and pancreas (Fig. 18-11). The spleen is attached to the stomach by the gastrosplenic ligament. Behind the stomach lies the pancreas, along the upper border of which passes the splenic artery. Thus, a malignancy in the posterior wall of the stomach may erode posteriorly into the pancreas or even cause severe hemorrhaging to occur from the splenic artery. The duodenum curves around the head of the pancreas, and the pancreas lies anterior to the bile duct (Fig. 18-11). An ulcer of the duodenal wall may thus perforate into the pancreas, or it may result in the release of intestinal contents into the upper region of the peritoneal cavity which may then pass down the right lateral paracolic gutter to the right iliac fossa. Enlargement of the pan-

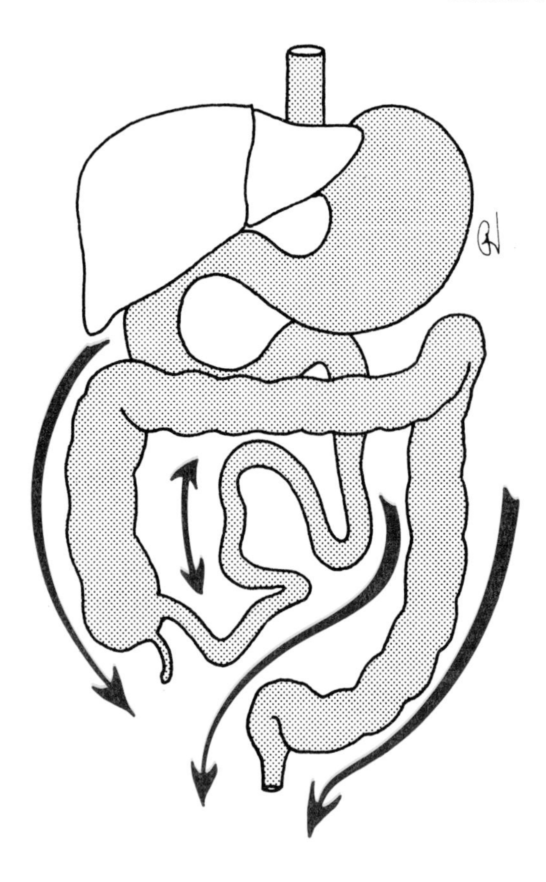

Fig. 18-10. The paracolic gutters, anterior view, along which fluid can pass as indicated by the *arrows*. (Modified after Grant.)

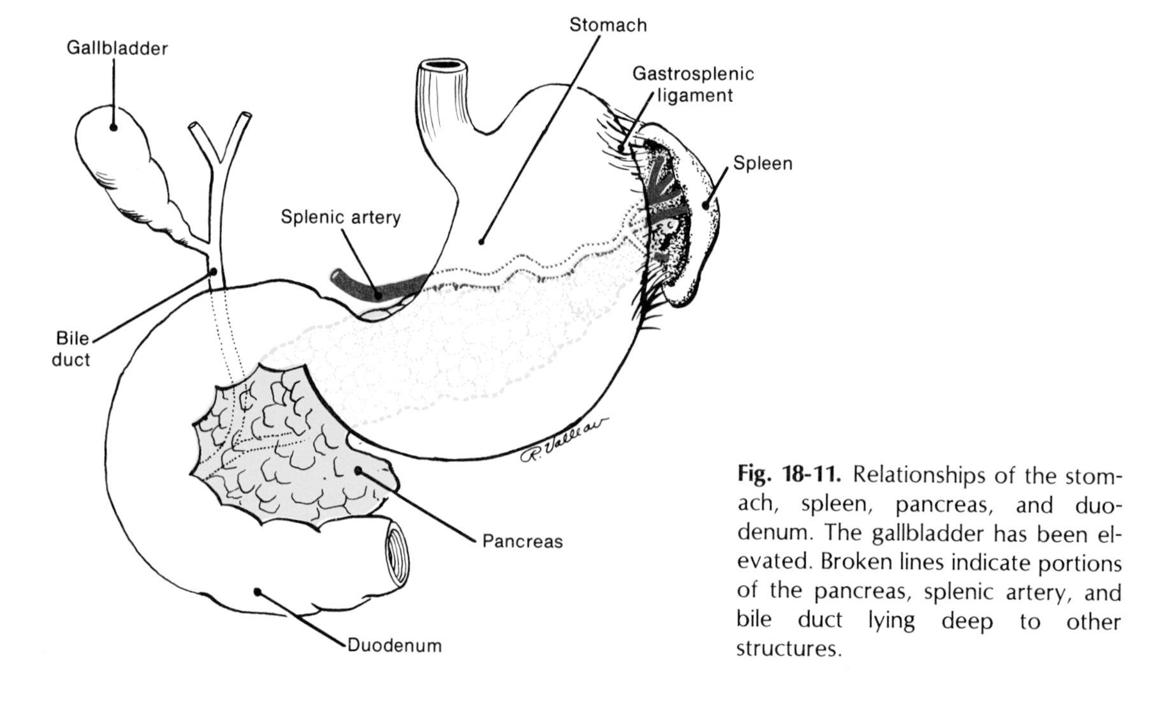

Fig. 18-11. Relationships of the stomach, spleen, pancreas, and duodenum. The gallbladder has been elevated. Broken lines indicate portions of the pancreas, splenic artery, and bile duct lying deep to other structures.

creas can obstruct the bile duct thereby producing jaundice, or it may compress the portal vein behind it.

The gallbladder, duodenum, and colon also show a close relationship to one another. The gallbladder projects downward in front of the duodenum and transverse colon near the right flexure of the colon (Fig. 18-12). A gallstone can thus penetrate through the wall of the gallbladder and perforate the wall of the duodenum behind the gallbladder or the wall of the colon near the colic flexure.

The loops of the jejunum and ileum are highly mobile because of their rather loose attachment via the mesentery to the posterior abdominal wall. These loops fill the abdominal cavity and much of the pelvic cavity (Fig. 18-2). Because of their mobility, they may occasionally slip into one of the fossae of the peritoneal cavity (for example, the lesser sac) or into the inguinal canal. Such herniations of the intestinal loops are especially dangerous should they become obstructed or if their blood supply is compromised (strangulation). In contrast, the ascending and descending colon are relatively fixed and immobile. The transverse colon, however, moves freely on its mesentery and can slip downward a considerable distance and even into the pelvis.

The viscera of the posterior abdominal wall deserve special attention because of their anatomical relationships to more anteriorly placed organs. One should keep in mind that the abdominal cavity is heart-shaped in cross section because the bodies of the vertebrae project a considerable distance anteriorly (Fig. 18-13). Thus structures near the midline of the posterior abdominal wall, such as the aorta and inferior vena cava, lie in a plane anterior to that of structures along the lateral regions of the posterior abdominal wall. Indeed, the lumbar vertebrae as well as pulsations of the abdominal aorta may sometimes be palpated through the anterior abdominal wall in thin individuals.

The aorta lies to the left of the inferior vena cava. Because of this relationship the proximal portion of the right common iliac artery crosses over the proximal portion of the left common

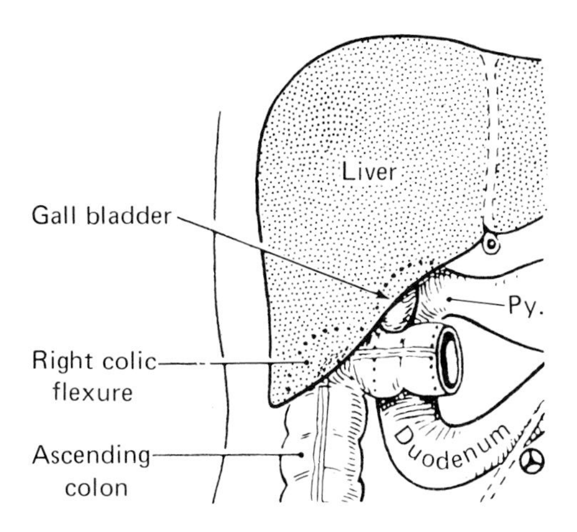

Fig. 18-12. Relationships of the gallbladder, duodenum, and transverse colon. (From E. K. Sauerland, *Grant's Dissector,* Ed. 7, The Williams & Wilkins Co., Baltimore, 1974.)

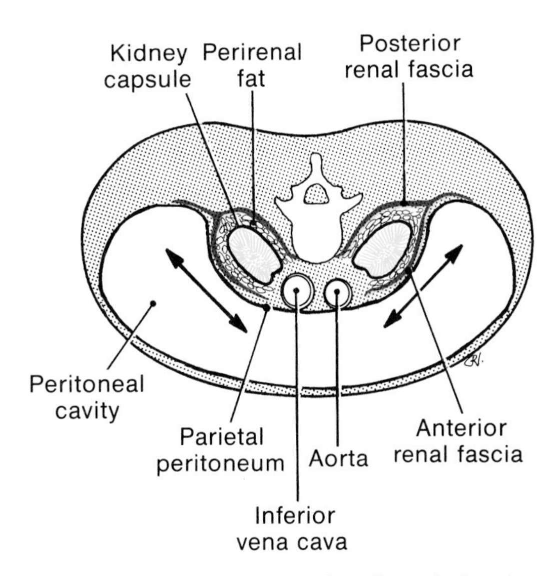

Fig. 18-13. A transverse section through the abdominal cavity showing proximity of some posterior midline structures to the anterior abdominal wall. *Arrows* indicate oblique orientation of the kidneys. The renal fascia is indicated in red.

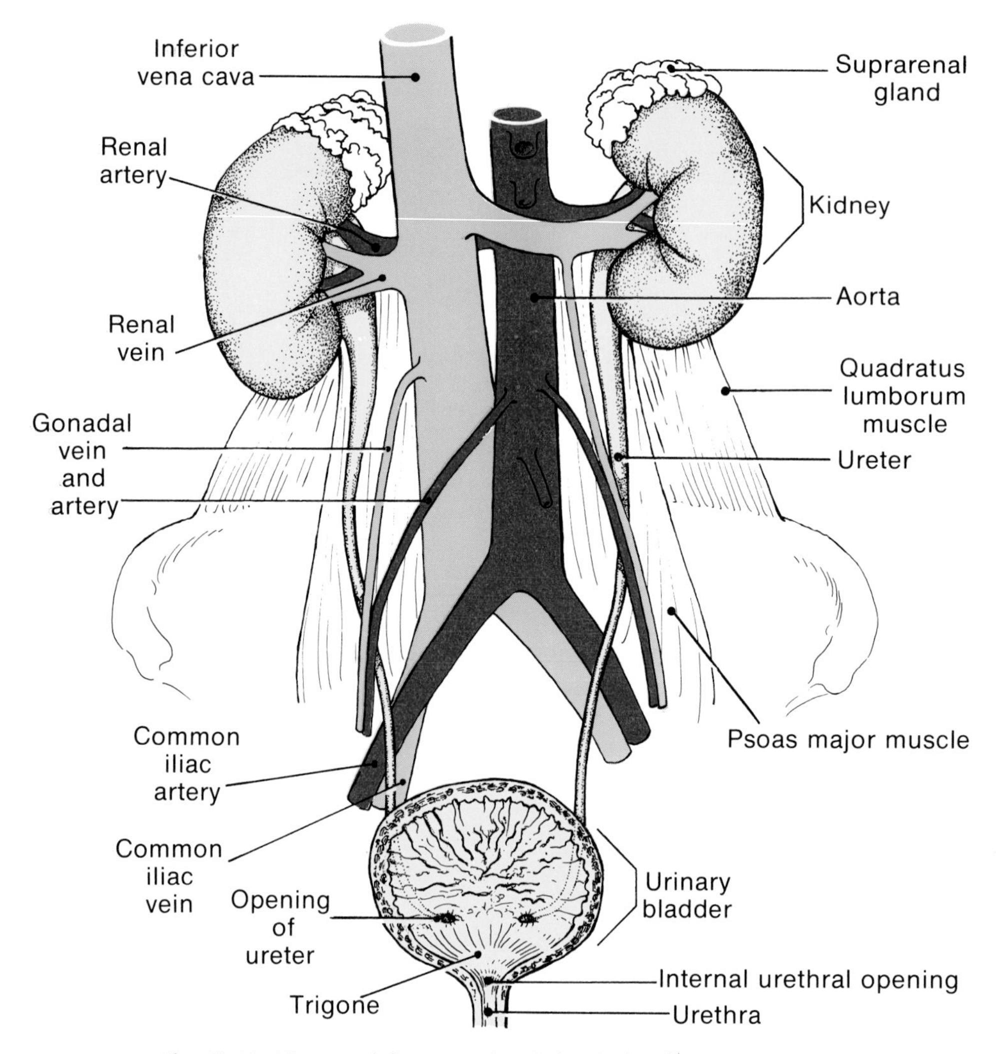

Fig. 18-14. Viscera of the posterior abdominal wall, anterior view.

iliac vein (Fig. 18-14). It is thus possible for the vein to become compressed, with the result that venous drainage from the lower limb may be impaired. Also, because of the right-sided position of the inferior vena cava, the left renal vein is longer than the right one and must pass anterior to the aorta to reach the vena cava.

The sympathetic trunks are situated behind the peritoneum along the lateral surfaces of the vertebral bodies. The right trunk underlies the right border of the inferior vena cava and the left one lies behind the left border of the aorta. Each trunk enters the pelvis by passing posterior to the iliac vessels.

In addition to the retroperitoneal portions of the gastrointestinal tract (pancreas, duodenum, ascending colon, and descending colon), the posterior abdominal wall also contains several paired organs: the suprarenal (adrenal) glands, kidneys, and ureters. The suprarenal glands are tucked under the diaphragm and sit atop the kidneys. The right gland is situated behind the liver; the left one is situated partly behind the pancreas. Since the

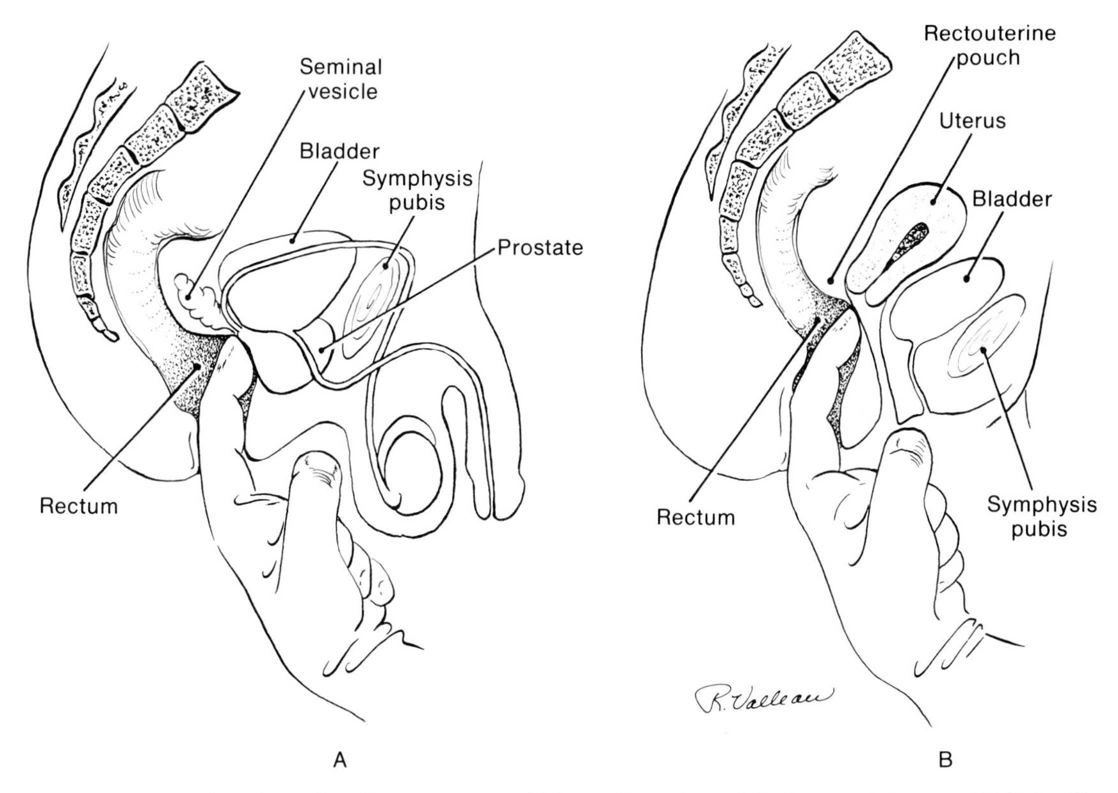

Fig. 18-15. Sagittal sections showing structures which can be palpated during a rectal exam. (A) Male, (B) female.

kidneys and suprarenal glands are closely related to the diaphragm, they move slightly with each respiratory movement. The kidneys are vulnerable to injury during surgical procedures on structures lying anteriorly, particularly the pancreas and duodenum. The kidneys themselves are approached surgically from the posterolateral abdominal wall usually by means of an oblique incision below the twelfth rib. Since the kidneys and adrenal glands are contained within their own compartments of fascia, either of these organs can be manipulated and even removed without affecting the other.

The abdominal portion of each ureter travels obliquely behind the peritoneum along the anteromedial surface of the psoas muscle. During their course both ureters are crossed anteriorly by the gonadal arteries and veins (Fig. 18-14). At the pelvic brim each ureter crosses anterior to the common iliac artery and vein.

The pelvic portion of each ureter runs along the lateral wall of the pelvis and finally passes medially to enter the urinary bladder. In the female the pelvic course of the ureter lies close to the uterine artery and is thus quite vulnerable during some pelvic procedures such as removal of the uterus (hysterectomy). Conversely, the uterine artery may be damaged by manipulations involving the ureter where it crosses below the uterine artery. In the male the pelvic portion of the ureter is crossed by the ductus deferens.

A knowledge of the disposition of organs in the pelvis is of use in diagnosing pelvic pathology, since many of these structures can be palpated by a rectal or vaginal examination. The cavity of the true pelvis is bounded above by the pelvic brim (sometimes called the pelvic inlet) and below by the pelvic diaphragm consisting of the levator ani and coccygeus mus-

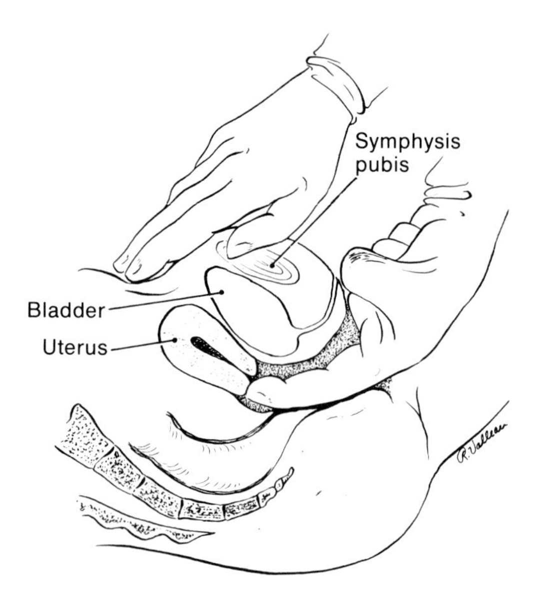

Fig. 18-16. Sagittal section showing structures which can be palpated during a vaginal exam.

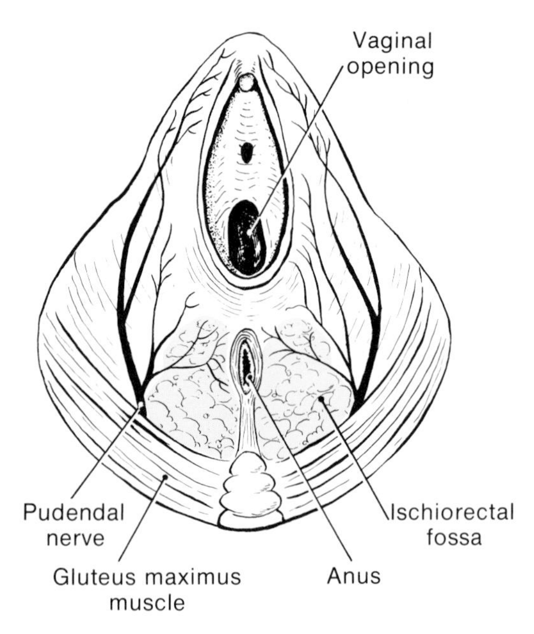

Fig. 18-17. The ischiorectal fossa in the female, viewed from below. The skin has been removed to expose the fat (yellow) which fills the fossa.

cles. The pelvic diaphragm is perforated in the midline by the rectum and urethra (in the male), or by the rectum, vagina, and urethra (in the female). These terminal regions of the digestive, reproductive, and urinary systems are situated so closely to one another that a disorder in one structure frequently has a marked effect on the others. In both sexes the rectum lies in front of the sacrum and coccyx, both of which can be palpated during a **rectal exam** (Fig. 18-15). In the male an enlargement or hardening of the prostate gland can be felt anteriorly via the rectum. In the female the cervix of the uterus can be palpated by means of the rectum, and this can be of considerable use in assessing the degree of cervical dilation during labor. An abnormal mass may also be detected such as an enlarged ovary bulging into the rectouterine pouch between the uterus and rectum.

In a bimanual **vaginal exam** the finger of one hand is placed in the vagina while the other hand is placed against the anterior surface of the lower abdominal wall. The urethra, urinary bladder, and symphysis pubis lie anterior to the vagina (Fig. 18-16). The cervix can be felt, and the size and position of the uterus can be ascertained. The ovary and uterine tubes lie laterally but usually cannot be felt unless enlarged or unless the ligamentous supports of the ovaries have been stretched by previous pregnancies. In such cases the ovaries may project downward into the rectouterine pouch.

The size of the pelvis can also be determined vaginally in order to ascertain whether it is sufficient to permit parturition. Of particular importance is the distance between the symphysis pubis and the sacrum.

Inferior to the pelvic diaphragm is the perineum. This area contains not only the external genitalia but also includes the anal portion of the digestive tract. Stretching and tearing which can occur in this region during childbirth can thus cause disturbances in urination and defecation because of damage to the pelvic diaphragm and sphincter muscles.

A deep pocket, the **ischiorectal fossa** occurs beneath the skin in the area of the anal triangle (Fig. 18-17). This fossa is filled with fat and frequently is the site of abscesses which form as a result of infection from fissures or lesions of the anal canal or from irritations of the perianal skin. The central area of the fossa can be incised and drained without risk to deeper structures. Since the **pudendal nerve** runs in the **pudendal canal** along the lateral wall of the fossa, local anesthetics may be injected into this area to help alleviate pain from the perineum during difficult childbirth (Fig. 18-17).

The lymphatic drainage of the abdomen follows several pathways. In general, the abdominal and pelvic organs are drained by lymphatic vessels which pass directly to lumbar nodes along the aorta, and finally to the lower end of the thoracic duct (Fig. 10-1). In contrast, the lymphatics of the anterior abdominal wall take a different pathway. Those of the upper abdominal wall drain upward to the axillary nodes and then to the right lymphatic duct or thoracic duct. Lymphatics of the lower portion of the abdominal wall, including the scrotum, pass downward to the inguinal nodes and then upward to the lumbar nodes. The testicular lymphatics, however, travel upward in company with the testicular veins and pass directly to the lumbar nodes.

19

The Limbs

The upper and lower limbs are structurally similar to one another, although they show modifications based on their function. The upper limb is highly mobile and capable of performing very complex and intricate movements, whereas the lower limb is adapted primarily for bearing weight and for locomotion. The upper and lower limbs are attached to the trunk by means of bones, muscles, tendons, and ligaments. Each limb consists of three general regions: the upper limb contains the arm (brachium), forearm, and hand, whereas the lower limb contains the thigh, leg, and foot.

During embryonic development the upper and lower limbs consist of paddle-shaped structures projecting outward from the lateral body wall (see Chapter 5, Fig. 5-11). The limbs then undergo complex rotations, particularly the lower limb in which the big toe and tibia become situated medially. The arm becomes quite mobile at the shoulder joint, whereas the thigh is less mobile at the hip joint. The forearm acquires capacity for the movements of pronation and supination; the leg lacks this ability. The digits of the hand, particularly the thumb, gain considerable mobility, whereas the digits of the foot remain less agile. In humans, the big toe shows far less range of movement than the thumb.

UPPER LIMB

Scapular Region

The scapular region (including the shoulder) is actually a transitional zone where bones and muscles attach the upper limb to the trunk. The muscles which move the scapula originate from nearby structures and insert on relatively limited portions of the bone. For example, the trapezius muscle which elevates and adducts (retracts) the scapula medially toward the vertebral column originates from the skull and vertebral column and inserts along the spine and acromion of the scapula (Fig. 19-1). The serratus anterior muscle which abducts (protracts) the scapula laterally from the vertebral column originates anteriorly on the thoracic cage and inserts along the vertebral border of the scapula (Fig. 19-2).

The scapula itself contains the origins of muscles which move the upper limb. Some of these muscles (such as the supraspinatus, infraspinatus, teres minor, and teres major) occupy much of the surface of the scapula (Fig. 19-3). Other muscles (such as the deltoid, coracobrachialis, biceps, and long head of the triceps brachii) take origin from a more limited region on the scapula and lie primarily over the arm. The muscles of the scapular and shoulder regions are richly supplied with blood vessels which form an extensive network with numerous interconnections (anastomoses) (Fig. 19-4). Thus, if one of these vessels becomes narrowed or occluded, other vessels can take over its area of supply.

Axilla

The axilla is a pyramid-shaped region situated inferior to the shoulder joint (Fig. 19-5). The base or floor of the axilla is commonly called the armpit and consists of loose skin and subcutaneous tissue. The apex of the axilla projects upward toward the neck. Anteriorly the axilla is bounded by the lateral portion of the pectoralis major muscle, posteriorly by the latissimus dorsi, teres major, and subscapularis muscles, medially by the upper ribs covered with the serratus anterior muscle, and laterally by the arm (brachium). The dimensions of the axilla thus change when the arm is moved.

The axilla contains blood vessels (axillary artery and vein) passing to and from the upper limb. It also houses the distal portions of the brachial plexus of nerves which innervate the upper limb. A cluster of lymph nodes (the axillary nodes) is situated here, and these may become palpable when they enlarge in response to infections. The axillary nodes receive afferent lymphatic vessels from the upper limb, lateral portion of the breast, anterior thoracic wall, and anterior abdominal wall (above the umbilicus). On the right side of the body efferent lymphatic vessels pass from the axillary nodes to the right lymphatic duct; on the left side they pass to the thoracic duct.

The axillary lymph nodes lie in loose connective tissue, whereas dense connective tissue binds the axillary vessels and nerves of the brachial plexus together into a neurovascular bundle. The brachial plexus can be damaged by a sharp blow to the axilla (for example from a crutch thrust suddenly upward), or if the upper limb is wrenched or pulled sharply (as may happen to an infant during birth or when young children are yanked upward by their arms). Vascular disorders of the upper limb can occur if the blood vessels become compressed in the axillary region.

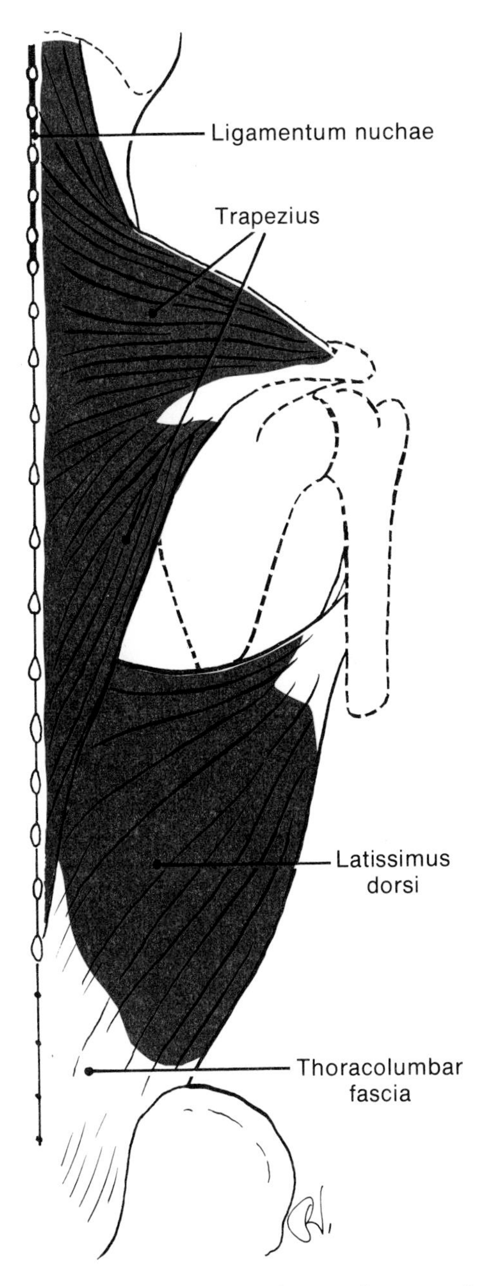

Fig. 19-1. Superficial muscles on the posterior surface of the neck and back, right side. Note the extensive vertebral origin of the trapezius muscle.

Arm

Although the term "arm" is commonly used to denote the entire upper limb, the stricter anatomical definition limits it to the portion between the shoulder and elbow. In the arm the anatomical relationships between the nerves and vessels deserve special attention. The major superficial veins are the cephalic and basilic. In the upper region of the arm the

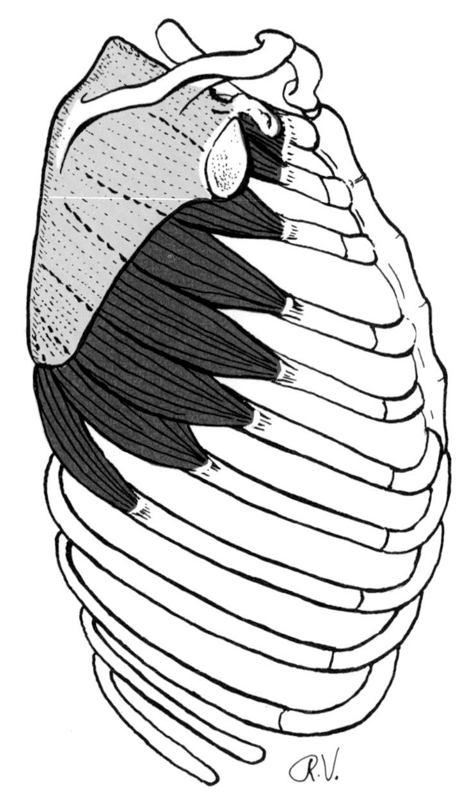

Fig. 19-2. Lateral view of the right serratus anterior muscle showing origin from the ribs and insertion on the medial border of the scapula.

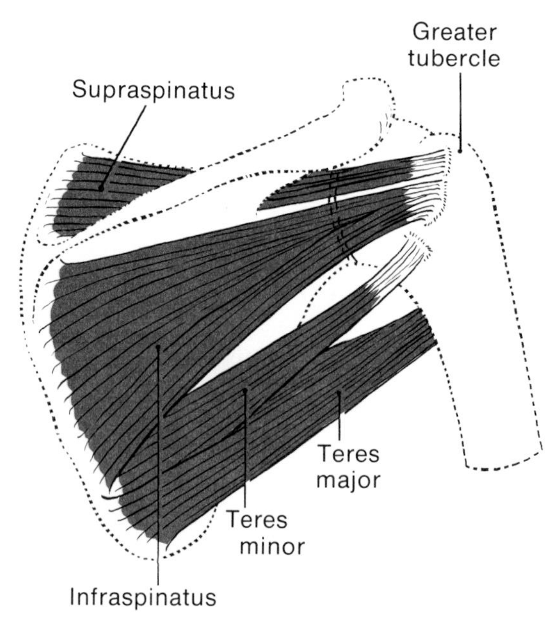

Fig. 19-3. Muscles on the posterior surface of the scapula. The teres minor has been separated and pulled downward from the infraspinatus muscle.

cephalic vein passes deeply and eventually joins the axillary vein, whereas the basilic vein first joins the brachial vein which in turn becomes the axillary vein (Fig. 19-6). The brachial vein accompanies the brachial artery, which follows a relatively superficial course along the medial aspect of the arm. It is here that the pulse may be felt and also where blood pressure can be measured. In the uppermost region of the arm three major nerves are closely associated with the brachial artery: the radial nerve lies posteriorly, the median nerve laterally, and the ulnar nerve medially (Fig. 19-6).

The radial nerve soon loses its association with the brachial artery and passes backward behind the humerus in order to send branches to the triceps brachii muscle. Fractures of the humerus thus pose a particular danger to this nerve. Although the median nerve begins its course lateral to the brachial artery, it crosses anteriorly over the artery near the middle of the arm, and then travels medial to it (Fig. 19-6). In contrast, the ulnar nerve loses its association with the brachial artery and passes downward and further medially toward the back of the elbow, thereby becoming vulnerable to injury if the bones at the elbow become dislocated or fractured.

Cubital Fossa

The anterior aspect of the elbow is often termed the cubital fossa and is the site at which blood is drawn or intravenous injections are made via superficial veins. The median cubital vein (which connects the basilic vein with the cephalic vein) is often used for these purposes, although any of several other superficial veins may be used (Fig. 19-6). Just deep to the median cubital vein is the bicipital aponeurosis (a thin sheet of connective tissue passing medially from the biceps tendon), and beneath the aponeurosis is the brachial artery with its companion, the median nerve. Thus, if a hypodermic needle penetrates too deeply and passes through the median cubital vein, it would be possible for the brachial artery to be pierced or the median nerve to be damaged. In the cubital

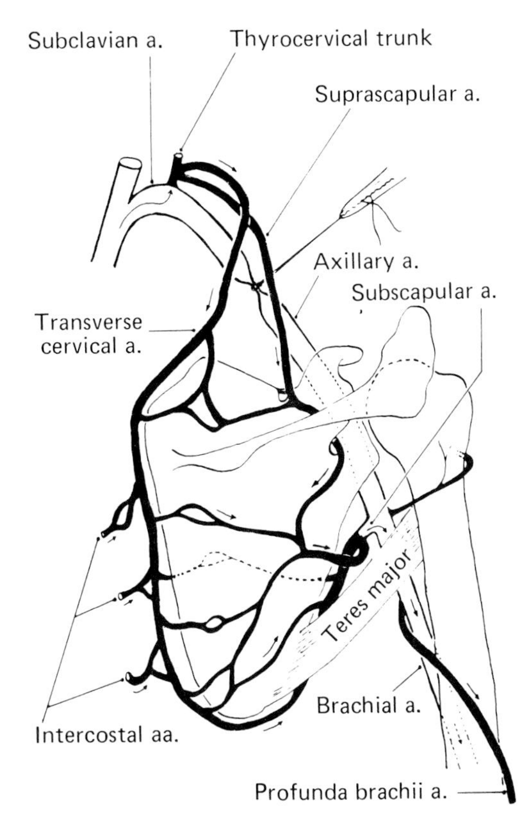

Fig. 19-4. Anastomoses of blood vessels around the shoulder and upper arm. (From E. K. Sauerland, *Grant's Dissector,* Ed. 7, The Williams & Wilkins Co., Baltimore, 1974.)

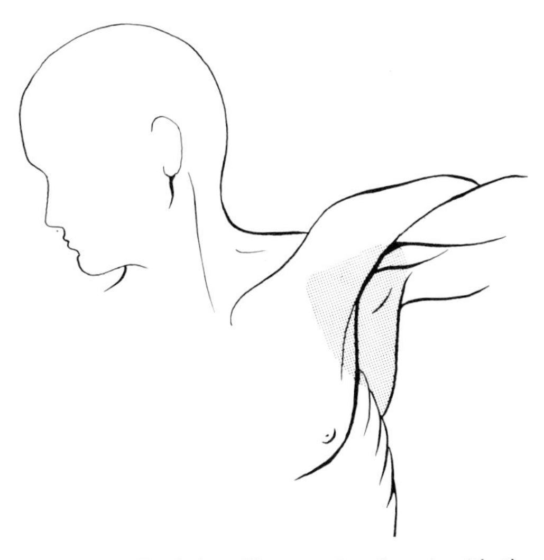

Fig. 19-5. The left axillary region (gray) with the arm raised.

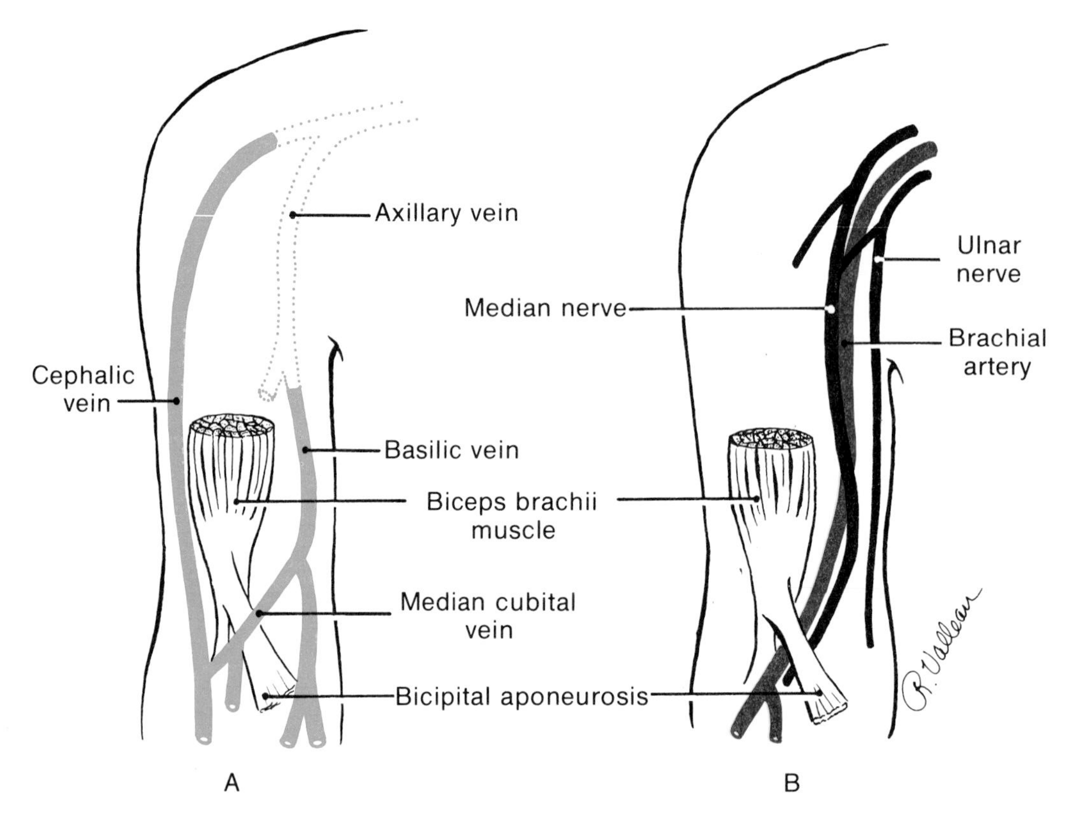

Fig. 19-6. Right arm and cubital region, anterior view. (A) Relationships of the superficial veins (solid blue) to the biceps brachii muscle, (B) the course of the brachial artery, median nerve, and ulnar nerve. (The radial nerve lies posteriorly and is not depicted here.)

fossa the brachial artery divides into its two terminal portions, the radial and ulnar arteries, which pass into the forearm.

Forearm and Wrist

The anterior region of the forearm contains a series of muscles flexing the wrist and fingers, as well as two muscles which pronate the forearm. The radial artery travels at first deep to the brachioradialis muscle along the lateral aspect of the forearm and then becomes superficial near the wrist where it lies just lateral to the tendon of the flexor carpi radialis muscle (Fig. 19-7). Here the pulse can be felt. The ulnar artery travels with the ulnar nerve along the medial side of the forearm under cover of the flexor carpi ulnaris muscle. Near the wrist the ulnar artery becomes superficial, and its pulsations can be felt just lateral to the tendon of the flexor carpi ulnaris muscle.

The median nerve runs along the midline of the anterior region of the forearm and is covered by the flexor digitorum superficialis muscle. When the median nerve reaches the wrist, it becomes superficial and passes just beneath the flexor retinaculum (the cufflike band of connective tissue which holds the tendons of the flexor muscles in place). The superficial position of the median nerve, ulnar artery, and radial artery makes them particularly vulnerable to injury from lacerations in the region of the wrist.

The posterior aspect of the forearm contains muscles which extend the wrist and fingers and one muscle which supinates the forearm. These muscles are innervated by the radial nerve. Damage to the radial nerve produces a striking disability known as **wrist drop,** in which the extensors of the wrist become paralyzed, and the unopposed action of the flexors keeps the wrist in the flexed position (Fig. 19-8).

The Hand

The hand is a remarkable instrument capable of great strength (as in grasping or squeezing objects) and of fine precision (as in playing the piano). The thenar eminence on the lateral side of the hand is particularly important since it contains the muscles which move the thumb (pollex). The thumb is essential for many of the skills performed by the hand; however, it is unfortunate that the nerve which supplies the thenar muscles (the recurrent branch of the median nerve) lies quite superficially and may be easily damaged (Fig. 19-7).

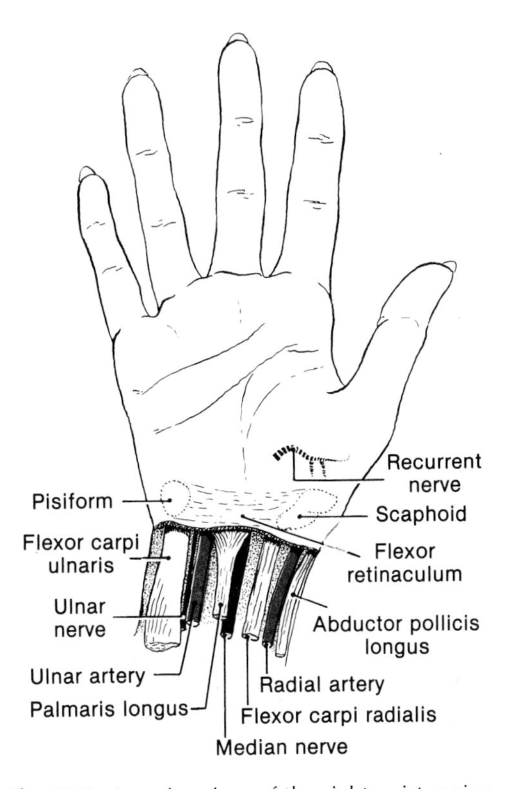

Fig. 19-7. Anterior view of the right wrist region, showing relationships of the arteries, nerves, and tendons. (Modified after Grant.)

The hand contains a complex series of compartments and synovial sheaths of tendons whereby some infections may be localized whereas others may spread from one region to another and even upward to the lower forearm. Infections which affect the synovial sheaths of tendons are particularly serious since they may impair muscle function.

The skin on the palmar surface of the hand is thick and firmly attached to an underlying layer of dense connective tissue, the palmar aponeurosis. In contrast, the skin on the dorsum (posterior surface) is thin and loosely attached to underlying layers of subcutaneous tissue. Hence, fluid and pus from deeper regions tend to accumulate more easily beneath the skin on the dorsum.

LOWER LIMB

Gluteal Region

This region (commonly called the buttocks) overlies the posterior aspect of the pelvic bones and may be considered more properly as a transitional zone between the trunk and lower limb. The gluteal muscles (gluteus maximus, gluteus medius, and gluteus minimus) act on the lower limb. When the limb is fixed, these

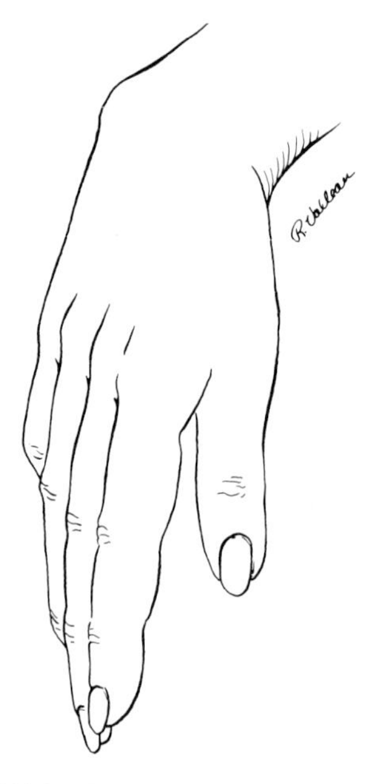

Fig. 19-8. Wrist drop, caused by damage to the radial nerve resulting in paralysis of extensor muscles.

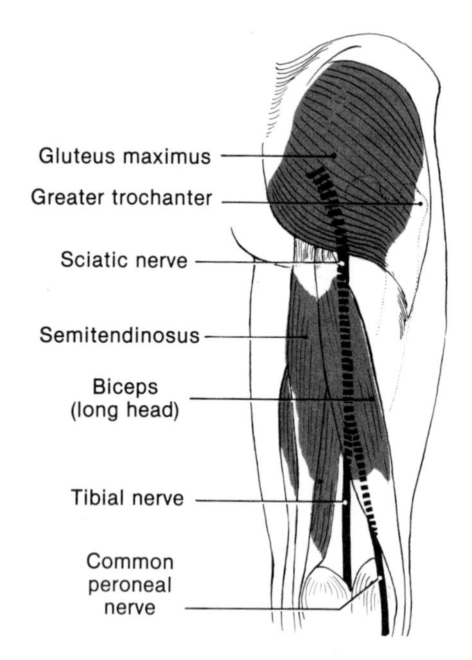

Fig. 19-9. The course and relations of the right sciatic nerve, posterior view. (Modified after Basmajian.)

muscles can also act on the pelvis and trunk. The gluteal subcutaneous tissue is invested with an abundant supply of fat which helps to cushion this region when one sits. Although the gluteus maximus muscles also provide bulk, they tend to be pushed laterally when the thighs are flexed, and the ischial tuberosities are exposed to and support the full weight of the body in the sitting position. The tuberosities may thus become sore with prolonged sitting.

The gluteus maximus muscle is a major extensor of the thigh during climbing and running. It also serves as a safe and common site for intramuscular injections, provided that these are administered in the upper outer quadrant so as to avoid injuring the sciatic nerve which travels under cover of the muscle (Fig. 19-9). The gluteus medius and gluteus minimus muscles not only abduct the thigh but are also extremely important during walking. When one lower limb is fixed on the ground, the gluteus medius and minimus of that limb prevent the opposite side of the pelvis from sagging as the opposite limb is swung forward. Most of the other muscles of the gluteal region act as lateral rotators of the thigh.

The gluteal muscles are sometimes surgically incised in order to approach the hip joint posteriorly. During these procedures care must be taken to avoid damage to the superior and inferior gluteal vessels and nerves which supply these muscles, as well as to the various nerves traversing the gluteal region on their way from the sacral plexus to the other areas of the body.

Inguinal Region

The inguinal (groin) region occurs anteriorly at the junction between the trunk and lower limb. An important landmark in this region is the inguinal ligament stretching between the anterior superior iliac spine and the pubic tubercle. Further details of this region are presented in Chapter 18.

Thigh

The thigh begins just below the inguinal ligament and extends downward to the knee. Behind and below the ligament is a compartment surrounded by a fibrous **femoral sheath** which transmits the femoral artery, femoral vein, and the femoral canal (Fig. 19-10). The **femoral canal** lies just medial to the femoral vein and ordinarily contains fat and a few lymphatic vessels. Although its upper end is separated from the peritoneal cavity by a layer of peritoneum, straining or increased abdominal pressure can force intestinal loops downward from the abdominal cavity into the femoral canal, resulting in a **femoral hernia.** The canal tends to be slightly larger in females, who therefore have a higher incidence of femoral hernias than do males.

Pulsations can be felt in the femoral artery about one inch below the midinguinal point (roughly halfway between the anterior superior iliac spine and the symphysis pubis). Medial to this point a large superficial vein, the great saphenous vein, joins the femoral vein (Fig. 19-11).

The lymphatic vessels from the lower limb and from the gluteal region drain into superficial and deep inguinal nodes. The superficial inguinal nodes are located along the upper end of the great saphenous vein and below the inguinal ligament (Fig. 19-11). The deep inguinal nodes are situated medial to the femoral vein. The superficial and deep nodes are drained by efferent lymphatic vessels passing to the external iliac nodes along the external iliac artery.

The femoral nerve originates from the lumbar plexus, passes into the thigh lateral to the femoral sheath, and innervates the massive, powerful muscle on the anterior thigh, the quadriceps femoris muscle. The muscles on the medial aspect of the thigh belong to the adductor group and are innervated by the obturator nerve. In the upper region of the thigh the femoral artery and vein are somewhat superficially located, but then pass deep to the sartorius muscle which arches over them forming the roof of a passageway termed the **adductor (subsartorial) canal** (Fig. 19-10). At the lower end of the canal the vessels pierce the adductor magnus muscle and pass to the posterior aspect of the limb.

The posterior aspect of the thigh contains the "hamstring" muscles (biceps femoris mus-

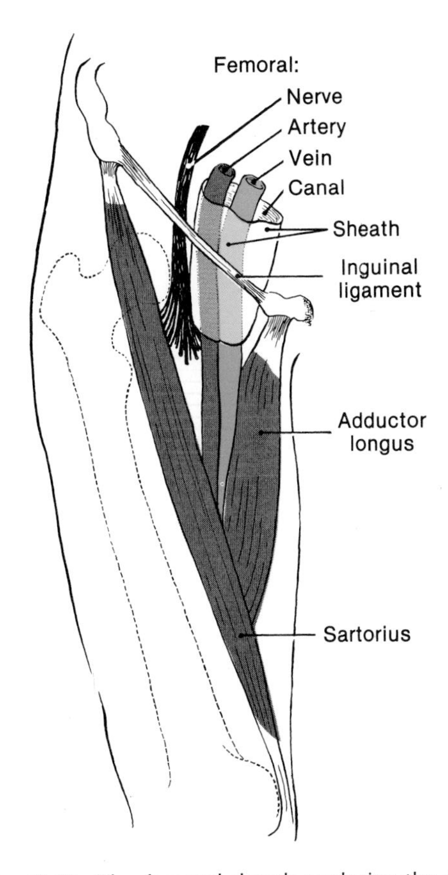

Fig. 19-10. The femoral sheath enclosing the femoral artery, vein, and femoral canal. Note that the femoral nerve lies outside the sheath. The femoral artery and vein pass deep to the sartorius muscle which forms the roof of the adductor (subsartorial) canal.

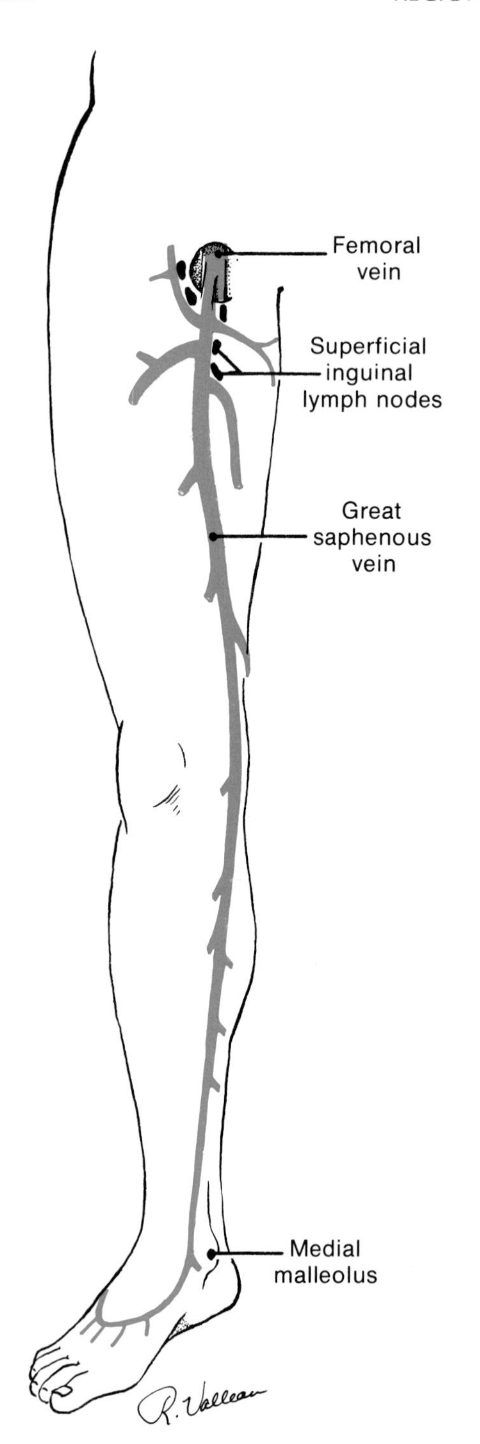

Fig. 19-11. Course of the great saphenous vein.

cle laterally and the semimembranosus and semitendinosus muscles medially). These muscles are innervated by branches of the sciatic nerve which travels along the midline of the thigh. In the lower third of the thigh the sciatic nerve subdivides into the tibial and common peroneal nerves.

Popliteal Fossa

This region is the counterpart of the cubital fossa of the upper limb, except that the latter faces anteriorly whereas the popliteal fossa is located posteriorly at the back of the knee.

The popliteal fossa is a diamond-shaped area bounded above by the biceps femoris muscle laterally and the semimembranosus and semitendinosus muscles medially, and below by the two heads of the gastrocnemius muscle (Fig. 19-12). The lower end of the adductor canal communicates with the fossa and provides a passageway enabling the femoral artery and vein to pass posteriorly from the anterior region of the thigh. Within the fossa, these vessels assume the name popliteal artery and vein, respectively. The artery lies deep to the vein which in turn lies deep to the tibial nerve; hence the arterial pulse is not easily palpated in this region. The fossa also contains the common peroneal nerve laterally, the popliteus muscle anteriorly, and some small nerves and vessels, lymph nodes, and fat. Anterior to the popliteal fossa is the knee joint which includes the condyles of the femur and tibia, and the patella.

Leg

Although the term "leg" is often used to denote the entire lower limb, the anatomical definition is limited to the portion between the knee and the ankle joint. Of the two leg bones (tibia and fibula) the tibia is the more massive; however, its anterior and medial aspects are subcutaneous and thus vulnerable to injury. Although the fibula is clothed with muscles, it is a long and slender bone likewise subject to fractures. These can be particularly dangerous in the upper region because of possible damage to the common peroneal nerve which winds around the head of the fibula (Fig. 19-13). Indeed, even a plaster cast compressing this area can damage the nerve.

One of the two terminal branches of the common peroneal nerve is the deep peroneal nerve innervating muscles which extend the toes (extensor digitorum longus, extensor hallucis longus) and a muscle which dorsiflexes and inverts the foot (tibialis anterior). The other branch of the common peroneal nerve is the superficial peroneal nerve which innervates muscles responsible for everting the foot (peroneus longus and peroneus brevis). Damage to the common peroneal nerve (and thus the deep peroneal nerve) can result in "foot drop" whereby the foot flaps downward and cannot be dorsiflexed sufficiently to clear the ground when walking.

The anterior and lateral leg muscles receive their blood supply from the anterior tibial artery which branches from the popliteal artery at the back of the knee and which then passes forward to travel down the anterior aspect of the leg. This vessel is accompanied by a pair of anterior tibial veins and by the deep peroneal nerve (Fig. 19-13).

The posterior aspect of the leg contains the massive "calf muscles" which are innervated by the tibial nerve. This nerve leaves the popliteal fossa, passes under cover of the posterior muscles, and supplies branches to the plantar flexor muscles (gastrocnemius and soleus), flexors of the toes (flexor digitorum and flexor hallucis longus) and the chief invertor of the foot (tibialis posterior). Damage to the tibial nerve can affect the calf muscles so that the heel cannot be raised off the ground for walking.

The muscles on the back of the leg receive their blood supply from the posterior tibial artery which, like the anterior tibial artery, is a terminal branch of the popliteal artery. The posterior tibial artery gives off the peroneal artery laterally and travels along with a pair of posterior tibial veins and the tibial nerve (Fig. 19-14).

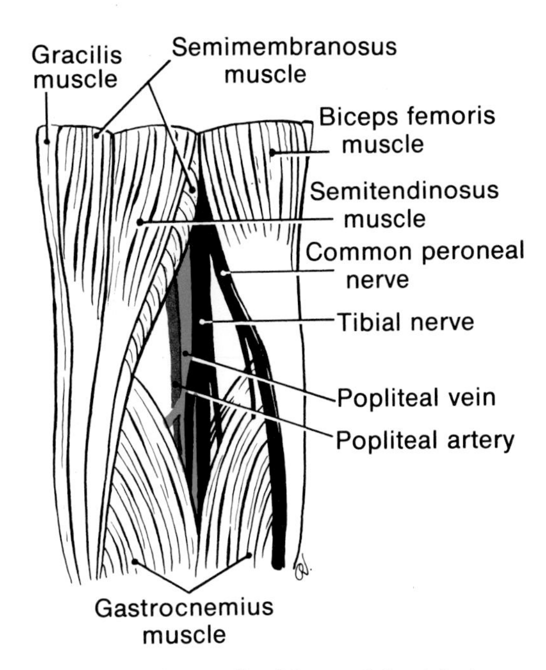

Fig. 19-12. The popliteal fossa of the right lower limb. The popliteal artery lies deep to the popliteal vein. The tibial nerve lies most superficially.

Foot

The anatomical relationships of structures in the foot are quite similar to those in the

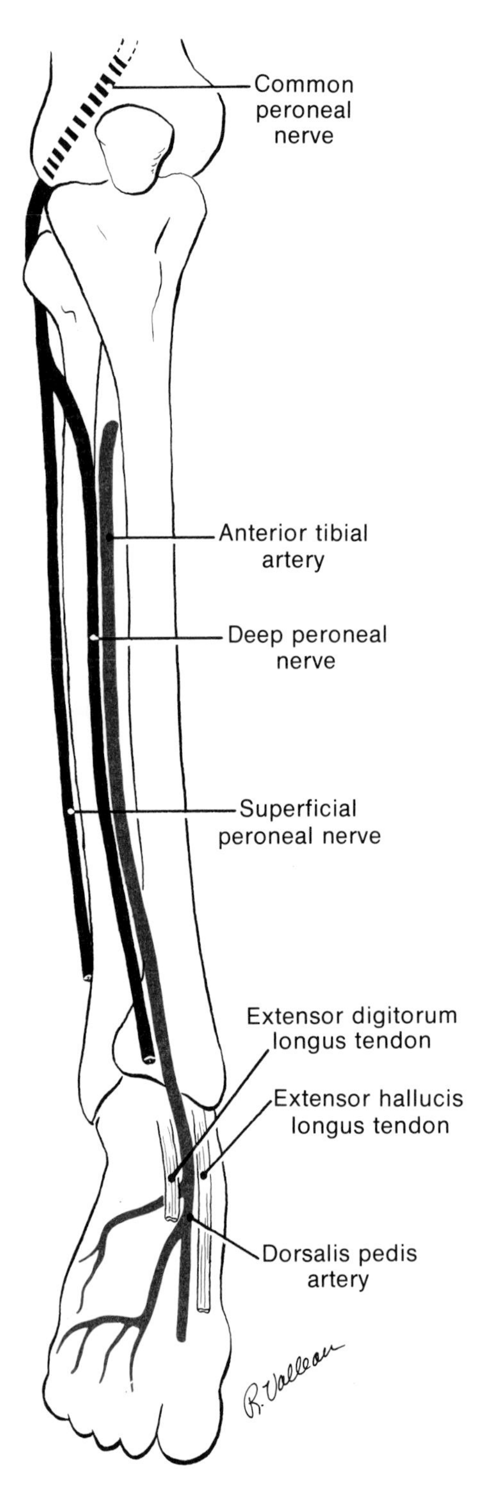

Fig. 19-13. Course of the anterior tibial artery, and the common peroneal, deep peroneal, and superficial peroneal nerves. *Broken black line* represents the course of the common peroneal nerve posterior to the femur.

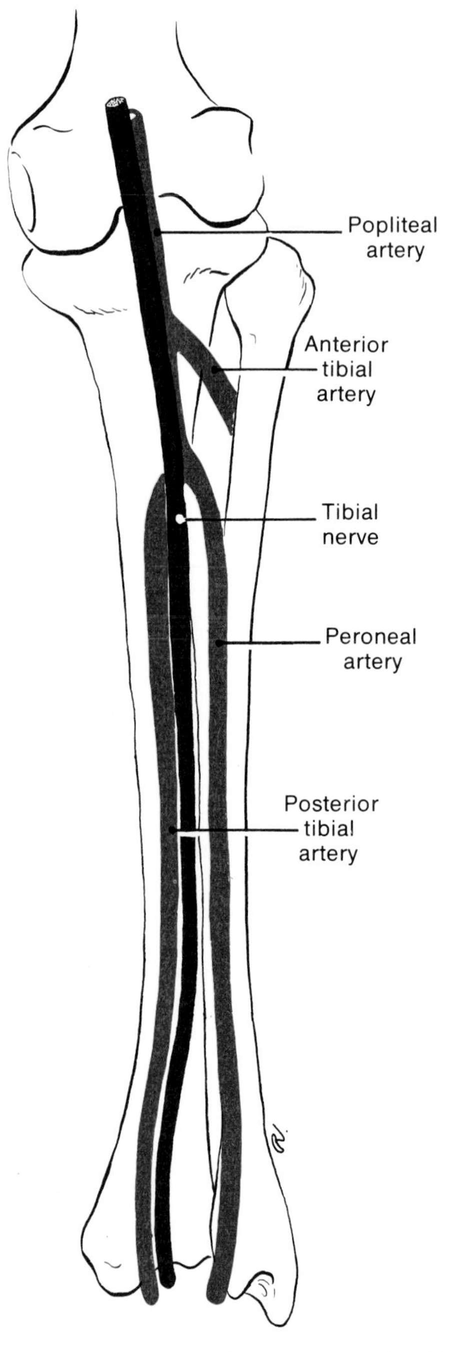

Fig. 19-14. The peroneal artery, posterior tibial artery, and tibial nerve, as seen in the right leg, posterior view.

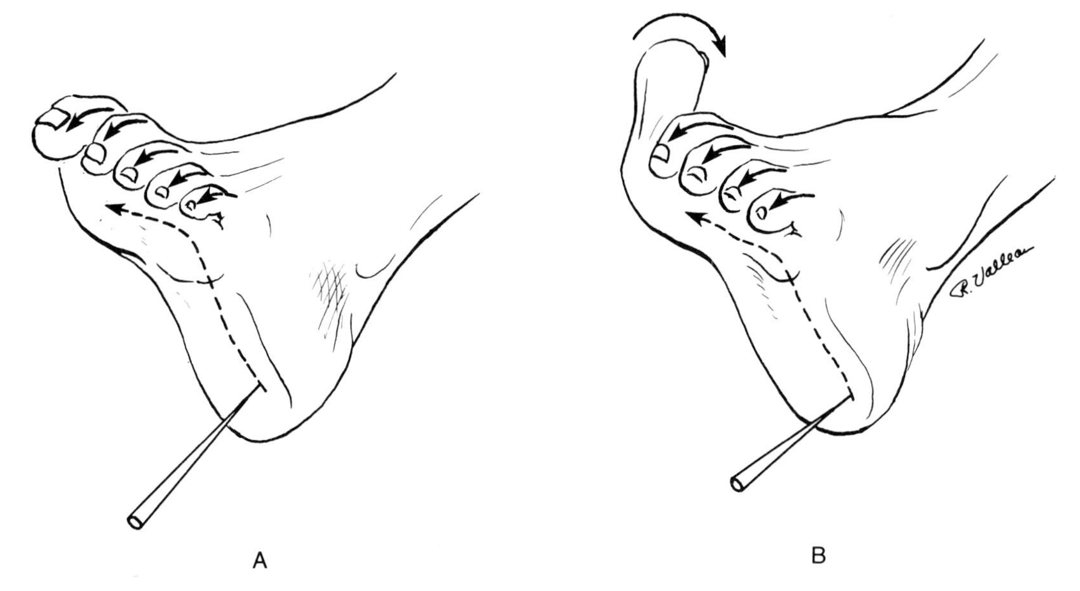

Fig. 19-15. The plantar reflex. *Dashed arrows* show direction of stroke; *solid arrows* show direction of movement. (A) Normal, (B) Babinski (abnormal).

hand, even though the foot is modified for supporting weight and lacks the dexterity of the hand. As a result, the skin of the sole is extremely thick, as is the dense connective tissue of the subcutaneous layer. The latter also contains a considerable amount of fat to help cushion areas of weight support.

Although the foot exhibits a series of compartments and tendon sheaths, these do not intercommunicate as extensively as do those in the hand. Thus the tendons of the foot are not as vulnerable to the spread of infection as are their counterparts in the hand.

The arteries of the foot include the dorsalis pedis artery (a continuation of the anterior tibial artery) where the pulse can be felt between the tendons of the extensor digitorum longus and extensor hallucis longus muscles (Fig. 19-13). The medial and lateral plantar arteries (terminal divisions of the posterior tibial artery) are the major source of blood supply to the foot, and these are accompanied by deep veins of the same name. The superficial veins of the foot are highly variable; however, the great saphenous vein shows a relatively constant position in the ankle region where it passes in front of the medial malleolus. It is here that transfusions are sometimes administered (Fig. 19-11).

The medial and lateral plantar arteries and veins travel along with the medial and lateral plantar nerves, respectively. These nerves are branches of the tibial nerve and innervate the intrinsic muscles of the foot. An injury to the tibial nerve or to these branches not only affects the intrinsic muscles, but also produces loss of sensation on the sole. This sensory loss can be quite serious, since walking becomes difficult when one cannot ascertain the extent of contact between the sole of the foot and the ground.

The sole of the foot also shows an interesting **plantar reflex** whereby the toes flex in response to light stroking of the lateral aspect of the sole. However, in infants and in individuals in which there are disturbances in certain motor pathways of the brain and spinal cord, stroking produces dorsiflexion of the big toe and a spreading apart of the other toes. This abnormal response is known as the **Babinski reflex** and is often tested in routine physical or neurological examinations (Fig. 19-15).

References

Listed below are textbooks, atlases, and dictionaries which provide more extensive and detailed information on various aspects of human anatomy.

Gross Anatomy

Basmajian, J. V., *Grant's Method of Anatomy*, Ed. 10, The Williams & Wilkins Co., Baltimore, 1980.

Clemente, C. D., *Anatomy: A Regional Atlas of the Human Body*, Ed. 2, Lea & Febiger, Philadelphia, 1981.

Ellis, H., *Clinical Anatomy*, Ed. 6, J. B. Lippincott Co., Philadelphia, 1977.

Gardner, E. D., Gray, D. J., and O'Rahilly, R., *Anatomy*, Ed. 4, W. B. Saunders Co., Philadelphia, 1975.

Anderson, J. *Grant's Atlas of Anatomy*, Ed. 7, The Williams & Wilkins Co., Baltimore, 1978.

Hamilton, W. J., Simon, G., and Hamilton, S. G. I., *Surface and Radiological Anatomy*, Ed. 5, Heffer & Sons, Cambridge, 1971.

McMinn, R. M. H., and Hutchings, R. T., *Color Atlas of Human Anatomy*, Year Book Medical Publishers, Inc., Chicago, 1977.

Moore, K. L., *Clinically Oriented Anatomy*, The Williams & Wilkins Co., Baltimore, 1980.

Netter, F. H., *CIBA Collection of Medical Illustrations*, Vols. 1–6, CIBA, Summit, N.J. 1962–1974.

Williams P. L., and Warwick R., *Gray's Anatomy*, Ed. 36, W. B. Saunders Co., Philadelphia, 1981.

Woodburne, R. T., *Essentials of Human Anatomy*, Ed. 6, Oxford University Press, 1978.

Yokochi, C., *Photographic Anatomy of the Human Body*, Ed. 2, University Park Press, Baltimore, 1978.

Microscopic Anatomy

Bergman, R. A., and Afifi, A. K., *Atlas of Microscopic Anatomy*, W. B. Saunders Co., Philadelphia, 1974.

Bloom, W. and Fawcett, D. W., *A Textbook of Histology*, Ed. 10, W. B. Saunders Co., Philadelphia, 1975.

Copenhaver, W. M., Kelly, D. E., and Wood, R. L., *Bailey's Textbook of Histology*, Ed. 7, The Williams & Wilkins Co., Baltimore, 1978.

DiFiore, M. S. H., *An Atlas of Human Histology*, Ed. 5, Lea & Febiger, Philadelphia, 1981.

Dodd, E., *Atlas of Histology*, McGraw-Hill Book Co., New York, 1979.

Fawcett, D., *The Cell*, Ed. 2, W. B. Saunders Co., Philadelphia, 1981.

Ham, A. W., and Cormack, D. H., *Histology*, Ed. 8, J. B. Lippincott, Philadelphia, 1979.

Kessel, R. G., and Kardon, R. H., *Tissues and Organs: A Text-Atlas of Scanning Electron Microscopy*, W. H. Freeman & Co., San Francisco, 1979.

Leeson, C. R., and Leeson, T. S., *Histology*, Ed. 4, W. B. Saunders Co., Philadelphia, 1981.

Reith, E. J., and Ross, M. N., *Atlas of Descriptive Histology*, Ed. 3, Harper & Row, New York, 1977.

Rhodin, J. A. G., *Histology: A Text and Atlas*, Oxford University Press, New York, 1976.

Developmental and Pediatric Anatomy

Carlson, B. M., *Patten's Foundations of Human Embryology*, Ed. 4, McGraw-Hill Book Co., New York, 1981.

Crowley, L. V., *An Introduction to Clinical Embryology*, Year Book Medical Publishers, Inc., Chicago, 1974.

Hamilton, W. J., and Mossman, H. W., *Hamilton, Boyd, and Mossman's Human Embryology*, Ed. 4, Heffer & Sons, Cambridge, 1972.

Hopper, A. F., and Hart, N. H., *Foundations of Animal Development*, Oxford University Press, New York, 1980.

Langman, J., *Medical Embryology*, Ed. 4, The Williams & Wilkins Co., Baltimore, 1981.

Moore, K. L., *The Developing Human*, Ed. 3, W. B. Saunders Co., Philadelphia, 1982.

Neuroanatomy

Barr, M. L., *The Human Nervous System*, Ed. 3, Harper & Row, New York, 1979.

Carpenter, M. B., *Human Neuroanatomy*, Ed. 7, The Williams & Wilkins Co., Baltimore, 1976.

Gardner, E. D., *Fundamentals of Neurology*, Ed. 6, W. B. Saunders Co., Philadelphia, 1975.

Noback, C. R., *The Human Nervous System*, Ed. 3, McGraw-Hill Book Co., New York, 1981.

Dictionaries

Dorland's Medical Dictionary: Shorter Edition, W. B. Saunders Co., Philadelphia, 1980.

Stedman's Medical Dictionary, Ed. 24, The Williams & Wilkins Co., Baltimore, 1982.

Index

Structures in this index are listed primarily under the nouns. For example, the radial nerve is listed under Nerve(s). Page references in **bold face** indicate illustrations.

UNITS OF MEASURE

Linear

1 meter (m) = 39.37 inches
1 centimeter (cm) = 0.01 m
1 millimeter (mm) = 0.001 m
1 micrometer (μm) or micron (μ) = 0.001 mm
1 nanometer (nm) or millimicron (mμ) = 0.001 μm
1 Ångstrom (Å) = 0.1 nm

Weight

1 kilogram (kg) = 2.205 pounds
1 gram (gm) = 0.001 kg
1 milligram (mg) = 0.001 gm
1 microgram (μg) = 0.001 mg

Average Linear Measurements and/or Weights of Various Structures

Structure	Linear Measurement	Weight
Ribosome	150–250 Å (diameter)	——
Red blood cell	7 μm (diameter)	——
Oocyte	0.1 mm (diameter)	——
Pineal gland (body)	8 mm (length)	140 mg
Testis	4–5 cm (length)	25 gm
Kidney	12 cm (length)	150 gm
Pancreas	23 cm (length)	110 gm
Heart	——	275 gm
Lung: Right	——	450 gm
Left	——	375 gm
Brain	——	1300 gm

PREFIXES, SUFFIXES, AND ROOT WORDS

ab — away, from
ad — to, toward
alb — white
ambi — both
an — not, without
andr — man
ante — before
anti — opposite, opposed
arthr — joint
auto — self
bi — two, twice
brachi — arm
brachy — short
bucc — cheek
cardi — heart
cele (coele) — chamber
cephal — head
chondr — cartilage
chrom — color
circum — around
clas — break
cleid — clavicle
co — with, together
contra — opposite
corp — body
cost — rib
crani — skull
cut — skin
cyst — bladder
cyto — cell
derm — skin
di — two, twice
dis — apart
dys — bad
ect — outside
emia — blood
encephal — brain
endo — in, into
enter — intestine
epi — above, on, upon
ex — out
extra — outside of
-ferent — carry
gastr — stomach
glosso — tongue
gyn — woman
hemi — half
hemo — blood
hepat — liver
hetero — other
hist — tissue
hydr — water
hyper — over, more than
hypo — under, less than
infra — beneath
inter — between
intra — within
-itis — inflammation
kine — move
later — side
leuk — white
logy — study of
lysis — dissolve
macro — large
mal — bad
mast — breast
melan — black
meso — middle
meta — beyond
micro — small
mono — one
multi — many
myo — muscle
nephr — kidney
neur — nerve
-oid — like
-ole — small
olig — few
oo — egg
oss — bone
osteo — bone
ot — ear
ovi (ovo) — egg
para — beside, near
per — through
peri — around, near
pod — foot
poiesis — make
poly — many
post — after, behind
pre — before, in front
pro — before
pseud — false
pulmo — lung
pyel — basin
re — back, again
ren — kidney
retro — backward
sarco — muscle, flesh
sclero — hard
scopy — examine
semi — half
somat — body
sten — narrow
sub — below, under
supra — above
syn, sym — together
-tomy — cut into
trache — windpipe
trans — beyond, through
troph — nourish
ultra — beyond
vas — vessel
ventro — belly, front